MEDICAL CARE OF THE SURGICAL PATIENT

DAVID R. GOLDMANN, M.D., *Assistant Professor, University of Pennsylvania Department of Medicine; Hospital of the University of Pennsylvania, General Medicine Section, Philadelphia, PA*

FRANK H. BROWN, M.D., *Assistant Professor, University of Pittsburgh Department of Medicine; Presbyterian University Hospital, Pittsburgh, PA*

WILLIAM K. LEVY, M.D., *Assistant Physician and Staff Cardiologist, Abington Memorial Hospital, Abington, PA*

GAIL B. SLAP, M.D., *Assistant Professor, University of Pennsylvania Department of Medicine; Hospital of the University of Pennsylvania, General Medicine Section, Philadelphia, PA*

ELLIOT J. SUSSMAN, M.D., *Assistant Professor, University of Pennsylvania Department of Medicine; Hospital of the University of Pennsylvania, General Medicine Section, Philadelphia, PA*

With 49 additional contributors

MEDICAL CARE OF THE SURGICAL PATIENT

A Problem-Oriented Approach to Management

 J. B. LIPPINCOTT COMPANY

PHILADELPHIA & TORONTO

Sponsoring Editor: Richard Winters
Manuscript Editor: Martha Hicks-Courant
Indexer: Ellen Murray
Production Supervisor: N. Carol Kerr
Production Assistant: Susan A. Caldwell
Compositor: Hampton Graphics
Printer/Binder: R. R. Donnelley & Sons Company

The authors and publisher have exerted every effort to ensure that drug selection and dosage set forth in this text are in accord with current recommendations and practice at the time of publication. However, in view of ongoing research, changes in government regulations, and the constant flow of information relating to drug therapy and drug reactions, the reader is urged to check the package insert for each drug for any change in indications and dosage and for added warnings and precautions. This is particularly important when the recommended agent is a new or infrequently employed drug.

Library of Congress Cataloging in Publication Data
Main entry under title:

Medical care of the surgical patient.

Includes index.
1. Therapeutics, Surgical. 2. Surgery—Complications
and sequelae. I. Goldmann, David R. [DNLM: 1. Preoperative care. 2. Postoperative care. 3. Intraoperative care. WO 181 M489]
RD49.M4   617'.01   82–6605
ISBN 0–397–50485–3

1   3   5   6   4   2

CONTRIBUTORS

ELIAS ABRUTYN, M.D.
Associate Professor and
Assistant Chairman
Department of Medicine
Medical College of Pennsylvania;
Assistant Chief of Medicine
Chief of Infectious Diseases
Veterans Administration Hospital;
Adjunct Associate Professor
of Medicine
University of Pennsylvania
School of Medicine
Philadelphia, Pennsylvania

PAUL C. ATKINS, M.D.
Associate Professor of Medicine
University of Pennsylvania
School of Medicine;
Chief, Allergy-Immunology Clinic
Hospital of the University of
Pennsylvania
Philadelphia, Pennsylvania

MAURICE F. ATTIE, M.D.
Assistant Professor of Medicine
University of Pennsylvania
School of Medicine
Philadelphia, Pennsylvania

WILLIAM M. BATTLE, M.D.
Assistant Clinical Professor
of Medicine
University of Pennsylvania
School of Medicine;
Attending Staff
Jeanes Hospital and
Nazareth Hospital;
Associate Staff
American Oncologic Hospital
Philadelphia, Pennsylvania

LAURENCE H. BECK, M.D.
Associate Professor of Medicine
and Vice-Chairman
Department of Medicine
University of Pennsylvania
School of Medicine;
Chief, Medical Service
Philadelphia Veterans Administration
Medical Center
Philadelphia, Pennsylvania

BONNIE J. BLATT, M.D.
Acting Director, Emergency Department
Temple University Hospital;
Instructor in Internal Medicine
Temple University School of Medicine
Philadelphia, Pennsylvania

GORDON P. BUZBY, M.D.
Assistant Professor of Surgery
University of Pennsylvania
School of Medicine
Philadelphia, Pennsylvania

JAIME CARRIZOSA, M.D.
Associate Professor of Medicine
Medical College of Pennsylvania
Philadelphia, Pennsylvania

JEFFREY L. CARSON, M.D.
Assistant Professor of Medicine
College of Medicine and Dentistry
of New Jersey
Rutgers Medical School at Camden
Camden, New Jersey

RANDALL D. CEBUL, M.D.
Assistant Professor of Medicine
Section of General Medicine
Hospital of the University of Pennsylvania
Philadelphia, Pennsylvania

MALCOLM COX, M.D.
Assistant Professor of Medicine
Renal-Electrolyte Section
Department of Medicine
Philadelphia Veterans Administration
Medical Center and
University of Pennsylvania
School of Medicine
Philadelphia, Pennsylvania

JULIUS J. DEREN, M.D.
Professor of Medicine
University of Pennsylvania;
Director of Gastroenterology and
Nutrition
Graduate Hospital of the University
of Pennsylvania
Philadelphia, Pennsylvania

JOHN M. EISENBERG, M.D.
Sol Katz Associate Professor
of General Medicine
Chief, Section of General Medicine
Department of Medicine
University of Pennsylvania
Philadelphia, Pennsylvania

MICHAEL A. GEHEB, M.D.
Assistant Professor of Medicine
Renal-Electrolyte Section
Department of Medicine
Philadelphia Veterans Administration
Medical Center and
University of Pennsylvania
School of Medicine
Philadelphia, Pennsylvania

PHILIP P. GERBINO, PHARM. D.
Associate Professor of Clinical Pharmacy
Philadelphia College of
Pharmacy and Science
Philadelphia, Pennsylvania

STANTON L. GERSON, M.D.
Fellow, Hematology-Oncology Section
Hospital of the University of
Pennsylvania
Philadelphia, Pennsylvania

STEPHEN J. GLUCKMAN, M.D.
Chief, Infectious Diseases Section
Pennsylvania Hospital;

Clinical Assistant Professor of
Medicine
University of Pennsylvania
Philadelphia, Pennsylvania

STANLEY GOLDFARB, M.D.
Associate Professor of Medicine
University of Pennsylvania
School of Medicine
Philadelphia, Pennsylvania

**FRANCISCO GONZALEZ-
SCARANO,** M.D.
Assistant Professor of Neurology
University of Pennsylvania
School of Medicine
Philadelphia, Pennsylvania

ARTHUR GREENBERG, M.D.
Assistant Professor of Medicine
Renal-Electrolyte Division
Department of Medicine
School of Medicine
University of Pittsburgh
Pittsburgh, Pennsylvania

ALDEN H. HARKEN, M.D.
Associate Professor of Surgery
University of Pennsylvania
Philadelphia, Pennsylvania

DAVID H. HENRY, M.D.
Major, USAF, MC
Staff, Hematology-Medical Oncology
Wilford Hall USAF Medical Center
Lackland AFB, Texas

ROBERT A. HIRSH, M.D.
Chairman, Department of Anesthesiology
Jeanes Hospital;
Adjunct Assistant Professor
Department of Anesthesia
University of Pennsylvania
Philadelphia, Pennsylvania

JOHN W. HIRSHFELD, Jr., M.D.
Associate Professor of Medicine
University of Pennsylvania
School of Medicine;
Director, Cardiac Catheterization Laboratory
Hospital of the University of Pennsylvania
Philadelphia, Pennsylvania

RICHARD S. HOROWITZ, M.D.
Attending Staff
St. Francis Heart Hospital
Roslyn, New York

HOWARD I. HURTIG, M.D.
Associate Professor of Neurology and
Chairman, Department of Neurology
Graduate Hospital of the
University of Pennsylvania
Philadelphia, Pennsylvania

JERRY C. JOHNSON, M.D.
Director, Geriatric Physician
Fellowship Program
Philadelphia Veterans Administration
Medical Center;
Assistant Professor of Medicine
University of Pennsylvania
Philadelphia, Pennsylvania

MARK A. KELLEY, M.D.
Associate Chairman and
Assistant Professor
Department of Medicine
University of Pennsylvania
School of Medicine
Philadelphia, Pennsylvania

WILLIAM G. KUSSMAUL, M.D.
Cardiology Section
Hospital of the University of
Pennsylvania
Philadelphia, Pennsylvania

PAUL N. LANKEN, M.D.
Assistant Professor of Medicine
Cardiovascular-Pulmonary Division
Department of Medicine
University of Pennsylvania;
Medical Director, Respiratory
Therapy Department
Associate Director, Medical
Intensive Care Unit
Hospital of the University of
Pennsylvania
Philadelphia, Pennsylvania

GARY M. LEVINE, M.D.
Chief, Gastrointestinal Section
Albert Einstein Medical Center
Philadelphia, Pennsylvania

FRANCIS E. MARCHLINSKI, M.D.
Assistant Professor of Medicine
Cardiovascular Section
Department of Medicine
University of Pennsylvania
Philadelphia, Pennsylvania

JOEL MORGANROTH, M.D.
Professor of Medicine
Hahnemann University of the
Health Sciences;
Director, Sudden Death Prevention
Program
Likoff Cardiovascular Institute
Philadelphia, Pennsylvania

JAMES L. MULLEN, M.D.
Associate Professor of Surgery
University of Pennsylvania
School of Medicine;
Chief, Surgical Service
Philadelphia Veterans Administration
Medical Center;
Director, Nutrition Support Service
Hospital of the University of
Pennsylvania
Philadelphia, Pennsylvania

THOMAS G. MURRAY, M.D.*
Assistant Professor of Medicine
Director of Dialysis Programs
University of Pennsylvania
School of Medicine
Philadelphia, Pennsylvania

GREGORY R. OWENS, M.D.
Assistant Professor of Medicine
University of Pittsburgh
School of Medicine;
Director, Exercise Physiology Laboratory
Co-Director, Pulmonary Function Laboratory
Presbyterian University Hospital
Pittsburgh, Pennsylvania

**BERNADETTE MARIE
PASTEWSKI,** PHARM. D.
Assistant Professor of Clinical Pharmacy
Philadelphia College of
Pharmacy and Science
Philadelphia, Pennsylvania

*Deceased

MICHAEL J. REICHGOTT, M.D., Ph.D.
Associate Professor of Medicine and
Pharmacology
Department of Medicine
University of Pennsylvania
School of Medicine
Philadelphia, Pennsylvania

GARY C. RICHTER, M.D.
Clinical Assistant Professor of Medicine
School of Medicine at
Morehouse College
Atlanta, Georgia

JOHN A. SCARLETT, M.D.
Associate Investigator and
Clinical Research Fellow
Departments of Medicine
Veterans Administration Medical Center
and University of Colorado
Health Sciences Center
Denver, Colorado

ALAN D. SCHREIBER, M.D.
Associate Professor of Medicine
University of Pennsylvania
School of Medicine
Philadelphia, Pennsylvania

YIH-FU SHIAU, M.D., Ph.D.
Chief, Gastrointestinal Section
Philadelphia Veterans Administration
Medical Center
Philadelphia, Pennsylvania

STEVEN A. SILBER, M.D.
Assistant Professor of Medicine
Graduate Hospital
University of Pennsylvania
School of Medicine
Philadelphia, Pennsylvania

PETER J. SNYDER, M.D.
Associate Professor of Medicine
University of Pennsylvania
School of Medicine
Philadelphia, Pennsylvania

ARTHUR P. STADDON, M.D.
Clinical Assistant Professor
University of Pennsylvania
School of Medicine;
Associate in Hematology-Oncology
Presbyterian University of
Pensylvania Medical Center and
Graduate Hospital of the
University of Pennsylvania
Philadelphia, Pennsylvania

JAMES L. STINNETT, M.D.
Director, Psychiatric Consultation Service
Hospital of the University of
Pennsylvania;
Associate Professor
Department of Psychiatry
University of Pennsylvania
School of Medicine
Philadelphia, Pennsylvania

GEORGE HARRISON TALBOT, M.D.
Assistant Professor of Medicine
Infectious Diseases Section
University of Pennsylvania
School of Medicine;
Hospital Epidemiologist
Hospital of the University of
Pennsylvania
Philadelphia, Pennsylvania

JOSEPH VERBALIS, M.D.
Assistant Professor of Medicine
University of Pittsburgh
School of Medicine
Pittsburgh, Pennsylvania

SANKEY V. WILLIAMS, M.D.
Henry J. Kaiser Family Foundation
Faculty Scholar;
Section of General Medicine
Department of Medicine
Hospital of the University of
Pennsylvania
Philadelphia, Pennsylvania

FOREWORDS

Reading this volume, *Medical Care of the Surgical Patient,* made me wish it had been available 45 years ago when I first was asked to see surgical patients in consultation. It is a most remarkable collection of useful and important information in this area. Perusal of the table of contents and reference lists reflects its extensive scope.

There are 38 chapters written by over 50 physicians, many from the University of Pennsylvania School of Medicine. They discuss the problems a medical consultant might meet when called to see a surgical patient. Many of the authors became interested in this subject during their medical residencies, when they served a period of duty as medical consultants. Since their residencies, many of the authors have had special training that has allowed them to expand their knowledge in the areas about which they write. These facts about the authors and the genesis of this book explain to some extent why it is so reliable, authentic, comprehensive, and coherent.

My interest and earliest experience in consultations on surgical patients resulted when Dr. Alexander Randall asked me to see patients on his urology service before and after operation. Nothing makes you realize more clearly what you don't know and what you need to know than being called at 2 A.M. to see a very sick postoperative patient. I soon learned how well most elderly patients come through serious operations. One of my teachers once said, "You worry too much about these old people. If they weren't tough, they wouldn't have lived so long." I found that the cardiovascular competence of an elderly patient to withstand an operation is often easily determined by asking him about his ability to lead a normal life and walking with him down the hall and, if possible, up a flight or two of stairs. His endurance may surpass your own!

Incidentally, surgeons as well as internists could learn a great deal from reading this book. If they could absorb and retain all of it, they would not need many medical consultations. I am proud to have been asked to write this foreword. This is the best book on the subject that it has been my privilege to read.

Francis C. Wood, M.D.
Emeritus Frank Wister Thomas
Professor of Medicine
University of Pennsylvania
School of Medicine
Philadelphia, Pennsylvania

The stated objective of this timely book was to bring together the widely scattered information necessary to provide effective medical care to the surgical patient. This objective has been achieved with solid success. The authors have outlined the essentials of preoperative preparation, as well as transoperative and postoperative management for a wide variety of medical disorders. Perioperative medical hazards and major postoperative complications for virtually the entire range of common surgical procedures are considered.

For many years, the surgeon was sometimes looked upon, perhaps often unjustly, as largely a technician with little understanding of physiology. After World War II, a new era of surgical investigation and learning resulted in a much more pervasive education throughout the surgical environment with respect to the metabolic preparation of the patient for surgery and the management of transoperative and postoperative metabolic alterations. In recent years, a still further orientation has developed, in that it is commonly recognized that the busy surgeon, even one with extensive experience with metabolic parameters, cannot always provide his patient with optimal treatment without the consultation and active assistance of those in other disciplines, especially internal medicine. Close cooperation between the surgeon and the internist in a difficult case can only result in better treatment for the patient. While this is not to say that the surgeon should not have a comprehensive grasp of what is required for successful surgical therapy, it does acknowledge that medical information is expanding too rapidly to be assimilated by any single specialist.

One of the major strengths of *Medical Care of the Surgical Patient* is the specificity with which the diagnosis and treatment of the many medical problems is presented. Care has been taken to detail "how much, of what, how fast" when such precise therapeutic information is appropriate. Further, a concise summary appears at the end of each chapter.

It is safe to predict that this book will be highly useful both to internists and to surgeons. For the consulting internist, it may serve as a refresher course for a highly specialized physician who needs to know more about medical problems in fields other than his own. For the surgeon, it will afford comprehensive and immediately useful information regarding the management of medical problems in his patient. And for both, it can pave the way for maximally fruitful collaboration in providing optimal medical–surgical care.

It is a privilege to have been invited to write this foreword.

James D. Hardy, M.D.
Professor and Chairman
Department of Surgery
University of Mississippi
Medical Center
Jackson, Mississippi

PREFACE

Patients undergoing surgery frequently have medical problems that influence their course in the perioperative period. The interactions of medical and surgical illnesses are complex and may complicate management. Many questions, even those that arise most commonly, remain unanswered. What are the risks of surgery and general anesthesia in patients with a given set of medical illnesses? What are the predictors of these risks? Can they be reduced by preoperative measures? How should medical problems be managed before and after surgery? What complications might be expected? How should problems common to the perioperative period be approached diagnostically and therapeutically?

The information necessary to answer these questions is scattered throughout the literature and is never systematically addressed during medical school or house-staff training. *Medical Care of the Surgical Patient: A Problem-Oriented Approach to Management* began with a critical review of this literature to help senior residents at the Hospital of the University of Pennsylvania who serve as consultants to surgical services. Although the book was originally conceived to meet the needs of the training program, its potential usefulness to all those caring for surgical patients became apparent. It is not a textbook of medicine dealing with diagnosis and treatment of medical illnesses or a textbook of surgery discussing indications for surgery or techniques and complications. Rather, it is our intention to assemble existing data from diverse sources in readily accessible form, to review critically what is known, to indicate deficiencies in current knowledge, and to identify areas for future research. Internists, surgeons, anesthesiologists, family practitioners, and trainees can use this book to formulate a comprehensive approach to perioperative patients.

Medical Care of the Surgical Patient: A Problem-Oriented Approach to Management stands as the concerted effort of many physicians and pharmacologists, nearly all of whom are or were affiliated with the Department of Medicine at the University of Pennsylvania School of Medicine. We gratefully acknowledge the contributions of our medical and surgical colleagues. We acknowledge the generous support of the Robert Wood Johnson Foundation. We thank Barbara Mihatov and Pamela Wagner for their technical assistance and our publishers for their invaluable advice. Finally, we thank Dr. Lawrence Earley and Dr. Arnold S. Relman, present and past Chairman of the Department of Medicine, respectively, for their inspiration.

David R. Goldmann, M.D.
Frank H. Brown, M.D.
William K. Levy, M.D.
Gail B. Slap, M.D.
Elliot J. Sussman, M.D.

CONTENTS

MEDICAL CARE OF THE SURGICAL PATIENT

The Physiologic Response to Surgery and Anesthesia

ALDEN H. HARKEN
ELLIOT J. SUSSMAN

Since Claude Bernard first perceived the constancy of the "milieu interieur" and Walter Cannon initially described "bodily changes in pain, hunger, fear and rage," substantial progress has been made in delineating the physiologic response to surgery and anesthesia. The resultant metabolic approach to the care of the surgical patient has permitted the thoughtful physician to minimize the insult necessarily inflicted by surgery.

This chapter is an overview of the physiologic changes that occur in response to anesthesia and surgery in the normal patient. These changes include myocardial depression, hemodynamic derangement, respiratory compromise, alteration in oxygen delivery, negative nitrogen balance, acid–base deregulation, glucose intolerance, hyperaldosteronism, inappropriate antidiuretic hormone (ADH) secretion, and hypercortisolism. Most are well tolerated when managed properly.

CARDIOVASCULAR SYSTEM

General anesthesia and surgical manipulation modify the response of the heart and blood vessels to many physiologic and pharmacologic stimuli. Much of the available data on cardiovascular physiology and pharmacology is derived from animal experiments usually conducted with the subjects anesthetized and their chests open. Circulatory responses to physiologic and pharmacologic interventions in this setting frequently differ in magnitude and direction, depending upon experimental design; this often results in data that are difficult to interpret and extrapolate to the patient.

Cardiac Output

All general anesthetics are myocardial depressants.[1,2] Halothane, the most commonly used agent, causes a reduction in cardiac contractility with a 30% reduction in cardiac index.[3] This depressant effect is directly related to both the concentration of halothane and the duration of its administration. Halothane does not affect venous return; however, sodium thiopental, which is commonly used for induction, does markedly lower both venous return and mean systemic arterial pressure.[4,5] Both sodium thiopental and pentobarbital reduce myocardial contractility and induce a reflex tachycardia. Studies of myocardial contractility using cat papillary muscle indicate that anesthetic preparations in order of decreasing depressant effect are ethrane, halothane, penthrane, cyclopropane, and diethylether.[6]

Anesthetics also indirectly affect myocardial contractility by influencing the carotid sinus reflex. In the unanesthetized subject, carotid sinus hypotension produces tachycardia and increases inotropy, whereas carotid sinus hypertension causes bradycardia and reduces contractility. In the anesthetized subject, the increase in heart rate resulting from carotid sinus hypotension causes a disproportionate increase in myocardial contractility.

Acute increases in preload during anesthesia produce variable changes in heart rate. An abrupt increase in afterload produces an acute increase in left ventricular end diastolic volume, resulting in a positive inotropic effect. Left ventricular end diastolic volume then shortly returns to normal.

General anesthetics also alter the inotropic action of other drugs. Ouabain produces more inotropy in anesthesized than in conscious dogs, probably by causing coronary vasodilatation; coronary vasoconstriction is predominantly observed in animals that are awake. Sympathomimetic drugs like norepinephrine, dopamine, and dobutamine may produce more inotropy in open-chest anesthetized dogs than they do in closed-chest anesthetized animals or conscious animals. It is clear that anesthetic–drug interactions must therefore be viewed in the experimental context before clear conclusions can be drawn.

Cardiac output normally increases in the postoperative state because of increased catecholamine output and metabolic demands. Increased metabolism requires greater blood flow, especially since the oxyhemoglobin curve is shifted to the left in post-traumatic alkalosis, although this finding has recently been challenged.[7]

Volume

The body responds to acute volume reduction with transient changes in blood flow and tissue perfusion. In the unanesthetized subject, there is a compensatory increase in arterial pressure and renal vasodilatation. In the anesthetized subject, the response to volume loss is intense vasoconstriction of the mesenteric, muscular, and renal vascular beds. General anesthetics may affect the function of arterial baroreceptors and impair the defense of arterial pressure in response to hemorrhage. If tissue perfusion is insufficient for a prolonged period, irreversible shock ensues. Any acute stress or injury invariably leads to a redistribution of blood flow to vital organs (Fig. 1-1) and relative ischemia of other tissue beds. The brain, heart, and liver are the major beneficiaries of this redistribution. Because cells cannot effectively store oxygen, they shift from an energy-productive and efficient aerobic to an anaerobic metabolism.[8,9]

As oxygen availability inside the cell decreases, various intracellular redox systems shift toward a more reduced state.[10] All of these biochemical systems, except the lactic acid dehydrogenase system, are intimately interrelated, and products of one reaction become substrates for the next. A decrease in the activity of one of these reactions therefore retards the whole sequence of energy metabolism. In a hypoxic cell, the oxidation of nicotinamide adenine dinucleotide ($NADH_2$) to NAD^+ through the electron-carrier system decreases, and lactic acid dehydrogenases

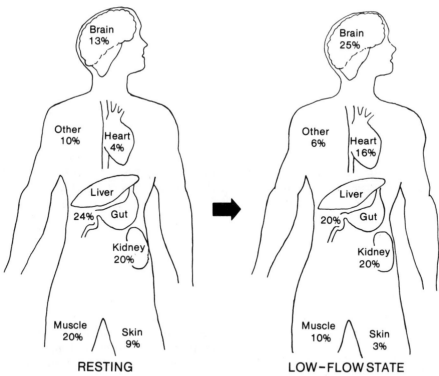

Fig. 1-1. The distribution of cardiac output under stable, resting conditions and during a low-flow state. Acute stress leads to a redistribution of blood flow toward vital organs and transient ischemia of less-favored tissue beds.

assume the responsibility for this oxidation. Because lactic acid is not a substrate in any other intracellular reaction, its accumulation has no influence on any other system.[11] Thus, as the lactic dehydrogenase system takes over the oxidation of $NADH_2$ to NAD^+, the serum lactate level rises. Serum lactate is a reflection of the cellular struggle for electrochemical homeostasis and survival.

Hemorrhage is the most common cause of volume reduction. Venous hemorrhage of 10% to 20% of total blood volume results in a net flow of water, salt, and protein into the intravascular space over a 20- to 40-hr period. Initially, the intravascular volume expands by as much as 2 ml/min.

Although this continues until volume is restored, compositional ratios remain altered.[12] Other responses to acute volume reduction are discussed below.

With surgery, there are also more subtle forms of volume reduction or redistribution. General anesthesia is characteristically administered with positive-pressure ventilation. The resultant increase in intrathoracic pressure produces a decrease in venous return and in cardiac output.[13] Similarly, a thoracotomy effects an increase in the normally negative pleural pressure to atmospheric levels with a resultant decrease in venous return and cardiac output.[14] These clinical conditions are analogous to MacLean's "hypovolemic" shock and should respond to volume replacement.[15]

Compensation for progressive hypovolemia through neurohumoral reflexes not only protects the patient but may mask the shock syndrome during its early phases. The decrease in arterial blood pressure is sensed by carotid and aortic baroreceptors. These receptors initiate reflex vasoconstriction with an attendant increase in heart rate and left ventricular contractility.[16] Decreased stretch on the atrial and caval receptors stimulates pituitary secretion of ADH and renal release of renin. The latter results in an increase in angiotensin II production and, subsequently, in aldosterone secretion.[17] The reflex elaboration of aldosterone and ADH mediated by atrial afferent receptors promotes maintenance of vascular volume and systemic arterial pressure.

Regional Blood Flow

The amount of blood flow to any organ is determined by the difference between arterial and venous pressures in the vasculature supplying that organ and by vascular resistance within the organ. Most regulation of flow occurs by changes in vessel caliber at the level of the small arteries and arterioles. These changes are mediated by neural influences and by hormonal, metabolic, and chemical substances produced locally or carried in the blood. Vasodilatation occurs in response to hypoxia or increases in P_{CO_2}. Vasoconstriction generally occurs as a result of increased sympathetic tone. The distribution of cutaneous, skeletal muscle, renal, splanchnic, hepatic, carotid, and coronary perfusion is mediated by rich alpha-adrenergic innervation in the vascular beds supplying these organs.[16,18] In normal low-flow states, relative blood flow is altered, as seen in Figure 1-1. Collapse of this distributional system, an unusual form of hemodynamic compromise, may result from inhalational or local anesthetics.

Anesthetics more commonly produce a differential effect on regional vascular resistance and blood flow. Halothane dilates the renal and iliac beds and constricts the mesenteric bed. All inhalational anesthetics are direct cerebral vasodilators. The accumulation of CO_2 through anesthetic-induced ventilatory depression further increases cerebral vasodilatation.

Anesthetics may also affect the response of vascular beds to other drugs. For example, cardiac glycosides cause mesenteric vasodilatation in the conscious animal and mesenteric vasoconstriction in the anesthetized animal. In addition, conscious and anesthetized animals manifest different coronary circulation responses to sympathomimetic agents.[19]

RESPIRATORY SYSTEM

Pulmonary Function

A complex array of stimuli compromise pulmonary function during and after surgery. Identifiable pulmonary dysfunction after operation has been reported in 21% to 80% of patients.[20] Although all surgical patients are at risk, those undergoing thoracic or upper abdominal surgery face the highest risk.[21,22] Moore and associates have described the loss of compliance and the ventilation–perfusion imbalance that are characteristic of post-traumatic or surgical pulmonary insufficiency.[23]

Even before surgery, however, commonly used medications may predispose the surgical patient to respiratory complications. Mucosal-drying agents and central nervous system depressants decrease ciliary motility, reflex responses to respiratory stimuli, and deep-breathing.

Tracheal intubation may lead to hoarseness, glottal edema, and reflex sympathetic stimulation with subsequent tachycardia, hypertension, and arrhythmias.[24,25] Women are more prone to complications than are men. Other risk factors for postintubation complications include prolonged anesthesia, upper airway infection, traumatic intubation, high-pressure cuffs, and large tubes.[26] Aspiration may occur even with the tube in place and extubation may precipitate prolonged laryngospasm.[27] Late complications of endotracheal intubation are uncommon but include vocal-cord paralysis and tracheal stenosis.[28,29]

Even brief intubation results in some desquamation of epithelium from the upper respiratory tract. Dogs intubated for 2 hr exhibit areas denuded of cilia along the path of passage of the tube. Inflated cuffs produce similar changes, which require at least a week to resolve. These findings correlate well with results of human autopsy studies.[30]

When anesthetic agents are administered to intubated patients, normal respiratory patterns and mechanisms of gas exchange are altered. Many anesthetics, including halothane, cause significant hypoventilation and depress the normal sighing mechanism, predisposing patients to atelectasis and hypoxemia. General anesthetics also diminish the respiratory response to carbon dioxide by blunting the response of the respiratory center in the central nervous system to hydrogen ions. Anesthetics also promote a vagally mediated increase in mucosal secretions from the tracheobronchial tree.

After surgery, patients may exhibit an abnormal ventilatory pattern with shallow breathing and no deep sighs. In animals, long-term shallow breathing leads to reduced surfactant, microatelectasis, and a progressive decrease in functional residual capacity (FRC) to levels below the closing volume with subsequent ventilation–perfusion mismatch.[31] Vital capacity, forced expiratory volume in 1 sec (FEV_1), and FRC all decrease after upper abdominal surgery by 25% to 66%.[32] FRC decreases 20% in patients in the supine position. Postoperative conditions are therefore optimal for gas trapping and pulmonary shunting.

Maldistribution of ventilation due to small-airway and alveolar closure is exacerbated by muscle weakness, chest wall and abdominal pain, ileus, abdominal distention, and narcotic drugs. Dependent pulmonary congestion, incipient left ventricular failure due to fluid overload, and platelet and white cell emboli may further exacerbate this problem. Maldistribution of pulmonary blood flow due to local release and activation of vasoactive hormones such as prostaglandins, serotonin, and kinins further promotes ventilation–perfusion mismatch.[33] Atelectasis and increased lung water due to pneumonia or pulmonary edema increase the elastic resistance of the lungs and decrease compliance.

In the late 1950s, Mead and Collier noted a decrease in pulmonary compliance in anesthetized dogs and excised dog lung during quiet breathing; this decrease was prevented by periodic sigh maneuvers.[34] Ferris and Pollard confirmed this observation in humans.[35] Bendixen and co-workers demonstrated an average decrease in oxygen tension of 22% and in pulmonary compliance of 15% during an average of 76 min of surgery with general anesthesia and controlled ventilation.[36]

Gamsu and co-workers used powdered tantalum to examine mucociliary clearance after laparotomy in 18 patients.[37] Abnormal pooling of tantalum-labeled mucus and accompanying x-ray evidence of atelectasis were noted in 14 of the 18 patients. Mucociliary clearance was depressed further by codeine, morphine, atropine, barbiturates, halothane, and increased inspired oxygen concentrations.

Surgery clearly affects respiration, and respiratory complications clearly affect surgical outcome. Perioperative measures designed to prevent or diminish postoperative pulmonary dysfunction are discussed in Chapter 23.[20]

Oxyhemoglobin Affinity

In 1904, Bohr first described the sigmoid shape of the oxyhemoglobin dissociation curve.[38] The curve is shifted to the right by increases in hydrogen ion concentration, P_{CO_2} temperature, organic phosphates such as 2,3-DPG, ATP, and pyridoxal phosphate, and hemoglobin concentration. Halothane, ethrane, nitrous oxide, and cyclopropane all reduce oxyhemoglobin affinity.[39] Many drugs used perioperatively have been reported to influence hemoglobin affinity for oxygen; these include propranolol,[40] aluminum hydroxide,[41] androgens,[42] prostaglandin E_2,[43] aldosterone,[44] cortisol,[45] methylprednisone,[46] acetazolamide,[45] and dipyridamole.[47]

Aste-Salazar and Hurtado were the first to suggest that the rightward shift of the oxyhemoglobin dissociation curve at high altitude might constitute an adaptive mechanism to permit increased oxygen unloading at the tissue level.[48] However, it has been difficult to relate the oxyhemoglobin affinity of blood to the oxygen uptake of individual cells. Chance and associates have studied cellular oxygen utilization and determined that the cytochrome system can function with ambient oxygen tensions measured in fractions of a torr.[49]

There is evidence that oxyhemoglobin affinity has real physiologic significance in humans. Lenfant agreed that a decrease in oxyhemoglobin affinity augments oxygen unloading[50] but believed that the shift in oxyhemoglobin affinity during acclimatization to altitude is of negligible significance.[51] Harken and Woods showed that oxygen uptake differs when an isolated canine tissue bed is perfused with autologous blood of different oxyhemoglobin affinities.[52] Bowen and Fleming studied massive human transfusion of stored blood with high oxyhemoglobin affinity.[53] Increased venous oxygen extraction and cardiac output compensated for the increase in oxyhemoglobin affinity. Oski and co-workers examined the influence of hemoglobin function in two patients with inherited defects in erythrocyte metabolism.[54] One patient, who had a pyruvate kinase deficiency, had high levels of 2,3-DPG and a markedly rightward-shifted oxyhemoglobin dissociation curve. The other, who had a hexokinase deficiency, showed low levels of 2,3-DPG and a leftward-shifted curve. After exercise, the child with low oxyhemoglobin affinity and a rightward-shifted curve was able to maintain high oxygen consumption with a significantly lower cardiac output. This was presumably due to facilitated oxygen unloading in the tissues.

The surgical patient is subjected to many agents and stresses that alter hemoglobin function. In most cases, however, the effect on tissue oxygen supply is small.

ENDOCRINE SYSTEM

Catecholamines

Even minor tissue injury or fluctuations in blood volume are associated with increased levels of circulating epinephrine and norepinephrine. Catecholamines, which are neurotransmitters in the central nervous system, mediate peripheral sympathetic nervous system activity in controlling visceral tissues. Neural signals prompt rapid release of stored catecholamines, which are then rapidly cleared from the extracellular fluid.

The hemodynamic and metabolic expression of sympathoadrenal activation may be modulated by the influence of these hormones on adrenergic receptor function and by catecholamine clearance.[55] In addition, catecholamines directly affect the metabolism of carbohydrates, lipids, and proteins. Epinephrine inhibits the production of insulin and stimulates glycogenolysis and lipolysis. Catecholamines activate the entire neuroendocrine machinery by directly stimulating the pituitary to produce adrenocorticotropic hormone (ACTH), which in turn promotes the release of glucocorticoids and aldosterone.

Epinephrine is produced solely in the adrenal medulla. Norepinephrine is released throughout the body at nerve synapses. Bilateral adrenalectomy completely eliminates epinephrine from the body but has no influence on blood and urine norepinephrine levels.[56] The intricate interdependence of epinephrine and norepinephrine and other hormones is emphasized by the fact that a basal level of glucocorticoid is essential for catechol-amines to have an effect on peripheral vasomotor activity.[56]

Glucocorticoids

For many years, physiologists have emphasized the concept of a unified neuroendocrine response to psychosocial stress, or the "alarm reaction," so called by Selye.[57] Before and during surgery, serum corticosteroid levels are very high. Tissue injury results in a maximal ACTH–glucocorticoid response.

Direct neural stimulation and catecholamines from sympathetic nerve endings and the adrenal medulla combine to increase the release of ACTH from the pituitary gland. ACTH stimulates the adrenal cortex to produce cortisol. Corticosteroids, together with glucagon and catecholamines, facilitate gluconeogenesis. This provides glucose at a time when it is lacking in the diet and supplies low-molecular-weight nitrogen compounds for collagen synthesis in the healing wound.[58]

In clean, elective surgical procedures, corticosteroid levels may increase tenfold immediately after surgery and return to normal within 24 hr.[59] With complex multiorgan injury or concurrent sepsis, adrenocortical output may remain elevated for weeks or months. Prolonged adrenal stimulation characteristically causes glandular hypertrophy. Hypotension with intraadrenal hemorrhage or infection rarely produces adrenal hypofunction.

Aldosterone

General and regional anesthesia may cause peripheral vasodilatation, which decreases renal perfusion and right-heart filling pressure. Isotonic volume loss, as in pure hemorrhage, promotes the redistribution of cardiac output away from the kidney, reducing its share from the usual 20% to 10%.[60] Decreased renal blood flow is sensed by cells adjacent to the glomerulus; they respond by secreting renin, thereby activating the renin–angiotensin system to produce angiotensin II. Angiotensin II acts as a vasoconstrictor 50 times as potent as norepinephrine and directly stimulates the adrenal cortex to produce aldosterone.[61] Aldosterone promotes renal resorption of sodium in exchange for potassium and hydrogen ions in the distal tubule.

Because of transient hyperaldosteronism, the surgical patient typically produces acid urine, which is high in potassium and low in sodium and contributes to the common postoperative alkalemia.[62] Urine in the early postoperative period is so low in sodium—always below 40 mEq/liter and frequently less than 10mEq/liter—that measurement of urine sodium concentration has become a useful clinical test of renal function. A value higher than 40 mEq/liter signifies renal dysfunction or acute tubular necrosis.

Aldosterone supports plasma and interstitial fluid volume by promoting renal sodium conservation. The associated release of the potent pressor angiotensin and transient perioperative hyperaldosteronism appropriately aids in maintaining circulating intravascular volume and perfusion of vital organs.

Antidiuretic Hormone

Stress and trauma promote the production of antidiuretic hormone (ADH) in the hypothalamus and its release from the posterior pituitary.[63] An isotonic decrease in blood volume, as seen with hemorrhage, stimulates ADH release, the response being greater if the plasma becomes hypertonic. Preoperative water deprivation, tissue trauma, and administration of narcotics all stimulate ADH production.[63] Postoperative water administration does not appropriately inhibit ADH and leads to hypotonicity and hyponatremia. Free water clearance may be decreased for hours or even days as a result of inappropriate ADH secretion.[56]

Insulin

Pancreatic islet cells are exquisitely sensitive to changes in blood glucose concentration.[55] Insulin not only favors glucose utilization by facilitating its entry into cells but also inhibits the release of amino acids from muscle and minimizes the hydrolysis of fat to free fatty acids. With surgical stress, the release and availability of circulating glucose is increased for several days.[64] Catecholamines induce hyperglycemia by accelerating hepatic glucose production (glycogenolysis and gluconeogenesis) and reducing glucose clearance from the circulation. The latter is primarily responsible for the typical prolonged posttraumatic hyperglycemia.[65] Glucagon and corticosteroids act synergistically to maximize the production of glucose from protein stores and suppress insulin secretion. Catecholamines directly depress pancreatic release of insulin and blunt peripheral insulin activity.[66,67] Thus, conditions of surgical stress are accompanied by inappropriately low insulin concentrations, rising glucagon levels for as long as 5 days after surgery, increased gluconeogenesis, high catecholamine levels, and decreased peripheral insulin action. This process causes glucose intolerance and, if prolonged, leads to characteristic patterns of postoperative catabolism.

Thyroid Hormone

The serum concentration of T_4 may increase after surgery, depending on the anesthetic agent used. T_3 levels fall, and those of reverse T_3 rise. Although these changes may persist for up to 6 days after surgery, patients remain clinically euthyroid.

METABOLISM

Surgical Catabolism

A healthy patient undergoing elective surgery is equipped to handle the combined insults of starvation, hemorrhage, tissue injury, and emotional anxiety. Indeed, differences in nitrogen flux and metabolism are sufficiently small to permit controversy over whether clean surgical procedures impose an additional metabolic insult over simple starvation (Fig. 1-2). Approximately 5% of fat-free body mass may be lost with routine elective surgical intervention.

Moore and Brennan have described three overlapping phases of starvation.[68] They emphasize that, particularly in gastrointestinal surgery, patients have been starving for weeks or months before the procedure. During the first 2 to 4 days, blood glucose requirements are met by gluconeogenesis, since hepatic glycogen stores are small and muscle glycogen cannot be converted to glucose because of the lack of the enzyme glucose-6 phosphatase in muscle. Gluconeogenesis takes place mainly in the liver and the kidney, with alanine and glutamine as their respective substrates. Although all endogenous proteins, including liver polypeptides, serum albumin, and digestive enzymes, are used, skeletal muscle is the chief contributer.[69]

Urinary nitrogen increases from 5 to 10 g/day.

During the second phase, 3 to 6 weeks after surgery, protein is conserved, and urinary nitrogen excretion decreases while fat oxidation increases to a maximum. Lipolysis, perhaps triggered by low serum insulin, releases free fatty acids and glycerol. Free fatty acids do not participate directly in gluconeogenesis but lead to energy production by providing acetyl coenzyme A for the tricarboxylic acid cycle in the liver. Glycerol is readily converted to glucose, but only 18 to 20 g/day of glucose are produced from this source.[69]

During the third phase, nitrogen losses further decrease as tissues that normally utilize glucose fully adapt to the use of ketone derivatives of both protein and fat.[70] Metabolism of triglycerides leads to an elevation of serum ketone bodies, and starvation ketosis may signal a reduction in alanine synthesis by muscle and trigger conversion to ketone-body metabolism in the central nervous system.[41]

Major trauma disrupts this energy-efficient system. Long-term structural goals are sacrificed in favor of immediate energy production. There is profligate use of body protein; administered carbohydrate has only a minor protein-sparing effect. Body-fat oxidation accelerates. Water and salt conservation is profound. Exogenous nitrogen substrate is ignored in favor of immediate energy production from carbohydrate. After severe surgical injury, glycogen may be depleted in as little as 12 hr, and deficit protein spending ensues. Skeletal muscle yields polypeptides to the extracellular fluid for transamination into carbohydrate, producing a negative nitrogen balance.

Clean elective surgery, like starvation,

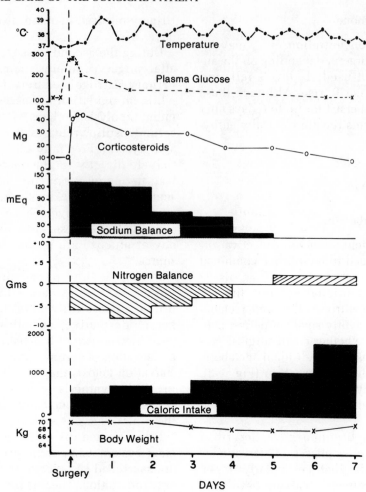

Fig. 1-2. A diagram of the metabolic response to surgery. Temperature (°C), plasma glucose, corticosteroids (Mg.), positive sodium balance (mEq.), negative and positive nitrogen balance (Gms.), caloric intake, and body weight (Kg.) were charted for a week following cholecystectomy.

does not lead to such metabolic disruption. With refeeding, the orderly phases of the adaptive process are readily reversible. In this setting, healing of the incision occurs and wound tensile strength increases even in the face of general energy and nitrogen catabolism.[68,71]

Acid–Base Regulation

Typical postoperative alkalosis with a serum pH of 7.50 to 7.60 is the result of transient hyperaldosteronism. There is a decrease in the excretion of sodium in urine, sweat, saliva, and perhaps even distal small bowel. With sodium retention, potassium and hydrogen ions either are lost or move into cells, with resultant extracellular alkalosis. In contrast, with sodium loss, potassium and hydrogen ions are retained or move out of cells, with resultant acidosis and hypokalemia. Postoperatively, the patient does not excrete sodium bicarbonate, despite a circulating alkalosis. The resultant hydrogen ion and potassium excretion by the distal tubule in exchange for sodium leads to the typical postoperative paradoxic aciduria.

Other factors exacerbate postoperative alkalosis. Nasogastric suction removes gastric acid. Citrate contained in transfused blood is oxidized to bicarbonate. Hyperventilation, either spontaneous or mechanical, produces respiratory alkalosis. Maintenance of intravascular volume through aldosterone production is more important for the health of the patient than acid–base neutrality.

Although respiratory compensation for metabolic acidosis is well recognized, respiratory compensation through hypoventilation for metabolic alkalosis is often overlooked.[72] Indeed, minute ventilation is an almost linear function of cerebrospinal fluid hydrogen ion concentration.[73] This is important to know when weaning an alkalotic patient from the ventilator. As the patient begins to breathe spontaneously, his Pa_{CO_2} should rise above 40 torr until the serum bicarbonate returns to normal. In this instance, hypercapnea is not necessarily an indication for reintubation.

CENTRAL NERVOUS SYSTEM

Physiology and Anesthetic Effects

Perivascular hydrogen ion concentration plays a major role in determining cerebro-vascular resistance and cerebral blood flow (CBF). Local metabolites such as adenine, potassium, osmolarity, and changes in P_{CO_2}, PO_2, and blood pressure also alter CBF. Normal CBF is 45 to 50 ml/100 g of tissue. The cerebral metabolic rate (CMR) is 5 to 6 mg of glucose/100 g of tissue/min. Physiologic needs are met by changes in flow.

The overall effect of anesthetics on CBF and CMR vary. Assuming that PO_2, P_{CO_2}, and blood pressure are maintained relatively constant under anesthesia, halothane causes a doubling of CBF and a 25% decrease in CMR, with a resultant increase in intracranial pressure.[74] Enflurane, isoflurane, and methoxyflurane have similar but less marked effects. Nitrous oxide causes an even greater increase in CBF than halothane and a marked increase in CMR. All intravenous anesthetics, including morphine, barbiturates, and diazepam, cause a decrease in CBF and CMR.[75]

The concentration of volatile anesthetic is directly proportional to the increase in CBF within a blood pressure range of 50 to 150 torr. Anesthetics also alter the response of CBF to changes in P_{CO_2}. If hypercapnia, hypoxia, elevated cerebral venous pressure, or elevated arterial pressure persist, increased intracranial pressure with decreased cerebral perfusion pressure occurs and may result in neurologic damage. Increases in intracranial pressure have been reported with all inhalational anesthetics.

Stages of Anesthesia

The function of all anesthetics is to depress the function of the central nervous system after crossing the blood-brain barrier. The clinical signs of nervous system depression are listed below. The use of preanesthetic agents and other adjuncts may make some clinical signs difficult to interpret.

Stage 1 **Analgesia**	Consciousness is retained but altered
	Motor and reflex functions remain intact
Stage 2 **Delirium**	Amnesia and analgesia are present
	There are uninhibited muscle movements and exaggerated reflexes
	Respiration is irregular, ocular movements are erratic, and pupils are dilated
	Blood pressure and pulse rate are increased
Stage 3 **Surgical** **anesthesia**	There are no spontaneous muscle movements
	Respirations are regular
	Reflexes are depressed or absent
Stage 4 **Medullary** **paralysis**	Respirations and all reflexes are absent
	Circulation is depressed

(After Jenkins LC: General Anesthesia and the Central Nervous System. Baltimore, Williams & Wilkins, 1969)

Effects on Electroencephalogram

The effects of anesthesia on the electroencephalogram (EEG) differ widely. Cyclopropane, at one end of the spectrum, causes progressive slowing. When given in increasing doses, enflurane causes spike-and-dome complexes alternating with electrical silence and, finally, frank seizure activity.[76] Halothane causes an initial fast-frequency, low-voltage pattern that changes to slow waves of moderate amplitude as anesthesia deepens and to even slower waves of increased amplitude as surgical anesthesia is reached.[77]

SUMMARY

This chapter has reviewed physiologic changes that occur in healthy patients perioperatively. The details of these changes and their effects on patients with underlying disease are addressed in subsequent chapters. Advanced technology has made surgery a therapeutic option for those who in the past were believed to present an unacceptable risk. It is thus the responsibility of all who care for surgical patients to fully understand these complex physiologic and pathophysiologic changes in order to prepare patients optimally for a safe procedure and to manage postoperative complications, should such complications arise.

REFERENCES

1. Ngai SH, Mark LC, Papper EM: Pharmacologic and physiologic aspects of anesthesiology. Anesthesiology 282:479, 1970
2. Rehder K, Sessler AD, Marsh HM: General anesthesia and the lung. Amer Rev Resp Dis 112:541, 1975
3. Filner BE, Karliner JS: Alterations of normal left ventricular performance by general anesthesia. Anesthesiology 45:610-621, 1976
4. Eckstein JW, Hamilton WK, McCammond JM: The effect of thiopental on peripheral venous tone. Anesthesiology 22:525, 1961
5. Lurie AA: Anesthesia and the systemic venous circulation. Anesthesiology 24:368, 1963
6. Brown BR, Crout JR: A comparative study of five general anesthetics on myocardial contractility. Anesthesiology 34:236, 1971

7. Harken AH: The surgical significance of the oxyhemoglobin dissociation curve. Surg Gynecol Obstet 144:935, 1977

8. Harken AH, Barlow CH, Harden WR et al: Two and three dimensional display of myocardial ischemic "borderzone" in dogs. Am J Cardiol 42:954, 1978

9. Harken AH, Lillo RS, Haut MJ: The depressant influence of extracellular fluid hyperoxis on liver slice oxygen uptake. J Lab Clin Med 89:1269, 1977

10. Harken AH: Lactic acidosis. Surg Gynecol Obstet 142:593, 1976

11. Taradash MR, Jacobson LB: Vasodivasor therapy of idiopathic lactic acidosis. N Engl J Med 293:468, 1975

12. Moore FD: The effects of hemorrhage on body composition. N Engl J Med 273:567, 1965

13. Harken AH, Brennan MF, Smith BS et al: The hemodynamic response to positive end expiratory ventilation in hypovolemic patients. Surgery 76:786, 1974

14. Kinley CE, Marble AE: Some changes in cardiovascular function accompanying thoracotomy. Can J Surg 15:260, 1972

15. MacLean LD, Duff JH, Scott HM et al: Treatment of shock in man based on hemodynamic diagnosis. Surg Gynecol Obstet 120:1, 1965

16. Sobel BE: Cardiac and non-cardiac forms of acute circulatory collapse (shock). In Braunwald E (ed): Heart Disease: A Textbook of Cardiovascular Medicine. Philadelphia, WB Saunders, 1980

17. Linden RJ: Function of cardiac receptors. Circulation 48:463, 1973

18. Green HD, Kepchar JH: Control of peripheral resistance in major systemic vascular beds. Physiol Rev 39:617, 1959

19. Vatner SF, Braunwald E: Cardiovascular control mechanisms in the conscious state. N Engl J Med 293:970, 1975

20. Jung R, Wight J, Nusser R et al: Comparison of three methods of respiratory care following upper abdominal surgery. Chest 78:31, 1980

21. Harmon E, Lillington G: Pulmonary risk factors in surgery. Med Clin North Am 63:1289, 1979

22. Rehder K, Jessler A, March HM: General anesthesia and the lung. Amer Rev Respir Dis 112:541, 1975

23. Moore FD, Lyons JH Jr, Pierce EC et al: Post-traumatic Pulmonary Insufficiency. Philadelphia, WB Saunders, 1969

24. Campbell D: Trauma to larynx and trachea following intubation and tracheostomy. J Laryngol Otol 82:981, 1968

25. Baron SH, Kohlmoos HW: Laryngeal sequelae of endotracheal anesthesia. Annals Otol Rhinol Laryngol 60:767, 1961

26. Appelbaum EL, Bruce DL: Tracheal Intubation. Philadelphia, WB Saunders, 1976

27. Mehta S: The risk of aspiration in presence of cuffed endotracheal tubes. Br J Anaesth 44:601, 1972

28. Holley HS, Gilder JE: Vocal cord paralysis after tracheal intubation. JAMA 215:281, 1971

29. Rainer WG, Sanchez M, Lopez L: Tracheal stricture secondary to cuffed tracheostomy tubes. Chest 59:115, 1971

30. Klainer AS, Turndorf H, Wu WH et al: Surface alterations due to endotracheal intubation. Am J Med 58:674, 1975

31. Tisi GM: Preoperative evaluation of pulmonary function. Amer Rev Respir Dis 119:293, 1979

32. Meyers JR, Lembeck L, O'Kane H: Changes in functional residual capacity of the lung after operation. Arch Surg 110:576, 1975

33. Addonizio VP, Harken AH: Current research review: The surgical implications of non-respiratory lung function. J Surg Res (in press)

34. Mead Jr, Collier C: Relation of volume history of lungs to respiratory mechanics in anesthetized dogs. J Appl Physiol 14:669, 1959

35. Ferris BG, Pollard DS: Effect of deep and quiet breathing on pulmonary compliance in man. J Clin Invest 39:143, 1960

36. Bendixen HH, Hedley-Whyte J, Lever MB: Impaired oxygenation in surgical patients during general anesthesia with controlled

ventilation. N Engl J Med 269:991, 1963

37. Gamsu G, Singer MM, Vincent HH: Postoperative impairment of mucous transport in the lung. Amer Rev Respir Dis 114:673, 1976

38. Bohr C: Theoretische Behandlung der quantitativen Verhältnisse bei der Sauerstoffaufnahme des Hemoglobins. Zentralbl Physiol 17:682, 1903

39. Smith TC, Colton ET, Behar MG: Does anesthesia alter hemoglobin dissociation? Anesthesiology 32:5, 1970

40. Pendleton RG, Newman DJ, Sherman S: Effect of propranolol upon the hemoglobin-oxygen dissociation curve. J Pharmacol Exp Ther 180:647, 1972

41. Sherwin RS, Hendler RG, Felig P: Effect of ketone infusion on amino acid and nitrogen metabolism in man. J Clin Invest 55:1382, 1975

42. Parker JP, Beirne GJ, Desai JN: Androgen induced increase in red cell 2,3-diphosphoglycerase. N Engl J Med 287:381, 1972

43. Rorth M: Hemoglobin interactions and red cell metabolism. Ser Haematol 5:1, 1972

44. Bauer C, Rathschlag-Schaefer AM: The influence of aldosterone and cortisol on oxygen affinity and cation concentration of the blood. Respir Physiol 5:360, 1968

45. Eliot RS, Holsinger JW, Hawkins HM et al: Relief of myocardial ischemia associated with increased blood oxygen release. Clin Res 20:67, 1972

46. Bryan-Brown CW, Baek S, Markabali G et al: Consumable oxygen; availability of oxygen in relation to oxyhemoglobin dissociation. Crit Care Med 1:17, 1973

47. Zachara B: The effect of persantin on the phosphate compounds in erythrocytes during blood conservation. Acta Haematol 48:164, 1972

48. Aste-Salazar H, Hurtado A: Affinity of hemoglobin for oxygen at sea level and at high altitudes. Am J Physiol 142:733, 1944

49. Chance B, Thurman RJ, Josalvez M: Oxygen affinities of cellular respiration. Forvars Medicim 5:235, 1969

50. Lenfant C, Torrance J, English E: Effect of altitude on oxygen binding by hemoglobin and on organic phosphate levels. J. Clin Invest 47:2652, 1968

51. Lenfant C, Torrance JD, Reynafar JE: Shift of the O_2-Hb dissociation curve at altitude; mechanism and effect. J Appl Physiol 30:625, 1971

52. Harken AH, Woods M: The influence of oxyhemoglobin affinity on tissue oxygen consumption. Ann Surg 183:130, 1976

53. Bowen JC, Fleming WH: Increased oxyhemoglobin affinity after transfusion of stored blood. Ann Surg 180:760, 1974

54. Oski FA, Marshal BE, Cohen PJ et al: Exercise with anemia; the pole of the left-shifted or right-shifted oxygen hemoglobin equilibrium curve. Ann Intern Med 74:44, 1971

55. Cryer PE: Physiology and pathophysiology of the human sympathoadrenal neuroendocrine system. N Engl J Med 303:436, 1980

56. Moore FD: Homeostasis: Bodily changes in trauma and surgery. In Sabiston D (ed): Textbook of Surgery. Philadelphia, WB Saunders, 1977

57. Selye H: General adaptation syndrome and diseases of adaptation. J Clin Endocrinol Metab 6:117, 1946

58. Moore FD: La Maladie Post-Operatoire: Is there order in variety? Surg Clin North Am 56:803, 1976

59. Hume DM, Bell CC, Baster FM: Direct measurement of adrenal secretion during operative trauma. Surgery 52:174, 1962

60. Gordon RJ, Ravin MB, Daicoff GR: Cardiovascular Physiology for Anesthesiologists. Springfield, CC Thomas, 1979

61. Addonizio VP, Harken AH: Current research review: The surgical implications of non-respiratory lung function. J Surg Res 28:86, 1980

62. Skillman JJ, Lauler DP, Hickler RB et al: Hemorrhage in normal man: Effect on renin, cortisol, aldosterone and urine composition. Ann Surg 166:865, 1967

63. Shuayb WA, Moran WH Jr, Zimmerman B: Studies of the mechanism of anti-diuretic hormone secretion and the post-commissurotomy dilutional syndrome. Ann Surg 162:690, 1965

64. Giddings AEB: The control of plasma glucose in the surgical patient. Br J Surg 61:787, 1974

65. Rizza RA, Cryer PE, Haymond MW et al: Adrenergic mechanisms for the effects of epinephrine on glucose production and clearance in man. J Clin Invest 65:682, 1980

66. Schade DS, Eaton RE: The regulation of plasma ketone body concentration by counter-regulatory hormones in man. III. Effects of norepinephrine in normal man. Diabetes 28:5, 1979

67. Wilmore DW, Long JM, Mason AD et al: Catecholamines: Mediator of the hypermetabolic response to thermal injury. Ann Surg 180:653, 1974

68. Moore FD, Brennan MF: Surgical injury: Body composition, protein metabolism and neuroendocrinology. In Balinger WF (ed): Manual of Surgical Nutrition, p 169. Philadelphia, WB Saunders, 1975

69. Grant JD: Handbook of Total Parenteral Nutrition, p 81. Philadelphia, WB Saunders, 1980

70. Hanson EL, Brennan MF, O'Connell RC et al: Response of glucose, insulin, free fatty acid and human growth hormone to norepinephrine and hemorrhage in normal man. Ann Surg 117:453, 1973

71. Levenson SM, Geever EF, Crowley LV et al: The healing of rat skin wounds. Ann Surg 161:293, 1965

72. Harken AH, Gabel RA, Fencl V: Hydrochloric acid in the correction of metabolic alkalosis. Arch Surg 110:819, 1975

73. Fencl V, Miller TB, Pappenheimer JR: Studies on the respiratory response to disturbances of acid-base balance, with deductions concerning the ionic composition of cerebral interstitial fluid. Am J Physiol 210:459, 1966

74. Shapiro HM, Aidinis JT: Neurosurgical anesthesia. Surg Clin North Am 55:913, 1975

75. Shapiro HM: Neuroanesthesia: Physiologic and pharmacologic principles. In 1980 ASA Annual Refresher Lectures. American Society of Anesthesiologists, 1980.

76. Dripps RD, Eckenhoff JE, Vandam LD: Introduction to Anesthesia, p 133. Philadelphia, WB Saunders, 1977

77. Gain EA, Petetz SG: An attempt to correlate the clinical signs of flurothane anesthetic with the electroencephalographic levels. Can Anaesth Soc J 4:289, 1957

The Preoperative Screening Examination

JEFFREY L. CARSON
JOHN M. EISENBERG

Although it is generally agreed that a medical history and physical examination should be obtained preoperatively from a patient who is to undergo surgery, there is a great deal of controversy regarding the additional benefit of preoperative screening tests. This chapter assesses the role and extent of preoperative evaluation in the asymptomatic patient undergoing elective surgery. The sensitivity, specificity, and predictive value of screening tests are reviewed, and recommendations are made regarding the preoperative evaluation.

In this chapter, the term "screening" refers to the search for unsuspected disease in preoperative patients whose symptoms relate only to their surgical problems. In this regard, a more appropriate term might be "case finding," since this implies the search for disease in a person who already has a relationship with the physician or surgeon. In contrast, the traditional definition of screening denotes the search for disease in large unselected general populations of asymptomatic persons. Obtaining a chemistry profile for a patient undergoing an appendectomy is an example of case-finding, whereas performing such a profile for every person in a community constitutes screening. This chapter does conform to the common use of the term "screening" to describe multiphasic testing in the hospitalized patient.

It is seldom necessary to repeat screening tests that have been performed recently, unless there is reason to suspect onset of disease in the meantime. It should be noted that this chapter does not address the evaluation of patients who have specific symptoms or who require emergency surgery.

In 1961, Dripps and co-workers proposed a classification system for preoperative patients to predict the risk of surgical mortality.[1] This system, which is outlined below, has become widely accepted and has been adopted by the American Society of Anesthesiologists (ASA).[2]

Physical Status I	A normal, healthy patient
Physical Status II	A patient with mild systemic disease
Physical Status III	A patient with severe systemic disease that limits activity but is not incapacitating

| Physical Status IV | A patient with an incapacitating systemic disease that is a threat to life |
| Physical Status V* | A moribund patient not expected to survive 24 hr even with operation |

*In the event of emergency operation, the Dripps–ASA system prefaces the number with an "E."

Vacanti and associates confirmed the excellent correlation between mortality and preoperative status as determined by the Dripps–ASA criteria but did not describe the causes of death in their patients.[3] The American College of Surgeons' Critical Incident Study of Surgical Deaths and Complications showed that, in 12 specific surgical situations, myocardial infarction, pulmonary embolus, infection, and heart failure were the most frequent causes of death.[4] Although these problems were also responsible for significant morbidity, infection and bleeding were the most common causes of morbidity. Hence, an effective preoperative screening program should define the risk of these complications in patients who are classified as "physical status I" by the Dripps–ASA criteria.

Major surgery textbooks and manuals recommend various sets of laboratory tests for preoperative screening. In Sabiston's *Textbook of Surgery*, Polk suggests a chest radiograph, electrocardiogram, urinalysis, and blood urea nitrogen and creatinine tests.[5] In *Current Surgical Diagnosis and Treatment*, Wilson recommends a complete blood count, urinalysis, serology, and chest radiograph for all patients and an electrocardiogram, stool for occult blood, and undefined "blood chemistries" for those over 40.[6] In the *Manual of Surgical Therapeutics*, Wright's routine preoperative recommendations include a complete blood count, electrolytes, blood urea nitrogen or creatinine, glucose, total protein, albumin, calcium, prothrombin time, partial thromboplastin time, chest radiograph, electrocardiogram, and urinalysis for all patients and, the addition of a sickle-cell preparation for those who are black.[7] None of these textbooks provides data to support its recommendations. Moreover, Schwartz's *Principles of Surgery* and the American College of Surgeons' *Manual of Preoperative and Postoperative Care* provide no formal recommendations for preoperative testing.[8,9]

Robbins and Mushlin recently considered preoperative screening in asymptomatic patients and recommended a hematocrit and urinalysis for each patient and a pregnancy test for women of childbearing age.[10] Tests considered of uncertain value were the electrocardiogram, blood urea nitrogen or creatinine, serum glutamic oxaloacetic transaminase (SGOT), tuberculin skin test, serum glucose, and platelet count. Tests thought not to be indicated were chest radiograph, tonometry, and partial thromboplastin time.

In order to determine which diagnostic tests are actually performed in preoperative patients, the Professional Activities Study of the Commission on Professional and Hospital Activities studied a sample of 45,871 patients discharged from 40 hospitals in the North Central United States.[11] In 1968, electrocardiograms were performed for 42% of surgical patients; by 1974, this number had increased to 53.4%. In 1974, chest radiographs were performed for 69.1%, blood glucose determinations for 75.2%, and blood urea nitrogen tests for 76%.

PRINCIPLES OF SCREENING

In deciding which tests to do for the preoperative patient, it is useful to review the characteristics of the ideal screening test. A synthesis of several criteria proposed by the World Health Organization,[12] Robbins and Mushlin,[10] Frame and Carlson, and others mandates that (1) the patient is asymptomatic, with no evidence on history or physical examination of the condition for which he is being screened; (2) the condition will potentially alter the outcome of surgery; (3) preoperative diagnosis will aid perioperative management; (4) the prevalence and severity of the condition are great enough to warrant the expense of screening; and (5) the tests are sufficiently sensitive to allow detection and specific enough to avoid overdiagnosis.[10,12,13]

To understand these criteria, it is important that the terms "sensitivity," "specificity," and "prevalence" be explained. *Sensitivity* is defined as that percentage of patients with a disease who have an abnormal test. *Specificity* is that percentage of healthy patients who have a normal test. Hence, an ideal test will give positive results in all diseased subjects (100% sensitivity) and negative results in all healthy subjects (100% specificity).[14] *Prevalence* is that percentage of patients with the disease at the time of the study, whereas *incidence* is the number of new cases over a certain period of time, such as a year.

The *predictive value* of a test is also important. The predictive value of a positive test is the percentage of positive results obtained that are true positives (i.e., that are obtained from patients who have the disease in question). Positive results may also be obtained from some patients who do not have the disease; such results are called false positives. In contrast, the predictive value of a negative or normal test is defined as the percentage of negative results that are true negatives (i.e., that are obtained from patients who are free of the disease in question). False-negative results may also be obtained from some patients who have the disease in question.

The relationship between prevalence and predictive value is important. The predictive value of a test varies directly with the prevalence of the disease in the population studied. Table 2-1 shows that, if the sensitivity and specificity of a test are both 95%, the predictive value of the test varies considerably with different levels of prevalence. When the test is applied to a population of a 50% prevalence of disease, its positive predictive value is 95%; however, if the prevalence is 1%, the positive predictive value is only 16%, implying that 84% of all positive test results will be false-positive ones.

The routine partial thromboplastin time determination serves to illustrate the clinical relevance of predictive value. Because surgery may be postponed in patients with abnormal results, the proportion of true positives and false positives is important. The prevalence of hemostatic disease is low in the asymptomatic population; therefore, although some persons may actually have hemostatic abnormalities, most are normal, and the number of

Table 2-1. Predictive Value and Prevalence for a Test with 95% Sensitivity and Specificity

Prevalence of Disease (%)	Predictive Value of a Positive Test (%)
0.1	1.9
1	16.1
2	27.9
5	50.0
50	95.0

false-positive tests that occur is relatively high. This means that the positive predictive value of the test is low, and surgery may be postponed or cancelled unnecessarily. The test inconveniences both patient and surgeon and leads to additional expense by necessitating further evaluation. In an aysmptomatic, otherwise healthy patient population, the prevalence of disease is low, and most tests will be of little value. For many diseases for which screening is performed, prevalence increases with the age of the patient, making the test more valuable in older populations. Moreover, the presence of other clinical characteristics also indicates a higher prevalence of disease in a screened population. Hence, in an evaluation of the value of a test, it is crucial to consider the likelihood of finding disease in the population.

Because the normal limits of a test are often defined as those values 2 standard deviations (SD) above and below the mean in a population of healthy people, a small proportion of normal individuals, typically 4.5%, will have an abnormal result. Some false-positive results are therefore inevitable. The greater the number of tests carried out in a healthy individual, the greater the likelihood that a false-positive result will occur (Table 2-2).

In evaluating screening tests, it is important to consider whether they provide information that would not have been suspected on the basis of history and physical examination and whether they uncover new problems that necessitate a change in patient care. One study assessed the diagnostic yield of the medical history alone in the evaluation of 200 preoperative patients by five anesthesiologists.[15] Answers to a set of simple questions predicted fitness for operation in 96% of the cases. A more extensive his-

Table 2-2. Probability of Obtaining an Abnormal Result in a Multiphasic Screening Battery

Number of Independent Tests	Abnormal Results Found (%)
1	5
2	10
4	19
6	26
10	40
20	64
50	92
90	99

(Galen RS, Gambino SR: Beyond Normality: The Predictive Value and Efficiency of Medical Diagnosis. New York, John Wiley & Sons, 1975)

tory, physical examination, and laboratory investigation provided little additional useful information. This said, the remainder of this chapter addresses the utility of several common preoperative tests in elective surgical patients.

PREOPERATIVE CARDIAC EXAMINATION AND THE ELECTROCARDIOGRAM

Cardiac disease is the most common cause of mortality and morbidity postoperatively.[4] Goldman and co-workers prospectively evaluated 1001 consecutive patients undergoing noncardiac surgery for cardiac risk factors and complications.[16] All patients were 40 years of age or older and were admitted for elective procedures. All underwent a history and physical examination, an electrocardiogram, and a chest radiograph. Most had complete blood counts and serum creatinine and liver enzyme determinations. Patients were evaluated postoperatively if cardiac symptoms developed, and all had a routine postoperative electrocardiogram 5 days after surgery.

In the group of 59 patients who died, a

cardiac cause was held responsible in 19. Eighteen additional patients suffered a myocardial infarction, and five of these (28%) died. Fourteen patients died from cardiac causes without documented myocardial infarctions; five had sudden cardiac deaths, and nine died with refractory cardiogenic shock. Goldman and associates found that five factors were associated with a significantly higher risk than normal of developing a postoperative myocardial infarction: (1) age greater than 70; (2) dyspnea, orthopnea, or edema; (3) mitral regurgitant murmur of grade 2/6 or louder; (4) more than 5 premature ventricular contractions per minute; and (5) tortuous or calcified aorta on chest radiograph.

Thirty-six patients investigated by Goldman developed postoperative congestive heart failure. The preoperative factors in these patients that correlated most closely with postoperative heart failure were the presence of a mitral regurgitant murmur of grade 2/6 or louder and evidence of aortic regurgitation, mitral stenosis, or aortic stenosis. However, 21 of these 36 patients had no history of heart failure, and all but two were older than 60. Factors that were correlated with postoperative death by multivariate analysis included jugular venous distention, S_3 gallop, myocardial infarction within the past 6 months, rhythm other than sinus, more than 5 premature ventricular contractions per minute, significant aortic stenosis, age greater than 70, emergency surgery, and a reduction in blood pressure by 33% or more for longer than 10 min during surgery.

Although Goldman and associates have provided the most comprehensive evaluation to date of perioperative cardiac risk, their conclusions are drawn from a relatively small number of adverse outcomes—19 cardiac deaths, 18 myocardial infarctions, and 36 episodes of postoperative congestive heart failure. For example, the conclusion that surgery within 6 months of a myocardial infarction is no safer than surgery within 6 weeks of infarction is based upon a comparison that included only seven deaths. These conclusions need to be confirmed by other studies. Not only were the risk factors not prospectively validated, but nearly all of them can be identified by a thorough history and physical examination. Although confirmation of the presence of premature contractions or a rhythm other than sinus may require an electrocardiogram, the finding of a regular rhythm on cardiac auscultation should be adequate screening for nearly all arrhythmias.

Other studies investigating the value of preoperative electrocardiograms are flawed in design. In 1958, Wang and Howland studied 482 patients between the ages of 40 and 90 who had preoperative electrocardiograms.[17] They found "little definitive" correlation between preoperative electrocardiographic abnormalities and postoperative complications, except in two categories. Of 6 patients with evidence of an old myocardial infarction on the electrocardiogram, 1 died, 2 had major surgical complications, and 1 had a minor complication. Among 4 patients with premature atrial contractions, there were 1 death and 2 major complications. However, the investigators did not demonstrate that the surgical complications were related to the electrocardiographic abnormalities or the history of a previous infarction. Furthermore, it is likely that a physical examination would have raised the possibility of premature atrial contractions, and a history would have identified most of the patients with an old myocardial infarction.

In a more recent study, Cooperman and co-workers retrospectively analyzed cardiovascular risk factors in 566 patients undergoing major vascular surgery, excluding those with ruptured aortic aneurysm and those undergoing carotid endarterectomy.[18] Five risk factors were correlated with postoperative complications: (1) a prior myocardial infarction; (2) congestive heart failure; (3) arrythmia; (4) an abnormal electrocardiogram (including bundle-branch block); and (5) a previous cerebrovascular accident. Most of these risk factors could have been detected by careful history and physical examination. Although an abnormal electrocardiogram was considered a risk factor in the study, the criteria for abnormality were not defined. In contrast, two other studies have found that, in patients with right bundle-branch block and left axis deviation, the risk of developing complete heart block after surgery is nearly zero.[19,20]

In another recent study, Ferrer reviewed the preoperative electrocardiograms of 1068 surgical patients and found abnormalities in 19%, with t-wave changes the most common finding.[21] The prevalence of abnormal results varied with age. In patients 35 to 45 years old, 8% to 10% were abnormal; in those 71 to 85, 43% to 71% were abnormal. Ferrer suggested that an electrocardiogram be performed for all preoperative surgical patients; however, no correlation was found between abnormal electrocardiograms and the perioperative course.

The sensitivity and specificity of an electrocardiogram for detecting cardiac disease have been reported to be only 27% and 81% respectively.[10] Because of the relatively low prevalence of cardiac dis-ease in the asymptomatic population, the positive predictive value is also low.[22] Hence, the electrocardiogram has only limited value as a screening test and adds little to a history and physical examination. Although the argument may be made that a preoperative electrocardiogram is potentially valuable as a baseline study against which to compare subsequent postoperative electrocardiograms, there is no evidence to support this contention. In fact, a related study of the value of baseline electrocardiograms in assessing the significance of chest pain in patients in the emergency room showed such a baseline test to be of little use.[23]

CHEST RADIOGRAPH

Chest radiographs account for more than 50% of the radiography performed in the United States[24] and are often included in the preoperative evaluation of surgical patients. In patients who are to undergo cardiopulmonary surgery and who are known to have disease in the thorax, the chest radiograph confirms the diagnosis, aids in assessing operative risk, and provides a baseline for postoperative comparison. It does not serve as a screening test in these patients.

The value of the preoperative chest radiograph has been questioned for patients undergoing other surgical procedures. In an investigation sponsored by the Royal College of Radiologists, 10,619 patients undergoing nonacute elective surgery other than cardiopulmonary procedures were studied.[25] Radiographs were ordered for 29.7% of these patients with no apparent consideration of the underlying disease, age of the patient, or procedure planned. Preoperative radiographs did not alter the choice of anesthesia or the decision to operate and were of little value as a baseline study against which to judge subsequent radiographs. Rees and associates studied 607 consecutive patients undergoing elective nonacute noncardiopulmonary surgery in a large hospital in Wales.[26] There were 126 significant abnormalities reported, 54% of which consisted of cardiomegaly and 19% of which were due to chronic respiratory disease. Most patients had received a chest radiograph within the preceding 3 years, and the maximum marrow dose had been exceeded in 12.5% of the study population. The authors found that history and clinical examination are more sensitive detectors of disease than radiographs, except in tuberculosis. However, tuberculin skin testing was not evaluated. Finally, Petterson and Janover found that the routine chest film was helpful in only 2 of 1393 preoperative patients.[27] In both cases, surgery was postponed because of the presence of interstitial lung disease.

It appears that the frequency of abnormalities detected on chest radiograph is related to the age of the patient. Loder studied 1000 preoperative radiographs and, among 437 patients under the age of 30, found 5 with abnormalities.[28] Only one abnormality could not have been predicted by history or physical examination. In the study by Rees and colleagues, normal chest radiographs were obtained for all patients under 20[26] and did not change the original diagnosis in those under 30. Similarly, Sagel and co-workers discovered no new abnormalities through chest radiograph in 521 patients under 20 and only 9 abnormalities in 894 patients under 30.[29] Findings on preoperative chest radiograph had little or no effect on the operative management of these patients.

Farnsworth and associates studied 350 pediatric surgical patients and found that the routine preoperative chest radiograph is of limited value in children and infants as well.[30] In these cases, surgery was never cancelled, and the preoperative diagnosis was never modified because of findings on the preoperative chest radiograph. Of 31 abnormal radiographs, 25 could have been suspected on the basis of history and physical examination, and 5 were questionable or clinically inconsequential. One patient was found to have a mediastinal mass, but the authors did not describe the clinical outcome. Brill and co-workers detected no abnormalities requiring treatment among 1000 healthy children seen in a pediatric preventive health clinic.[31]

However, Sane and colleagues studied preoperative chest radiography in 1500 patients from birth to 19 years of age and found at least one abnormality in 7.5%.[32] Moreover, 4.7% of chest radiographs demonstrated entirely unsuspected radiographic abnormalities. In 3.8% of the patients, surgery was postponed or cancelled or the choice of anesthesia was changed as a result of the radiographic findings. In 41 instances, pneumonia or atelectasis was identified. There were no clinical or auscultative findings in many of these patients. Three unsuspected asymptomatic mediastinal masses were identified. The authors did not determine the frequency of false-positive findings or of those resulting in new diagnoses; however, among the abnormalities noted on chest radiographs were patent ductus arteriosus, ventricular septal defect, mediastinal tumors, and scoliosis. The authors concluded that preoperative chest radiographs are justified in children.

Arriving at a recommendation regarding the use of preoperative chest radiographs is difficult, given the ambiguous results in the available literature. It seems reasonable to propose that chest radiographs not be obtained for patients under 30 years of age who have no suspected cardiac or pulmonary disease, despite the study by Sane and co-workers suggesting that children be screened. It is likely that a single view is sufficient and that the lateral chest radiograph may be eliminated as a preoperative test. It is important to recall that the purpose of this examination is to detect disease that will alter preoperative or perioperative care, not to serve as a routine screening test. The Bureau of Radiological Health has recognized the difficulty facing physicians with regard to preoperative chest radiographs and is sponsoring two studies designed to provide additional data upon which recommendations may be based.

Further discussion of the preoperative evaluation of patients with pulmonary disease may be found in Chapter 23.

CHEMICAL AND HEMATOLOGIC PROFILES

Biochemical profiles are performed for many patients entering the hospital, particularly since multichannel analyzers provide panels of clinical chemistry tests that obviate the need for the physician to decide which ones to order. Although the multiphasic profile is convenient for the physician and supposedly inexpensive for the patient, its true value depends upon its contribution to detecting disease in the asymptomatic patient. This is particularly important if the discovery of disease will influence clinical care during the perioperative period. The true cost of

the profile includes the price of handling possible complications of follow-up testing to evaluate abnormal screening tests.

The yield of the screening clinical chemistry profile has been extensively studies. Daughaday and associates found at least one abnormal test in 60% of all hospitalized patients studied with the frequency of abnormalities varying according to the admitting service.[33] Only 8% of obstetric and gynecological patients showed abnormalities, in contrast to 55% of medical patients and 19% of surgical patients. The frequency of "significant" abnormalities varied with the patient's age. Abnormalities were found in 14% of patients up to 40 years of age but in 43% of patients over 70. As expected, the frequency of significant abnormalities was less than that of all abnormalities, and the frequency with which new diagnoses were made was even lower. Only 65 new diagnoses attributable to the tests were made.

Newman discovered new disease on the basis of serum calcium in 0.4% of patients, cholesterol in 0.5%, glucose in 5.5%, alkaline phosphatase in 1.9%, uric acid in 1.8%, and serum glutamic oxaloacetic transaminase (SGOT) in 3.9%.[34] Whitehead and Wootton studied the results of profiles performed on in-patients admitted to the Queen Elizabeth Medical Centre in Birmingham, England.[35] Of 31,439 tests performed in 2,071 patients, only 0.7% gave abnormal results that had been unsuspected and that provided new diagnostic information.

Finding an abnormal test result or making a new diagnosis may not necessarily be beneficial to the patient. Korvin and co-workers evaluated 1000 patients undergoing 20 chemical and hematologic tests.[36] Of the 2235 abnormal results obtained,

675 were predictable on clinical grounds, 1325 yielded no new information, and the remaining 223 led to 83 new diagnoses. In the authors' opinion, recognition of only one of these diagnoses proved beneficial to the patient. Durbridge and colleagues compared a group of 500 patients undergoing admission testing with two control groups for which admission multiphasic testing was not available.[37] They found no significant difference in the quality of care provided these patients. The use of routine admission testing did not shorten the hospital stay, but it did increase the total cost of hospital care by 5%, probably because of a greater number of follow-up tests and consultations.

Glucose

Abnormalities in serum glucose are the most frequently detected dysfunctions found in patients given biochemical profiles. Of 57 new diagnoses made in Korvin's series, 17 were diabetes mellitus.[36] Newman found an elevated glucose level in 5.5% of his patients.[34] In a series reported by Galloway and Shuman, the initial diagnosis of diabetes mellitus was made on the basis of a preoperative glucose test in 100 of 467 patients; 40 of the 100 had serum glucose determinations greater than 200 mg/dl.[38] However, the authors pointed out that diabetes mellitus might have been suspected in 70 of the 100 patients from careful review of the history and physical examination. Difficulty arises in interpreting these statistics because of differences in the criteria used for diagnosing diabetes mellitus; Galloway and Shuman used 120 mg/dl and Korvin used 150 mg/dl as their cut-off values. Serum glucose may rise postoperatively because of stress, anesthesia, and intravenous fluids administered.[39,40]

Postoperative hyperglycemia can cause an osmotic diuresis and dehydration or impair white-cell function. In one study, diabetics had a surgical mortality rate of 3.6% and a morbidity rate of 17%. Although knowing whether the preoperative serum glucose is elevated is of undecided value, most clinicians feel that this measurement is useful.

Creatinine

The ability to metabolize and excrete drugs and anesthetics is important in the clinical course of the surgical patient. Although serum creatinine does not rise until renal function has been compromised by more than 50%,[41] this determination is less expensive and more easily obtained than a 24-hr creatinine clearance. However, the prevalence of renal insufficiency among asymptomatic patients with no history of renal disease is only 0.3%.[42] Despite this low prevalence, most clinicians check either serum blood urea nitrogen or creatinine before surgery.

Calcium

The availability of panels of clinical chemistry tests is thought to be responsible for the increased detection of asymptomatic hypercalcemia or hyperparathyroidism.[43,44] In Rochester, Minnesota, the average age-adjusted incidence of primary hyperparathyroidism is 27.7 ± 5.8 per 100,000.[43] Boonstra and Jackson found 50 cases of hypercalcemia among 50,000 clinic patients.[45] Williamson and Van Peenev found that 4 of 4727 in-patients screened with serum calcium determinations had unsuspected hyperparathyroidism.[46] These studies imply that the likelihood of finding hypercalcemia among asymptomatic patients is low and that the serum calcium determination is therefore not a useful preoperative screening test.

Urinalysis

Little data are available regarding the value of a preoperative urinalysis. Heimann and co-workers examined the records of 400 patients admitted to Vancouver General Hospital and found that 116 patients (29%) had abnormalities on routine urinalysis.[47] Of these, 22 (5.5%) had abnormalities in protein, glucose, or bilirubin, 56 (14%) in the sediment, and 38 (9.5%) in both. Despite these relatively high frequencies, physicians recognized the abnormalities in only 51% of the cases, and it is not clear whether care was influenced by the findings. Therefore, in the asymptomatic patient with normal renal function, the value of a routine preoperative urinalysis must be questioned.

Liver Function

Tests of liver function, including liver enzyme determinations, may be important in detecting underlying hepatic disease, which may influence the metabolism of drugs or anesthetic agents, increase their toxicity, or affect coagulation. In Korvin's study, 22 of 1000 patients had unsuspected elevated serum bilirubin determinations, and 19 had elevated liver enzyme determinations leading to information possibly important to their care.[36] Altogether, definitive disease was diagnosed in 30 of the 1000 patients. However, 7 were alcohol abusers, and 4 were thought to have Gilbert's disease and therefore did not benefit from the screening tests. One patient was found to have liver damage due to halothane anesthesia.

Similarly, Daughaday and colleagues suspected liver enzyme abnormalities and subsequently confirmed liver function impairment in 5 of 1869 patients.[33] Elevations in serum total bilirubin occurred only in cases of clinically suspected hepatic or biliary disease, except for one case of presumptive Gilbert's disease. Although Belliveau and co-workers did not assess ultimate changes in outcome, they found abnormalities in serum alkaline phosphatase in 4.8% of patients, SGOT in 13.5%, lactic dehydrogenase in 12.3%, and total bilirubin in 5.8%.[48] On the basis of these abnormal results, 6 new cases of cirrhosis were discovered among 1046 patitents admitted to a community hospital.

It appears from these results that, before surgery involving potentially hepatotoxic anesthesia is undertaken, it may be reasonable to obtain a test of hepatocellular function such as SGOT or serum glutamic pyruvate transaminase (SGPT) and a test of hepatobiliary function such as alkaline phosphatase.

Complete Blood Count

A complete blood count is traditionally performed before surgery. Although the white-cell count has not been evaluated as a screening test and is unlikely to be useful, thrombocytopenia is potentially important in the patient undergoing surgery. The history and physical examination may be of only limited value in screening for thrombocytopenia; however, the prevalence of this disorder in an asymptomatic population is only 0.005%, making identification of a single case expensive.[42]

A hematocrit of at least 30% or a hemoglobin level of greater than 10 g/dl is recommended by most authors as a prerequisite for elective surgery. An average level of 9 g/dl was given by 1249 American hospitals that replied to a questionnaire requesting the minimum acceptable hemoglobin level for patients undergoing elective surgery.[49] As noted in Chapter 30, anemia may be a relevant risk factor for surgical patients. In patients with chronic anemia, cardiac output increases when the hemoglobin level falls below 8.0 g/dl. Hypoxia in the perioperative period is common, and the induction of anesthesia may cause a 20% to 30% reduction in cardiac output. These factors decrease the delivery of oxygen to peripheral tissues and increase cardiac workload.

Despite these theoretical considerations, it is important to consider whether the presence of anemia results in a poor surgical outcome. Rawston retrospectively analyzed 145 patients with hemoglobin levels below 10 g/dl and compared them to a control group of 412 with normal hemoglobin levels.[49,50] There was no difference in perioperative complications in the two groups. Although four anemic patients died, Rawston concluded that the cause of death was not related to anemia. In contrast, Gillies found the frequency of major complications to be 16% in a group of anemic patients and only 6% in the control group.[51]

The clinician's ability to make the diagnosis of anemia clinically is limited until the hemoglobin level drops to 7 g/dl. The hemoglobin determination is usually necessary for detection of mild to moderate anemia, and the prevalence of anemia in an asymptomatic population is estimated to be about 1%. This relatively high prevalence and the limited sensitivity of the physical exam speak in favor of the routine carrying out of a preoperative hemoglobin determination.

Prothrombin Time and Partial Thromboplastin Time

The prothrombin time and partial thromboplastin time to detect coagulation disorders have been evaluated in several recent studies. Clark and Eisenberg studied the prevalence of prolonged prothrombin and partial thromboplastin times in surgical patients without evidence of a bleeding disorder on history or physical examination and assessed the consequences of abnormalities not being detected.[52] They defined patients with an increased risk of bleeding as those with (1) a history of anticoagulant use; (2) a history or physical examination suggestive of liver disease; (3) active bleeding; or (4) a history or physical examination indicative of bleeding. In 467 patients with no risk of bleeding, they found 13 (2.8%) abnormal coagulation tests, in contrast to 25 (18%) of 139 with defined risk. Of the 13 patients with abnormal results but seemingly not at risk, 4 had repeat tests that were normal, 8 underwent surgery without further investigation and experienced no bleeding complications, and 1 underwent an emergency cesarean section. The latter patient subsequently became hypotensive, at which time the prothrombin and partial thromboplastin times were normal; at exploration, a pumping artery was found. The investigators concluded that preoperative testing is necessary only in those patients previously identified as having an increased risk of bleeding.

Eika and associates studied 101 patients undergoing elective surgery in whom platelet count, bleeding time, normotest and thrombotest (similar to prothrombin time), thromboplastin time, partial thromboplastin time, fibrinogen, thrombin time, and fibrin degradation products were determined.[53] On the basis of the tests, two hematologists assigned each patient to one of three groups of no, possible, or definite bleeding risk. Of 8 patients with definite risk, 2 developed significant bleeding. Of 9 with a possible risk of bleeding, 2 developed significant bleeding, and 1 had possibly increased bleeding. Finally, of 84 patients judged to be at no increased risk of bleeding, 13 had significant bleeding, and 9 had possible surgical bleeding. The authors concluded that preoperative bleedings tests are not helpful in distinguishing patients likely to develop bleeding.

Robbins and Rose studied 1025 patients in whom partial thromboplastin testing was done and found 143 (14%) with abnormal values.[54] On chart review, it was found that each of these patients had an underlying process that could explain the abnormality. The authors concluded that abnormal results occur in patients who have a clinically predictable bleeding risk. These data suggest that neither a prothrombin time nor a partial thromboplastin time test is of value in the asymptomatic patient undergoing surgery.

PREADMISSION TESTING AND LENGTH OF HOSPITAL STAY

Preadmission testing has been purported to reduce the cost and length of the hospital stay by identifying unexpected problems that may lead to delay or cancellation of surgery; however, two studies cast doubt on this contention. Barbaro, Shuman, and Swinkola compared length of stay in hospitals in Western Pennsylvania in which preadmission testing was used with that in all other hospitals in Allegheny County.[55] After eliminating the effects of case mix, these investigators found that the duration of the preoperative period was directly affected by coordination of admission and surgery scheduling, regardless of whether testing was used. Adoption of preadmission testing ensured neither efficient scheduling in the operating room nor ready availability of results on the chart. The investigators concluded that length of stay for surgical

patients was more dependent on efficient hospital operation than on preadmission testing.

A similar investigation was conducted by Dumbaugh and Neuhauser, who studied the effect of preadmission testing in surgical patients on length of stay in a group of Massachusetts hospitals.[56] They found that the difference in preoperative period between patients receiving and patients not receiving preadmission testing was less than 0.5 days. Postoperative length of stay did not differ. In addition, patients who underwent preadmission testing had more laboratory tests performed during their hospital stay than those who did not. Available evidence indicates that screening for disease in surgical patients before their admission does not help to contain the cost of hospitalization.

The national Blue Cross/Blue Shield organization has encouraged its local plans to require that admission testing for hospitalized patients be ordered specifically by the physician instead of being routine. Because of concern that routine admission testing for all patients is not cost-effective, many Blue Cross plans now deny payment for admission screening panels not ordered by the physician.

SUMMARY

1. A thorough and detailed *history* and *physical examination* are the most important factors in the evaluation of the surgical patient. They constitute the best possible screening process and provide nearly all the clinical data necessary for detection of diseases that may affect surgical outcome.

2. *Electrocardiogram.* Available data

fail to demonstrate that an electrocardiogram is more effective in predicting cardiovascular morbidity or mortality than a history and physical examination. The electrocardiogram is a poor predictor of ischemic heart disease. It is therefore not routinely recommended for young adults. However, it may be useful for the geriatric population.

3. *Chest radiograph.* A chest radiograph should be performed for patients undergoing cardiopulmonary surgery and for those with cardiopulmonary risk factors. There is conflicting evidence on the usefulness of preoperative chest radiographs for all other patients.

4. *Hemoglobin or hematocrit.* This simple, inexpensive test should be carried out for all patients undergoing surgery. The 1% prevalence of anemia in asymptomatic patients is relatively high, and the physical examination is limited in its sensitivity for detecting anemia.

5. *Creatinine or blood urea nitrogen.* One of these tests should be considered for all patients receiving drugs excreted by the kidneys. Their major limitation as preoperative screening tests is the low prevalence of renal insufficiency and the resulting high cost of detecting a significant abnormality.

6. *Serum glucose.* It is uncertain how management or surgical outcome is affected by knowledge that the serum glucose level is elevated preoperatively; however, because the prevalence of disease is high and the test is inexpensive, serum glucose determination is recommended.

7. *Platelet count.* There is no adequate data on the value as a screening test of either a quantitative platelet count or an estimate on blood smear. The main limitation of such a test is the very low prevalence of unsuspected thrombocytopenia in the asymptomatic population.

8. *Prothrombin time and partial thromboplastin time.* Prothrombin and partial thromboplastin time determinations are of no demonstrated value in the preoperative patient. A careful history and physical examination can identify nearly all patients with a risk of bleeding.

9. *Urinalysis.* There is little available data to determine the utility of a preoperative urinalysis. Despite the high prevalence of abnormalities, a urinalysis is unlikely to contribute significantly to the care of the patient.

10. *Calcium.* Although detection of hypercalcemia is important because of the disorder's diagnostic implications, its prevalence in the asymptomatic population is too low to warrant a screening test.

11. *Liver function tests.* Hepatic dysfunction has significant implications for perioperative care; however, the prevalence of liver enzyme abnormalities is low. A test of hepatocellular function, such as SGOT or SGPT, and a test of the hepatobiliary system, such as a bilirubin or alkaline phosphatase assay, are reasonable but of uncertain value in the patient undergoing anesthesia that is potentially hepatoxic.

REFERENCES

1. Dripps RD, Lamont A, Eckenhoff JE: The role of anesthesia in surgical mortality. JAMA 178:261, 1961

2. New classification of physical status. Anesthesiology 24:111, 1963

3. Vacanti CJ, Van Houten RJ, Hill RC: A statistical analysis of the relationship of physical status to postoperative mortality in 68,388 cases. Anesth Analg (Cleve) 49:564, 1970

4. Surgery in the U.S., p 2132. Chicago, American College of Surgeons, 1976

5. Polk HC: Principles of preoperative preparation of the surgical patient. In Sebiston DC (ed): Textbook of Surgery, 11th ed. Philadelphia, WB Saunders, 1977

6. Wilson JL: Preoperative care. In Dunphy JE, Way LW (eds): Current Surgical Diagnosis and Treatment, 4th ed. Los Altos, Lange Medical Publications, 1979

7. Wright R: Preoperative and postoperative care. In Condon RD, Nyhus LM (eds): Therapeutics, 4th ed. Boston, Little, Brown & Co, 1978

8. Schwartz SI: Principles of Surgery. New York, McGraw-Hill, 1979

9. Saltzman EW: Hemorrhagic disorders. In American College of Surgeons: Manual of Preoperative and Postoperative Care, 2nd ed. Philadelphia, WB Saunders, 1971

10. Robbins JA, Mushlin AI: Preoperative evaluation of the healthy patient. Med Clin North Am 63:1145, 1979

11. The Professional Activities Study of the Commission on Professional and Hospital Activities: Testing to uncover medical conditions in surgical patients. Hosp Prac 9:97, 1974

12. World Health Organization: Mass health examinations. Public Health Pap 45:50, 1971

13. Frame PS, Carlson SJ: A critical review of periodical health screening using specific screening criteria. J Fam Pract 2:29, 1975

14. Galen RS, Gambino SR: Beyond Normality: The Predictive Value and Efficiency of Medical Diagnosis. New York, John Wiley & Sons, 1975

15. Wilson ME, Williams NB, Baskett PJF et al: Assessment of fitness for surgical procedures and the variability of anesthetists' judgments. Br Med J 1:509, 1980

16. Goldman L, Caldera DL, Southwick FS et al: Cardiac risk factors and complications in non-cardiac surgery. Medicine (Baltimore) 57:375, 1978

17. Wang KC, Howland WS: Cardiac and pulmonary evaluation in elderly patients before elective surgical operations. JAMA 166:993, 1958

18. Cooperman M, Pflug B, Martin EW et al: Cardiovascular risk factors in patients with peripheral vascular disease. Surgery 84:505, 1978

19. Rooney SM, Godinger PL, Muss E: Relationship of right bundle branch block and marked left axis deviation to complete heart block during general anesthesia. Anesthesiology 44:64, 1976

20. Pastore JO, Yurchak PM, Janis KM et al: The risk of advanced heart block in surgical patients with right bundle branch block and left axis deviation. Circulation 57:677, 1977

21. Ferrer MI: The value of obligatory preoperative electrocardiograms. J Am Med Wom Assoc 33:459, 1978

22. Margolis JR, Kannel WB, Feinleib M: Clinical features of unrecognized myocardial infarction—silent and symptomatic. Am J Cardiol 32:1, 1973

23. Rubenstein LZ, Greenfield S: The baseline ECG in evaluation of acute cardiac complaints. JAMA 244:2536, 1980

24. Bureau of Radiological Health: Chest x-ray screening practices: An annotated bibliography. Washington DC, HEW Publication (FDA) 78–8067, 1978

25. Royal College of Radiologists: Preoperative chest radiology. Lancet 2:83, 1979

26. Rees NM, Roberts CJ, Bligh AS et al: Routine preoperative chest radiography in non-cardiopulmonary surgery. Br Med J 1:1333, 1976

27. Petterson SR, Janover ML: Is the routine preoperative chest film of value? Appl Radiol 6:70, 1977

28. Loder RE: Routine preoperative chest radiography. Anaesthesia 33:972, 1978

29. Sagel SS, Evans RG, Forrest JV et al: Efficacy of routine screening and lateral chest

radiographs in a hospital-based population. N Engl J Med 291:1001, 1974

30. Farnsworth PB, Steiner E, Klein RM et al: The value of routine preoperative chest roentgenograms in infants and children. JAMA 244:582, 1980

31. Brill PW, Ewing ML, Dunn AA: The value (?) of routine chest radiography in children and adolescents. Pediatrics 52:156, 1973

32. Sane SM, Worsing RA, Weins CW et al: Value of preoperative chest x-ray examinations in children. Pediatrics 60:669, 1977

33. Daughaday WH, Erickson MM, White W et al: Evaluation of routine 12-channel chemical profiles on patients admitted to a university general hospital. In Benson ES, Standjord PE (eds): Multiple Laboratory Screening, p 18. New York, Academic Press, 1969

34. Newman HF: Chemical screening. NY State J Med 78:2172, 1978

35. Whitehead TP, Wootton IDP: Biochemical profiles for hospital patients. Lancet 2:1439, 1974

36. Korvin CC, Pearce RH, Stanley J: Admissions screening: Clinical benefits. Ann Intern Med 83:197, 1975

37. Durbridge TC, Edwards F, Edwards RG et al: An evaluation of multiphasic screening on admission to hospital. Med J Aust 1:703, 1976

38. Galloway JA, Shumen CR: Diabetes and surgery. Am J Med 34:177, 1963

39. Clark RSJ: Anesthesia and carbohydratic metabolism. Br J Anaesth 45:237, 1973

40. Fletcher J, Langman MJS, Kellock TD: Effect of surgery on blood sugar levels in diabetes mellitus. Lancet, 1:52, 1965

41. Brenner BM, Hostetter TH: Disturbances of renal function. In Isselbacher KJ (ed): Principles of Internal Medicine. New York, McGraw-Hill, 1980

42. Vital and Health Statistics Series 10, Number 109. Washington, DC, HEW Service Resources Administration, 1973

43. Heath H, Hodgson SF, Kennedy MA: Primary hyperparathyroidism. N Engl J Med 302:189, 1980

44. Editorial: Mild asymptomatic hyperparathyroidism. Br Med J 2:174, 1980

45. Boonstra CE, Jackson CE: Serum calcium survey for hyperparathyroidism. Am J Clin Pathol 55:523, 1971

46. Williamson E, Van Peenev HJ: Patient benefit in discovering occult hyperparathyroidism. Arch Intern Med 133:430, 1974

47. Heimann GA, Frohlich J, Bernstein M: Physicians' response to abnormal results of routine urinalysis. Can Med Assoc J 115:1094, 1974

48. Belliveau RE, Fitzgerald JE, Nikerson DA: Evaluation of routine profile chemistry screening of all patients admitted to a community hospital. Am J Clin Pathol 53:447, 1970

49. Kowalyshyn TJ, Prager D, Young J: A review of the present status of preoperative hemoglobin requirements. Anesth Analg (Cleve) 51:75, 1972

50. Rawston ER: Anaemia and surgery. A retrospective clinical study. Aust NZ J Surg 39:425, 1970

51. Gillies IDS: Anemia and anesthesia. Br J Anaesth, 46:589, 1974

52. Clark JR, Eisenberg JM: Screening for coagulation disorders in surgical patients. Clin Res (in press)

53. Eika C, Havig D, Godal HC: The value of preoperative hemostatic screening. Scand J Haematol 21:349, 1978

54. Robbins JA, Rose SD: Partial thromboplastin time as a screening test. Ann Intern Med 90:796, 1979

55. Barbaro DM, Shuman LJ, Swinkola RB: An evaluation of various presurgical testing procedures. Inquiry 14:369, 1977

56. Dumbaugh K, Neuhauser D: The effect of preadmission testing on length of stay. Inquiry (Suppl) 1:13, 1976

An Approach to Assessing Perioperative Risk

ROBERT A. HIRSH

The term risk refers to the chance or probability of injury, damage, or loss. *Operative risk* refers to the probability of adverse outcomes, illness and death, associated with surgery and anesthesia. Implicit in the decision to accept risk is the probability of gain or benefit from a therapeutic intervention resulting in amelioration or cure of disease, restoration of function, or relief of pain. Decisions to proceed with therapy are based on conceptualized risk:benefit ratios. The possibility of gain or benefit balanced against the urgency or elective nature of the operation are central to whether a given risk is acceptable.

The overall risk of perioperative death is 1.52%.[1] In 1981, 1 person in 15, or 15 million Americans, had surgery. Estimates of risk are accurate only when they are applied to groups and insofar as they are based on the experience of groups of comparable patients undergoing similar procedures. Estimates of risk for individuals within a group are not reliable.[2]

It is often difficult to categorize the cause of perioperative death as the underlying disease, the surgical procedure, or anesthesia. About 30 years ago, Beecher and Todd ascribed 78% of postoperative deaths on surgical services in ten university hospitals to patients' diseases, 18% to surgical management, and 3% to anesthetic management.[3] Today, a higher percentage of mortality might be ascribed to surgical and anesthetic causes than to the underlying disease, since our understanding of the pathophysiology of disease and the physiologic effects of surgical intervention and anesthetic drugs has improved. However, the patients who come to operation now are sicker than those of 30 years ago.

The internist's advice is often sought when patients come to surgery. The anesthesiologist and surgeon look to the medical consultant to provide answers to the following questions: (1) Does the patient have cardiac, pulmonary, renal, or other systemic disease? (2) If so, has the patient achieved maximum benefit from medical therapy? (3) If further improvement in the patient's medical condition is possible, what additional therapy should be given? Such questions should be explicitly asked by the physician requesting consultation and specifically addressed by the consultant. Statements by the medical consultant pointing to "high risk" or providing "medical clearance" for surgery serve no useful purpose; neither do recommendations regarding the preferred type of anesthesia, surgical incision, or procedure. Anesthetic and surgical plans are legitimate topics for discussion among the internist, anesthesiologist, and surgeon. The three can reach a consensus regarding the timing of surgery, the relative merits of different anesthetic and surgical techniques, and anticipated perioperative complications and their management. In this way, rational planning for patient care and professional satisfaction prevail.

DETERMINANTS OF PERIOPERATIVE RISK

The risks associated with anesthesia and surgery can be classified as patient-related risks, procedure-related risks, provider-related risks, and anesthetic agent-related risks.

Patient-Related Risks

The patient brings to surgery a chronological age, gender, race, surgical disease, related or unrelated medical disease(s), drug history, socioeconomic status, and nutritional state. Many of these variables are interdependent, such as age, the prevalence of cardiovascular disease, and associated drug therapy with digitalis derivatives, antihypertensive agents, and diuretics. Some variables, such as socioeconomic status, may determine the type and quality of the institution in which the patient obtains medical care or the experience of the surgeon.[4] Ewy and his coworkers have devised a logistic function to estimate operation-specific mortality on the basis of patient-control variables.[5]

Most investigators have found that perioperative mortality is a U-shaped function with the nadir in death rate in the 15- to 25-year-old age group.[3,6,7,8,9] Dripps and Deming made a similar observation re-

garding the association between age and the incidence of postoperative atelectasis and pneumonia after upper abdominal surgery.[10] In two major studies of anesthesia-related deaths, women had lower death rates than men.[3,9] Beecher and Todd found no relation between perioperative death rate and race.[3]

The patient's overall physical status can be simply described according to the American Society of Anesthesiologists' (ASA) Physical Status Scale (PSS), seen in Table 3-1. Although the ASA's physical status classification was not originally designed as a predictor of risk or outcome, it does correlate with surgical outcome. Both anesthesia-related mortality (Table 3-2) and postoperative mortality (Table 3-3) rise as physical status classification moves from I to V.[7,9,11-13] Anesthetic and surgical mortality double in the case of emergency surgery for patients in physical status categories I, II, and III. Emergency surgery does not confer an additional risk of death for patients in physical status groups IV and V.[14,15]

Drug therapy may also be associated with specific perioperative risks. Diuretic drugs may produce hypokalemia, which potentiates the effects of nondepolarizing neuromuscular blocking agents like tubocurarine, gallamine, and pancuronium and sometimes results in prolonged muscle paralysis. Aminoglycoside antibiotic therapy, particularly with neomycin, may have the same effect. Echothiophate eyedrops impair plasma pseudocholinesterase activity and prolong the neuromuscular blockade of succinylcholine, a commonly used, short-acting depolarizing muscle relaxant. Chronic steroid therapy may compromise the patient's ability to respond to stress.

Most drug therapy poses no significant risk for anesthetic management beyond that established by the disease for which

Table 3-1. The American Society of Anesthesiologists' Physical Status Classification

Class I. No organic, physiologic, biochemical, or psychiatric disturbance. The pathologic process for which operation is to be performed is localized and does not entail a systemic disturbance. Examples: inguinal hernia in a fit patient; fibroid uterus in an otherwise healthy woman.

Class II. Mild to moderate systemic disturbance caused either by the condition to be treated surgically or by other pathophysiologic processes. Examples: non- or only slightly limiting organic heart disease; mild diabetes; essential hypertension; anemia. Some might choose to list the extremes of age here, the neonate and the octogenarian, even though no discernible systemic disease is present. Extreme obesity and chronic bronchitis may be included in this category.

Class III. Severe systemic disturbance or disease from whatever cause, even though it may not be possible to define the degree of disability with finality. Examples: severely limiting organic heart disease; severe diabetes with vascular complications; moderate to severe degrees of pulmonary insufficiency; angina pectoris; healed myocardial infarction.

Class IV. Severe systemic disorders that are already life-threatening and not always correctable by operation. Examples: organic heart disease with marked signs of cardiac insufficiency, persistent anginal syndrome, or active myocarditis; advanced degrees of pulmonary, hepatic, renal, or endocrine insufficiency.

Class V. Moribundity with little chance of survival. Examples: burst abdominal aneurysm with profound shock; major cerebral trauma with rapidly increasing intracranial pressure; massive pulmonary embolus. Most patients of this class require operation as a resuscitative measure with little if any anesthesia.

Emergency Operation (E). Any patient in one of the classes listed above who is operated upon as an emergency is considered to be in poorer physical condition than normal. The letter E is placed beside the numeric classification. Thus, the patient with a hitherto uncomplicated hernia now incarcerated and associated with nausea and vomiting is classified as IE.

(After Hallen B: Acta Anaesthet Scand Suppl (52:5, 1973)

it is prescribed. The two drugs that constitute exceptions to this generalization are insulin and monoamine oxidase inhibitors. Potentially fatal hypoglycemia may go unnoticed in an anesthetized diabetic patient; management of surgical patients with diabetes is discussed in Chapter 11.

Table 3-2. Anesthetic Death Rate by Physical Status

Physical Status	Death Rate [Number of Deaths/ 10,000 Operations (%)]*	
	Dripps et al[11]	*Marx et al*[8]
I	0/16,192 (0)	2/18,320 (1)
II	12/12,154 (1)	1/10,609 (1)
III	27/4,070 (66)	11/3,820 (29)
IV	33/720 (458)	9/1,073 (75)
V	8/87 (920)	5/323 (155)
Total	80/33,224 (24)	27/34,145 (8)

*Includes "definite" and "possible" anesthesia deaths. There were 0, 7, 11, 17, and 4 "definite" anesthesia deaths among class I, II, III, IV, and V patients, respectively.

Monoamine oxidase inhibitors may have unpredictable cardiovascular effects and usually cause hypertension, particularly in patients given meperidine or vasopressors. This can lead to cerebral edema, hemorrhage, and death. However, patients who use monoamine oxidase inhibitors may receive morphine with no apparent ill effects. If possible, it is best that these agents be discontinued two weeks before surgery; if they are not, surgery should be performed under local anesthesia without epinephrine. Even spinal anesthesia and peridural anesthesia may be dangerous, because vasopressors may be required to treat hypotension, which sometimes results from these techniques. Chlorpromazine or promethazine may be used as sedatives, and atropine may be used in the usual dosages. Inhalational anesthesia with halothane or enflurane may be tried if local anesthesia is not feasible. Muscle relaxants do not appear to be contraindicated.[16]

Table 3-3. Postoperative Death Rate by Physical Status

Physical Status	Death Rate [Number of deaths/10,000 operations (%)]		
	Vacanti[13] 48-Hour Mortality	*Marx et al*[8] 7-Day Mortality	*Hallen*[7]* 30-Day Mortality
I	43/50,703 (8.5)	11/18,320 (6)	7/8,672 (10)
II	34/12,601 (27)	50/10,609 (47)	42/4,388 (100)
III	66/3,616 (182)	168/3,820 (440)	51/1,367 (370)
IV	66/1,850 (780)	252/1,073 (2,345)	35/195 (1,800)
V	57/608 (940)	164/323 (5,080)	*
Unknown			5/566 (90)
Total	266/68,388 (39)	645/34,145 (189)	140/15,188 (92)

*Hallen has no risk group 5. His four risk groups may not correspond precisely to the physical status categories with the same numbers. The criteria for his risk group classification are not stated.

Procedure-Related Risks

The operative procedure itself is an important determinant of perioperative mortality. In the National Halothane Study, operations were classified by the mortality level of the procedure standardized for age, gender, and physical status.[17] The death rate for each mortality level of operation is presented in Table 3-4. Procedures associated with a high death rate include craniotomy, heart surgery, exploratory laparotomy, and large bowel surgery. Those with a low death rate are cystoscopy, dilitation and curettage, eye surgery, procedures in and around the mouth, hysterectomy, herniorrhaphy, and plastic surgery. All others have an intermediate death rate. There is significant variation in mortality rate within each category. It should be noted that this study included patients who had general anesthesia only. Other investigators have found higher death rates associated with procedures on the head and neck and intra-abdominal, intrathoracic, and cardiac operations.[8,9,11] Crude operation-specific death rates based on over 4 million hospital discharges in the United States in 1969 have been published for the 50 most common operations.[1]

Provider-Related Risks

Institutional differences in perioperative death rate have been documented for both university medical centers and comparable nonuniversity medical centers.[3,17] Moses and Mosteller found a 3- to 24-fold difference in postoperative death rate among 34 participating institutions. They concluded that "there are real differences in institutional death rates for which neither the data taken in the study (age, sex, physical status, operation, etc.) nor sampling error furnish an explanation. . ." They implied that differences in quality of medical care may be one explanation for the observed differences in institutional death rate. Other factors noted in-

Table 3-4. Death Rate by the Mortality Level of Operation Standardized for Physical Status, Age, and Gender

Mortality Level of Operation	Death Rate
Low	0.27%
Middle	1.76%
High	9.48%
All operations	1.91%

These data from the National Halothane Study include patients who had general anesthesia only.
(Beecher HK, Todd DP: Ann Surg 140:2, 1954)

Table 3-5. Cholecystectomy Mortality

Hospital Size Group	Number of Hospitals	Number of Patients	Actual Mortality Rate*	Expected Mortality Rate*	Difference
Small	353	10,672	21.3	16.5	+4.8
Medium-Small	278	23,673	17.4	16.5	+0.9
Medium-Large	201	27,653	14.7	15.7	−1.0
Large	144	29,972	14.1	15.7	−1.6
All Hospitals	976	91,970	16.0	16.0	0.0

*Per 1000 patients.
(Kinkaid WH: PAS Reporter 9 (12):1, 1971)

cluded differing nutritional levels in the population, willingness of surgeons to operate on poor-risk patients, and the percentage of referred cases.[18]

Beecher and Todd noted a threefold difference in surgical rates among ten university medical centers.[3] Differences in case mix did not account for the observed differences in mortality. Ament and co-workers found that mortality for cholecystectomy was higher than expected in small hospitals with fewer than 5,000 annual discharges and lower than expected in large hospitals with more than 15,000 annual discharges.[19] These data, which are summarized in Table 3-5, show that the death rate was 40% higher in the small hospitals than in the large hospitals. They do not reveal the underlying reasons for the observed differences in mortality and do not elucidate the patterns of operative mortality with respect to respiratory, cardiovascular, renal, or infectious causes.

Ewy reported a fourfold difference in

standardized mortality rate among 1213 hospitals.[20] He found no relationship between hospital size and postoperative death rate. However, he reported a strong correlation between good surgical outcome and the amount of money expended per patient day within each hospital size class. This association was stronger for smaller hospitals than for very large hospitals. Similarly, hospitals with high nursing labor intensity had low mortality rates.

The experience of an institution and its providers with a particular technique or operation also has an effect on outcome. Mortality for coronary artery bypass surgery decreases as institutional experience increases.[21] Hotchkiss found that teaching hospitals had lower mortality rates for both ligation and division procedures for patent ductus arteriosus than nonteaching hospitals (Table 3-6).[22] Teaching hospitals performed 4 times as many ligations and 11 times as many divisions as nonteach-

Table 3-6. Mortality from Ligation and Division of Patent Ductus Arteriosus in Teaching and Non-Teaching Hospitals

	Ligation No. of deaths/No. of patients (%)	Division No. of deaths/No. of patients (%)
Teaching Hospitals	38/1476 (2.6%)	63/2212 (2.75%)
Non-Teaching Hospitals	12/320 (3.75%)	18/188 (9.55%)

(Ament RP, Gustafson PG, Holtz CL: PAS Reporter 8:1, 1970)

ing hospitals. Luft and co-workers found that mortality rates for open-heart, major vascular, and transurethral surgery were 25% to 41% lower in institutions performing 200 or more of these operations annually than in hospitals with lower volumes.[23]

The experience of an anesthesiologist with new drugs has also been shown to have an effect on mortality. Dripps and associates showed that deaths associated with the use of muscle relaxants were due to errors of omission or commission.[11] This finding and two decades of subsequent experience refute the hypothesis of Beecher and Todd that such deaths are due to the inherent toxicity of muscle relaxants. This controversy demonstrates that it is sometimes difficult to determine the cause of adverse outcomes and that associations do not necessarily imply causation.

Forrest found no difference in morbidity among hospitals in which primarily anesthesiologists or primaily certified registered nurse anesthetists provided anesthesia care.[24] Gilbert concluded from a study of perioperative morbidity and mortality at the Massachusetts General Hospital that surgical outcome is not a function of the training and experience of the anesthetist.[15] This is most likely due to close supervision of inexperienced personnel, a factor that might also explain Forrest's results.

Cooper and his co-workers have used a modification of Flanagan's critical incident technique in an attempt to define the etiologic factors involved in preventable anesthetic mishaps.[25,26] They examined incidents that would have led to severe illness and death had they not been discovered in time, as well as incidents with adverse outcomes, the rationale being that the same factors are involved in both cases. The former occurs much more often

than the latter and is more likely to be reported. Of the 359 incidents studied, one-third had no effect on the patient, and one-sixth had "more than a transient effect." Of the preventable incidents, such as breathing circuit disconnections, inadvertent changes in gas flow, and drug-syringe errors, 82% were due to human error. Overt equipment failures accounted for 14% of the incidents. However, equipment design, inadequate experience, and insufficient familiarity with equipment or with the specific surgical procedure carried out were important contributors.

Anesthetic Agent-Related Risk Factors

None of the studies of anesthesia-related and anesthesia-caused death has established that one of the major modes of anesthesia—regional (spinal, peridural, nerve block) or general—is safer than the other. Indeed, Dornette reported anesthetic deaths associated with overdoses of local anesthesia, and the Baltimore Anesthesia Study Committee ascribed two deaths to anesthetic management when no anesthetic agent was used.[9,27] In the latter cases, the committee felt that "more adequate preparation and the contribution of an anesthetic might have enhanced the patient's chances of surviving the operative intervention."

In this regard, it is worthwhile to remember that the primary priority of the anesthetist is life-support. The second priority is good operating conditions for the surgeon. The third priority is patient comfort. The specific agent used by the anesthetist is never as important as these priorities.

Conclusions similar to those described above have been documented for postoperative pulmonary morbidity. Greene concludes, "All controlled studies demonstrate that in the absence of prophylactic measures or if the anesthesia is given by relatively untrained personnel, the incidence of postoperative pulmonary complications will be higher following general anesthesia than following spinal anesthesia. But if the quality of medical care is high in the two groups, there is no difference that can be ascribed to the anesthesia."[28]

There are three rare problems that dictate specific anesthesia management: malignant hyperpyrexia, halogenated hydrocarbon-induced hepatitis, and hyperkalemic cardiac arrest after the administration of succinylcholine to patients who have received a spinal cord injury within the last year or who have active neurologic disease. Only the last of these is consistently predictable and avoidable.

EMERGENCY SURGERY

Patients facing emergency surgery have a higher risk of dying than those undergoing elective surgery.[11,13] Intravascular hypovolemia predisposes to renal, cardiac, and cerebral hypoperfusion resulting from the myocardial depressant and vasodilatory effects of anesthetic agents. Emergency patients are likely to have full stomachs and may aspirate regurgitated gastric contents. These patients often have acid–base, extracellular fluid volume and electrolyte abnormalities secondary to diuretic therapy, prolonged vomiting or diarrhea, intestinal obstruction, and prolonged bed rest.

It is important, and perhaps life-saving, that electrolyte and particularly potassium abnormalities be corrected, that the euvolemic state be established with appropriate monitoring or central blood volume and left ventricular function, and that a full stomach be decompressed be-fore surgery. However, if there is uncontrolled bleeding, as from a ruptured aorta or ectopic pregnancy, delaying surgery is unjustified, since controlling the bleeding vessel is the definitive resuscitative measure.

High-risk patients are more sensitive than normal to the effects of hypotension, cardiac depression, and blood gas and acid–base derangements. One strategy for managing such patients is to monitor these parameters at frequent intervals. Electronic monitoring equipment makes it possible to obtain an electrocardiogram, arterial pressure, and central pressures continuously in the perioperative period. The rationale for such monitoring and the acceptance of the attendant expense and risk is that early recognition of abnormalities will lead to prompt correction. It is often advisable to transfer high-risk patients to tertiary care centers before surgery when specialized problems such as prolonged respiratory or hemodynamic support, hemodialysis, or care of spinal cord and head trauma are anticipated.

Most castastrophes are furthered by the absence of a plan of treatment, the lack of an identifiable chain of command, and a lack of communication. Sound patient care necessitates not only satisfactory physiologic evaluation, but also provision for communication among physicians rendering concurrent care. Treatment strategies should be established before surgery and before the development of the crises that frequently beset high-risk surgical patients.

SUMMARY

1. **Most operative illness and death result from the patient's concurrent underlying physiologic dysfunction.**
2. **Anesthetic deaths are most often due**

to human error. However, anesthetic deaths account for only 5% to 10% of the total perioperative mortality rate.

3. The goal of preoperative preparation is not to reach an absolute level of function but to achieve the optimal level of function for a particular patient. Disease states and medications that may cause problems should be identified so that complications can be anticipated and treated in a timely fashion in both elective and emergency surgery.

REFERENCES

1. Kinkaid WH (ed): Hospital deaths following surgery. PAS Reporter 9 (12):1, 1971
2. Goldstein A, Keats AS: The risk of anesthesia. Anesthesiology 33:130, 1970
3. Beecher HK, Todd DP: A study of the deaths associated with anesthesia and surgery. Ann Surg 140:2, 1954
4. Egbert LD, Rothman IL: Relation between the race and economic status of patients and who performs their surgery. N Engl J Med 279:90, 1977
5. Ewy W: Important patient control variables in outcomes of surgery and anesthesia. In Hirsh RA, Forrest WH, Orkin FK et al (eds): Health Care Delivery in Anesthesia, p. 85. Philadelphia, George F. Stickley, 1980
6. Graff TD, Phillips OC, Benson DW, et al: Baltimore Anesthesia Study Committee: Factors in pediatric mortality. Anesth Analg (Cleve) 43:407, 1964
7. Hallen B: Computerized anesthesia record-keeping. Acta Anaesthesiol Scand (Suppl) 52:5, 1973
8. Marx GF, Mateo CV, Orkin LR: Computer analysis of postanesthesia deaths. Anesthesiology 39:54, 1973
9. Phillips OC, Frazier TM, Graff TD et al: The Baltimore Anesthesia Study Committee: Review of 1024 postoperative deaths. JAMA 174:2015, 1960
10. Dripps RD, Deming MV: Postoperative atelectasis and pneumonia. Ann Surg 124:94, 1946
11. Dripps RD, Lamont A, Eckenhoff JE: The role of anesthesia in surgical mortality. JAMA 778:261, 1961
12. Lewin I, Lerner AG, Green SH et al: Physical class and physiologic status in the prediction of operative mortality in the aged sick. Ann Surg 174:2, 1971
13. Vacanti CJ, Van Houten RJ, Hill RC: A statistical analysis of the relationship of physical status to postoperative mortality in 68,388 cases. Anesth Analg (Cleve) 49:564, 1970
14. Dripps RD, Eckenhoff JE, Vandam LD: Introduction to Anesthesia, 5th ed. Philadelphia, W B Saunders, 1977
15. Gilbert JP: Outcome—Experience and training of the anesthetist. In Hirsh RA, Forrest WH, Orkin FK et al (eds): Health Care Delivery in Anesthesia, p 143. Philadelphia, George F. Stickley, 1980
16. Perks ER: Monomine oxidase inhibitors. Anaesthesia 19:376, 1964
17. Bunker JP, Forrest WH, Mosteller F et al: The National Halothane Study. NIH:NIGMS. Bethesda MD, U.S. Government Printing Office, 1969
18. Moses LE, Mosteller F: Institutional differences in postoperative death rates. JAMA 203:492, 1968
19. Ament RP, Gustafson PG, Holtz CL et al: Cholecystectomy mortality. PAS Reporter 8:1, 1970
20. Ewy W: Hospital death and morbidity studies. In Hirsh Ra, Forrest WH, Orkin FK et al (eds): Health Care Delivery in Anesthesia, p 49. Philadelphia, George F. Stickley, 1980
21. Mundth ED, Austen WG: Surgical measures for coronary heart disease. N Engl J Med 293:13, 75, 125, 1975
22. Hotchkiss WS: Patent ductus arteriosus and the occasional cardiac surgeon. JAMA 173:244, 1960

23. Luft HS, Bunker JP, Enthoven AC: Should operations be regionalized? The empirical relation between surgical volume and mortality. N Engl J Med 301:1364, 1979

24. Forrest WH: Outcome—The effect of the provider. In Hirsh RA, Forrest WH, Orkin FK et al (eds): Health Care Delivery in Anesthesia, p 137. Philadelphia, George F. Stickley, 1980

25. Cooper JB, Newbower RS, Long CD, et al: Preventable anesthetic mishaps: A study of human factors. Anesthesiology 49:399, 1978

26. Flanagan JC: The critical incident technique. Psychol Bull 51:327, 1954

27. Dornette WHL, Ortho OS: Death in the operating room. Anesth Analg (Cleve) 35:545, 1956

28. Greene N: Physiology of Spinal Anesthesia, 2nd ed, p 130. Baltimore, Williams & Wilkins, 1969

Antibiotic Prophylaxis of Infective Endocarditis

FRANK H. BROWN

Prophylactic use of antibiotics to prevent infective endocarditis is one of the most common reasons for preoperative consultation. The physician must frequently evaluate patients with heart murmurs, decide whether endocarditis prophylaxis is warranted, and choose appropriate drug regimens. Surveys have indicated that considerable confusion exists among practitioners concerning the use of antibiotics for this purpose.[1]

The rationale for prophylaxis against infective endocarditis began with Paget's observation that endocarditis most frequently develops in patients with pre-existing valvular heart disease.[2] Osler noted that endocarditis frequently follows operative, puerperal, or traumatic septicemia.[3] Janeway was the first to directly relate endocarditis to the asymptomatic bacteremia induced by diagnostic or therapeutic procedures.[4] Lewis and Grant later suggested that transient bacteremia occurs frequently and, although of no consequence to normal patients, serves as the source of infection of abnormal valves.[5]

Following Horder's suggestion that the oval cavity is the most frequent portal of entry for the infecting organism, many clinicians noted a temporal relationship between dental extraction and the occurrence of endocarditis.[6–13] In 1935, Okell and Elliott documented streptococcal bacteremia after dental extraction in 60% of all patients.[14] Burket and Burn confirmed that extraction induces bacteremia by applying cultures of pigmented Serratia to the gingival crevices before extraction and subsequently isolating the organism from blood cultures after the procedure.[15] In 1944, Taran reported that 52% of 350 children with rheumatic heart disease developed bacteremia after extraction and that 4, or 1.1%, subsequently died of endocarditis.[16]

These observations led to a search for methods of preventing bacteremia. Initial attempts relied on physical methods such as cautery and curettage. With the discovery of sulfonamides, chemoprophylaxis before dental extraction was begun for patients with valvular heart disease.[17–21] Subsequent studies, however, showed that sulfaprophylaxis did not decrease the frequency of postextraction bacteremia, and reports of endocarditis occurring despite prophylaxis appeared.[22–24] The increasing availability of the bactericidal antibiotic penicillin prompted its use for endocarditis prophylaxis, and a variety of prophylactic regimens were proposed by individual experts.[25–28] It was not until

1965 that the American Heart Association (AHA) published guidelines for prophylaxis.[29] These guidelines remained essentially unchanged until 1977, when revisions provoked considerable controversy and a re-examination of the concept of endocarditis prophylaxis.[30-36]

Despite the controversy over the efficacy of prophylaxis, there is widespread acceptance of endocarditis prophylaxis. It is recommended in all major medical, cardiology, and infectious disease texts. Surveys of practitioners confirm this acceptance, and the AHA recommendations have been referred to as the "currently recognized standard of practice."[1,37] Prevention of the consequences of endocarditis remains the most important reason for accepting endocarditis prophylaxis.

Even with appropriate antibiotic treatment, the mortality rate of endocarditis remains high. The complications of the disease can be catastrophic, and, even after successful treatment, long-term sequelae can cause significant illness. However, there is no definitive clinical documentation of the efficacy of prophylactic antibiotics in preventing endocarditis in humans.[35] The only direct comparison of a group of susceptible patients who received prophylaxis and another group who did not was reported by Taran in 1944.[16] The study was not randomized, used historical controls, and lacked statistical analysis. It provided no information about the effectiveness of prophylaxis as currently practiced.

Theoretically, antibiotic prophylaxis might be effective in reducing the risk of endocarditis by decreasing the frequency or magnitude of bacteremia and eliminating bacteria that have gained access to the bloodstream before endocarditis has been established.[32,38] Indirect evidence that prophylaxis is effective is derived largely from three sources. First, the administration of penicillin before a dental procedure decreases the incidence of positive blood cultures after the procedure, even with addition of penicillinase to the culture medium to inactivate residual drug.[39-42] Secondly, proponents of prophylaxis point to the relative paucity of reports of prophylaxis failure as evidence of its effectiveness. When such reports are examined, it is clear that few use adequate prophylaxis as defined by current standards. However, there are 30 reported cases of endocarditis in patients who received prophylaxis, indicating that some regimens are not totally effective.[43] The third source of evidence is the rabbit model of endocarditis initially developed by Garrison and Freeman.[44] In this model, a polyethylene catheter is passed transvenously across the tricuspid valve or transarterially across the aortic valve, traumatizing the endocardium and allowing thrombus to form at the site of contact. Injected viable bacteria localize in the thrombus and multiply, leading to the formation of the typical vegetations of infective endocarditis.[45] Various prophylactic regimens have been shown to prevent endocarditis in this experimental model.[46-48]

Despite the indirect evidence that endocarditis prophylaxis might be effective, questions of its value for the individual patient and as health care policy still exist. Transient bacteremia is ubiquitous, occurring frequently after activities such as brushing of teeth or chewing of candy (see Table 4-1). Given the frequency of bacteremia and the relatively low incidence of endocarditis, establishment of endocardial infection must be exceedingly uncommon.

The only direct estimates of the risk of developing endocarditis after a procedure likely to induce bacteremia come from two studies performed in the preantibiotic era. Both suggest a relatively low risk. In

1942, Schwartz and Salman studied 98 patients with rheumatic heart disease undergoing a total of 403 extractions and found no cases of endocarditis.[49] Various estimates of risk appearing in the literature range from 1 in 533 to fewer than 1 in 100,000 for susceptible patients.[38,50,51] Although these estimates are extrapolations based on a number of assumptions, the risk appears to approximate that of an anaphylactic reaction to the prophylactic penicillin.[52]

Even if antibiotic prophylaxis were undoubtedly effective, it would have relatively little impact on the overall incidence of endocarditis. Between 40% and 60% of patients have no previously recognized heart disease and would not receive prophylaxis. Furthermore, current prophylaxis regimens are directed against streptococci, the frequency of which as the causative organism has fallen in most series, currently accounting for only 65% of all cases of endocarditis. In 80% of cases, the source of bacteremia is unknown, with no clearly identifiable procedure preceding the illness. Kaye therefore calculated that only 7% of cases of endocarditis would be prevented if prophylaxis regimens were 100% effective and compliance were perfect.[33] In a series of 125 patients at the University of Washington, 10% of cases were felt to be potentially preventable.[53]

The effectiveness of prophylaxis may be limited by several other factors. Surveys indicate that 60% to 80% of susceptible patients are unaware of the need for prophylaxis.[54–56] Furthermore, many practitioners do not aggressively recommend prophylaxis. Of 113 susceptible patients from a total of 2069 attending a dental clinic, 64% indicated that the dentist did not inquire about heart disease, and 77% of 424 procedures involving these patients were done without prophylactic antibiotics.[56] Recent studies suggest that an increasing proportion of endocarditis is found among drug addicts, who obviously do not receive prophylaxis.

Several authors point out that there has been no change in the incidence of endocarditis since the preantibiotic era, implying that antibiotic prophylaxis is not effective.[57] However, such a conclusion may be erroneous. Because infective endocarditis is not a reportable illness, estimates of its incidence are derived largely from mortality statistics. Secondly, the incidence of endocarditis may have increased as the number of operations and invasive diagnostic procedures has multiplied. Finally, if problems in compliance and patient education are considered, lack of decline in the incidence of endocarditis in the antibiotic era does not necessarily imply that prophylaxis is ineffective.

The controversy surrounding prophylaxis became more heated than previously when the AHA revised its recommendations in 1977. The new guidelines emphasize parenteral and longer courses of antibiotic therapy. Petersdorf has characterized these recommendations as "hyperaggressive," emphasizing that their cost and inconvenience are likely to decrease compliance.[36] Administration of parenteral penicillin also increases the likelihood of significant adverse reactions.

The revisions of the AHA guidelines were largely based on evidence derived from the rabbit model that showed several of the 1972 regimens to be ineffective in preventing experimental endocarditis. However, there are serious objections to applying data from this model to antibiotic prophylaxis in humans. To achieve an ID_{100}, or adequate infecting dose, in rabbits, 10^8 colony-forming units were injected into the animals, more than that seen in transient bacteremia following dental extraction or other procedures in humans. In these settings, only 5 to 20 CFU/ml enter the bloodstream, and the bacteremia lasts less than 30 min.[58] In addition, in the rabbit studies, the presence of the catheter and thrombus lowers the size of inoculum required to initiate infection and makes the infection harder to eradicate. Because of this, some feel that the rabbit model is more comparable to established endocarditis or the presence of a prosthetic valve.[59,60] Finally, rabbits excrete most antibiotics more rapidly than humans at comparable doses per unit weight. Although these objections are valid, the rabbit model is clearly valuable in confirming the usefulness of in vitro sensitivity data to the formulation of prophylaxis regimens and allowing comparison of the relative efficacies of various regimens. The model provides a rigorous test of any given antibiotic regimen and probably guarantees a wide margin of safety when results are extrapolated to humans.

A randomized controlled trial would be helpful in resolving much of the controversy surrounding prophylaxis. However, Durack calculated that 10,000 patients with valvular heart disease would be required to demonstrate statistical significance if the risk of developing endocarditis were 1 in 500 and prophylaxis were 90% effective.[60] Furthermore, current ethical standards would probably preclude the withholding of prophylaxis from a control group, although, in such a trial, 50% of susceptible patients would receive prophylactic antibiotics, considerably more than the figures reported in current surveys of compliance.[34] The American Heart Association is currently attempting to approach the problem from another perspective by establishing a formal registry of prophylaxis failures. It is hoped that these data will provide further information about the effectiveness of current regimens.[52]

Although the issues surrounding the use of antibiotics to prevent endocarditis are clearly not resolved, the weight of the evidence continues to support prophylaxis. The clinician is therefore faced with three basic questions in patient management: (1) For which procedures should prophylactic antibiotics be given? (2) For which types of heart disease should prophylactic antibiotics be given? (3) What drug regimens should be employed?

PROCEDURES REQUIRING PROPHYLAXIS

The desirability of administering prophylactic antibiotics before a given procedure is proportional to the risk of endocarditis developing after the procedure. It is impossible to assess the magnitude of risk directly; it can only be inferred from the reported incidence of endocarditis after the particular procedure to which the endocarditis is presumably causally related. An approximation of the risk can also be made from the following information.

Incidence of Bacteremia After a Given Procedure

The incidence of bacteremia after various procedures has been reported by numerous investigators; the results of many of these studies are summarized in Table 4-1.[31,32] The wide variation in the reported incidence of bacteremia for many procedures reflects considerable diversity in

Table 4-1. Incidence of Bacteremia With Common Procedures

Procedure	Incidence (%)	Reference
Dental and Upper Respiratory Tract		
Dental extraction	18–92	31,32,37
Tooth cleaning	0–40	61–63
Tooth brushing	0–40	63–65
Oral irrigation	7–50	65–67
Chewing of hard candy or gum	0–22	63,68
Tonsillectomy	20–38	69–71
Nasotracheal intubation	16	72
Orotracheal intubation	0	72
Rigid bronchoscopy	15	73
Fiberoptic bronchoscopy	0	74,75
Nasotracheal suctioning	16	76
Gastrointestinal		
Endoscopy	2–12	77–81
Esophageal dilation	0–100	81,82
Endoscopic retrograde cholangiopancreatography	4	83
Sigmoidoscopy	0–9.5	84–87
Colonoscopy	0–27	79,88–93
Barium enema	11–23	94–96
Percutaneous liver biopsy	3–14	97,98
Peritoneoscopy	0	99
Rectal exam	0–4	100,101
Urologic		
Urethral catheterization	8	102
Cathetar removal	2–30	103
Urethral dilation	10–33	102–105
Transurethral Prostatic Resection	32–46	102,106,107
sterile urine	11	
infected urine	58	
Retropubic prostatectomy	68	108,109
sterile urine	13	
infected urine	82	
Cystoscopy	0–22	102,105
Transrectal prostate biopsy	76	110
Obstetric–Gynecologic		
Vaginal delivery	0–5	111–116
Punch biopsy of cervix	0	117
Intrauterine device	0–6	118
Suction abortion	85	119
Surgical		
Burn surgery	21–46	120,121
Abscess drainage	25–54	122
Appendectomy	21	122
Cholecystectomy	17	122
Hemorrhoidectomy	8	123
Miscellaneous		
Peritoneal dialysis	2–4	124,125
Hemodialysis	2–8	126
Cardiac catheterization	0	127,128
Angiography	0	129

the timing and number of cultures and the sophistication of microbiologic techniques employed in different studies.

Magnitude and Duration of Bacteremia

The magnitude and duration of bacteremia are important determinants in the rabbit model, in which the occurrence of endocarditis is proportional to the size of the inoculum. In addition, measures such as reticuloendothelial blockade that decrease the clearance of organisms and prolong the duration of bacteremia increase the incidence of endocarditis. In most studies in patients undergoing diagnostic or therapeutic procedures, bacteremia has been shown to be of low magnitude and short duration.

Types of Organisms Involved

Although anaerobes and gram-negative bacilli are probably the most frequent organisms in bacteremia in humans, they seldom cause endocarditis in naturally diseased valves. Gram-positive cocci, in particular streptococci, appear to have an unusual predilection for attacking these valves and account for most cases of the disease. This clinical observation has been corroborated by both *in vivo* and *in vitro* experimental data. In the rabbit model, a much larger inoculum is required of gram-negative bacteria, like *Escherichia coli*, than of gram-positive bacteria to ensure an ID_{100}.[130] Using human and canine aortic valve tissue, Gould and his co-workers demonstrated that streptococci, enterococci, and staphylococci were more adherent than most gram-negative bacilli.[131] They also showed that the adherence ratio for each strain tested remained constant with different concentrations of bacteria and concluded that the number of bacteria adhering to a valve is related to the duration and magnitude of bacteremia as well as to the ability of the bacteria to adhere. The mechanism of the increased ability of the gram-positive cocci to adhere to damaged valves and cause endocarditis is not well understood. The role of surface dextrans has been investigated and found to be unimportant.[132] It has been suggested that the ability of these organisms to induce platelet aggregation may be important.[133]

Although no definitive statement can be made about which procedures require prophylaxis, the relative risk of a susceptible patient developing endocarditis can be inferred from reports of cases attributed to a given procedure and a knowledge of the incidence, type, duration, and magnitude of bacteremia following the procedure. Procedures can therefore be divided into three broad categories of risk, as follows:

Procedures requiring prophylaxis in all
    susceptible patients
        Dental and upper respiratory tract
            procedures
        Gasrointestinal and biliary tract sur-
            gery
        Genitourinary manipulation or sur-
            gery
        Manipulation of septic foci
        Cardiac surgery
Procedures requiring prophylaxis only in
    patients with prosthetic valves
        Sigmidoscopy
        Colonoscopy
        Barium enema
        Liver biopsy
        Endoscopy
        Dilatation and curettage
Procedures not requiring prophylaxis
        Intrauterine device insertion or re-
            moval

Cervical biopsy
Vaginal delivery
Fiberoptic bronchoscopy
Cardiac catheterization and angiography

HEART DISEASE REQUIRING PROPHYLAXIS

There is no uniformity of opinion about which cardiac lesions make a patient sufficiently susceptible to endocarditis to require antibiotic prophylaxis. Evidence of relative susceptibility is derived from the frequency with which endocarditis is reported to occur in patients with a given lesion and from experimental studies of the hemodynamic characteristics of lesions susceptible to endocarditis. Most of this information comes from Rodbard's elegant demonstration that susceptible valvular lesions are generally characterized by a high pressure source driving blood through a narrow orifice into a low-pressure sink, producing jet and Venturi effects that account for the distribution of endocarditis foci.[134] These studies help explain several epidemiologic observations, including the greater susceptibility of left-sided than right-sided valves to both naturally occurring and experimental endocarditis, the greater susceptibility of regurgitant than other lesions, the susceptibility of arteriovenous fistulas, the rarity of endocarditis in uncomplicated atrial septal defects, the greater susceptibility of small than large ventricular septal defects, and low susceptibility in valvular disease and concurrent atrial fibrillation or congestive heart failure.

The most common cardiovascular lesions can be divided into three categories of relative risk, as outlined below.

A. Cardiac lesions requiring prophylaxis
   1. Rheumatic valvular disease
   2. Congenital heart disease
      a. Ventricular septal defect
      b. Patent ductus arteriosus
      c. Tetralogy of Fallot
      d. Pulmonic stenosis
      e. Coarctation of the aorta
      f. Bicuspid aortic valve
      g. Systemic pulmonary shunts
   3. Degenerative valvular disease
   4. Marfan's syndrome with aortic insufficiency
   5. Luetic aortic insufficiency
   6. Asymmetric septal hypertrophy
   7. Prior infective endocarditis
   8. Prosthetic valve or patch
B. Cardiovascular lesions possibly requiring prophylaxis
   1. Mitral valve prolapse
   2. Hemodialysis shunts
   3. Transvenous pacemakers
   4. Ventriculojugular shunts
C. Cardiac lesions not requiring prophylaxis
   1. Uncomplicated ostium secundum atrial septal defect
   2. Coronary bypass grafting
   3. Patent ductus arteriosus 6 months after closure
   4. Atrial septal defect 6 months after suture closure

Several of these lesions are of sufficient interest or have provoked sufficient controversy to warrant specific mention.

Mitral Valve Prolapse

The question of whether to administer prophylactic antibiotics to patients with mitral valve prolapse is even more controversial than the issue of endocarditis prophylaxis itself. Although there are some data suggesting that these patients may have a higher risk than normal of developing endocarditis, the disease occurs in 5% to 7% of the adult population, making routine administration of prophylaxis impractical and suggesting that the risk is very low.[135,136]

Most of the data concerning the risk of endocarditis in these patients is derived from three series. In 1974, Allen and his co-workers reported on their long follow-up of 62 patients with late systolic murmurs or systolic clicks and late systolic murmurs.[137] Five patients, or 8% developed endocarditis. Although the authors made no recommendations concerning prophylaxis, this study has been widely used to support the use of antibiotics in patients with prolapse. However, the study is confounded by the fact that 14 of the patients reportedly had a history of rheumatic fever and 2 had Marfan's syndrome, which may account for their susceptibility to endocarditis.

Lachman and associates reported ten cases of endocarditis in patients with presumed mitral valve prolapse and advised prophylaxis.[138] However, the diagnosis was made by auscultation alone, and there was an unusually high incidence (80%) of staphylococcal endocarditis. Since staphylococci can cause endocarditis in even normal valves and would not be prevented by prophylactic antibiotics, the recommendation is suspect.

In 1977, Corrigall and colleagues reported a series of 25 patients with mitral valve prolapse and endocarditis.[139] Twenty-two of these patients presented with holosystolic murmurs, the unusually high incidence of which may have been due to deterioration of valve function caused by endocarditis or may suggest that patients with holosystolic mumurs and high degrees of regurgitant flow are more susceptible than normal to endocarditis. None of the 25 had isolated clicks, suggesting that

patients with such clicks may have lower risk. These authors recommend prophylaxis for patients with mitral valve prolapse and murmurs of mitral regurgitation.

At least 10 cases of endocarditis have been reported in patients with isolated systolic clicks. LeBauer and co-workers reported the first case in 1967 and stated that "consideration must be given to prophylaxis for endocarditis even when these mid- to late systolic clicking sounds occur without any accompanying late systolic murmur."[140] There have been no reported cases of endocarditis in patients with "silent prolapse," that is, in patients without systolic clicks or murmurs found incidentally to have evidence of prolapse on echocardiogram or ventriculogram.

Other studies of the natural history of mitral valve prolapse suggest that the risk of endocarditis is quite low. Koch and Hancock followed 40 patients for 10 years and found no cases of endocarditis.[141] Similarly, Appelblatt reviewed his experience with 69 patients followed for 10 to 40 years and encountered no cases of endocarditis.[142] Mills and colleagues noted a somewhat higher risk, reporting 3 cases of endocarditis in 53 patients with the syndrome followed for a mean of 13.7 years.[143]

In view of the high prevalence, inconclusive data, and apparently low risk, it would seem that prophylactic antibiotics should be mandatory only in patients with regurgitant murmurs.

Arteriovenous Fistulas

A higher than normal incidence of bacterial endocarditis has been reported in patients with arteriovenous (AV) fistulas for hemodialysis.[144,145] The presence of experimental AV fistulas in dogs is associated with a high incidence of spontaneous infective endocarditis, and experimental endocarditis can be produced with a small inoculum of bacteria in this setting.[146,147] Because of this, Kaye has recommended that prophylactic antibiotic be given to patients with AV fistulas even if they do not have valvular heart disease.[148]

Degenerative Valvular Disease

Osler was the first to note that degenerative valvular disease is susceptible to infection.[3] Degenerative valvular disease has become an increasingly important predisposing lesion as the elderly population has increased in size and has undergone more invasive procedures. It has accounted for as much as 25% of the predisposing heart disease in some series and as much as 50% in patients over 60 years of age.[149] An aggressive approach to the problem was proposed by Lichtman and Master, who noted anatomic evidence of valvular disease in 234 of 406 consecutive autopsies on patients over age 50.[150] Because clinical evidence of this disease was frequently absent, the investigators suggested consideration of routine prophylaxis for all patients over 50 years old. This is obviously impractical and unwarranted, but clinical evidence of degenerative valve disease should be sought in elderly patients, and, when it is found, prophylaxis should be administered.

Asymmetric Septal Hypertrophy

Infective endocarditis has now been reported in a sufficient number of patients with obstructive asymmetric septal hypertrophy (ASH) that prophylaxis for such patients appears warranted.[151–153]

Previous Infective Endocarditis

Patients successfully treated for an initial episode of endocarditis have an 8% to 10% chance of suffering a second episode, and 25% of those will suffer a third.[38,154,155] Therefore, all patients who have recovered from endocarditis should receive prophylactic antibiotics even if there is no evidence on physical examination of residual valvular disease.

Prosthetic Valves

Early prosthetic valve endocarditis might be expected to provide a model that would clearly document the efficacy of prophylactic antibiotics and to provide a microcosm of the entire prophylaxis debate. Prosthetic valve implantation is a common procedure; it serves as a clearly defined precipitating event in a controlled environment and uses valves known to be highly susceptible to infection. Despite this, definitive evidence of benefit from antibiotics in preventing early prosthetic valve endocarditis (PVE) is lacking. Nevertheless, documentation of the frequency of bacteremia during cardiopulmonary bypass, the frequency of staphylococcal endocarditis in patients not receiving perioperative antibiotics, and the exceedingly high mortality of PVE have led to the routine use of prophylactic antibiotics during the insertion of prosthetic valves.[156,157]

Several early studies reported an overall decrease in early PVE with the use of prophylactic antibiotics, but none was adequately controlled or randomized.[158,160] Staphylococcal endocarditis continues to account for approximately 50% of early PVE even with the prophylactic use of antistaphylococcal antibiotics. Controlled studies have been inconclusive. Fekety and co-workers compared a placebo, penicillin, and methicillin in bypass procedures and found no difference in postoperative infection.[161] Prosthetic valve endocarditis did not occur, precluding analysis of this complication. Goodman and associates compared a placebo, a combination of penicillin and streptomycin, and oxacillin alone.[162] The control group was discontinued during the course of the study after the development of two cases of pneumococcal endocarditis. Five cases of PVE occurred in the antibiotic groups. Although the numbers were too small to permit statistical analysis, the authors concluded that antibiotic regimens do not appear to alter the frequency of postoperative infection but may play a role in selecting more resistant organisms.

Thus, the available data show no clearly definable benefit of antibiotic prophylaxis in the prevention of early endocarditis after prosthetic valve placement. PVE continues to occur, often with staphylococci and other sensitive organisms. Prophylactic antibiotics apparently shift the spectrum of infection to more resistant organism, increasing the frequency of gram-negative rod and fungal endocarditis. The rate of mortality from PVE due to these organisms is equal to or greater than that due to staphylococcal endocarditis.

The patient with a prosthetic valve also has a continued risk of developing late PVE. Actuarial estimates of the risk have been calculated to be 0.7%/year for patients with a prosthetic aortic valve and 1.1%/year for those with a prosthesis in the mitral position.[38] Because of the high risk of infection in these patients and the high mortality rate of PVE, use of prophylactic antibiotics should be most aggressive in this group.

DRUG REGIMENS FOR ENDOCARDITIS PROPHYLAXIS

The 1977 drug regimens recommended by the American Heart Association are presented in Tables 4-2 and 4-3.[30] They require larger doses than the previous guidelines and emphasize the use of parenteral drugs. Petersdorf has proposed modifications of these guidelines, reserving parenteral prophylaxis against *Streptococcus viridans* only for high-risk patients, such as those with prosthetic valves.[36] He also recommends shortening the course of prophylactic antibiotics to three doses after the initial loading dose, emphasizing that, in the rabbit model, most successful programs prevented infection after a single dose only. These modifications may enhance compliance and, based on currently available data, are certainly reasonable.

Several other points regarding antibiotic regimens deserve mention. Experimental evidence indicates that bacteriostatic agents, even when given in large doses for prolonged periods, are ineffective in preventing endocarditis. The same results were obtained when the agents were tested against susceptible organisms and serum concentrations well in excess of the minimum inhibitory concentration were achieved. Bacteriostatic agents have no role in the prophylaxis of endocarditis.[163]

Prophylactic courses of antibiotics should be started shortly before the planned procedure in order for high serum levels to be achieved and the selection of relatively resistant organisms to be minimized. Cates and his co-workers reported a case of S. viridans endocarditis in a patient who had received penicillin for 36 to 84 hr before multiple tooth ex-

Table 4-2. Antibiotic Prophylaxis for Dental Procedures and Surgery of the Upper Respiratory Tract in Adults

Regimen A: Susceptible Naturally Occurring Heart Disease

1. Parenteral–oral combined:

    Aqueous crystalline penicillin G (1 million U IM) mixed with procaine penicillin G (600,000 U IM). Give 30 min to 1 hr prior to procedure and then give penicillin V, 500 mg orally every 6 hr for 8 doses.

2. Oral

    Penicillin V (2 g orally) 30 min to 1 hr prior to the procedure and then 500 mg orally every 6 hr for 8 doses.

    For patients allergic to penicillin, use

    Vancomycin (see Regimen B)

or

    Erythromycin (1 g orally) 1½ to 2 hr prior to the procedure and then 500 mg orally every 6 hr for 8 doses.

Regimen B: Susceptible Naturally Occurring Heart Disease or Prosthetic Valves

    Aqueous crystalline penicillin G (1 million U)

mixed with

    Procaine penicillin G (600,000 U IM)

plus

    Streptomycin (1 g IM)

    Give 30 min to 1 hr prior to the procedure and then give penicillin V, 500 mg orally every 6 hr for 8 doses.

    For patients allergic to penicillin, use

    Vancomycin (1 g IV over 30 min to 1 hr). Start initial vancomycin infusion ½ to 1 hr prior to procedure, and then give erythromycin, 500 mg orally every 6 hr for 8 doses.

(American Heart Association Committee Report: Circulation 56:139A, 1977)

Table 4-3. Antibiotic Prophylaxis for Gastrointestinal and Genitourinary Tract Surgery and Instrumentation in Adults

Aqueous crystallin penicillin G (2 million U IM or IV)

    or

Ampicillin (1 g IM or IV)

    plus

Gentamicin [1.5 mg/kg (not to exceed 80 mg) IM or IV]

    or

Streptomycin (1 g IM)

Give initial doses 30 min to 1 hr prior to procedure. If gentamicin is used, then give a similar dose of gentamicin and penicillin (or ampicillin) every 8 h for 2 additional doses. If streptomycin is used, then give a similar dose of streptomycin and penicillin (or ampicillin) every 12 hr for 2 additional doses.

For patients allergic to penicillin, use

Vancomycin (1 g IV given over 30 min to 1 hr) plus streptomycin (1 g IM). A single dose of these antibiotics begun 30 min to 1 hr prior to the procedure is probably sufficient, but the same dose may be repeated after 12 hr.

(American Heart Association Committee Report: Circulation 56:139A, 1977) tractions.[164] The causative organism was unusually resistant to penicillin. Garrod and Waterworth have shown that the population of penicillin-sensitive streptococci in the saliva decreases after 24 hr of penicillin therapy and is replaced by more resistant organisms after 48 hr of therapy.[165] Thus, premature initiation of antibiotics is unnecessary and costly and may select resistant organisms.

The doses of penicillin used to prevent recurrence of rheumatic fever are inadequate to prevent endocarditis. Furthermore, because patients with rheumatic fever have been receiving oral penicillin chronically, they frequently harbor relatively resistant alpha-hemolytic streptococci in the oral cavity. Therefore, such patients should receive erythromycin, vancomycin, or penicillin in combination with an aminoglycoside for endocarditis prophylaxis.[30]

The use of erythromycin in the prophylaxis of endocarditis, although recommended by the AHA, appears to be less certain than other regimens. When initially tested in the rabbit model under standard conditions, erythromycin was found to be ineffective. Only when the inoculum size was reduced was the drug effective.[132] Although it is probably reasonable to use the drug for prophylaxis, the margin of safety with erythromycin may not be as great as with other regimens tested. Furthermore, Hunt and associates have reported resistance to erythromycin in many strains of streptococci isolated from the oral cavity.[166]

The combination of penicillin or ampicillin and gentamicin may be more effective than penicillin and streptomycin and probably should be considered the regimen of choice for prevention of enterococcal endocarditis. This recommendation is based on in vitro data showing that 40% of enterococci are not inhibited by the penicillin–streptomycin combination.[36] Drug dosages should be modified as necessary for patients with severely compromised renal function.[30]

"Prophylactic" antibiotics cannot be given after the fact. Drug regimens that are effective in preventing experimental endocarditis are ineffective when first given 6 hr after the inoculum of bacteria.[132] This is not surprising; in experimental models, viable bacteria can be recovered from the catheter-induced thrombus within minutes of injection.

There are no formal AHA guidelines regarding antibiotic prophylaxis for patients undergoing cardiac surgery or for susceptible patients undergoing procedures on infected or contaminated tissues, such as soft tissue abscesses. The choice of antibiotic in these settings should be influenced by available culture and sensitivity data. In general, antibiotic combinations that include a penicillinase-resistant penicillin or a cephalosporin to provide adequate antistaphylococcal coverage should be employed.[30]

It is important to re-emphasize the warning included in the most recent AHA recommendations:

The committee recognizes that it is not possible to make recommendations for all possible clinical situations. Practitioners should exercise their clinical judgment in determining the duration and choice of antibiotic(s) when special circumstances apply. Furthermore, since endocarditis may occur despite antibiotic prophylaxis, physicians and dentists should maintain a high index of suspicion in the interpretation of any unusual clinical events following the above procedures. Early diagnosis is important to reduce complications, sequelae, and mortality.[30]

ANCILLARY MEASURES

It is just as important to emphasize ancillary measures to minimize the risk of endocarditis in patients with valvular heart disease as to give prophylactic antibiotics. Unnecessary risks imposed by water irrigation and intrauterine devices should be avoided. The highest level of dental hygiene should be maintained, and endodontic procedures rather than extraction should be performed. All patients undergoing prosthetic valve placement should first have a complete dental evaluation. Patients with a high risk of endocarditis should have orotracheal rather than nasotrachel intubation and fiberoptic rather than rigid bronchoscopy. In-dwelling urethral and intravascular catheters should be avoided. Urine should be sterilized before urinary tract instrumentation. These and other obvious steps will help to protect the susceptible patient.[31,32]

SUMMARY

The efficacy of prophylactic antibiotics in the prevention of bacterial endocarditis has been neither proved nor disproved. There appears to be sufficient indirect clinical evidence to support the continued use of antibiotics before procedures known to induce bacteremia in order to prevent endocarditis in susceptible patients. Based on the available data, the most recent AHA recommendations and Petersdorf's proposed modifications serve as rational guidelines.

REFERENCES

1. Durack DT: Current practice in prevention of bacterial endocarditis. Br Heart J 37:478, 1975
2. Paget J: On obstruction to the branches of the pulmonary artery. Medico-chirurgical Transactions 27:167, 1844
3. Osler W: Malignant endocarditis. Lancet 1:415, 459, 505, 1885
4. Janeway EG: Certain clinical observations upon heart disease. Medical News 75:257, 1899
5. Lewis T, Grant RT: Observations relating to subacute infective endocarditis. Heart 10:21, 1923
6. Horder TJ: Infective endocarditis with an analysis of 150 cases and with special reference to the chronic form of the disease. Q J Med 2:289, 1909
7. Rushton MA: Subacute endocarditis following extraction of teeth. Guy's Hospital Reports, 80:391, 1930
8. Abrahmson L: Subacute bacterial endocarditis following removal of septic foci. Br Med J 2:8, 1931
9. Bernstein M: Subacute bacterial endocarditis following extraction of teeth. Report of a case. Ann Intern Med 5:1138, 1932
10. Feldman L, Trace IM: Subacute bacterial endocarditis following removal of teeth and tonsils. Ann Intern Med 11:2124, 1938
11. Sale L: Some tragic results following extraction of teeth. J Am Dent Assoc 26:1647, 1939
12. Geiger AJ: Relation of fatal subacute bacterial endocarditis to tooth extraction. J Am Dent Assoc 29:1023, 1942
13. Weiss H: Relation of portals of entry to subacute bacterial endocarditis. Arch Intern Med 54:710, 1934
14. Okell CC, Elliott SD: Bacteraemia and oral sepsis with special reference to the aetiology of subacute endocarditis. Lancet 2:869, 1935
15. Burket LW, Burn CG: Bacteremia following dental extraction—Demonstration of source of bacteria by means of a nonpathogen (Serratia Marcescens). J Dent Res 16:521, 1937
16. Taran LM: Rheumatic fever in its relation to dental disease. NYJ Dent 14:107, 1944
17. Long PH, Bliss EA: The Clinical and Ex-

perimental Use of Sulfanilamide, Sulfa-pyridine, and Allied Compounds. New York, Macmillan, 1939

18. Kolmer JA: Progress in chemotherapy of bacterial and other diseases, with special reference to protonsil, sulfanilamide, and sulfapyridine. Arch Intern Med 65:671, 1940

19. Kolmer JA, Turt L: Clinical Immunology Biotherapy, and Chemotherapy. Philadelphia, WB Saunders, 1941

20. Spink WW: Sulfonamides and Related Compounds in General Practice. Chicago, Year Book Publishers, 1941

21. Paquin O Jr: Bacteremia following removal of diseased teeth. J Am Dent Assoc 28:79, 1941

22. Northrup PM, Crowley MC: Prophylactic use of sulfathiazole in transient bacteremia following extraction of teeth—Preliminary Report. J Oral Surg 1:19, 1943

23. Pressman RE, Bender IB: Effect of Sulfonamide Compounds on Transient Bacteremia Following Extraction of Teeth—Sulfanilamide. Arch Intern Med 74:346, 1944

24. Clement DH, Montgomery WR: Subacute bacterial endocarditis—Report of a case with apparent failure of sulfonamide prophylaxis complicated by massive hemoperitoneum. Ann Intern Med 22:274, 1945

25. Anderson DG, Keefer CS: The treatment of non-hemolytic streptococcus subacute bacteria endocarditis with penicillin. Med Clin North Am 29:1129, 1945

26. Loewe L: The combined use of penicillin and heparin in the treatment of subacute bacterial endocarditis. Can Med Assoc J 52:1, 1945

27. Hunter TH: The treatment of subacute bacterial endocarditis with antibiotics. Am J Med 1:83, 1946

28. Medical Annotation. Infective Endocarditis. Lancet 1:913, 1947

29. American Heart Association Committee Report. Prevention of rheumatic fever and bacterial endocarditis. Circulation 31:953, 1965

30. American Heart Association Committee Report. Prevention of bacterial endocarditis. Circulation 56:139A, 1977

31. Everett ED, Hirschman JV: Transient bacteremia and endocarditis prophylaxis. Annu Rev Med 56:61, 1977

32. Sipes JN, Thompson RL, Hook EW: Prophylaxis of infective endocarditis—A reevaluation. Annu Rev Med 28:371, 1977

33. Kaye D: Prophylaxis Against Bacterial Endocarditis—A dilemma. In Kaplan EL, Taranta AV (eds): Infective Endocarditis, p 67. American Heart Association Monograph Series No. 52, 1977

34. Hilson GRF: Is chemoprophylaxis necessary? Proc R Soc Med 63:267, 1970

35. Editorial: Prophylaxis of bacterial endocarditis—Faith, hope, and charitable interpretations. Lancet 1:519, 1976

36. Petersdorf RG: Antimicardial prophylaxis of bacterial endocarditis—Prudent caution or bacterial overkill? Am J Med 65:220, 1978

37. Wyse DG, McAnultz JH, Rahimtoola SH: Antibiotic prophylaxis in patients with rheumatic heart disease and prosthetic devices. Clin Cardiol 1:112, 1978

38. Hook EW, Kaye D: Prophylaxis of bacterial endocarditis. J Chronic Dis 15:635, 1962

39. Schirger A, Martin WJ, Roger RQ et al: Bacterial invasion of blood after oral surgical procedures. J Lab Clin Med 55:326, 1960

40. Elliot RH, Dunbar JM: Streptococcal bacteremia in children following dental extractions. Arch Dis Child 43:451, 1968

41. Glazer RJ, Dankner A, Mathes SB et al: Effect of penicillin on the bacteremia following dental extraction. Am J Med 4:55, 1948

42. Bender IB, Pressman RS, Tashman SG: Comparative effects of local and systemic antibiotic therapy in the prevention of postextraction bacteremia. J Am Dent Assoc 57:54, 1958

43. Bisno AL, Durach DT, Fraser DW et al: Letter: Failure of prophylaxis for bacte-

rial endocarditis. Ann Intern Med 91:493, 1979

44. Garrison PK, Freedman LR: Experimental endocarditis. I. Staphylococcal endocarditis in rabbits resulting from placement of a polyethylene catheter in the right side of the heart. Yale J Biol Med 42:394, 1970

45. Durack DT, Beeson PB, Petersdorf RG: Experimental bacterial endocarditis. III. Production and progress of the disease in rabbits. Br J Exp Pathol 54:142, 1973

46. Durack DT, Petersdorf RG: Chemotherapy of experimental streptococcal endocarditis. I. Comparison of commonly recommended prophylactic regimens. J Clin Invest 52:592, 1973

47. Pelletier LL Jr, Durack DT, Petersdorf RG: Chemotherapy of experimental streptococcal endocarditis. IV. Further observations on prophylaxis. J Clin Invest 56:319, 1975

48. Durack DT, Starkebaum MS, Petersdorf RG: Chemotherapy of experimental streptococcal endocarditis. VI. Prevention of enterococcal endocarditis. J Lab Clin Med 90:171, 1977

49. Schwartz SP, Salman I: The effects of oral surgery on the course of patients with disease of the heart. Am J Orthod 28:331, 1942

50. Kelson SR, White PD: Notes on 250 cases of subacute bacterial (streptococcal) endocarditis studied and treated between 1927 and 1939. Ann Intern Med 22:40, 1945

51. Pogrel MA, Welsby PD: The dentist and prevention of infective endocarditis. Br Dent J 139:12, 1975

52. Rudolph AH, Price EV: Penicillin reactions among patients in venereal disease clinics. JAMA 223:499, 1973

53. Pelletier LL Jr, Petersdorf RG: Infective endocarditis. A review of 125 cases from the University of Washington Hospitals. 1963–72. Medicine (Baltimore) 56:287, 1977

54. Harvey WP, Capone MA: Bacterial endocarditis related to cleaning and filling of teeth with particular reference to the inadequacy of present day knowledge and practice of antibiotic prophylaxis for dental procedures. Am J Cardiol 7:793, 1961

55. Munroe Company, Lazarus TL: Prevention of infective endocarditis. J Can Dent Assoc 42:483, 1976

56. McGowan DA, Tuoky O: Dental treatment of patients with valvular heart disease. Br Dent J 124:519, 1968

57. Wilkinson M: Bacterial endocarditis and focal infection. Dental Practitioner 17:201, 1967

58. Bennett IL Jr, Beeson PB: Bacteremia: A consideration of some experimental and clinical aspects. Yale J Biol Med 26:241, 1954

59. Editorial: Preventing endocarditis. Brit Med J 4:1564, 1977

60. Durack DT: Experience with prevention of experimental endocarditis. Kaplan EL, Taranto AV (eds): Infective Endocarditis. American Heart Association Monograph Series No. 52, 1977

61. Hurwitz GA, Speck WT, Keller GB: Absence of bacteremia in children after prophylaxis. Oral Surg 32:891, 1971

62. DeLeo AA, Schoenknecht FD, Anderson MW et al: The incidence of bacteremia following oral prophylaxis on pediatric patients. Oral Surg 37:36, 1974

63. Cobe HM: Transitory Bacteremia. Oral Surg 7:609, 1954

64. Rise E, Smith JF, Bell J: Reduction of bacteremia after oral manipulations. Arch Otolaryngol 90:106, 1969

65. Berger SA, Weitzman S, Edberg SC et al: Bacteremia after the use of an oral irrigation device. Ann Intern Med 80:510, 1974

66. Felix JE, Rosen S, App GR: Detection of bacteremia after the use of an oral irrigation device in subjects with periodontitis. J Periodontol 42:785, 1971

67. Romans AR, App GR: Bacteremia, a result from oral irrigation in subjects with gingivitis. J Periodontol 42:757, 1971

68. Diener J, Schwartz SM, Sheianski M et

al: Bacteremia and oral sepsis with particular reference to the possible reduction of systemic disease originating from the oral cavity. J Periodontol 35:236, 1964

69. Elliot SD: Bacteremia following tonsillectomy. Lancet 2:589, 1939
70. Fischer J, Gottdenker F: Transient bacteremia following tonsillectomy. Experimental, bacteriological and clinical studies. Laryngoscope 51:271, 1941
71. Rhoads PS, Sibley JR, Billings CE: Bacteremia following tonsillectomy. JAMA 157:877, 1955
72. Berry FA Jr, Blankenbaker WL, Ball CG: A comparison of bacteremia occurring with nasotracheal and orotracheal intubation. Anesth Analg (Cleve) 52:873, 1973
73. Burman SO: Bronchoscopy and bacteremia. J Thorac Cardiovasc Surg 40:635, 1960
74. Kane RC, Cohen MH, Fossieck BE Jr et al: Absence of bacteremia after fiberoptic bronchoscopy. Am Rev Respir Dis 111:102, 1975
75. Pereira W, Kovnat DM, Khan MA et al: Fever and pneumonia after flexible fiberoptic bronchoscopy. Am Rev Respir Dis 112:59, 1975
76. LeFrock JL, Klainer AS, Wu WH et al: Transient bacteremia associated with nasotracheal suctioning. Clin Res 22:646, 1974
77. Shull HJ Jr, Greene BM, Allen SD et al: Bacteremia with upper gastrointestinal endoscopy. Ann Intern Med 83:212, 1975
78. Baltch AL, Buhac I, Agrawal A et al: Bacteremia following endoscopy. Abstract 165, presented at the 15th Interscience Conference on Antimicrobial Agents and Chemotherapy, Washington, DC Sept, 1975
79. Liebermann TR: Bacteremia and fiberoptic endoscopy. Gastrointest Endosc 23:36, 1976
80. Baltch AL, Buhac I, Agrawal A et al: Bacteremia after upper gastrointestinal endoscopy. Arch Intern Med 137:594, 1977

81. Stephenson PM, Dorrington L, Harris OD et al: Bacteremia following oesophageal dilatation and oesphago-gastroscopy. Aust NZ J Med 7:32, 1977
82. Raines DR, Branche WC, Anderson DL et al: The occurrence of bacteremia after esophageal dilatation. Gastrointest Endosc 22:86, 1975
83. Seagel JH, Berger SA, Sable RA et al: Low incidence of bacteremia following endoscopic retrograde cholangiopancreatography. Am J Gastroenterol 71:465, 1979
84. Unterman D, Milberg MB, Kranis M: Evaluation of blood cultures after signoidoscopy. N Engl J Med 257:773, 1957
85. Buchman E, Berglund EM: Bacteremia following signoidscopy. Am Heart J 60:863, 1960
86. LeFrock JL, Ellis CA, Turchick JB et al: Transient bacteremia associated with sigmoidoscopy. N Engl J Med 289:467, 1975
87. Engeling ER, Eng BF, Sullivan-Sigler N: Letter: Bacteremia after sigmoidoscopy: Another view. Ann Intern Med 85:77, 1976
88. Norfleet RG, Mulholland DD, Mitchell PD et al: Does bacteremia follow colonoscopy? Gastroenterology 70:20, 1976
89. Dickman MD, Farrell R, Higgs RH et al: Colonoscopy-associated bacteremia. Surg Gynecol Obstet 142:173, 1976
90. Hartong WA, Barnes WG, Calkins WG: The absence of bacteremia during colonoscopy. Am J Gastroenterol 67:240, 1977
91. Coughlin GP, Butler RN, Alp MH et al: Colonoscopy and bacteremia. Gut 18:678, 1977
92. Pelican G, Hentges D, Butt J et al: Bacteremia during colonoscopy. Gastrointest Endosc 23:33, 1976
93. Schwesinger WH, Levine BA, Ramos R: Complications of colonoscopy. Surg Gynecol Obstet 148:270, 1979
94. LeFrock J, Ellis CA, Klainer AS et al: Transient bacteremia associated with barium enema. Arch Intern Med 135:835, 1975
95. Schimmel DH, Hanelin LG, Cohen S et al: Bacteremia and the barium enema. Am J Roentgenol 128:207, 1977

96. Butt J, Hentges D, Pelican G et al: Bacteremia during barium enema study. Am J Roentgenol 130:715, 1978

97. McCloskey RV, Gold M, Weser E: Bacteremia after liver biopsy. Arch Intern Med 132:213, 1973

98. LeFrock JL, Ellis CA, Turchik JB et al: Transient bacteremia associated with percutaneous liver biopsy. J Infect Dis (Suppl) 131:S104, 1975

99. Zwelling LA, Mandell GL, Young RC: Peritoneoscopy: An invasive procedure without bacteremia. Ann Intern Med 87:454, 1977

100. Tandberg D, Reed WP: Blood cultures following rectal examination. JAMA 239:1789, 1978

101. Hoffman BI, Kobasa W, Kaye D: Bacteremia after rectal examination. AIM 88:658, 1978

102. Sullivan NM, Sutter VL, Mims MM et al: Clinical aspects of bacteremia after manipulation of the genitourinary tract. J Infect Dis 127:49, 1973

103. Slade N: Bacteremia and septicemia after urological operations. Proc R Soc Med 51:331, 1958

104. Barrington FJF, Wright HD: Bacteremia following operations on the urethra. J Pathol Bacteriol 33:871, 1930

105. Powers JH: Bacteremia following instrumentation of the infected urinary tract. NY State J Med 36:323, 1936

106. Biorn CL, Browning WH, Thompson L: Transient bacteremia immediately following transurethral prostatic resection. J Urol 63:155, 1950

107. Creevy CD, Feeney MJ: Routine use of antibiotics in transurethral prostatic resection: A clinical investigation. J Urol 71:615, 1954

108. Marshall A: Bacteremia following retropubic prostatectomy. Br J Urol 33:25, 1961

109. Steyn JH, Logie NJ: Bacteremia following prostatectomy. Br J Urol 34:459, 1962

110. Ashby EC, Rees M, Dowding CH: Prophylaxis against systemic infection after transrectal biopsy for suspected prostatic carcinoma. Br Med J 2:1263, 1978

111. Lein JN, Stander RW: Subacute bacterial endocarditis following obstetric and gynecologic procedures. Obstet Gynecol 13:568, 1959

112. Burwell CS, Metcalfe J: Heart Disease and Pregnancy: Physiology and Management, p 277. Boston, Little, Brown & Co, 1959

113. Redleaf PD, Fadell EJ: Bacteremia during parturition. JAMA 169:1284, 1959

114. Baker TH, Hubbell R: Reappraisal of a symptomatic puerperal bacteremia. Am J Obstet Gynecol 97:575, 1967

115. McCormack WM, Rosner B, Lee YH et al: Isolation of genital mycoplasmas from blood obtained shortly after vaginal delivery. Lancet 1:596, 1975

116. Fleming HA: Antibiotic prophylaxis against infective endocarditis after delivery. Lancet 1:144, 1977

117. Regetz MJ, Starr SE, Dowell VR Jr et al: Absence of bacteremia after diagnostic biopsy of the cervix: Chemoprophylactic implications. Chest 65:223, 1974

118. Everett ED, Reller LB, Droegemueller W et al: Absence of bacteremia after insertion or removal of intrauterine devices. Obstet Gynecol 47:207, 1976

119. Ritvo R, Moore P, Andriale VT: Transient bacteremia due to suction abortion: Implications for SBE antibiotic prophylaxis. Yale J Biol Med 50:471, 1977

120. Beard CH, Ribeiro CD, Jones DM: The bacteraemia associated with burns surgery. Br J Surg 62:638, 1975

121. Sasaki TM, Welch GW, Hendon DN et al: Burn wound manipulation—Induced bacteremia. J Trauma 19:46, 1979

122. Seifert E: Über Bakterien Befunde im Blut nach Operationen. Arch Klin Chir 138:565, 1925

123. Bonardi RA, Rosin JD, Stowesifer GL Jr et al: Bacteremias associated with routine hemorrhoidectomies. Dis Colon Rectum 19:233, 1976

124. Stevens RE, Baskin S, Greene JA et al: Peritoneal dialysis in the management of

chronic renal failure. J Am Med Assoc 190:102, 1964

125. Montgomerie J, Kalmonson GM, Guze LB: Renal failure and infection. Medicine 47:1, 1968

126. Robinson PJA, Rosen SM: Pyrexial reactions during haemodialysis. Br Med J 1:528, 1971

127. Kreidberg MB, Chernoff HL: Ineffectiveness of penicillin prophylaxis in cardiac catheterization. J Pediatr 66:286, 1965

128. Sande MA, Levison ME, Lukas DS et al: Bacteremia associated with cardiac catheterization. N Engl J Med 281:1104, 1969

129. Shawker TH, Kluge RM, Ayella RJ: Bacteremia associated with angiography. JAMA 229:1090, 1974

130. Freedman LR, Valone J: Experimental infective endocarditis. Prog Cardiovasc Dis 22:169, 1979

131. Gould K, Ramez-Rands CH, Holmes RK et al: Adherence of bacteria to heart valve in vitro. J Clin Invest 56:1364, 1975

132. Petersdorf RG, Pelletier LL, Durack DT: The 1976 Paul B. Beeson Lecture: Some observations on experimental endocarditis. Yale J Biol Med 50:67, 1977

133. Weinstein L, Schlesinger JJ: Pathoanatomic, pathophysiologic, and clinical correlations in endocarditis. N Engl J Med 91:832, 1974

134. Rodbard S: Blood velocity and endocarditis. Circulation 27:18, 1963

135. Procacci PM, Savian SV, Schreiter SL et al: Prevalence of clinical mitral valve prolapse in 1169 young women. N Engl J Med 294:1086, 1976

136. Darsee JR, Mikolich R, Nicoloff NB et al: Prevalence of mitral valve prolapse in presumably healthy young men. Circulation 59:619, 1979

137. Allen A, Harris A, Leatham A: Significance and prognosis of an isolated late systolic murmur. Br Heart J 36:525, 1974

138. Lachman AS, Bramwell-Jones DM, Lakier JB et al: Infective endocarditis in the billowing mitral leaflet syndrome. Br Heart J 37:326, 1975

139. Corrigall D, Bolen J, Hancock EW et al: Mitral valve prolapse and infective endocarditis. Am J Med 63:215, 1977

140. LeBauer EJ, Perloff JK, Keliher TF: The isolated systolic click with bacterial endocarditis. Am Heart J 73:534, 1967

141. Koch FH, Hancock EW: Ten year follow-up of forty patients with the midsystolic click/late systolic murmur syndrome. Am J Cardiol 37:149, 1976

142. Appelblatt NH, Willis PW, Lenhart JA et al: Ten to forty year follow-up of 69 patients with systolic click with or without late systolic murmur. Am. J. Cardiol. 35:119, 1975

143. Mills P, Rose J, Hollingsworth J: Long-term prognosis of mitral valve prolapse. N Engl J Med 297:13, 1977

144. King LH, Bradley KP, Shires DL et al: Bacterial endocarditis in chronic hemodialysis patients: A complication more common than previously suspected. Surgery 69:554, 1971

145. Ribot S, Ruthfeld D, Frankel HJ: Infectious endocarditis in maintenance hemodialysis patients: A report of four episodes among three patients. Am J Med Sci 264:183, 1972

146. Lillihei LC, Robb JRR, Visscher MB: The occurrence of endocarditis with valvular deformities in dogs with arteriovenous fistulae. Ann Surg 132:577, 1950

147. Lillihei LC, Shaffer JM, Spink WW et al: Role of cardiovascular stress in the pathogenesis of endocarditis and glomerulonephritis. Arch Surg 63:421, 1951

148. Kaye D: Bacterial endocarditis in the presence of arteriovenous fistulae. Am J Med Sci 264:189, 1972

149. Uwaydah MM, Weinberg AN: Bacterial endocarditis—A changing pattern. N Engl J Med 273:1231, 1965

150. Lichtman P, Master AM: The incidence of valvular heart disease in people over fifty and penicillin prophylaxis of bacterial endocarditis. NY State J Med 49:1693, 1949

151. Vecht RJ, Oakley CM: Infective endocar-

ditis in three patients with hypertrophic obstructive cardiomyopathy. Br Med J 2:455, 1968

152. Cardelia JU, Befeler B, Hildmen FJ et al: Hypertrophic subaortic stenosis complicated by aortic insufficiency and subacute bacterial endocarditis. Am Heart J 81:543, 1971

153. Habibzadeh MA, Curd GW, Zeller NH: Subacute bacterial endocarditis superimposed on idiopathic hypertrophic subaortic stenosis. Ariz Med 33:793, 1976

154. Morgan WL, Bland EF: Bacterial endocarditis in the antibiotic era. Circulation 19:753, 1959

155. Pankey GA: Subacute bacterial endocarditis at the University of Minnesota Hospital, 1939 through 1959. Ann Intern Med 55:550, 1961

156. Blakemore WS, McGarrity GS, Thurer RJ et al: Infection by airborne bacteria with cardiopulmonary bypass. Surgery 70:830, 1971

157. Ankeney JL, Parker RF: Staphylococcal endocarditis following open-heart surgery related to positive intraoperative blood cultures. In Brewer LA, III (ed): Prosthetic Heart Valves, p 719. Springfield, Ill., C.C. Thomas, 1969

158. Nelson RM, Jenson LB, Peterson CA et al: Effective use of prophylactic antibiotics in open-heart surgery. Arch Surg 90:731, 1965

159. Amoury RA, Bowman FO Jr, Malm JR: Endocarditis associated with intracardiac prostheses: Diagosis, management, and prophylaxis. J Thorac Cardiovasc Surg 51:36, 1966

160. Stein PD, Harken DW, Dexter L: The nature and prevention of prosthetic valve endocarditis. Am Heart J 71:393, 1966

161. Fekety FR, Cluff LE, Sabiston DE et al: A study of antibiotic prophylaxis in cardiac surgery. J Thorac Cardiovasc Surg 57:757, 1969

162. Goodman JS, Schaffner W, Colllins HA et al: Infection after cardiovascular surgery: Clinical study including examination of antimicrobial prophylaxis. N Engl J Med 278:117, 1968

163. Southwick FS, Durack DT: Chemotherapy of experimental streptococcal endocarditis. III. Failure of a bacteriostatic agent (tetracycline) in prophylaxis. J Clin Pathol 27:261, 1974

164. Cates JE, Christie RB, Garrod LP: Penicillin-resistant subacute bacterial endocarditis treated by a combination of penicillin and streptomycin. Br Med J 1:653, 1951

165. Garrod LP, Waterworth PM: The risks of dental extraction during penicillin therapy. Br Heart J 24:39, 1962

166. Hunt DE, King TJ, Fuller GE: Antibiotic susceptibility of bacteria isolated from oral infections. J Oral Surg 36:527, 1978

Arrhythmias and Conduction Disturbances in Surgical Patients

FRANCIS E. MARCHLINSKI

The perioperative management of patients with cardiac arrhythmias is an important part of the internist's practice. The incidence of arrhythmias during anesthesia and surgery approaches 84%, but most of these disorders are transient and clinically insignificant.[1,2] However, 5% of general surgical patients develop significant intraoperative or postoperative tachyarrhythmias or bradyarrhythmias, and patients undergoing thoracic or cardiac surgery have an even greater incidence of these rhythm disorders.[3–7] The recognition of preoperative clinical and electrocardiographic markers of serious rhythm disturbances is essential.

This chapter reviews (1) information on the incidence of various arrhythmias, (2) preoperative electrocardiographic markers that may predict the development of arrhythmias, (3) intraoperative and postoperative factors that precipitate their occurrence, and (4) the value of prophylactic treatment. A practical approach to the management of the surgical patient with a rhythm or conduction system disturbance will follow.

ARRHYTHMOGENIC EFFECTS OF SURGERY AND ANESTHESIA

With the advent of continuous monitoring systems, detailed analysis of electrocardiographic activity throughout surgery was made possible. Kuner and co-workers reviewed the electrocardiographic recordings of 154 patients undergoing surgery and found that 95 of the 154 patients had 195 cardiac arrhythmias.[1] Most of these were slow supraventricular dysrhythmias (128 patients), including sinus bradycardia, wandering atrial pacemakers, isoarrhythmic atrioventricular dissociation, and nodal rhythm. Another large group of patients had premature ventricular (28 patients) and supraventricular (19 patients) depolarizations. A smaller group had supraventricular (9 patients) and ventricular tachycardia (5 patients). Patients undergoing neurosurgical and thoracic procedures, endotracheal intubation, and operations lasting more than 3 hr had a significantly greater incidence of arrhythmias. Precipitating factors included the use of general anesthesia, hyperventilation, and intubation. Other investigators have similarly noted the high frequency, up to 84%, of transient supraventricular bradyarrhythmias and premature atrial and ventricular depolarizations but low incidence of serious arrhythmias during surgery.[2,8]

Clinical and experimental data suggest that hypercapnia, hypoxia, hypokalemia, and hyperkalemia increase arrhythmogenic potential, especially when they are associated with general anesthesia.[9] Alterations in the autonomic nervous system that occur with endotracheal intubation, such as ocular pressure, traction on the extraocular muscles, and central nervous system stimulation, also play a causative role in arrhythmogenesis. Cyclopropane can independently produce arrhythmias during deep levels of anesthesia, probably by altering catecholamine release and/or by stimulating the central nervous system, but halothane and enflurane are much less likely to induce arrhythmias even in excessive concentrations.[9] Diethylether and nitrous oxide induce arrhythmias even more rarely. Succinylcholine, which may alter potassium flux, and vasopressor agents can increase the potential for serious arrhythmias.[10–13]

In summary, although cardiac rhythm disturbances during anesthesia are common, serious arrhythmias requiring treatment are relatively infrequent.[9] The occurrence of any rhythm disturbance, however, should provoke a search for precipitating factors and an immediate reassessment of all ongoing pharmacologic and physical manipulations.

SUPRAVENTRICULAR TACHYCARDIA

In order to determine the need for electrocardiographic monitoring and prophylactic antiarrhythmic therapy, the physician must recognize preoperative historical and electrocardiographic information that predict the occurrence of arrhythmias. Among patients undergoing noncardiac surgery, supraventricular tachycardia has been reported to occur most frequently in those over the age of 70, those with preoperative pulmonary rales, and those undergoing intra-abdominal, intrathoracic, or major vascular surgery.[14] A history of heart disease, evidence of chronic obstructive pulmonary disease, or the presence of premature atrial depolarizations on routine electrocardiograms do not, however, predict the occurrence of supraventricular tachycardia.[14] Rogers and colleagues also noted that an antecedent history of heart disease or electrocardiographic evidence of premature depolarizations does not correlate with the subsequent development of supraventricular tachycardia.[15] Of 50 patients who developed supraventricular tachycardia intraoperatively (10) or postoperatively (40), 21 had no known heart disease and only 3 had preoperative premature atrial depolarizations.

There are no well-recognized electrocardiographic markers that predict intraoperative or postoperative development of supraventricular arrhythmias. However, Buxton and associates have reported preliminary data on P wave duration as a predictor of postoperative atrial arrhythmias in 38 patients undergoing coronary artery bypass surgery. They noted that atrial fibrillation or flutter developed only in patients with intra-atrial conduction delay, which was defined as a P wave duration equal to or greater than 110 msec. Of 28 patients with evidence of an intra-atrial conduction delay, 10 developed atrial flutter or fibrillation, suggesting that P wave duration may have predictive value. Supraventricular tachycardia, primarily atrial fibrillation or flutter, is particularly common after cardiac or thoracic surgery, with an incidence reported to be as high as 30%.[4-7] The high frequency of atrial arrhythmias has been attributed in part to pericardial and myocardial inflammation, which develops after the surgical procedure.[7,17]

The prophylactic use of digoxin to prevent supraventricular tachycardia in patients undergoing thoracic or cardiac surgical procedures is controversial. In a retrospective nonrandomized study, Shields and co-workers reported a decreased incidence of post-thoracotomy atrial flutter and fibrillation in patients who received a total dose of 2 to 3 mg of digoxin 2 to 3 days before surgery followed by a daily maintenance dose of 0.25 mg.[18] In a prospective, randomized study of 120 patients undergoing coronary bypass grafting, Johnson and associates also found a significant decrease in supraventricular arrhythmias with no evidence of drug toxicity in digitalized patients.[19]

In contrast, Juler and co-workers noted an increased complication rate without a decrease in the incidence of atrial fibrillation or flutter in digitalized patients undergoing thoracotomy. Furthermore, Tyras and colleagues found that prophylactic digitalization did not prevent the postoperative occurrence of supraventricular tachycardia in 141 consecutive patients undergoing coronary artery bypass grafting.[21] Others have also recommended a cautious approach to the use of prophylactic digitalis derivatives.[22] They point out that electrolyte shifts, hypoxia, and decreased creatinine clearance are frequently assoicated with surgical procedures and predispose patients to digitalis toxicity. In addition, certain automatic atrial tachycardias seen after thoracotomy may mimic digitalis toxicity, leaving the clinician uncertain as to whether to use more digoxin to control ventricular rates.

A study by Stephenson and associates reported that 10 mg of propranolol administered orally every 6 hr from the time of transfer from the intensive care unit was associated with a significant decrease in the incidence of postoperative arrhythmias in patients who had undergone coronary artery bypass surgery.[23] Confirmation of these results and determination of their possible applicability to the general surgical population await further testing. The prophylactic use of digoxin and propranolol could therefore be limited to carefully defined high-risk groups. Atrial premature depolarizations do not appear to warrant specific prophylactic antiarrhythmic therapy to prevent the occurrence of postoperative supraventricular tachycardia.

Data clearly suggest that, when the postoperative course is complicated by concurrent medical problems, the patient is at increased risk for the development of new arrhythmias. Goldman recently reported on 35 patients who developed new postoperative supraventricular tachycardia after noncardiac operative procedures.[14] Of the 35, 22 developed atrial flutter or fibrillation, 3 had multifocal atrial tachycardia, and 6 had a regular supraventricular tachycardia without discernible P waves, most likely either AV nodal re-entrant tachycardia or automatic junctional (His bundle) tachycardia. An additional 4 patients exhibited a rhythm disturbance that was labeled as paroxysmal atrial tachycardia. Of the 35 patients, 18, or 52%, developed their supraventricular tachycardia by the third postoperative day. Thirty-one, or 91%, had identifiable factors that could have precipitated the arrhythmia. These factors included major infection, acute cardiac events related to ischemia or pump dysfunction, metabolic derangements, medications, hypotensive events, and abnormal temperature elevation without documented infection. Of the 3 patients without associated abnormalities, 2 had a preoperative history of supraventricular tachycardia.

Goldman emphasized the seriousness of concurrent medical problems in patients who developed supraventricular tachycardia postoperatively. Seventeen patients died, but no patient died as a direct consequence of his arrhythmia. Fourteen patients reverted to normal sinus rhythm without any new antiarrhythmic intervention. All patients with arrhythmias that persisted for more than 6 hr remained hemodynamically stabilized, the ventricular response to the atrial arrhythmia being controlled with digoxin or propranolol. The significance of associated postoperative complications was similarly emphasized in a report by Rogers and co-workers.[15]

Prompt recognition and treatment of postoperative tachyarrhythmias minimizes the disorder's hemodynamic effects and the tendency to progress to further electrical instability. Over the last ten years, the use of intracardiac recordings and programmed electrical stimulation has led to greater understanding of the electrocardiographic features and basic physiologic mechanisms of supraventricular and ventricular tachycardias.[24-27] This has resulted in a reclassification of supraventricular tachyarrhythmias and a more rational approach to the diagnosis and therapy of all arrhythmias.[28-33]

The physician's approach to the patient with a sustained tachyarrhythmia remains the same during all phases of the perioperative period. Prompt assessment of hemodynamic stability is of crucial importance. A careful search for precipitating factors that may have initiated the rhythm disturbance should be undertaken. Such factors include the following:

Medications
    Antiarrhythmias
    Pressors
    Bronchodilators
    Digoxin
Hypo- or hyperkalemia
Hypoxia
Acidosis
Anemia
Infection
Myocardial ischemia
Congestive heart failure
Hypotension
Elevated temperature without infection
Pulmonary emboli
Pericarditis

Precise electrocardiographic diagnosis of the arrhythmia is essential. The regularity of the rhythm, morphology of the P wave and QRS complexes, location of the P wave axis, frequency of atrial depolarizations, temporal relation of atrial depolarization to the QRS complex, and presence of capture or fusion beats or of atrioventricular dissociation should be rapidly determined.

Intraesophageal and intracardiac leads can provide crucial information not readily apparent on surface electrocardiograms, and they are invaluable in defining the type of atrial arrhythmia and in distinguishing between a wide complex supraventricular tachycardia and a ventricular tachycardia (Figs. 5-1 and 5-2). Intracardiac electrodes can also be used to terminate the tachyarrhythmia by appropriate pacing modalities. An esophageal electrogram can be obtained by passage of a bipolar electrode catheter or a 12-gauge nasogastric tube filled with electrocardiogram paste through the nasopharynx to the level of the midesophagus. Intracardiac electrograms recording right atrial activity can be safely obtained at the bedside by passage of a bipolar electrode

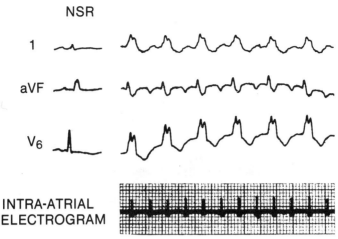

Fig. 5-1. Atrial electrode used to diagnose atrial flutter during a wide complex tachycardia. Narrow QRS complex associated with sinus rhythm and wide QRS complex associated with regular tachycardia (rate, 140) are illustrated. The bottom panel is an intra-atrial electrogram recorded during the tachycardia. It clearly demonstrates regular atrial activity at 280/min, leading to a diagnosis of atrial flutter with a 2:1 ventricular response and aberrant conduction and ruling out a diagnosis of ventricular tachycardia.

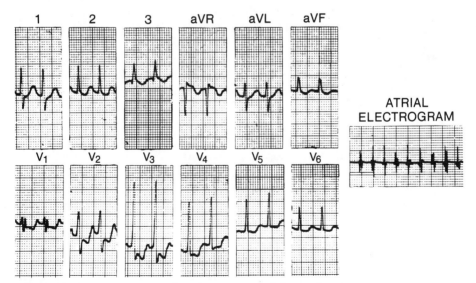

Fig. 5-2. Atrial electrode used to diagnose atrial flutter during a narrow complex tachycardia. A twelve-lead ECG demonstrates regular, narrow, complex tachycardia with an unclear atrial mechanism. An atrial electrogram recorded during tachycardia demonstrates regular atrial activity at 300/min, leading to a diagnosis of atrial flutter as the basic mechanism.

catheter transvenously to the right atrium, a procedure that can usually be done without fluoroscopy. A classification of supraventricular arrhythmias based on electrocardiographic appearance and underlying mechanisms is provided in Table 5-1.

Therapy of supraventricular tachycardia should initially be aimed at controlling the rate of ventricular response. When the origin of the supraventricular arrhythmia is located above the level of the atrioventricular node (atrial fibrillation, atrial flutter, automatic atrial tachycardia), atrioventricular nodal conduction can be slowed acutely with intravenous propranolol or digoxin. Propranolol is preferred because increased catecholamine activity in a patient in the postoperative state antagonizes the blocking effect of digitalis on atrioventricular nodal conduction and enhances its effect on automatic pacemakers. Verapamil, a calcium channel blocker, markedly decreases atrioventricular nodal conduction and may become the agent of choice now that it is available for general use in this country.[24–36] Multifocal atrial tachycardia should be managed by aggressive treatment of the underlying medical condition, primarily pulmonary dysfunction. Digoxin can be cautiously used as supplemental therapy, particularly if there is evidence of myocardial pump dysfunction.

A second group of supraventricular tachycardias involves a re-entrant mechanism that often incorporates the atrioventricular node in at least one limb of the re-entrant circuit. Control of the ventricular response is usually synonymous with termination of the arrhythmia. Initial therapy is again aimed at slowing atrioventricular nodal conduction and includes vagal maneuvers, edrophonium, propranolol, or digoxin. Persistent tachy-

cardia warrants treatment with agents that slow conduction in the other limb of the re-entrant circuit to terminate the tachycardia, and procainamide is the drug of choice. Its ease of administration as an intravenous preparation and its effect on slowing conduction in atria, ventricles, accessory pathways, and probably the retrograde limb of dual atrioventricular nodal pathways make it suitable for this purpose.

A third group of frequent postoperative supraventricular arrhythmias includes the automatic junctional tachycardias. These may or may not be due to digitalis toxicity. The tachycardia probably originates below the atrioventricular node in the bundle of His. Treatment should be directed at decreasing catecholamine enhancement of automaticity with propranolol and decreasing automaticity with procainamide. If digitalis toxicity is suspected, the digoxin should be withheld, electrolyte balance maintained, and treatment with lidocaine or procainamide attempted if indicated by the rate of the tachycardia and hemodynamics.

Rarely, cardioversion will be necessary to convert a supraventricular tachycardia to normal sinus rhythm. The urgency of this intervention obviously depends on the symptomatic and hemodynamic status of the patient at the time of the arrhythmia. Potentially serious tachyarrhythmias and bradyarrhythmias can occur with cardioversion, and 1 to 2 mg of atropine, 1 to 3 μg/min of isoproterenol, and 100 mg of lidocaine should be available for intravenous administration.

VENTRICULAR ARRHYTHMIAS

Treatment of ventricular premature depolarizations is based on the assumption that these arrhythmias predict life-threatening ventricular tachycardia or fibrillation and that treatment of ventricular ectopic activity prevents these potentially lethal ventricular rhythm disorders. Although ventricular ectopic activity has long been considered a marker for more serious ventricular arrhythmias, critical analysis of available medical and surgical data fails to support this assumption.

Ventricular ectopic activity, observed in 62% of 283 overtly healthy middle-aged ambulatory men monitored for 6 hr, is common in the general population. Furthermore, ventricular premature depolarizations unaccompanied by clinical heart disease or other electrocardiographic abnormalities do not significantly influence mortality.[37–39] Kennedy and co-workers demonstrated that only 5 of 25 asymptomatic patients with complex ventricular ectopy had coronary artery disease.[40] They also noted that no deaths occurred in the patient group during an average follow-up period of 34 months.

Ventricular ectopic activity does not appear to be a specific predictor for the occurrence of clinical ventricular tachycardia or sudden death in patients with coronary artery disease, at least 84% of whom develop such arrhythmias.[41] Moss and his co-workers reported that complex ventricular arrhythmias in the postinfarction period were associated with a significantly high cardiac death rate but did not specifically determine the incidence of sudden death.[42] However, Ruberman and colleagues have reported preliminary data on patients who had myocardial infarctions and have shown that runs of two or more ventricular ectopic depolarizations and early, R-on-T, premature depolarizations observed on 1-hr Holter monitor recordings were independent predictors of sudden death in patients followed for a 5-year period.[43] Because of the short period of electrocardiographic monitoring in this study and spontaneous variations in arrhythmias, these results need confirmation.[44]

It has been suggested that the importance of ventricular ectopic activity lies in its reflection of severe underlying coronary artery disease and in the degree to which there is left ventricular dysfunction.[45] Goldman and his colleagues reported that the occurrence of ventricular premature depolarizations with a frequency of greater than 5 per minute documented any time before operation is an independent, significant risk factor for a variety of life-threatening cardiac complications, though not of ventricular tachycardia per se.[3,46] Ventricular tachycardia occurred in only 12 of 1001 patients undergoing noncardiac surgery and was not associated with the presence of ventricular ectopy observed on a preoperative electrocardiogram. These data also suggest that ventricular ectopic activity may be a marker for underlying cardiac disease and not a specific predictor for sustained ventricular arrhythmias.

The potential toxicity of antiarrhythmic drugs, including life-threatening arrhythmias, has been well documented.[47–50] Caution should be exercised in the use of prophylactic antiarrhythmic drugs in situations in which their efficacy has not been demonstrated. The current body of evidence indicates that prophylactic therapy for ventricular arrhythmias should be used in patients who have had an ischemic episode within 48 hr before emergency surgery. In this setting, therapy should be instituted regardless of the degree of ventricular ectopic activity.[51–55] In addition, antiarrhythmic therapy should probably be carried out in patients with known or suspected coronary disease who

Table 5-1. Diagnostic Features and Management of Supraventricular Tachyarrhythmias in the Surgical Patient

Arrhythmia	P Wave Frequency Per Minute	Ventricular Response	P Wave Morphology/ Axis	First-Choice Therapy	Alternative Therapy	Comment
Atrial fibrillation	Greater than 350	Variable	No distinct P waves	Propranolol, 0.1 mg/ kg at rate of 0.5–1 mg q3–5 min IV titrated to control ventricular response	Digoxin, 0.5 mg IV followed by 0.25 mg IV q2 hr titrated to ventricular response	Both digoxin and propranolol may result in conversion to NSR. Procainamide can be used to convert rhythm to normal sinus if ventricular response has been controlled.
Atrial flutter	250–350	Usually 2:1	Classical saw-toothed pattern in the inferior leads with superior axis	Propranolol, 0.1 mg/ kg at rate of 0.5–1 mg q3–5 min titrated to ventricular response; cardioversion, particularly if any hemodynamic embarrassment (less than 25 watt/sec is usually successful)	Digoxin, 0.5 mg IV followed by 0.25 mg q2 hr titrated to ventricular response to a total dose of 1.0–1.5 mg	Rapid atrial pacing is frequently effective, safe therapy.
Multifocal atrial tachycardia (MAT)	100–200	Variable frequent APP that block in atrioventricular node	At least 3 different P-wave morphologies	Digoxin, 1 mg over 24 hr followed by maintenance therapy		Digitalis should be used cautiously.

Automatic atrial tachycardia (AAT)	150–200	Usually 1:1	Axis and morphology depend on site of focus; P wave usually before QRS	Propranolol, 0.1 mg/kg at rate of 0.5–1 mg q3–5 minutes IV	Procainamide, 0.5–1 g IV over 30 min followed by infusion of 1–4 mg/min	Digitalis toxicity should be considered, especially in the face of variable atrioventricular conduction.
Junctional His bundle (NPJT)	120–200	1:1	P wave buried in QRS			
Reentrant supraventricular tachyarrhythmia through the atrioventricular	150–200	1:1	P wave usually buried in QRS; when visible, usually follows QRS; superiorly directed axis	Vagal maneuvers; edrophonium, 10 mg IV; propranolol, 0.1 mg/kg at rate of 1 mg/min IV; vagal maneuvers repeated after each intervention	Procainamide, 0.5–1 g IV over 20–30 min	If blood pressure is relatively decreased, metaraminol, 10 µg/min IV titrated to a systolic blood pressure of 150, may be effective; vagomimetic effect of digoxin is potentially effective.
Reentrant supraventricular tachyarrhythmia through an accessory pathway	175–250	1:1	P wave different from sinus; usually superiorly directed and/or negative in lead 1			

NSR = normal sinus rhythm; APD = atrial premature depolarization have frequent, multifocal, or runs of two or more ventricular premature depolarizations. The risk of developing ventricular tachycardia and the efficacy of prophylactic antiarrhythmic intervention in this subset of surgical patients have not yet been documented. Other patients who have not had documented sustained arrhythmias or symptoms attributable to tachyarrhythmias do not, on the basis of their ventricular ectopic activity, appear to warrant the risk of antiarrhythmic therapy. Electrocardiographic monitoring is indicated.

The therapy of choice for preventing ventricular tachycardia is lidocaine, an intravenous injection of 100 to 200 mg at the onset of the surgical procedure followed by the infusion of 1 to 4 mg/min. An alternative treatment is procainamide, an intravenous injection of 0.5 to 1.0 g over 30 min before the operation followed by the infusion of 1 to 4 mg/min. It has been documented that the use of intravenous procainamide is well tolerated even in patients with significant myocardial dysfunction.[56, 77] Patients already taking antiarrhythmic medication for ventricular arrhythmias need to have their therapy continued during surgery. Intravenous procainamide, because of its ease of administration and demonstrated effectiveness in controlling recurrent ventricular arrhythmias, is usually the drug of choice.

Ventricular tachyarrhythmias are poorly tolerated because of hemodynamic compromise resulting from the loss of atrial contraction, less efficient ventricular contraction due to the abnormal sequence of activation, and decreased diastolic filling due to rapid heart rate. Initial antiarrhythmic therapy consists of lidocaine, an intravenous injection of 75 to 200 mg followed by the continuous infusion of 1 to 4 mg/min to prevent recurrent arrhythmias. Procainamide is the drug of second choice for immediate treatment and subsequent prevention of recurrence; 500 to 1000 mg of procainamide should be infused over 20 min with continuous electrocardiographic monitoring for QRS widening and QT interval prolongation and frequent blood pressure determinations. The initial dose should be followed by an infusion of 1 to 4 mg/min. Because of frequent associated hemodynamic embarrassment noted with ventricular tachycardia, immediate cardioversion is frequently necessary.

BRADYARRHYTHMIAS AND CONDUCTION DISTURBANCES

Preoperative management of the asymptomatic adult patient with sinus bradycardia or chronic bifascicular conduction disease is controversial. The asymptomatic patient with sinus bracycardia should not be assumed to have sinus node dysfunction. Heart rates of less than 60 beats/min have been observed on electrocardiograms in one-third of all males and one-sixth of all females admitted to a general medical service.[58] Moreover, the resting heart rate tends to decrease with age. Agruss and associates assessed the significance of chronic sinus bradycardia (a heart rate of 41 to 51) in elderly patients.[59] Autonomic function and response to exercise were evaluated in these patients and compared to those in an age-matched control group. The investigators demonstrated that sinus bradycardia is not incompatible with normal cardiac performance. Josephson and colleagues emphasized the role that autonomic tone plays in determining sinus rate, suggesting that an isolated heart rate of less than

60 beats/min should not be considered abnormal unless it is persistent and inappropriate for physiologic circumstances.[60] They and others have noted a blunted heart rate response to atropine in patients with significant sinus node dysfunction.[61] Clinical evaluation of sinus node function with atropine and exercise appears to predict reserve response to stress in patients with sinus bradycardia.[62]

Patients with sinus bradycardia should be questioned for a history of palpitations followed by periods of dizziness or syncope, this being one of the most common clinical presentations of the sick sinus syndrome. Presence of the sick sinus syndrome requires the insertion of a temporary pacemaker before surgery. In the asymptomatic patient, persistent marked sinus bradycardia that cannot be readily explained by apparent alterations in autonomic tone warrants further evaluation. The response to atropine (0.02 mg/kg) should be assessed. With atropine, caution is mandatory, and the drug should be avoided in any patient who has angina at rest or with minimal exertion. An increase in heart rate to greater than 90 beats/min suggests that the sinus node is normal and that the heart rate will be able to increase appropriately to meet the demands of surgery. A good response to atropine also provides the anesthesiologist with information about the drug's potential use during surgery. In the event of an abnormal response to atropine, further electrophysiologic study should be undertaken.[63] If this is not possible, temporary pacing at the time of surgery is indicated.

Patients with chronic bifascicular conduction disturbances on surface electrocardiograms are felt to be at higher than normal risk for progression to complete heart block, but the risk still appears to be low. Kulbertus and co-workers followed 106 patients who had evidence of right bundle-branch block with left axis deviation on routine screening electrocardiograms.[64] After a mean follow-up of 3 years, only 2 patients developed heart block. Rothman and Triebwasser followed 249 asymptomatic Air Force personnel, 125 of whom had left bundle-branch block and 124 of whom had right bundle-branch block.[65] After a 10 year mean follow-up, only 1% had developed complete heart block. In a large prospective study of 452 patients with chronic bifascicular block, Dhingra and colleagues reported a cumulative incidence of spontaneous atrioventricular block after 5 years of only 7%.[66] Less than half of these cases had the block at or below the His bundle. Assessment of His–Purkinje conduction by measurement of H–V conduction intervals appears to increase predictability of which patients will progress to complete heart block, but, even in patients with H–V prolongation, the incidence of progression to complete heart block is small.[67] Markedly prolonged H–V intervals, a block below the His bundle during atrial pacing, and marked H–V prolongation and/or infra-His block after the administration of procainamide are electrophysiologic features that identify those patients who have the highest risk for developing complete heart block.[60,67–70]

There has been concern about the potential of patients with chronic bifascicular conduction disease for developing advanced heart block during the stress of anesthesia and surgery.[71] The results of numerous studies appear to negate the need for standby cardiac pacemaker therapy in patients who have these electrocardiographic abnormalities but have no previous evidence of advanced heart block.[3,72–77] Only 1 of 291 patients with bifascicular block reported from seven studies progressed to complete heart block with surgery. This episode of heart block was transient, was associated with intubation, and was preceded by PR prolongation, strongly suggesting that the block occurred at the level of the atrioventricular node and not in the His–Purkinje system.

Electrocardiographic evidence of PR prolongation in addition to chronic bifascicular disease is not associated with an increased risk of developing complete heart block during surgery.[3,72,74] This is consistent with the observation that, during long follow-up periods, PR prolongation does not predict advancement to complete heart block in patients with bifascicular disease.[66,68] The number of patients found to have right bundle-branch block and left posterior hemiblock before surgery has been small.[3,76] However, of 12 patients reported with this conduction disturbance, none developed heart block during surgery.[3,67] Furthermore, large prospective studies have indicated that the risk of development of advanced heart block during long-term follow-up in patients with right bundle-branch block and left posterior hemiblock is also small, similar to that in other forms of bifascicular disease.[66,68]

Bellocci and co-workers assessed the significance of a prolonged H–V interval in 98 patients with chronic bifascicular block undergoing surgery.[76] Of 51 patients with H–V prolongation, none developed advanced heart block postoperatively, however, H–V interval prolongation was associated with a higher incidence than normal of cardiac disease and cardiac complications.

Patients with a clinical history of syncope or dizziness and electrocardiographic evidence of bifascicular disease warrant special consideration. It has been recommended that prophylactic pacemakers be placed in these patients;[78] however, this view is not uniformly accepted. Berg and Kotler suggest that patients with bifascicular disease and syncope in whom no previous evidence of advanced heart block has been noted be observed closely without temporary pacing.[72] Although the total number of patients studied is small, there has been no demonstration of an increased risk of advanced heart block in surgical patients with bifascicular disease and syncope without previously documented atrioventricular block.[72–76] Moreover, it has been stressed that syncope in patients with bifascicular disease is multifactorial. Dhingra and associates were able to attribute syncope to bradyarrhythmias in only 6 of 30 such patients, 5 with intermittent heart block and 1 with sinus exit block.[79] Of the 24 remaining patients, 2 had orthostatic hypotension, 3 had seizure disorders, 9 had ventricular arrhythmias, 1 had acute blood loss, and 9 had no documented etiology for syncope and no recurrent symptoms. Thus, only 20% of the patients required pacemaker intervention.

In the patient without a pacemaker, the occurrence of hemodynamically significant bradyarrhythmias during the intraoperative or postoperative period requires prompt attention. Reversal of physical or pharmacologic factors that increase vagal tone is the first priority. The possibility of acute myocardial ischemia should be considered. Electrocardiographic assessment of the site of the conduction disturbance should be undertaken. Atropine (0.6 mg) should be given intravenously, and this should be repeated at increasing doses. If an adequate initial response does not occur after a total dose of 3 mg, an isoproterenol infusion, starting at a dose of 1 μg/min and titrated to the heart rate response, may increase the heart rate, particularly with His–Purkinje escape rhythms, which do not respond to atropine.[86] The increase in heart rate may provide enough hemodynamic stability to allow life-saving insertion of a transvenous electrode catheter for pacing. For atrial kick to be preserved, atrial pacing may be attempted in patients with bradyarrhythmias in whom atrioventricular nodal conduction is intact. With fluoroscopic guidance, the catheter can frequently be placed in the coronary sinus or right atrial appendage to provide catheter stability. If atrioventricular conduction is not intact or a stable position for pacing the atrium cannot be attained, the catheter must be advanced into the right ventricle for pacing.

PACEMAKERS

Indications for the insertion of a permanent pacemaker have been the subject of many reviews.[81–86] The generally accepted bradyarrhythmias and conduction system disturbances that warrant pacemaker intervention are listed below.

Symptomatic cardioinhibitory carotid
   sinus hypersensitivity
Sinus node dysfunction
     Sinus pauses greater than 3 sec or
       those resulting in symptoms
     Symptomatic* sinus bradycardia
Atrioventricular nodal block
     Symptomatic* second-degree heart
       block (Mobitz I)
     Symptomatic* complete heart block
Infranodal block

---

*Symptoms include evidence of cerebral hypoperfusion, cardiac ischemia, congestive heart failure or increased ventricular irritability, and precipitation of tachyarrhythmias.

New bifascicular conduction system
   disease (right bundle-branch block
   and left axis deviation, right bundle-branch block and left posterior
   hemiblock, alternating bundle-branch block) associated with acute
   ischemia
Second-degree heart block (Mobitz II)
Complete heart block

Patients with any of the above disorders require temporary pacing at the time of surgery if permanent pacing has not yet been established. Before the development of the pacemaker, Vandam and McLemore documented the occurrence of circulatory arrest in the operating room in 6 of 22 patients with chronic complete heart block, illustrating the extremely high risk that exists without pacing intervention.[87]

Asymptomatic patients with bifascicular conduction disturbances are not at increased risk for the development of bradyarrhythmias during surgery. Prophylactic pacing is not indicated. An exception to this policy is the case of a patient with left bundle-branch block in whom a Swan–Ganz catheter is needed. Catheter-induced right bundle-branch block may occur and result in complete heart block.[88]

Patients with symptoms of syncope or dizziness and bifascicular conduction abnormalities deserve careful evaluation before temporary pacemaker insertion. As previously discussed, of the symptomatic patients currently reported who have undergone surgical procedures, none has developed complete heart block. Syncope in patients with chronic bifascicular block is not usually related to heart block. Indeed, syncope may be secondary to ventricular tachyarrhythmias. Therefore, patients with bifascicular conduction system abnormalities and previous symptoms of syncope or dizziness do not appear to warrant temporary pacing during surgery unless documentation of previous advanced heart block exists or the syncope has been recurrent. Electrocardiographic monitoring for the occurrence of ventricular arrhythmias is important. Further investigation to determine the risk of advanced heart block during surgery, markers for the increased risk, and the predictive value of preoperative electrophysiologic testing in this subset of patients is clearly needed.

In patients in whom temporary pacing is prophylactically employed, care must be taken to recognize and avoid potential complications. Temporary pacing can usually be performed with a low incidence of complications.[89] However, Nolewajka and co-workers reported venographically demonstrated deep venous thrombosis in approximately 37% of 30 consecutive patients who had had a wire placed through the femoral vein for temporary pacing.[90] The frequency of deep venous thrombosis was increased further in a subgroup of patients with hemodynamic compromise, 6 of 7 such patients developing deep venous thrombosis, as evidenced by venography. The clinical significance of these reported radiologic findings needs to be assessed. The risk of significant complications appears to increase if the pacemaker is left in place more than 72 hr. Pacing catheters inserted through the femoral vein have been associated with an increased risk of sepsis and pulmonary emboli.[91] In experienced hands, insertion of the pacing catheter through the brachial, internal jugular, or subclavian vein is preferred.

Patients with permanent pacemakers should have normal pacing and sensing function documented before the surgical procedure. A patient with a demand unit may have pacing function evaluated by application of a magnet to the pacemaker for activation of the fixed rate mode.

Ventricular demand pacemakers are suppressed by spontaneously occurring R waves but may also detect and be suppressed by electrical activity from a source other than the heart. Electrocoagulation and electrosection used during surgery have both caused suppression of pacemaker activity.[92] Maintaining the pacemaker in a fixed rate mode and limiting the frequency and duration of electrocautery to 1-sec bursts 10 sec apart should prevent this complication.[93]

SUMMARY

1. **Antiarrhythmic prophylaxis is rarely indicated except in patients with a prior history of symptoms attributable to documented paroxysmal arrhythmias. Only the patient with a very recent ischemic episode and the patient with coronary artery disease and complex ventricular ectopy appear to warrant therapy to prevent ventricular arrhythmias.**

2. **Risk factors for the development of supraventricular tachycardia include age over 70, rales on preoperative physical examination, thoracic or cardiac surgery, and, possibly, intraatrial conduction delay on a surface electrocardiogram. Electrocardiographic monitoring is suggested, with prompt treatment of arrhythmias.**

3. **All patients who have an accepted indication for permanent pacemaker intervention require temporary pacing at the time of surgery. Asymptomatic sinus bradycardia rarely indicates a need for pacing intervention. Preoperative assessment of sinus node function and influence of vagal tone in pro-**

ducing sinus bradycardia can be made with atropine. Except for patients with left bundle-branch block in whom a Swan–Ganz catheter is to be inserted, asymptomatic patients with bifascicular conduction disturbances should not undergo temporary pacing. Even patients with a history of dizziness or syncope and bifascicular disease have not been shown to be at increased risk of developing advanced heart block if this disorder has not been previously documented. It therefore appears that temporary pacing should be reserved for patients with recurrent symptoms in whom a neurologic basis for these symptoms has not been demonstrated.

4. An organized approach to the diagnosis and management of the patient with an arrhythmia is crucial. Most arrhythmias that develop intraoperatively, with transient slow supraventricular rhythms and premature depolarizations being most frequent, require no specific antiarrhythmic therapy. Therapy for the arrhythmia should be based on an accurate electrocardiographic diagnosis, an understanding of electrophysiologic mechanisms, and an awareness of the enhanced catecholamine state of the postoperative patient.

5. The surgical patient with an arrhythmia should be assessed immediately for evidence of precipitating factors. Associated medical conditions that contribute to the development of arrhythmias should be searched for and treated.

REFERENCES

1. Kuner J, Enescu V, Utsu F et al: Cardiac arrhythmias during anesthesia. Dis Chest 52:580, 1967

2. Bertrand CA, Steiner NV, Jameson AG et al: Disturbances of cardiac rhythm during anesthesia and surgery. JAMA 216:1615, 1971

3. Goldman L, Caldera DL, Southwick FS et al: Cardiac risk factors and complications in non-cardiac surgery. Medicine 57:357, 1978

4. Ghosh P, Pakrashi BC: Cardiac dysrhythmias after thoracotomy. Br Heart J 34:374, 1972

5. Moury FM, Reynolds EW: Cardiac rhythm disturbances complicating resectional surgery of the lung. Ann Intern Med 61:688, 1964

6. Rose MR, Glassman L, Spencer FC: Arrhythmias following cardiac surgery: Relation to serum digoxin levels. Am Heart J 89:288, 1974

7. Southgand J: Cardiac arrhythmias following pneumonectomy. Thorax 24:568, 1969

8. Vanik PE, Davis HS: Cardiac arrhythmia during halothane anesthesia. Anesth Analg 47:299, 1968

9. Katz RL, Bigger JT: Cardiac arrhythmias during anesthesia and operation. Anesthesiology 33:193, 1970

10. Walker DE, Barry JM, Hodges CV: Succinylcholine-induced ventricular fibrillation in the paralyzed urology patient. Urol 113:111, 1975

11. Tolmie JD, Joyce TH, Mitchell GD: Succinylcholine danger in the burned patient. Anesthesiology 28:467, 1967

12. Gronest GA, Theye RA: Pathophysiology of hyperkalemia induced by succinylcholine. Anesthesiology 43:89, 1975

13. Katz RL, Epstein RA: The interaction of anesthetic agents and adrenergic drugs to produce cardiac arrhythmias. Anesthesiology 29:763, 1968

14. Goldman L: Supraventricular tachyarrhythmias in hospitalized adults after surgery. Chest 73:4, 1978

15. Rogers WR, Wrobleski F, LaDue JS: Supraventricular tachycardia complicating surgical procedures. Circulation 7:192, 1952

16. Buxton AE, Kastor JA, Josephson ME: Role

of P wave duration as a predictor of postoperative atrial arrhythmias. Chest (in press)

17. Logue RB, Robinson PH, Hatcher CR et al: Medical management in cardiac surgery. In Hurst JW, Logue RB, Schlant RC et al (eds): The Heart, p 1777. New York, McGraw-Hill, 1978

18. Shields TW, Ujiki GT: Digitalization for prevention of arrhythmias following pulmonary surgery. Surg Gynecol Obstet 126:743, 1968

19. Johnson LW, Dickestein RA, Fruehan CT et al: Prophylactic digitalization for coronary artery bypass surgery. Circulation 53:819, 1976

20. Juler GL, Stemmer EA, Connelly JE: Complications of prophylactic digitalization in thoracic surgical patients. J Thorac Cardiovasc Surg 58:352, 1969

21. Tyras DH, Stothert JC, Kaiser GC et al: Supraventricular tachyarrhythmias after myocardial revascularization: A randomized trial of prophylactic digitalization. J Thorac Cardiovasc Surg 77:310, 1979

22. Selzer A, Cohen KE: Some thoughts concerning the prophylactic use of digitalis. Am J Cardiol 26:215, 1970

23. Stephenson LW, MacVaugh H, Tomasello D et al: Propranolol for the prevention of postoperative cardiac arrhythmias. A randomized study. Ann Thorac Surg 29:113, 1980

24. Wu D, Denes P, Amant-y-Leon F et al: Clinical electrocardiographic and electrophysiologic observations in patients with paroxysmal supraventricular tachycardia. Am J Cardiol 41:1045, 1978

25. Farshidi A, Josephson ME, Horowitz LN: Electrophysiologic characteristics of concealed bypass tracts: Clinical and electrocardiographic correlates. Am J Cardiol 41:1052, 1978

26. Josephson ME: Paroxysmal supraventricular tachycardia: An electrophysiologic approach. Am J Cardiol 41:1123, 1978

27. Wellens HJ, Bar FW, Lie KI: The value of the electrocardiogram in the differential diagnosis of a tachycardia with a widened QRS complex. Am J Med 64:27, 1978

28. Peters RW, Scheinman MM: Emergency treatment of supraventricular tachycardia. Med Clin North Am 63:73, 1979

29. Josephson ME, Kastor JA: Supraventricular tachycardia: Mechanisms and management. Ann Intern Med 87:346, 1977

30. Winkle RA, Glantz SA, Harrison DC: Pharmacologic therapy of ventricular arrhythmias. Am J Cardiol 36:629, 1975

31. Lown B, Temte JV, Arter WJ: Ventricular tachyarrhythmias: Clinical aspects. Circulation 47:1364, 1973

32. Josephson ME, Horowitz LN: Recurrent ventricular tachycardia: An electrophysiologic approach. Med Clin North Am 63:53, 1979

33. Singh BN, Collett JT, Chew CY: New perspectives in the pharmacologic therapy of cardiac arrhythmias. Prog Cardiovasc Dis 22:243, 1980

34. Arono WS, Landa D, Plasencia G et al: Verapamil in atrial fibrillation and atrial flutter. Clin Pharmacol Ther 26:578, 1979

35. Rosen MR, Wit AL, Hoffman BF: Electrophysiology and pharmacology of cardiac arrhythmias. VI. Cardiac effects of verapamil. Am Heart J 89:665, 1975

36. Plumb VJ, Karp RB, Kouchoukes NT: Verapamil treatment of atrial fibrillation and atrial flutter after open heart surgery (abst). Circulation (Suppl) 62:84, 1980

37. Desai DC, Hershberg PI, Alexander S: Clinical significance of ventricular premature beats in an outpatient population. Chest 64:564, 1973

38. Hinkle LE, Carver ST, Stevens M: The frequency of asymptomatic disturbances of cardiac rhythm and conduction in middle-aged men. Am J Cardiol 24:629, 1969

39. Rodstein M, Wolloch L, Gubner RS: Mortality study of the significance of extrasystole in an insured population. Chest 64:564, 1973

40. Kennedy HL, Pescarmona JE, Bouchard RJ et al: Coronary artery status of apparently healthy subjects with frequent and complex ventricular ectopy. Ann Intern Med 92:179, 1980

41. Kotler MN, Tabtznik B, Mower NM et al: Prognostic significance of ventricular ec-

topic beats with respect to sudden death in the late post infarction period. Circulation 47:959, 1973

42. Moss AJ, Davis HT, DeCamille J et al: Ventricular ectopic beats and their relation to sudden and non-sudden cardiac death after myocardial infarction. Circulation 60:998, 1979

43. Ruberman W, Weinblatt E, Goldberg JD et al: Sudden death after myocardial infarction: Runs of ventricular premature beats and R on T as high risk factors (abst). Am J Cardiol 45:444, 1980

44. Morganroth J, Michelson EL, Horowitz LN et al: Limitations of routine long-term ambulatory electrocardiographic monitoring to assess ventricular ectopic frequency. Circulation 58:408, 1978

45. Schulze RA, Rouleau J, Rigo P et al: Ventricular arrhythmias in the late hospital phase of acute myocardial infarction: Relation to left ventricular function detected by gated blood pool scanning. Circulation 52:1006, 1975

46. Goldman L, Caldera DL, Southwick FS et al: Multifactorial index of cardiac risk in non-cardiac surgical procedures. N Engl J Med 297:845, 1977

47. Koster RW, Wellens HJ: Quinidine-induced ventricular flutter and fibrillation without digitalis therapy. Am J Cardiol 38:519, 1976

48. Meltzer RS, Robert EW, McMorrow M et al: Atypical ventricular tachycardias: A manifestation of disopyramide toxicity. Am J Cardiol 42:1049, 1978

49. Nicholson WJ, Martin CE, Gracey JG et al: Disopyramide induced ventricular fibrillation. Am J Cardiol 43:1053, 1979

50. Cohen IS, Jick H, Cohen SI: Adverse reactions to quinidine in hospitalized patients: Findings based on data from the Boston Collaborative Drug Surveillance Program. Prog Cardiovasc Dis 20:151, 1977

51. Lie KI, Wellens HJ, Van Capelle FJ et al: Lidocaine in the prevention of primary ventricular fibrillation. N Engl J Med 291:1324, 1974

52. Noneman JW, Rogers JF: Lidocaine prophylaxis in acute myocardial infarction. Medicine 57:501, 1978

53. Harrison DC: Should lidocaine be administered routinely to all patients after acute myocardial infarction? Circulation 58:581, 1978

54. Lie KI, Wellens HJ, Downar E et al: Observations on patients with primary ventricular fibrillation complicating acute myocardial infarction. Circulation 52:755, 1975

55. El-Sherif N, Myerburg RJ, Scherlag BJ et al: Electrocardiographic antecedents of primary ventricular fibrillation—Value of the R on T phenomenon in acute myocardial infarction. Br Heart J 38:415, 1976

56. Burton JR, Matthew MJ, Armstrong PW: Comparative effects of lidocaine and procainamide on acute impaired hemodynamics. Am J Cardiol 43:98, 1977

57. Lima JJ, Goldfarb AL, Conti DR et al: Safety and efficiency of procainamide infusions. Am J Cardiol 43:98, 1979

58. Kirk JE, Kvorning SA: Sinus bradycardia: A clinical study of 515 consecutive cases. Acta Med Scand (Suppl) 266:625, 1952

59. Agruss NS, Rosen EV, Adolph RJ et al: Significance of chronic sinus bradycardia in elderly people. Circulation 46:924, 1972

60. Josephson ME, Seides SF: Clinical Cardiac Electrophysiology: Techniques and Interpretations. Philadelphia, Lea and Febiger, 1979

61. Dhingra RC, Amat-y-Leon F, Wyndham C et al: Electrophysiologic effects of atropine on sinus node and atrium in patients with sinus node dysfunction. Am J Cardiol 38:848, 1976

62. Holder W, McAnulty JH, Rahimtoola S: Characteristics of heart rate response to exercise in the sick sinus syndrome. Br Heart J 49:923, 1978

63. Gann D, Tolentino R, Samet P: Electrophysiologic evaluation of elderly patients with sinus bradycardia. Ann Intern Med 90:24, 1979

64. Kulbertus HE, deLeval-Rutter F, Dubois M et al: Prognostic significance of left anterior hemiblock with right bundle branch

block in mass screening. Am J Cardiol 41:385, 1978

65. Rothman M, Triebwasser JH: A clinical and follow-up study of right and left bundle branch block. Circulation 51:477, 1975

66. Dhingra RC, Wyndham C, Amat-y-Leon F et al: Incidence and site of atrioventricular block in patients with chronic bifascicular block. Circulation 59:238, 1979

67. Rosen KM, Dhingra RD, Wyndham CR et al: Significance of HV interval in 513 patients with chronic bifascicular block (abstr). Am J Cardiol 45:405, 1980

68. Scheinman MM, Peter RW, Modin G et al: Prognostic value of infranodal conduction time in patients with chronic bundle branch block. Circulation 56:240, 1977

69. Dhingra RC, Wyndham C, Baurnfeind R et al: Significance of block distal to the His bundle induced by atrial pacing in patients with chronic bifascicular block. Circulation 60:1455, 1979

70. Tonkin AM, Heddle WF, Tornos P: Intermittent A-V block: Procainamide administration as a provocative test. Aust NZ J Med 8:594, 1978

71. Atlee JL, Alexander SC: Halothane effect on conductivity of the AV node and His–Purkinje system in the dog. Anesth Analg 56:378, 1977

72. Berg GR, Kotler MN: The significance of bilateral bundle branch block in the preoperative patient. Chest 59:62, 1971

73. Kundstadt D, Punga M, Cagin N et al: Bifascicular block: A clinical and electrophysiologic study. Am Heart J 86: 173, 1973

74. Venkataraman K, Madias JE, Hood WB: Indications for prophylactic preoperative insertion of pacemakers in patients with right bundle branch block and left anterior hemiblock. Chest 68:501, 1975

75. Pastore J, Yurchak PM, Janis KM et al: The risk of advanced heart block in surgical patients with right bundle branch block and left axis deviation. Circulation 57:677, 1978

76. Bellocci F, Santanelli P, DiGennano M et al: The risk of cardiac complication in surgical patients with bifascicular block: A clinical and electrophysiologic study in 98 patients. Chest 77:343, 1980

77. Rooney SM, Goldiner PL, Muss E: Relationship of right bundle branch block and marked left axis deviation to complete heart block during anesthesia. Anesthesiology 44:65, 1976

78. Logue RB, Kaplan JA: Medical management in non-cardiac surgery. In Hurst JW, Logue RB, Schlat RG et al: (eds): The Heart, p 1762. New York, McGraw-Hill, 1978

79. Dhingra RC, Denes P, Wu D et al: Syncope in patients with chronic bifascicular block. Ann Intern Med 81:302, 1974

80. Scherlag BJ, Lazzara R, Helfant RH: Differentiating A-V junctional rhythms. Circulation 38:304, 1973

81. Walter PF, Crawley IS, Dorney ER: Carotid sinus hypersensitivity and syncope. Am J Cardiol 42:396, 1978

82. Ferrer MI: The sick sinus syndrome. Circulation 47:635, 1973

83. Krishnaswami V, Geraci AR: Permanent pacing in disorders of sinus node function. Am Heart J 89:579, 1975

84. Furman S: Cardiac pacing and pacemakers. I. Indications for pacing bradyarrhythmias. Am Heart J 93:523, 1977

85. Kastor JA: Atrioventricular block. N Engl J Med 292:462, 572, 1975

86. Hindman MC, Wagner GS, Jaro M et al: The clinical significance of bundle branch block complicating acute myocardial infarction. II. Indications for temporary and permanent pacemaker therapy. Circulation 58:689, 1979

87. Vandam LD, McLemore GA: Circulatory arrest in patients with complete heart block during anesthesia and surgery. Ann Intern Med 47:518, 1957

88. Thomson IR, Dalton BC, Lappos DG et al: Right bundle branch block and complete heart block caused by the Swan–Ganz catheter. Anesthesiology 31:359, 1979

89. Campo I, Garfield G, Escher DJ et al: Com-

plications of pacing by pervenous subcla-vian semi-float electrodes including two extraluminal insertions. Am J Cardiol 26:627, 1970

90. Nolewajka AJ, Goddard MP, Brown TC: Temporary transvenous pacing and femoral vein thrombosis. Circulation 62:646, 1980

91. Austin JL, Preiss LK, Crampton RS et al: An analysis of malfunction and complications of temporary pacing (abstr). Am J Cardiol 45:459, 1980

92. Lerner SM: Suppression of a demand pacemaker by transurethral electrocautery. Anesth Analg 52:703, 1973

93. Simon AB: Perioperative management of the pacemaker patient. Anesthesiology 46:127, 1977

Hypertension in the Perioperative Patient

MICHAEL J. REICHGOTT

Management of the surgical patient with hypertension is a common problem in perioperative medicine. In the preoperative period, the risks of anesthesia and surgery for the hypertensive patient must be accurately assessed. Such an assessment must take into account the etiology, severity, and existing complications of the disease, the adequacy of blood pressure control, and the perioperative problems posed by specific therapeutic agents. In the postoperative period, blood pressure control per se is the most important consideration. The selection of parenteral antihypertensive agents and transition to oral agents are major management issues. In addition, it may be necessary to manage unanticipated hypertensive episodes in previously normotensive patients by identifying their causes and instituting appropriate therapy.

The intent of this chapter is to provide for decision-making. The preoperative and postoperative periods will be considered separately, since the basic considerations in each are different. Management of hypertension in the intraoperative period is usually not the province of the internist and is not discussed. The special case of the patient with pheochromocytoma is considered in Chapter 10.

RISK OF HYPERTENSION IN THE SURGICAL PATIENT

Hypertension is extremely common; as many as 28% of preoperative patients have a history of hypertension, are already under treatment, or are found to have elevated blood pressure.[1] Extensive population studies indicate that, although the majority of patients are aware that they have hypertension and a significant proportion may be taking antihypertensive drugs, only a minority of approximately 20% is adequately controlled.[2] Therefore, the surgical patient with hypertension is most often poorly controlled, despite the ingestion of some antihypertensive medication; less often, hypertension is newly discovered preoperatively.

Two classic studies from the early part of this century identified a significant increase in mortality rate among hypertensive surgical patients.[3,4] In Sprague's series, 30% died in the intraoperative or postoperative period, usually from cardiac failure, and many of these patients had no obvious evidence of complications due to their hypertension.[4]

The perioperative risk associated with elevated blood pressure was reiterated in more recent studies that demonstrated that untreated hypertensive patients exhibit greater lability of blood pressure and peripheral vascular resistance under anesthesia than age-matched normotensive persons or hypertensive patients under treatment.[5] Since the ability to maintain effective vascular autoregulation is impaired in hypertensive persons,[6] wide swings of blood pressure due to changes in peripheral resistance could result in significant cardiac or cerebral ischemia. These changes, compounded by depression of cardiac output due to the direct myocardial depressant effect of many anesthetic agents, could increase the risk of ischemia in the uncontrolled hypertensive patient.

Goldman and Caldera have shown that very poor control of hypertension, with diastolic blood pressures greater than 110 torr, confers high risk and is therefore a specific contraindication to surgery.[7] However, Prys-Roberts and his colleagues demonstrated that wide intraoperative swings in blood pressure in the uncontrolled hypertensive, rather than a given preoperative level of pressure, were responsible for death during anesthesia.[8,9] A majority of their untreated patients developed transient electrocardiographic abnormalities when intraoperative blood pressure fell to 50% of the preoperative levels. Goldman and Caldera identified the same phenomenon of intraoperative hypotension as one of two independent determinants of risk predicting perioperative cardiac complications in patients with or without a history of hypertension.[7]

These observations suggest that patients with uncontrolled hypertension and existing cardiovascular complications form a high-risk subgroup with surgical morbidity and mortality rates significantly higher than normal. It is therefore important that adequate blood pressure control be achieved before surgery in this group of patients, and, given the lack of unanimity in the literature, it is probably best for good preoperative blood pressure control to be the aim in all patients. Not all authors agree with this precept, and some believe that mild to moderate uncomplicated essential hypertension does not constitute a significantly increased risk for patients undergoing surgery.[10] Goldman and his colleagues[1,7] suggest that elevation of diastolic blood pressure to the range of 90 to 110 torr in itself confers no specific risk on the surgical patient. The presence of pre-existing cardiovascular disease is a far more important risk factor.[11] Data from patients who underwent emergency surgery to control malignant hypertension and among whom there were few reported cases of postoperative illness or death, despite significant blood pressure deviations, tend to support this position.[12] These data must be interpreted carefully because of the lack of a control population.

Risk related to hypertension is also dependent on the cause of the elevated blood pressure. Unanticipated pheochromocytoma is associated with intra- and postoperative mortality rates as high as 50%[13] In contrast, primary hyperaldosteronism probably confers no excess risk, provided that hypokalemia is identified and treated.

Surgery need not be postponed if renovascular disease is suspected unless blood pressure cannot be controlled or hypokalemia is present. Specific evaluation to confirm the suspected diagnosis can be delayed unless corrective renovascular surgery is planned. Arteriography provides the only reliable method of diagnosis.[14] Intravenous urography is not adequately specific and should not be used as a routine screening test in the evaluation of hypertension.[15] However, it can be useful when there are particular reasons to avoid more invasive procedures. The sampling of renal vein renin concentrations at the time of arteriography adds prognostic information for determining the potential value of renovascular surgery, but random determination of peripheral venous renin levels is not useful.

The risks of anesthesia and surgery for the patient with hypertension may be estimated by careful consideration of three issues: (1) the etiology of the hypertension; (2) the existing complications of the hypertension, specifically cardiovascular disease; and (3) the status of therapy.

PREOPERATIVE EVALUATION

Hypertension may be a manifestation of some definable disease process (secondary hypertension), but its etiology most often cannot be defined (primary or essential hypertension). The most common causes of hypertension and their incidences are listed in Table 6-1.[16-18] Categorizing hypertension according to etiology is relatively simple and can be accomplished through the steps outlined in the report of the Joint National Committee on Detection, Evaluation and Treatment of High Blood Pressure.[19] The history should focus on the duration of

Table 6-1. Most Common Causes of Hypertension

Cause	Reported Incidence (%)
Essential hypertension	89–94
Chronic renal disease	2–5
Renovascular disease	1–3
Coarctation of the aorta	0.1–1
Oral contraceptives	4
Primary hyperaldosteronism	0.1–0.5
Cushing's syndrome	0.2
Pheochromocytoma	0.2

(Data from Gifford RW Jr: Milbank Mem Fund Q 47(2):170, 1969; Burglund G, Anderson O, Wilhelmsen L: Br Med J 2:554, 1976; Ferguson RK: Ann Intern Med 82:761, 1975)

hypertension and the specifics of its treatment. The description of symptoms suggestive of disease processes causing secondary hypertension or cardiovascular complications should be carefully elicited. The physical examination should include careful blood pressure measurement by appropriate technique with a cuff of the proper size.[20] It is important that orthostatic hypotension be looked for, especially in patients receiving treatment. Examination for the presence of an abdominal bruit and for signs of endocrine disease as indicators of underlying etiology is crucial. Signs of the cardiovascular and cerebrovascular complications of hypertension should be sought. Minimal laboratory evaluation, including measurement of renal function with blood urea nitrogen and creatinine levels, serum potassium concentration, and careful urinalysis, including microscopic examination of the sediment of a fresh specimen, is required. More extensive testing may be necessary on the basis of the findings elicited from the history and physical examination. Surgery should be postponed only when diastolic blood pressure exceeds 110 torr.[7] If secondary hypertension or significant cardiovascular or cerebrovascular complications of hypertension add to the surgical risk, delay of the operation should be considered.

POSTOPERATIVE TREATMENT

Classic teaching advised that therapy for hypertension be stopped before surgery.[21] This recommendation was based on the presumed risks of hypotension thought to result from the interaction of antihypertensives and anesthetic agents.[22–24] However, more recent data clearly refute this position, indicating that adequate blood pressure control should be maintained up to the time of surgery and should be resumed as soon as necessary postoperatively.[25–27]

The sudden withdrawal of antihypertensive agents may be associated with adverse cardiovascular consequences.[29] Unstable angina and myocardial infarction have occurred after sudden withdrawal of the beta-blocker propranolol from patients with arteriosclerotic cardiovascular disease.[29,30] Within 24 hr of withdrawal of this drug, the patient shows autonomic hyperreactivity, manifested by increased heart rate and contractility.[32] The overshoot in contractility appears earlier than that in heart rate. Therefore, although there is no evidence that acute withdrawal of beta-blocking drugs results in rapid or dangerous changes in blood pressure, it is unwise to withdraw these agents suddenly from the hypertensive patient.[32] Arteriosclerotic cardiovascular disease may already exist, especially in the elderly, and sympathetic hyperreactivity, with its attendant demands on oxygen delivery, could precipitate unexpected symptoms. Moreover, withdrawal of propranolol and its subsequent autonomic hyperreactivity potentiate cardiovascular system lability during induction and recovery from anesthesia. Withdrawal hyperreactivity can persist for as long as 60 hr after the last dose.

Withdrawal syndromes have been described with several other antihypertensive agents as well.[32] Abrupt cessation of clonidine may produce sympathetic nervous system overactivity.[33–36] This can be inhibited by simultaneous alpha- and beta-blockade but may be exacerbated by the presence of beta-blockade only.[34–36] The symptoms of clonidine withdrawal are seen in some but not all patients.[24,36,37] Single case reports document a similar phenomenon with alpha-methyldopa; however, this is considered to be an idiosyncratic event.[38] Its occurrence is unpredictable, and there are no specific characteristics that identify patients at risk. It is therefore best for therapy with these drugs to be continued until the time of operation and for the anesthesiologist to be informed of the possibility of withdrawal symptoms so that appropriate plans for premedication, selection of an anesthetic agent, and intraoperative support and monitoring can be made.[39]

Following the recommendations of Goldman and Caldera, the physician would initiate or revise treatment in the mildly or moderately hypertensive patient without complications and proceed to surgery without delay.[7] In more severe hypertensives, or in those with complications, surgery should be delayed long enough for treatment to be initiated and an adequate response to be obtained. The guidelines of the "step-care" approach, outlined below, provide a proven effective sequence for treatment.

Step 1. Start all patients on a diuretic antihypertensive agent, usually a thiazide or thiazide derivative

Step 2. If the response is insufficient, add one of the following: clonidine, alpha-methyldopa, prazocin, propranolol, or rauwolfia alkaloid

Step 3. If the response is still insufficient, add a vasodilator, such as hydralazine

Step 4. If the response is still inadequate, add or substitute guanethedine (minoxidil may also be used at this step).[19]

Acute elevations of blood pressure are commonly seen in the immediate postoperative period. Defining such an elevation as a sustained increase in blood pressure to 160/95 or to a mean of 110 torr for a period of at least 10 min, Rever and his co-workers suggested that the incidence of postoperative hypertension varies from 4% in general surgical patients to a range of 8% to 32% in those undergoing cardiac valve replacement to as high as 13% to 73% in patients undergoing myocardial revascularization procedures.[38]

Defining high blood pressure as 190/100, Gel and Cooperman observed the incidence of postoperative hypertension to be 3.25% in a series of 1844 patients.[40] Thirty-five, or 58% of the patients had a history of hypertension before surgery. Most of them (33 of 35) were receiving antihypertensive therapy, although adequacy of blood pressure control was not documented. Twenty-two of the 35 preoperatively demonstrated evidence of end-organ effects. Blood pressure elevations were noted as soon as 10 min after completion of surgery and were sometimes extremely high. The mean duration of the hypertensive episode was 2 hr, and complications were confined to a group of 13 patients in whom blood pressure remained elevated for 3 hr or longer.

Factors contributing to acute postoperative hypertension are pain, emergence excitement, reaction to the endotracheal tube, hypercarbia with P_{CO_2} greater than 50 torr, hypothermia, volume overload, and hypoxia.[40] Complications associated with these hypertensive episodes include cardiac arrhythmia and congestive heart failure, increased bleeding, disruption of vascular suture lines, myocardial ischemia, and cerebrovascular accident.[38,40]

In summary, a variety of noxious stimuli can cause hypertension in the postoperative period, but complications are most likely to occur only in patients with prolonged significant blood pressure elevations. It is therefore important that the physician exclude possible external stimuli before initiating antihypertensive drug therapy, especially since postoperative patients often receive narcotics, which in themselves lower blood pressure. Removing noxious stimuli and the interaction of analgesic and antihypertensive medications can result in significant hypotension.

If postoperative hypertension cannot be corrected by removal of noxious stimuli, and especially if it is persistent, drug therapy should be initiated. Most often, this will require the use of parenteral medication (Table 6-2). As in the step-care approach, therapy involves the use of a combination of drugs indicated by the clinical situation.

Therapy can be initiated with the intravenous diuretic furosemide in doses of 20 to 40 mg if the patient is not volume-depleted. Should this prove inadequate, a second agent is added. Especially for patients with high risk of cardiac ischemia, it is probably safest to follow the diuretic with propranolol in small doses of 1 to 2 mg intravenously before the addition of a vasodilator. This will avoid the risks associated with reflex tachycardia and increased contractility that are seen with hydralazine. Although it may not be necessary if nitroprusside is selected, this precaution should still be considered. If trimethophan is used, there is no need for beta-blockade.

The only three commonly used antihypertensive agents available in both oral and parenteral preparations are alpha-methyldopa, propranolol, and hydralazine. Although rauwolfia is available in both forms, it is rarely used parenterally. Selection of one or a combination of these drugs for initiation of parenteral therapy will make transition to oral therapy simple. However, these drugs bring about somewhat slower blood pressure reduction than other parenteral agents. There-

fore, the choice of which drug to use will depend on the immediacy of the situation. There are no specific guidelines to dictate when immediately acting intravenous drugs should be used or when somewhat more slowly acting agents are appropriate. There are no specific doses that are right for all patients; each person requires a specifically tailored regimen. The usual dose ranges for most parenteral and oral agents are listed in Tables 6-2 and 6-3. Therapy should be started at the lower end of the range and doses increased stepwise until an adequate response is obtained.

The transition from intravenous to oral therapy is usually not difficult. Once the

Table 6-2. Parenteral Antihypertensive Drugs

	Route	Usual Dose Range	Time Until Onset of Action	Duration of Action	Major Side Effects
Drugs Acting Directly on Vascular Smooth Muscle					
Diazoxide	IV rapid bolus	300 mg	102 min	6 + hr	Hyperglycemia, flushing, nausea, vomiting
Sodium nitroprusside	IV drip	25–300 μg/ min	Acts immediately	Minutes	Nausea, vomiting, muscle twitching, possibly thiocyanate toxicity
Hydralazine	IV or IM	10–20 mg	15 min	2–6 hr	Palpitation, tachycardia, flushing, angina, headache
Drugs Acting on Sympathetic Nervous System					
Trimethaphan	IV drip	1–15 mg/min	Acts immediately	Minutes	Urinary retention, orthostatic hypotension, dry mouth, loss of accommodation ileus
Methyldopa	IV	250–1000 mg	30–60 min	2–8 hr	Drowsiness, liver abnormalities
Propranolol	IV	1–3 mg	2–5 min	3–6 hr	Bradycardia, hypotension
Diuretics					
Furosemide	IM or IV	40–80 mg	1–2 min	2 hr	Cramps, hypokalemia
Ethacrynic acid	IV Slow	50–100 mg	1–2 min	2 hr	Local irritation, cramps, hypokalemia

Table 6-3. Oral Antihypertensive Agents

Agent	Usual Dose Range (mg/day)	Time Until Onset of Effect	Time Until Peak Effect	Duration
Step 1				
Thiazide diuretics*	25–200 (100)†	2 hr	4 hr	6–12 hr
Spironolactone	25–400 (100)	2 hr	2–4 hr	12–24 hr
Step 2				
Clonidine	0.1–2.4 (0.2–0.8)	30 min	2–4 hr	6–8 hr
Methyldopa	200–2000 (750–1500)	30 min	4–6 hr	16–24 hr
Prazosin	1–20 (1–20)	30 min–1 hr	2–4 hr	12 hr
Propranolol	40–640 (80–240)	30 min	2–4 hr	10–12 hr
Rauwolfia	0.1–1.0 (0.1–0.25)	Hours		Days to weeks
Step 3				
Hydralazine	40–300 (100–200)	30 min	2–4 hr	6–8 hr
Step 4				
Guanethedine	10–100 (25–50)	Days		Days
Minoxidil	2.5–60 (20–40)	6 hr	12 hr	2–3 days

* There are many different thiazide diuretics, and hydrochlorothiazide is taken as the standard for comparison. The reader is referred to standard pharmacology texts for detailed discussion of other agents.
† Range (usual maintenance dose).

patient is able to tolerate oral drugs, an appropriate combination can be started. In a person who was under treatment before surgery, it is most appropriate to resume the previous regimen. Care should be taken to avoid additive effects of oral and parenteral drugs. Alpha-methyldopa is used in the same doses orally and parenterally because it is completely absorbed and bioavailable after oral administration. Dose intervals are also identical, since the kinetic characteristics of the drug are not influenced by the route of administration. However, propranolol and hydralazine are given in significantly larger oral than parenteral doses for the same effect. Both of these agents are rapidly, although incompletely metabolized during the absorbtive period. They also both begin to act at different times after oral or parenteral administration and exhibit slightly different durations of action.

When patients have required high doses of parenteral antihypertensive therapy, it is usually necessary to wean them on to oral medication. This is accomplished by the oral agent being started while the dose is decreased and the interval between doses of the intravenous drug is prolonged in a stepwise fashion. There is no specific formula for this transition; drug titration must be experimented with for each individual patient.

SUMMARY

1. Optimal blood pressure control is always desirable, but surgery need not be postponed if moderate blood pressure elevation exists and diastolic pressure is no greater than 110 torr.
2. Surgery should be postponed in patients with severe hypertension until adequate blood pressure control is achieved.
3. Antihypertensive medication should be continued up to the time of surgery. Exacerbation of ischemic heart disease may be precipitated by the abrupt

withdrawal of propranolol. With-drawal syndromes have also been de-scribed after the withdrawal of cloni-dine and alpha-methyldopa.

4. In the case of sustained postoperative hypertension, noxious stimuli should be identified and removed. If blood pressure does not fall to acceptable levels, therapy should be initiated with an intravenous diuretic, and, if necessary, parenteral propranolol or alpha-methyldopa should be added.

REFERENCES

1. Goldman L, Caldera DL, Mussbaum SR et al: Multifactorial index of cardiac risk in non-cardiac surgical procedures. N Engl J Med 297: 845, 1977
2. Hypertension: United States, 1974. Advance Data Report #2. Washington DC, U.S. Department of Health, Education and Welfare, 1974
3. O'Hare JP, Hoyt L: Surgery in nephritic and hypertensive patients. N Engl J Med 200: 1292, 1929
4. Sprague HB: The heart in surgery. An analysis of the results of surgery on cardiac patients during the past ten years at the Massachusetts General Hospital. Surg Gynecol Obstet 49:54, 1929
5. Prys-Roberts C, Meloche R, Foëx P: Studies of anesthesia in relation to hypertension. I Cardiovascular responses of treated and untreated patients. Br J Anaesth 43:122, 1971
6. Strandgaard S, Olesen J, Skinhof M et al: Autoregulation of brain circulation in severe arterial hypertension. Br Med J 1:507, 1973
7. Goldman L, Caldera DL: Risks of general anesthesia and elective operations in the hypertensive patient. Anesthesiology 50: 285, 1979
8. Prys-Roberts C: Hypertension and anesthesia. Fifty years on. Anesthesiology 50:281, 1979
9. Foëx P, Prys-Roberts C: Anesthesia and the hypertensive patient. Br J Anaesth 46:575, 1975
10. Breslin DJ, Swinton NW Jr: Elective surgery in hypertensive patients—Preoperative considerations. Surg Clin North Am 50: 585, 1970
11. Feigal DW, Blaisdell FW: The estimation of surgical risk. Med Clin North Am 63:1131, 1979
12. Bennett AH, Lazarus JM: Bilateral nephrectomy performed on an emergency basis for life-threatening malignant hypertension. Surg Gynecol Obstet 137:451, 1973
13. Apgar U, Papper EM: Pheochromocytoma: Anesthetic management during surgical treatment. Arch Surg 62:634, 1951
14. Maxwell MH: Evaluation of the patient suspected of secondary hypertension: New approaches. In Hunt JC (ed): Dialogs in Hypertension 1980, Hypertension Update, p171. Bloomfield NJ, Health Learning Systems, 1980
15. Bookstein JJ, Abrams HL, Buenger RE et al: Radiologic aspects of renovascular hypertension. II. The role of urography in unilateral renovascular disease. JAMA 220:1225, 1972
16. Gifford RW Jr: Evaluation of the hypertensive patient with emphasis on detecting curable causes. Milbank Mem Fund Q 47(2):170, 1969
17. Burglund G, Andersson O, Wilhelmsen L: Prevalence of primary and secondary hypertension: Studies in a random population sample. Br Med J 2:554, 1976
18. Ferguson RK: Cost and yield of the hypertensive evaluation. Ann Intern Med 82:761, 1975
19. Report of the Joint National Committee on Detection, Evaluation and Treatment of High Blood Pressure. JAMA 237:255, 1977
20. Benson H: Methods of blood pressure recording. In Onesti G, Moyer JH (eds): Hypertension: Mechanisms and Management, p1. New York, Grune and Stratton, 1973
21. Elwood CM: The management of surgery in the hypertensive patient. In Siegel JH,

Chodoff P (eds): The Aged and High Risk Surgical Patient, p 193. New York, Grune and Stratton, 1976

22. Osmundson PJ: Preoperative and postoperative management of patients with hypertension. Med Clin North Am 46:963, 1962

23. Coakley CS, Alpert S, Boling JS: Circulatory responses during anesthesia of patients on Rauwolfia therapy. JAMA 161:1143, 1956

24. Crandell DL: The anesthetic hazards in patients on antihypertensive therapy. JAMA 179:495, 1962

25. Katz RL, Weintraub HD, Patter EM: Anesthesia, surgery and Rauwolfia. Anesthesiology 25:142, 1964

26. Caranasos GJ: Drug reactions and interactions in the patient undergoing surgery. Med Clin North Am 63:1245, 1979

27. Miller RR, Olson HG, Amsterdam EA et al: Propranolol withdrawal rebound phenomenon. Exacerbation of coronary events after abrupt cessation of antianginal therapy. N Eng J Med 293:416, 1975

28. Katz JD, Cronlare LH, Barash PG: Postoperative hypertension: A hazard of abrupt cessation of antihypertensive medication in the preoperative period. Am Heart J 92:79, 1976

29. Alderman EL, Coltart DJ, Wettach GE et al: Coronary artery syndromes after sudden propranolol withdrawal. Ann Intern Med 81:625, 1974

30. Boudoulas H, Lewis RP, Kates RE et al: Hypersensitivity to adrenergic stimulation after propranolol withdrawal in normal subjects. Ann Intern Med 87:433, 1977

31. Garkas SB, Weber MA, Priest RT et al: The abrupt discontinuation of antihypertensive treatment. J Clin Pharmacol 19:476, 1979

32. Goldberg AD, Raferty EB, Wilkinson P: Blood pressure and heart rate and withdrawal of antihypertensive drugs. Br Med J 1:1243, 1977

33. Bailey RR, Neale TJ: Rapid clonidine withdrawal with blood pressure overshoot exaggerated by beta blockade. Br Med J 1:942, 1976

34. Hansson L, Hunyor SN, Julius S et al: Blood pressure crisis following withdrawal of clonidine: with special reference to arterial and urinary catecholamine levels, and suggestions for acute management. Am Heart J 85:605, 1973

35. Hunyor SN, Hansson L, Harrison TS et al: Effects of clonidine withdrawal. Possible mechanisms and suggestions for management. Br Med J 2:209, 1973

36. Whitsett TL, Chrysant SG, Dillard BL et al: Abrupt cessation of clonidine administration: A prospective study. Am J Cardiol 41:1285, 1978

37. Burden AC, Alexander CPT: Rebound hypertension after acute methyldopa withdrawal. Br Med J 1:104, 1976

38. Rever JG, Sheppard LC, Wallach R et al: Therapeutic uses of sodium nitroprusside and an automated method of administration. Int Anesthesiol Clin 16:51, 1978

39. Hickler RB, Vandam LD: Hypertension. Anesthesiology 33:214, 1970

40. Gel TJ, Cooperman LH: Hypertension in the immediate postoperative period. Br J Anaesth 47:70, 1974

Evaluation and Management of the Surgical Patient with Coronary Artery Disease

7

RICHARD S. HOROWITZ
JOEL MORGANROTH
WILLIAM K. LEVY

Because of the cardiovascular burdens imposed by surgery and anesthesia, the perioperative state may represent a period of instability for patients with ischemic heart disease. This chapter discusses the following issues: (1) cardiac effects of anesthesia and surgery; (2) determinants of perioperative cardiac risk; (3) perioperative management of common medications used in patients with coronary artery disease; and (4) recommendations for monitoring and for postoperative care. The evaluation and management of hypertension and arrhythmias, common problems in patients with coronary artery disease, are discussed in other chapters.

CARDIAC EFFECTS OF SURGERY AND ANESTHESIA

Numerous metabolic problems that may arise during surgery and anesthesia can upset the critical balance between myocardial oxygen supply and demand in the patient with ischemic heart disease. Oxygen supply can be reduced by hypoxemia, anemia, vagally induced bradyarrhythmias, and hypotension. Increased myocardial oxygen demand may result from sympathetic stimulation, sinus tachycardia due to fever, hypovolemia or pain, other tachyarrhythmias, and hypertension. Intubation and induction of anesthesia in particular represent a period of profound cardiovascular stress and may be associated with significant ischemia in patients with underlying ischemic heart disease.[1] In a study by Roy and co-workers, ischemia, as indicated by ST depressions on a lead V_5 monitor, occurred in 11 of 29 patients with coronary artery disease during noncardiac surgery. The occurrence of ischemia generally correlated with an increased rate–pressure product, and 73% of the patients who developed ischemia did so at the time of intubation.[2]

All anesthetics depress the myocardium and have variable effects on the autonomic nervous system.[3] The balance of these two effects determines the overall response of the circulatory system to anesthesia. Halothane, for example, produces a significant decrease in contractility as well as a decrease in sympathetic tone, leading to peripheral vasodilitation.[4,5] Enflurane has similar myocardial effects and even more vasodilitation.[1] Both of these agents may therefore cause hypotension. In contrast, ketamine and cyclopropane, although associated with some myocardial depression, cause sympathetic stimulation that tends to counterbalance the myocardial effects but may also result in tachycardia or hypertension.[4,5] Nitrous oxide has little depressant effect on the myocardium and minimal autonomic effect but may cause significant hypotension when combined with morphine sulfate.[6,7] The narcotic agents morphine sulfate and fentanyl cause minimal decreases in contractility; in contrast, meperidine has a more pronounced negative inotropic effect.[8] Spinal and epidural anesthesia generally cause no myocardial depression but, because of their sympathetic blockade, may cause significant hypotension.[9]

The anesthetic combination used for patients with ischemic heart disease depends on the manifestation of the disease in each patient. The patient who is prone to hypertension and ischemia but who demonstrates good ventricular function would probably benefit from agents with mild hypotensive and vasodilatory effects. The patient with a fixed low cardiac output due to poor ventricular function would probably do better with agents having balanced myocardial and autonomic effects. In most cases, however, the agent used is not as important as the close monitoring of blood pressure, cardiac rhythm, and volume status and the appropriate reaction to unfavorable changes.

DETERMINATION OF SURGICAL RISK

An important aspect of the preoperative evaluation of patients with coronary artery disease undergoing noncardiac surgery is the estimation of the risk of cardiovascular complications or death. Even more important is the identification of risk factors that can be mitigated either through deferral of the procedure or by active medical therapy before surgery. Early studies estimated that coronary artery disease leads to a two- or threefold increase in the morbidity and mortality rate for major surgery.[11,12] However, these studies were retrospective in design, often dealt with selected populations, and failed to consider potential interrelations among various risk factors. Furthermore, recent studies suggest that this increased risk may be quite variable, depending on the particular cardiovascular manifestations involved and on factors related to the operation itself.[13,14]

Previous Myocardial Infarction

Perhaps the most important cardiac risk factor is a history of previous myocardial infarction. Table 7-1 lists four large studies in which the incidence of perioperative infarction varied from 3% to 6.6% in patients with a history of previous infarctions.[14-17] Three of these studies compared the risk of perioperative infarction for patients with a history of previous infarction with the risk for members of a general population without a history of infarction. In the studies of Tarhan and associates and Topkins and co-workers, the incidence of perioperative infarction differed markedly between 0.13% and 0.66%, respectively, in control patients and 6.6% and 6.5%, respectively, in those with previous infarctions.[15,16] The study of Goldman and colleagues, involving a

Table 7-1. Incidence of Perioperative Myocardial Infarction in Surgical Patients with Previous Infarctions

Study	No. of Patients with Previous Myocardial Infarctions	Rate of Perioperative Reinfarction (%)	Mortality Rate of Perioperative Myocardial Infarction (%)
Topkins et al[15]	658	6.5	70
Tarhan et al[16]	422	6.6	54
Steen et al[17]	587	6.1	69
Goldman et al[13]	101	3	33

smaller number of patients, demonstrated a difference of only 2% to 3%.[14] In general, the mortality rate for a perioperative infarction is quite high, ranging from 27% to 70% in these studies. In Topkin's study, the mortality rate for a perioperative reinfarction (70%) was significantly higher than that for a first infarction (27%), but, in other studies, this significant difference was not found.

Patients undergoing surgery within 6 months of a recent myocardial infarction have a particularly high risk of perioperative infarction and cardiac death. Tarhan and co-workers and Steen and colleagues found the incidence of perioperative reinfarction to be 27% and 37%, respectively, when major surgery was performed within 3 months of a recent infarction.[16,17] In the 4- to 6-month period after infarction, they found the risk of perioperative reinfarction to be 16% and 11%, respectively. After 6 months, the rate of reinfarction stabilized at 4% to 6%. Fraser and associates found a reinfarction rate of 38% for patients undergoing major surgery within 3 months of a myocardial infarction.[18] Goldman and co-workers reported a rate of reinfarction or cardiac death of 27% when surgery was performed within 6 months of an infarction, compared to a rate of 4% when it was performed after the 6-month period.[14] In this study, patients with a history of infarction more than 6 months before surgery did not have a significantly higher risk of perioperative

infarction or cardiac death than patients with no history of previous infarction.

Perioperative myocardial infarction does not usually occur during surgery but most commonly in the week after the operation. In one study, the highest incidence was on the third postoperative day.[16] Furthermore, perioperative infarctions are frequently not accompanied by chest pain and may present as unexplained congestive heart failure, hypotension, arrhythmias, or cardiac arrest.[14,16,17]

Angina

The data on angina as a surgical risk factor are less extensive. In Goldman's series, stable angina did not represent a significant risk factor for cardiovascular morbidity and mortality.[14] In a study involving patients undergoing major vascular procedures, Cooperman and co-workers found that, although patients with angina had a higher cardiovascular complication rate (16%) than patients without angina (9%), the difference was not statistically significant.[19] Sapala and colleagues found that the combination of angina and a history of an old infarction, having a perioperative mortality rate of 14%, did represent a significant risk factor.[20] Unstable angina is generally felt by most authors to represent a strong preoperative risk factor, although actual data are few.[11,21]

Patients who have undergone recent coronary artery bypass grafting are not high-risk candidates, according to three recent studies. Scher and Tice studied 20 patients requiring noncardiac surgery 3 months to 5 years after bypass surgery.[22] No deaths were recorded in 16 elective procedures, and 1 death from noncardiac causes occurred in 4 emergency procedures. In a study by McCollum and colleagues, 60 patients underwent 77 noncardiac operations after coronary artery bypass.[23] Twenty-three had their noncardiac surgery 12 to 23 days after coronary bypass during the same hospitalization as the myocardial revascularization. Almost all involved high-risk procedures such as major vascular or intra-abdominal surgery. There were no perioperative deaths in the entire group and only 8 cardiac complications, including 7 episodes of easily controlled supraventricular tachycardia and 1 episode of pulmonary edema. Mahar and associates examined 99 patients with bypass grafts during 168 noncardiac operations and compared them to 49 patients with coronary artery disease without grafts.[24] The major difference between the two groups was a significantly higher perioperative infarction rate in the group without bypass grafts (5%) than in the group with the grafts (0%). It has not been proved that bypass grafting lessens perioperative risk in patients with coronary artery disease, although these studies suggest that this may be the case.

Congestive Heart Failure

Congestive heart failure, a common complication of ischemic heart disease, is in most studies a strong risk factor for perioperative illness and death. In Goldman's study, a previous history of congestive heart failure significantly increased the likelihood of perioperative heart failure or pulmonary edema.[14] Preoperative signs or symptoms of congestive heart failure were even stronger predictors of perioperative heart failure or pulmonary edema. Of patients with preoperative congestive heart failure, 16% developed perioperative pulmonary edema, and 21% experienced a worsening of their heart failure. In particular, an S_3 gallop or jugular venous distention was associated with perioperative pulmonary edema in 30% and a cardiac mortality rate of 20%. Perioperative pulmonary edema carried a poor prognosis with an overall mortality rate of 57%. Patients with a history of congestive heart failure under control at the time of surgery had a 6% incidence of perioperative pulmonary edema and a 5% incidence of cardiac death. These figures are higher than those for the general population but significantly lower than those for patients with evidence of congestive failure at the time of surgery.

Other studies have confirmed that congestive heart failure is a strong risk factor.[19–21] Skinner and Pearce reported a close correlation between perioperative mortality and functional class as determined by the New York Heart Association criteria. Mortality rates in this study were 4% for patients in class I (rare symptoms), 11% for those in class II (symptoms with increased exertion), 25% for those in class III (symptoms with minimal exertion), and 67% for those in class IV (rest symptoms).[21]

Preoperative Electrocardiogram

The preoperative electrocardiogram may also bear on cardiac risk. In Goldman's study, a preoperative electrocardiogram showing ischemic or nonspecific ST–T wave changes was associated with an increased risk of cardiac death, although such changes were not identified by multivariate analysis as independent risk factors.[14] The presence on the electrocardiogram of a cardiac rhythm other than sinus or premature atrial contractions or evidence of more than 5 premature ventricular contractions per minute were independent risk factors for cardiac death.[13] Other studies have also found increased surgical risk to be associated with abnormalities in the preoperative electrocardiogram, including rhythm disorders, conduction defects, and ST–T wave changes.[19–21] Further information on surgical risk for patients with arrhythmias and conduction defects can be found in Chapter 5.

Noncardiac Factors

There are several factors unrelated to cardiac history or function that have been reported to increase the risk of cardiovascular complications and death in patients with ischemic heart disease. The type and timing of surgery have a definite effect on cardiac morbidity and mortality. Patients undergoing emergency procedures are 4 times as likely to develop a postoperative myocardial infarction or suffer cardiac death than those undergoing elective procedures.[14] Patients undergoing major intra-abdominal (excluding cholecystectomy), intrathoracic, or aortic procedures have a higher risk of developing postoperative pulmonary edema or myocardial infarction and experiencing cardiac death than those undergoing less extensive procedures.[12,16,20]

Skinner and Pearce's retrospective analysis of 857 operations in which preoperative cardiac consultations were performed clearly demonstrated a correlation between operative procedure and risk in cardiac patients.[21] Carotid surgery appears to carry higher than normal risk of concomitant myocardial infarction in patients with coronary artery disease. In one series of 683 consecutive carotid endarterectomies, the incidence of documented myocardial infarction was 10 times greater in patients with a history of heart disease than in those with no such history.[25] This fact, coupled with the increased incidence of stroke in patients with extracranial carotid disease undergoing coronary artery bypass surgery, has led some physicians to pursue a surgical approach in which both carotid endarterectomy and coronary artery bypass graft surgery are performed concomitantly.

Transurethral urologic procedures in elderly patients prone to coronary artery disease appear to be relatively safe, having a low incidence of significant cardiovascular complications, even in patients with a recent myocardial infarction.[26,27] Thompson and co-workers demonstrated a mortality rate of 4.3% after transurethral prostatectomy in patients within 6 months of a myocardial infarction as compared to a rate of 4.7% in patients who had had an infarction more than 6 months earlier.[26] However, this margin of safety does not apply to all urologic procedures or even to prostatectomy performed by any but the transurethral approach.

Elective nonvascular ophthalmologic, otorhinolaryngologic, neurosurgical, and orthopedic procedures do not seem to be associated with undue cardiovascular risk. Retraction of the eye during an ophthalmologic procedure may increase vagal tone and result in an increased incidence of bradyarrhythmias and heart block. However, these occurrences do not alter cardiovascular mortality.[28]

The choice of anesthetic or technique has little effect on cardiovascular risk, despite differences in hemodynamic ef-

Table 7-2. Cardiac Risk Factors for Noncardiac Surgery

Factors	Relative Point Value
History	
1. Age greater than 70 years	5
2. Recent myocardial infarction (within 6 months)	10
Cardiac Exam	
3. Signs of congestive heart failure—S_3 gallop or jugular vein distention	11
4. Significant aortic stenosis	3
Electrocardiogram	
5. Preoperatively, rhythm other than sinus or premature atrial contractions	7
6. Documentation of 5 or more premature ventricular contractions per minute any time before surgery	7
General Medical Condition (any of the below)	3
7a. $PO_2 < 60$ or $P_{CO_2} > 50$	
b. Potassium <3, bicarbonate <20, BUN <50, creatinine <3.	
c. Abnormal SGOT or signs of chronic liver disease	
d. Bedridden state due to noncardiac causes	
Operation	
8. Emergency	4
9. Intraperitoneal, intrathoracic, or aortic	3

(Goldman L, Caldera DL, Nussbaum SR et al: N Engl J Med 297: 845, 1977)

fects.[10] Spinal or regional anesthesia is not significantly safer than general anesthesia.[12,14,16,17,21] Local anesthesia has a low incidence of cardiovascular complication but is generally used only for minor procedures.[9] The duration of anesthesia and surgery correlates with the incidence of cardiovascular complications in some studies but not in others.[14,16,17,21,29] Intraoperative hypotension has been associated with a higher risk than normal of perioperative infarctions, but hypotension may be the result rather than the cause of the infarction.[17,29]

Perhaps the best overall formula for assessing the risk of cardiovascular complications and death is that derived by Goldman and co-workers.[13] Through the use of multivariate discriminant analysis, they identified nine independent determinants of cardiac risk (Table 7-2). They assigned point values to each of these factors according to the strength of their correlation with cardiac complications and then added the point values to obtain an overall numeric index of cardiac risk. Goldman defined four subgroups according to the point totals. The incidence of cardiovascular complications and death for each group in their study is shown in Table 7-3. In class IV, the incidence of perioperative cardiac death was 56%, and that of nonfatal major complications was 22%. Furthermore, although only 18 patients, or 1.8% of the total, fell into class IV, over 50% of the cardiac deaths occurred in this group.

PERIOPERATIVE MEDICATION

Preoperative modification of cardiovascular risk in the surgical patient with cor-

Table 7-3. Cardiac Risk Index

Class	Point Total	No or Minor Complications	Life-Threatening Complications	Cardiac Deaths
I	0–5	532 (99%)	4 (0.7%)	1 (0.2%)
II	6–12	295 (93%)	16 (5%)	5 (2%)
III	13–25	112 (86%)	15 (11%)	3 (2%)
IV	≥26	4 (22%)	4 (22%)	10 (56%)

(Goldman L, Caldera DL, Nussbaum SR et al: N Engl J Med 297:845, 1977)

onary artery disease requires a critical understanding of a number of cardiovascular drugs, including digitalis preparations, beta-blocking agents, nitrates, anticoagulants, antiarrhythmics, and antihypertensive agents. Some of these drugs are discussed thoroughly in other chapters. Digitalis preparations, beta-blocking agents, and nitrates will be emphasized in this chapter.

Digitalis

Controversy surrounds the routine use of prophylactic preoperative digitalis in elderly patients with coronary artery disease. Some authors recommend the use of prophylactic digitalis in the asymptomatic patient with documented coronary artery disease or in the asymptomatic patient with cardiomegaly. This recommendation is based on the evidence that most anesthetic agents depress myocardial contractility and cardiac output.[30,31] In fact, congestive heart failure develops postoperatively for the first time in only about 5% of patients undergoing general anesthesia, whereas refractory or serious postoperative arrhythmias in digitalized patients is of frequent concern.[14] The potentiation of digitalis toxicity by certain anesthetic agents and numerous potential postoperative metabolic and electrolyte problems, including hypoxia and azotemia, constitute strong arguments against

prophylactic digitalization.[32] In patients without an increased left ventricular end-diastolic volume, digitalis increases myocardial oxygen requirements and can precipitate ischemia. Preoperative use of digitalis should therefore be reserved for specific indications such as significant left ventricular chamber enlargement with associated symptomatic congestive heart failure or a history of atrial tachyarrhythmias.

Nitrates

Nitrates and beta-blocking agents remain the pharmacologic mainstays of antianginal therapy. Standard sublingual nitroglycerin preparations of both short and long duration have been complemented by hemodynamically effective oral, topical, and intravenous preparations. Their mechanism of action remains unclear but includes venous dilatation, which decreases preload and myocardial oxygen needs. The potent preload reduction and hypotensive effect of nitrates must be carefully remembered when these drugs are used in patients on concomitant diuretic therapy, and it should be kept in mind that patients with postoperative volume depletion may be particularly sensitive. However, when careful attention is paid to volume status, nitrates can be used safely and effectively. The flexibility of topical and intravenous preparations renders them especially useful in the perioperative period. In a study by Fusciardi and co-workers, intravenous nitroglycerin was shown to reduce ischemia during noncardiac surgery in patients with severe angina.[33]

Beta-Blocking Agents

Nonselective beta-blocking agents such as propranolol and more selective longer-acting beta-blockers are important in the medical management of patients with severe coronary artery disease. Controversy has surrounded the preoperative use of these agents. The cardiac depressant and sympatholytic effects of these agents combined with the myocardial depressant effect of many anesthetics have made clinicians wary of using beta-blocking agents in the operative period.[34]

However, abrupt discontinuation of beta-blocking agents in the patient with coronary artery disease has occasionally been followed by distressing clinical events, including severe angina, myocardial infarction, and death.[35–37] One recent double-blind crossover study of the efficacy of propranolol in stable angina demonstrated untoward ischemic events in 10 of 20 patients within 2 weeks of the discontinuation of a dose of 160 to 320 mg/day.[35] A number of postulated but unsubstantiated mechanisms attempt to explain this withdrawal phenomenon.[38,39] They include changes in the affinity of hemoglobin for oxygen, increased platelet aggregation, denervation hypersensitivity, an increased number of beta-receptor binding sites, and increased receptor affinity for catecholamines.

It is rare for a patient to develop postoperative congestive heart failure owing solely to the preoperative use of beta-blockers. In fact, physiologic responses to perioperative stress such as intubation, fever, or pain are exaggerated by blocking, and this may be lifesaving to the patient with coronary heart disease.[40] Beta-blocking agents should therefore be continued before, during, and immediately after the operative procedure in patients who receive such agents for anginal control. The safety of this approach has been verified by a number of studies.[41,42]

MANAGEMENT

The following recommendations for the perioperative assessment and management of the patient with ischemic heart disease can be made on the basis of the preceding discussion of the literature. Preoperative evaluation should seek to identify factors that affect cardiac risk, especially those that can be modified before surgery, so as to improve the chances of a favorable surgical outcome. It is important to determine whether there is a history of myocardial infarction and especially whether the patient has had an infarction within 6 months of surgery. Because of the high incidence of reinfarction in patients with recent past infarctions, noncardiac surgery should be postponed if possible, at least until the 6-month period has passed.

In patients with angina, the severity of the symptoms must be assessed carefully. In particular, patients with an unstable pattern, offering a history of recent onset or increase in anginal symptoms or of angina occurring under conditions of rest or minimal exertion, should be identified. If possible, surgery should be deferred in order for optimal control to be achieved with therapy. In those in whom therapy with nitrates and beta-blocking agents is unsuccessful, cardiac catheterization and bypass surgery may be appropriate before the scheduled surgery. As discussed, some studies have reported good results for operations performed after successful coronary artery bypass procedures. For emergency procedures in patients with unstable angina or recent myocardial infarction, some authors have suggested use of the intra-aortic balloon pump to increase coronary perfusion.[32,43] Intravenous nitroglycerin may be another alternative for reducing ischemia during surgery for patients with unstable angina.[33]

Patients with stable angina do not clearly have a significantly higher than normal surgical risk. Patients receiving beta-blockers and nitrates should have these medications continued up to the morning of surgery and reinstituted immediately after surgery if hemodynamic status permits. Patients unable to take oral medications postoperatively can be treated with intravenous propranolol, the dose being titrated to the desired heart rate. Nitroglycerin ointment can be substituted for oral nitrates.

Congestive heart failure is an important complication of ischemic heart disease and constitutes a strong risk factor for perioperative cardiac complications and death. History, physical examination, and preoperative chest x-ray are adequate in most cases for the presence of congestive heart failure to be documented; however, other noninvasive techniques, such as echocardiography or radionuclide imaging for left ventricular function, may help in the evaluation of cardiac function in more difficult cases. Patients with congestive failure must be optimally treated before surgery. Digoxin, diuretics, preload-reducing drugs and afterload-reducing agents may be required. In many cases, surgery will have to be deferred or postponed in order for stable hemodynamics to be achieved. Rapid overnight correction of congestive failure in order for scheduled elective surgery to be carried out should be discouraged, because electrolyte abnormalities and intravascular depletion may result and lead to major perioperative problems.

Preoperative laboratory evaluation of patients with ischemic heart disease should be individualized. In general, all patients should have a preoperative electrocardiogram to serve as a baseline tracing in the evaluation of new ischemia or infarction after surgery. The baseline electrocardiogram may also reveal an unrecognized recent or old myocardial infarction as well as unsuspected rhythm disorders. There is evidence that an abnormal preoperative electrocardiogram may also carry prognostic implications. A chest x-ray should be obtained, as previously stated, to help the physician evaluate cardiac size and identify congestive heart failure. Routine blood studies, including a complete blood count and serum concentrations of blood urea nitrogen, creatinine, glucose, and electrolytes, are generally obtained in most institutions. In the patient with ischemic heart disease, these factors may be affected by myocardial dysfunction or cardiac medications. Significant abnormalities in these tests may predict perioperative cardiac complications.

Intraoperative monitoring of the patient with ischemic disease should include electrocardiographic monitoring of cardiac rhythm. Because hypotension during surgery is associated with an increased risk of perioperative ischemia, infarction, and death, the use of an intra-arterial line to monitor changes in blood pressure is indicated during any significant surgical procedure. In high-risk patients—those with a recent infarction or those with a history of significant congestive failure or severe angina—a Swan–Ganz catheter allows for optimal control of fluid status and filling pressures and thereby reduces hemodynamic stress.

The choice of anesthetic agent should be made by the anesthesiologist. Although the agents used have variable effects on myocardial performance, there is no evidence that one agent is preferable to another. Spinal anesthesia is in general no safer than well-controlled general anesthesia. However, some authors recommend spinal anesthesia for patients with significant congestive heart failure because, theoretically, spinal anesthesia has less of a myocardial depressant effect and promotes afterload reduction.

Postoperative monitoring is important in the patient with coronary artery disease; most perioperative infarctions occur in the first week after surgery and are often not accompanied by chest pain. Therefore, all patients considered to have a high risk of cardiac complications should be monitored postoperatively in an intensive care unit. It seems advisable for daily electrocardiograms to be obtained for at least three days for all high-risk patients.

The diagnosis of myocardial infarction after surgery may be difficult to establish. Evolution of Q waves on the electrocardiogram occurs only after transmural infarctions. The usual cardiac enzymes—lactic dehydrogenase (LDH), creatine phosphokinase (CPK), and serum glutamic oxaloacetic transaminase (SGOT)—may already be elevated by the trauma of surgery. The CPK–MB fraction is useful and is specific for myocardial damage; however, it may become negative 24 hr after infarction. If an electrocardiogram and CPK isoenzymes do not resolve the issue, radionuclide imaging with thallium or technetium pyrophosphate may be useful.

SUMMARY

1. **Patients with ischemic heart disease undergoing surgery and anesthesia with a high risk of complications include those with recent infarction (less than 6 months before surgery), congestive heart failure, and unstable angina. Surgery should be postponed if possible until adequate evaluation and treatment can be obtained.**
2. **Emergency procedures and major intra-abdominal, intrathoracic, and vascular procedures are the operations that carry the highest risk of cardiac complications.**
3. **Digoxin should not routinely be given to patients with ischemic heart disease in the perioperative period. It should be reserved for patients with cardiac enlargement or congestive heart failure or for patients with a history of atrial tachyarrhythmias.**
4. **Use of propranolol and nitrates should be continued through surgery, since these agents may protect against perioperative ischemia.**
5. **Intraoperative monitoring of patients with coronary artery disease should include close attention to cardiac rhythm and blood pressure. High-risk patients, especially those with significant cardiac dysfunction, should have pulmonary artery and capillary wedge pressure monitoring.**
6. **Perioperative myocardial infarctions occur most commonly in the first week after surgery. Since they are infrequently accompanied by chest pain, patients with significant coronary ar-**

tery disease should be followed carefully in the postoperative period with attention to the electrocardiogram, cardiac rhythm, and physical examination.

REFERENCES

1. Logue RB, Kaplan JA: Medical management in noncardiac surgery. In Hurst (ed): The Heart, p 1762. New York, McGraw Hill, 1978
2. Roy WL, Edelist G, Gilbert B: Myocardial ischemia during noncardiac surgical procedures in patients with coronary artery disease. Anesthesiology 51:393, 1979
3. Kaplan JA, Dunbar RW: Anesthesia for noncardiac surgery in patients with cardiac disease. In Kaplan JA (ed): Cardiac Anesthesia, p 377. New York, Grune and Stratton, 1979
4. Moffit EA: Anesthesia for patients early after infarction. Anesth Analg Curr Res 55:640, 1976
5. Stevens WC: Anesthetic management. Anesth Analg Curr Res 55:622,1976
6. Eisele JH, Smith NT: Cardiovascular effects of 40% nitrous oxide in man. Anesth Analg Curr Res 51:956, 1972
7. McDermott RW, Stanley TH: The cardiovascular effect of low concentrations of nitrous oxide during morphine anesthesia. Anesthesiology 41:89, 1974
8. Straner BE: Contractile responses to morphine, pitritramide, meperidine and fentanyl. Anesthesiology 37:304, 1972
9. Wolf MA, Braunwald E: General anesthesia and noncardiac surgery in patients with heart disease. In Braunwald E (ed): Heart Disease, p 1911. Philadelphia, WB Saunders, 1980
10. Rose SD, Corman LC, Mason DT: Cardiac risk factors in patients undergoing noncardiac surgery. Med Clin North Am 63:1271, 1979
11. Mattingly TW: Patients with coronary artery disease as a surgical risk. Am J Cardiol 12:279, 1963
12. Arkins R, Smessaert AA, Hicks RG: Mortality and morbidity in surgical patients with coronary artery disease. JAMA 190:485, 1964
13. Goldman L, Caldera DL, Nussbaum SR et al: Multifactorial index of cardiac risk in noncardiac surgical procedures. N Engl J Med 297:845, 1977
14. Goldman L, Caldera DL, Southwick FS et al: Cardiac risk factors and complications in noncardiac surgery. Medicine 57:357, 1978
15. Topkins MJ, Artusio JF: Myocardial infarction and surgery—A five-year study. Anesth Analg Curr Res 43:716, 1964
16. Tarhan S, Moffitt EA, Taylor WF et al: Myocardial infarction after general anesthesia. JAMA 220:1451, 1972
17. Steen PA, Tinker JH, Tarhan S: Myocardial re-infarction after anesthesia and surgery. JAMA 239:2566, 1978
18. Fraser JG, Ramachandran PR, Davis HS: Anesthesia and recent myocardial infarction. JAMA 199:96, 1967
19. Cooperman M, Pflug B, Martin EW et al: Cardiovascular risk factors in patients with peripheral vascular disease. Surgery 84:505, 1978
20. Sapala JA, Panka JL, Duvernoy WF: Operative and nonoperative risks in the cardiac patient. J Am Geriatr Soc 23:529, 1975
21. Skinner JF, Pearce ML: Surgical risk in the cardiac patient. J Chronic Dis 17:57, 1964
22. Scher KS, Tice DA: Operative risks in patients with previous coronary artery bypass. Arch Surg 111:807, 1976
23. McCollum CH, Garcia-Rinaldi R, Graham JM et al: Myocardial revascularization prior to subsequent major surgery in patients with coronary artery disease. Surgery 81:302, 1977
24. Mahar LJ, Steen PA, Tinker JH et al: Perioperative myocardial infarction in patients with coronary artery disease with and without aorto-coronary bypass grafts. J Thorac Cardiovasc Surg 76:533, 1978
25. Riles TS, Kopelman J, Imparato AM: Myocardial infarction following carotid endar-

terectomy: A review of 683 operations. Surgery 85:249, 1979

26. Thompson GJ, Panayotic PK, Connolly DC: Transurethral prostatic resection after myocardial infarction. JAMA 182:908, 1962

27. Erlik D, Valero A, Birkhan J et al: Prostatic surgery and the cardiovascular patient. Br J Urol 40:53, 1968

28. Reinikainen N, Pontinen P: Atrioventricular dissociation during surgery. Acta Med Scand (Suppl) 182:147, 1967

29. Mauncy FM, Ebert PA, Sabiston DC: Postoperative myocardial infarction: A study of predisposing factors, diagnosis and mortality in a high risk group of surgical patients. Ann Surg 172:497, 1970

30. Goldberg AH, Maling HM, Gaffney TE: The effect of digoxin pretreatment on heart contractile force during thiopental infusion in dogs. Anesthesiology 22:974, 1961

31. Goldberg AH, Maling HM, Gaffney TE: The value of prophylactic digitalization in halothane anesthesia. Anesthesiology 23:207, 1962

32. Hillis LD, Cohn PF: Noncardiac surgery in patients with coronary artery disease. Arch Intern Med 138:972, 1978

33. Fusciardi J, Daloz M, Cariat P et al: Prevention of myocardial ischemia by nitroglycerin in patients with severe coronary artery disease undergoing noncardiac surgery. Anesthesiology 53:S80, 1980

34. Viljoen JF, Estafanous G, Kellner GA: Propranolol and cardiac surgery. J Thorac Cardiovasc Surg 64:826, 1972

35. Miller RR, Olson HG, Amsterdam EA et al: Propranolol-withdrawal rebound phenomenon: Exacerbation of coronary events after abrupt cessation of anti-anginal therapy. N Engl J Med 293:416, 1975

36. Alderman ES, Coltart J, Wettach GE et al: Coronary artery syndrome after sudden propranolol discontinuation. Ann Intern Med 81:625, 1974

37. Harrison DC, Alderman EL: Discontinuation of propranolol therapy. Chest 69:1, 1976

38. Frishman W, Weksler B, Christondonlon J et al: Reversal of abnormal platelet aggregability and exchange in exercise tolerance in patients with angina pectoris following oral propranolol. Circulation 50:887, 1974

39. Oski FA, Miller LD, Delivoria-Papadopoulos M et al: Oxygen affinity in red cells: Changes induced by propranolol. Science 175:1372, 1972

40. Wynards JE: The high-risk cardiac patient undergoing general surgery. Can J Surg 21:475, 1978

41. Caralps JM, Mulek J, Wienke HR et al: Results of coronary artery surgery in patients receiving propranolol. J Thorac Cardiovasc Surg 67:526, 1974

42. Slogoff S, Keats AS, Ott E: Preoperative propranolol therapy and aorto-coronary bypass operation. JAMA 240:1487, 1978

43. Foster ED, Olsson CA, Rutenburg AM et al: Mechanical circulatory assistance with intra-aortic balloon counterpulsation for major abdominal surgery. Ann Surg 183:73, 1976

Surgery in the Patient with Valvular Heart Disease

JOHN W. HIRSHFELD, Jr.

Noncardiac surgery can be safely performed in virtually any patient with chronic valvular disease. However, the pathophysiology of the particular valvular lesion must be understood, sophisticated monitoring may often be necessary, and the hemodynamic and metabolic status of the patient must be carefully controlled.

The latitude for therapeutic error provided by a normal cardiovascular system is reduced in the patient with valvular heart disease. Consequently, unlike normal patients, those with valvular heart disease cannot compensate for errors in fluid and drug therapy and anesthetic management.

RISK OF SURGERY IN VALVULAR HEART DISEASE

The risk of noncardiac surgery in patients with significant valvular heart disease has not been carefully studied. Skinner and Pearce found a mortality rate after noncardiac surgery of 6% for patients with mitral stenosis and regurgitation.[1] Patients with aortic valve disease in this study had a mortality rate of 10% that increased to 20% when only intrathoracic or intra-abdominal procedures were considered.

In Goldman's study of cardiac risk factors in noncardiac surgery, patients with a mitral regurgitant murmur of grade II or greater had a mortality rate of 7%, significantly higher than those without the murmur. True aortic stenosis, with a mortality rate of 13%, was even more strongly associated with postoperative cardiac death and was also identified as an independent risk factor.[2] All of the major valvular abnormalities—aortic stenosis, aortic regurgitation, mitral stenosis, and mitral regurgitation—were associated with a 20% risk of new or worsening congestive heart failure in the postoperative period. Therefore, although large studies are lacking, there is evidence that valvular heart disease is a significant risk factor in noncardiac surgery.

These two studies represent pooled data from many patients. Valvular heart disease, however, is a heterogeneous group of disorders. Additionally, each disorder within the group varies from patient to patient with respect both to the hydraulic severity of the valvular defect and to the associated physiologic derangement it produces. Present-day diagnostic techniques enable the clinician to quantify the severity of a particular patient's cardiac disorder. Thus, the hazard to which a *particular* patient is exposed by a surgical procedure may be estimated with more precision than that given by the general figures cited above. Furthermore, most of the physiologic derangements produced by valvular disease are controllable, and appropriate perioperative management can lessen risk.

GENERAL PRINCIPLES

The safe conduct of noncardiac surgery in a patient with valvular heart disease requires control of intravascular volume or preload, cardiac rhythm, and systemic valvular resistance or afterload. Although it is generally true that patients with valvular heart disease provide less margin for error than normal patients, the amount of flexibility possible varies with both the type of lesion and its severity. For example, the problems involved in the management of a patient with critical aortic stenosis are entirely different from those involved in the management of a patient with moderately severe mitral regurgitation.

The hydraulic severity of a valvular defect is quantifiable, and severity correlates well with the degree of circulatory embarrassment that the defect may produce. Equally important is the response of the heart and circulation to the presence of the valvular lesion. Each defect imposes a different kind of hemodynamic burden on different chambers of the heart, and this determines the natural history of the valvular disease. It is therefore important to assess the functional integrity of the chambers of the heart, which are particularly affected by the defect.

In many types of valvular heart disease, cardiac rhythm profoundly influences hemodynamic status. Consequently, particular attention must be paid to correcting deviations from normal cardiac rhythm.

Stenotic Lesions

Stenotic valvular lesions as a group are more difficult to manage than regurgitant lesions. The patient with a stenotic valve is more fragile hemodynamically and more sensitive to changes in intervascular volume, systemic vascular resistance, and cardiac rhythm. This sensitivity to changes in hemodynamics is due to the quadratic relationship between the flow across a stenotic valve and the pressure gradient necessary to maintain that flow. For the flow rate across a stenotic cardiac valve to be doubled, the pressure gradient must be quadrupled. For example, a patient with aortic stenosis with a gradient of 80 torr at rest needs to generate a transvalvular gradient of 320 torr in order to double cardiac output. To do this while maintaining an acceptable arterial pressure requires a left ventricular pressure in excess of 400 torr. Since the left ventricle cannot develop this much pressure, the ability of the patient to increase cardiac output above the resting level is significantly impaired. Such patients do not tolerate vasodilatation because they are unable to increase cardiac output to compensate for a decrease in systemic vascular resistance.

The pressure gradient across a stenotic valve is also influenced by the time available for flow to take place. Changes in heart rate alter this time period and therefore influence the pressure gradient independently of any change in cardiac output. For example, since the time available for diastole decreases as heart rate increases, rapid heart rates are deleterious to patients with mitral stenosis. Patients with aortic stenosis tolerate tachycardias better because the time available for systolic ejection is not shortened and the pressure gradient is not increased.

Patients with stenotic valvular lesions are also exquisitely sensitive to changes in cardiac rhythm. For reasons outlined above, rapid atrial fibrillation can be deleterious to the patient with mitral stenosis because of a decrease in the time available for diastolic filling. It can also affect the patient with tight aortic stenosis because of the loss of the atrial contribution to ventricular filling. The hypertrophied left ventricle of aortic stenosis depends on atrial systole to provide the necessary diastolic myocardial fiber length to generate the elevated systolic pressure necessary for the left ventricle to eject against the stenotic aortic valve.

The impact of a stenotic lesion on the performance of the heart and circulation is closely correlated with the hydraulic severity of the stenosis. The more severe the stenosis, the more fragile the patient and the more likely he is to deteriorate when subjected to an adverse hemodynamic stress. It is therefore clear that patients with stenotic lesions are sensitive to changes in preload and tolerate intravascular volume depletion poorly. Careful attention must be paid to their intravascular volume status during all phases of perioperative management.

Regurgitant Lesions

Patients with regurgitant defects as a group are less difficult to manage than those with stenotic lesions. This discussion is confined to patients with chronic regurgitant valvular defects and specifically excludes patients with acute valvular regurgitation. The latter behave differently from the former; their cardiac disease overshadows all other medical or surgical problems and often requires immediate surgical correction of the valvular defect.

In patients with chronic regurgitant valvular defects, the determinants of systemic cardiac output are more complex than in those with stenotic lesions. Fortunately, systemic cardiac output is not rigidly fixed within a narrow range, and patients with chronic regurgitant lesions are in general better able to adapt to the stresses of anesthesia, surgery, and changes in intervascular volume than patients with stenotic lesions. Additionally, the physician can more readily influence both systemic cardiac output and left ventricular filling pressures by controlling preload, heart rate, and systemic vascular resistance.

In valvular stenosis, severity is determined principally by degree of stenosis. However, in valvular regurgitation, two factors determine severity: the quantitative severity of the regurgitation, and the state of left ventricular contractile function. The adaptive mechanisms of the left ventricle enable it to deal successfully with the increased volume load produced by valvular regurgitation and to maintain systemic cardiac output at acceptable filling pressures.

Symptoms generally appear as left ventricular contractile function deteriorates and not because of any change in the severity of the valvular defect. Patients with well-preserved left ventricular function can successfully deal with any hemodynamic perturbation, but their ability to do so decreases as left ventricular function deteriorates. However, it is important to realize that the correlation between symptomatic status and left ventricular contractile function is poor. The presence of only minimal symptoms does not guarantee that left ventricular contractile function is normal. Since left ventricular function is a major determinant of operative risk, it must be carefully assessed preoperatively as a guide to perioperative management.

AVAILABLE DIAGNOSTIC AND THERAPEUTIC TECHNIQUES

There are several diagnostic monitoring procedures available to aid in the management of patients with valvular heart disease in the perioperative period.

Right-Heart Pressure Monitoring

The Swan–Ganz balloon-tipped right-heart catheter, invaluable in the management of patients with valvular heart disease, can be employed with negligible risk and discomfort. Although right-heart pressure monitoring is not essential in all patients with valvular heart disease, it is vital in certain subsets.

Systemic Arterial Pressure Monitoring

Monitoring of systemic arterial pressure with an indwelling arterial cannula is virtually free of complications when performed by experienced people and maintained for less than 24 hr. In fragile cardiac patients, it provides continuous measurement of actual arterial pressure and is free from the ambiguities of the cuff method. Such ambiguities occur most often in low cardiac-output states, when accurate monitoring is most important.

Prophylactic Digitalization

In selected patients, prophylactic use of digitalis derivatives is useful in controlling cardiac rhythm, especially in preventing and controlling tachyarrhythmias. Its effect on inotropy is of no demonstrated value.

Determination of State of Hydration

Intravascular volume and state of hydration have a major influence on the patient's ability to tolerate surgery. There is a general tendency to err toward hypovolemia. Although this is desirable in some circumstances, in most patients with valvular heart disease, it is detrimental. Preoperative diagnostic and preparative procedures, poor diet, and medications can exacerbate this problem.

AORTIC STENOSIS

Aortic stenosis is the most common valvular lesion encountered in the noncardiac surgical patient. Patients with aortic stenosis are as a group the most fragile subset of patients with valvular heart disease. Failure to take appropriate precautions because of failure to recognize aortic stenosis may lead to an otherwise avoidable adverse outcome. Aortic stenosis is principally a disease of the elderly, and its differentiation from the omnipresent mid-systolic flow murmur is difficult in this age group. Most clinical findings consistent with aortic stenosis are related to alterations in the peripheral arterial pressure wave form caused by obstruction at the aortic valve. However, elderly patients have stiff, noncompliant great vessels, and the arterial wave form tends to feel normal, making recognition of the valvular lesion more difficult.

The presence of any of the following clinical signs strongly suggests the presence of significant aortic stenosis.[3,4] The absence of any of these clinical signs, however, does not exclude its presence.

1. The normal arterial wave form is distorted and has a low amplitude, slow upstroke, and sometimes a palpable shudder. When recognizable, the shudder can generally be felt only in the carotid vessels.
2. There is evidence of left ventricular pressure overload with palpable left ventricular hypertrophy of the pressure-overload type and a palpable fourth heart sound. This may or may not be accompanied by left ventricular hypertrophy on the electrocardiogram.
3. The systolic murmur of aortic stenosis, in contrast to the innocent systolic murmur found in elderly persons, is long in duration, frequently extending almost to the pulmonic component of the second sound. The aortic component of the second sound is usually absent.
4. The aortic valve is usually calcified, and calcification is occasionally visible on plain chest x-ray. Image-intensification fluoroscopy, an easy and safe technique, provides a highly sensitive means of detection.
5. Echocardiography demonstrates a hypertrophied left ventricle and a thickened distorted aortic valve. If other possible causes of left ventricular hypertrophy are excluded, this finding signifies the presence of significant aortic stenosis.

Preoperative Preparation

Patients with aortic stenosis face two basic problems. They have a limited, if not negligible, ability to increase cardiac output in response to stress. However, the hypertrophied left ventricle has diminished diastolic compliance. Consequently, these patients do not tolerate decreases in systemic vascular resistance and are highly dependent on diastolic preload as determined by intravascular volume.

When patients with aortic stenosis are assessed before surgery, particular attention must be paid to their state of hydration as an indicator of intravascular volume. In this circumstance, it is probably better to err on the side of minimal fluid overload than hypovolemia. Surgical patients are prone to hypovolemia due either to bleeding or to venous pooling, and those with aortic stenosis should go to the operating room with adequate left ventricular end-diastolic pressure. Although excessive intravascular volume and pulmonary vascular congestion can be dealt with easily in the preoperative period, the consequence of inadequate left ventricular filling pressure can be rapid, irremediable circulatory collapse.

Operative Management

Right-heart and systemic arterial pressure monitoring are important adjuncts to the operative management of patients with tight aortic stenosis. Since it is essential that optimal left ventricular filling pressures be maintained, right-heart pressure measurement enables the anesthesiologist to regulate the rate of fluid and blood administration optimally. If arterial pressure falls, this measurement reveals the cause and serves as a guideline for whatever corrective action is needed.

Systemic arterial pressure monitoring allows immediate recognition of changes in arterial pressure. In aortic stenosis, modest changes in systemic vascular resistance can produce substantial changes in arterial pressure and coronary artery blood flow. Since increased total myocardial metabolic demand requires greater coronary blood flow, the patient with aortic stenosis is highly dependent on diastolic arterial pressure to maintain coronary artery perfusion. If such a patient becomes hypotensive, coronary artery perfusion decreases, the left ventricle becomes ischemic and its systolic performance is impaired, arterial pressure falls further, and a vicious cycle is initiated. Consequently, it is crucial that arterial pressure be maintained within the normal range.

Because left ventricular stroke volume is dependent on diastolic fiber length, the patient with aortic stenosis is also sensitive to changes in cardiac rhythm. The loss of the atrial contribution to ventricular filling in atrial fibrillation does not significantly embarrass the normal circulatory system. However, if atrial fibrillation develops in a patient with aortic stenosis, abrupt circulatory deterioration may follow, and emergency cardioversion may be necessary. Even if circulation appears reasonably stable, it should be considered tenuous at best, and prompt aggressive efforts to control ventricular rate and restore sinus rhythm are indicated.

Intraoperative mangement should accordingly include attention to cardiac rhythm, left-heart filling pressures, and systemic vascular resistance. Spinal anesthetics should be avoided because of accompanying unpredictable vasodilatation.

Postoperative Management

Postoperative management of the patient with aortic stenosis can be difficult because of variable "third-space" fluid loss. In this setting, right-heart pressure measurements are especially useful in the planning of fluid therapy and blood replacement. Since hypovolemia may lead to circulatory collapse, if renal function is normal, it is safer to err toward over-replacement. Excess intravascular vol-

ume, if recognized promptly, can be easily handled with diuretics.

Atrial fibrillation should be promptly and aggressively managed, as during surgery. Moderate sinus tachycardia up to 120 is fairly well tolerated, since there is no resultant decrease in the time available for systolic ejection and cardiac output. The atrial contribution to left ventricular filling is preserved, allowing the ventricle to continue to eject from an acceptable diastolic myocardial fiber length. No effort need be made to slow the rate primarily, but a search for the cause should be undertaken and correctable causes addressed.

The increased basal metabolic rate that accompanies a significant fever increases the demand for cardiac output. Accordingly, aspirin or acetaminophen should be used to minimize temperature elevation. The value of cooling blankets for temperature reduction is debatable, and these should not be used for circulatory reasons alone.

MITRAL STENOSIS

Mitral stenosis is less common than aortic stenosis and is largely a disorder of middle-aged women, most of whom relate a past history of acute rheumatic fever in childhood or adolescence. It is a more chronic, insidiously progressive disease than aortic stenosis, and its symptoms, in contrast to those of aortic stenosis, correlate with the severity of the hydraulic defect. Significant mitral stenosis is thus rarely overlooked in routine preoperative evaluation. In addition to the history of acute rheumatic fever and symptoms, the cardiac silhouette on the chest x-ray is usually abnormal, even when the physical findings of mitral stenosis are difficult to appreciate. Difficulties in the perioperative period are directly related to the hydraulic severity of the mitral obstruction.[5] Since hydraulic severity correlates well with symptoms and other clinical findings, it is relatively easy to estimate the likelihood of problems.

In mitral stenosis, the left ventricle is inadequately preloaded. Because of valvular obstruction, abnormally elevated left atrial pressures are necessary for a satisfactory left ventricular end-diastolic pressure to be achieved. Lowering left atrial pressure toward normal produces an unacceptably low left ventricular end-diastolic pressure that may lead to a drop in cardiac output.

Patients with mitral stenosis can be divided into two groups, those with sinus rhythm and those with chronic atrial fibrillation.[6] The development of chronic atrial fibrillation is a well-recognized milestone in the natural history of mitral stenosis. Of the two groups, patients with sinus rhythm present earlier and have less severe obstruction.

All patients with significant mitral stenosis have evidence on physical examination of right ventricular enlargement and pulmonary hypertension. The intensity of the murmur varies from patient to patient and correlates poorly with the severity of the disorder. The degree of physiologic derangement can be more precisely estimated from evidence of pulmonary hypertension, tricuspid regurgitation, and low systemic cardiac output. Electrocardiographic findings are variable and also correlate poorly with severity. The chest x-ray reveals a characteristic distortion of the cardiac silhouette with enlargement of the left atrium, pulmonary artery, and right ventricle. These abnormalities, which correlate fairly well in degree with severity, may lead to the impairment of liver function, which, in turn, may deteriorate further with the stress of anesthesia and surgery.

Preoperative Preparation

Hydration and intravascular volume status are important determinants of a patient's ability to tolerate anesthesia and surgery. In patients with mitral stenosis, unlike those with aortic stenosis, it is preferable to err toward hypovolemia. Although these patients can be sensitive to changes in preload, it is easier to replete volume than to treat pulmonary edema. Small increases in intravascular volume may elevate left atrial pressure to unacceptable levels. Systemic arterial hypotension is not as dangerous in patients with mitral stenosis as it is in those with aortic stenosis, and it can be easily corrected with judicious use of fluids.

Many patients with mitral stenosis receive chronic diuretic therapy and may have depleted potassium stores. This becomes significant when digitalis is needed acutely to treat new atrial fibrillation or to control ventricular rate in chronic atrial fibrillation.

When a patient has chronic atrial fibrillation, the ventricular response rate should be well controlled before surgery. In mitral stenosis, tachycardia can be detrimental, because it reduces the time available for flow across the mitral valve and can lead to the sudden development of pulmonary edema.[7] When a patient has normal sinus rhythm, it may be appropriate to consider the prophylactic use of digitalis, which may prevent the development of a rapid ventricular response should atrial fibrillation develop.

Operative Management

Because it is virtually impossible to estimate changes in pulmonary capillary wedge pressure in the anesthesized patient, right-heart pressure monitoring is essential. Pulmonary capillary wedge pressure, greater than left ventricular filling pressure in patients with mitral stenosis, is usually in the range of 20 torr. Optimal pulmonary capillary wedge pressure varies with the severity of mitral obstruction, and a pressure of 10 torr to 12 torr in significant mitral stenosis represents hypovolemia. Since the response of pulmonary vasculature to mitral stenosis is also variable, pulmonary arterial pressure may not reliably reflect actual pulmonary capillary wedge pressure. Consequently, a concerted effort should be made to obtain an accurate and reproducible pulmonary capillary wedge pressure.

Patients with mitral stenosis are limited in their ability to increase cardiac output in response to changes in systemic vascular resistance. Accordingly vasodilating anesthetics should not be used. Since these patients also have a limited capacity to accept additional intravascular volume, acute volume expansion, such as that caused by the infusion of mannitol in neurosurgical procedures, is hazardous.

The development of atrial fibrillation or sinus tachycardia requires immediate action to re-establish normal sinus rhythm or slow ventricular response. If atrial fibrillation develops during surgery, immediate cardioversion is indicated. Sinus tachycardia should be recognized immediately and its cause sought and corrected. In certain circumstances, it may be wise to slow the ventricular response rate pharmacologically with intravenous propranolol in small dose increments.

Postoperative Management

In patients with mitral stenosis, as in those with aortic stenosis, the right-heart catheter is essential to guide postoperative fluid and blood infusion rates and should be maintained until major fluid shifts have ceased. Since mild hypovolemia has been deliberately sought and a significant amount of postoperative "third spacing" of fluid may be expected, there is danger of hypovolemic oliguria. Urine flow should therefore probably be maintained by diuretic administration and volume replacement in order for appropriate intravascular volume to be maintained.

Because of fixed obstruction to left atrial emptying, catecholamine stimulation in the hypotensive patient is usually ineffective and, if it produces tachycardia, may be counterproductive. Hypotension is not usually due to depressed left ventricular contractile function; more likely, it is caused by inadequate left ventricular filling because of hypovolemia, tachycardia, or some other hemodynamic change. Of course, control of fever and treatment of atrial fibrillation are important in this regard.

AORTIC REGURGITATION

Aortic regurgitation is more common than mitral stenosis but less common than aortic stenosis. Important causes of aortic regurgitation include rheumatic fever, infective endocarditis, congenital abnormalities of the valve, and disease of the ascending aorta. Since congenital defects of the aortic valve are more prevalent in males than females, aortic regurgitation occurs more commonly in males.[8]

In assessing the patient with aortic regurgitation, it is important to estimate not only the severity of regurgitation but also the quality of left ventricular function. Operative risk in the patient with aortic regurgitation is probably influenced more strongly by the quality of left ventricular function than by the severity of regurgitation. Isolated mild aortic regurgitation is essentially a trivial disorder and does not confer additional risk.

Aortic regurgitation is recognized by its characteristic blowing decrescendo diastolic murmur, which is heard maximally along the left sternal border. Severity is directly related to peripheral arterial findings and accompanying evidence of left ventricular volume overload. The abnormal arterial pressure pulse contour is expressed as Quinke pulses, pistol shot sounds heard over the femoral arteries, and a low diastolic arterial pressure (60 or less). Although peripheral signs such as an abnormal pulse contour and low diastolic blood pressure are useful in judging severity, they may be masked in patients with enlarged ascending aortas. The dilated ascending aorta functions as a damping chamber that decreases the amplitude of arterial pulsations.

Severity can also be judged from evidence of left ventricular volume loading. This is seen as an enlarged, diffuse, displaced left ventricular impulse on physical examination, as enlargement of the left ventricle on chest x-ray, and as an increase in the left ventricular end-diastolic diameter on an echocardiogram. Assembling these data should enable the physician to make an accurate quantitative assessment of the severity of the aortic regurgitation.

Assessment of the quality of left ventricular function is equally important. Left ventricular performance is probably a more important determinant of operative risk than regurgitation itself. Most pa-

tients with significant aortic regurgitation exhibit some electrocardiographic findings consistent with left ventricular hypertrophy. However, patients with major changes, including extensive repolarization changes, QRS intervals of greater than 100 msec, and abnormal P-wave vectors, are more likely to have depressed left ventricular function. Similarly, chest x-ray evidence of a greatly enlarged left ventricle suggests depressed left ventricular function. The echocardiogram provides the best assessment of left ventricular function.[9] Left ventricular end-diastolic diameters greater than 7 cm and end-systolic diameters greater than 5.5 cm correlate with substantially impaired left ventricular performance. Patients with these signs have high operative risk and require especially careful perioperative management.

Preoperative Preparation

Patients with aortic regurgitation are not as sensitive to changes in preload as those with aortic stenosis or mitral stenosis, and precise preoperative adjustment of intravascular volume is less crucial. However, these patients probably tolerate the stress of anesthesia and surgery better if their intravascular volume is slightly increased.

Operative Management

Right-heart pressure and arterial pressure monitoring are important only in high-risk patients with severely impaired left ventricular function; the majority of patients can be managed effectively without such measures. Vasodilating drugs are well tolerated, and, if pulmonary vascular congestion develops, vasodilator therapy may be valuable in reducing left atrial pressure. Reduction of systemic vascular resistance decreases the degree of aortic regurgitation and leads to a decrease in left ventricular end-diastolic volume and filling pressure and an increase in cardiac output.

Postoperative Management

Physiologic changes in the postoperative period are similar to those during surgery. In patients with severely impaired left ventricular function, moderate degrees of hypovolemia are well tolerated. If problems with pulmonary vascular congestion develop, vasodilator therapy is effective both in improving systemic cardiac output and in decreasing pulmonary vascular congestion. However, vasodilator therapy is best carried out with right-heart pressure monitoring. In extreme circumstances of low arterial pressure, low cardiac output, or pulmonary vascular congestion, inotropic stimulation of left ventricular contractility may be useful.

MITRAL REGURGITATION

Mitral regurgitation, like mitral stenosis, is more common in females than in males and, like aortic regurgitation, has many causes. In mitral regurgitation, the determinants of risk are the severity of regurgitation and the quality of left ventricular function.

Mitral regurgitation imposes a preload stress or volume load on the left ventricle without the afterload stress imposed by aortic regurgitation. Instead of having to eject its entire stroke volume against the relatively high impedance of the aorta, the left ventricle delivers the regurgitant fraction of mitral regurgitation into the relatively low impedance circuit of the left atrium. Compared to that in aortic regurgitation, afterload in mitral regurgitation is already somewhat reduced. Consequently, severe left ventricular dysfunction may be masked because of the relatively low impedance against which the left ventricle ejects.[10]

The presence of mitral regurgitation is easily recognized by the presence of a blowing systolic murmur that is loudest at the left ventricular apex. However, quantitative estimation of severity is complex. Important parameters include evidence of left ventricular dilatation on physical examination, chest x-ray, and echocardiogram. Patients with left ventricular dysfunction due to primary myocardial disease may develop moderate mitral regurgitation because of geometric distortion of the mitral apparatus.[11] These patients have physical signs similar to those of patients with primary mitral regurgitation. Left ventricular function is best assessed through measurement by echocardiography of cavity dimensions and wall excursion.

Preoperative Preparation

Preoperative preparation of the patient with mitral regurgitation is similar to that of the patient with aortic regurgitation. Hypovolemia should be avoided, and a normal or slightly increased intravascular volume is preferred. An exception to this general principle is the patient with preexisting right-heart failure and resultant liver function abnormalities. In such a patient diuresis sufficient to lower right atrial pressure to normal may enable the liver to better withstand the stress of anesthesia and surgery. In chronic atrial fibrillation, ventricular response should be well controlled with digoxin. Although beta-blockers may be useful in controlling ventricular response rate in mitral stenosis, they should never be used in mitral regurgitation because of their depressant effect on left ventricular function. Since patients with mitral regurgitation may require digitalis, maintenance of a normal serum potassium concentration is important.

Operative Management

Right-heart pressure monitoring is important only for patients who have severely depressed left ventricular function and in whom appropriate pulmonary capillary wedge pressure is about 20 torr. Some patients with mitral regurgitation have elevated pulmonary vascular resistance, and pulmonary artery pressure may not accurately reflect wedge pressure. It is therefore necessary for an accurate and reproducible pulmonary capillary wedge pressure to be obtained.

Patients with mitral regurgitation generally withstand vasodilatation well, and spinal anesthetics are well tolerated. If pulmonary vascular congestion develops, vasodilators such as nitroprusside are useful in relieving problems of both inadequate systemic cardiac output and elevated pulmonary capillary wedge pressure.[12]

Postoperative Management

Problems encountered in the postoperative management of patients with mitral regurgitation and the means for resolving them are similar to those for patients with aortic regurgitation. However, patients with severe mitral regurgitation and right-heart failure are more likely to develop hepatic insufficiency in the postoperative period.

IDIOPATHIC HYPERTROPHIC SUBAORTIC STENOSIS

Idiopathic hypertrophic subaortic stenosis (IHSS), or asymmetric septal hypertrophy (ASH), is a hypertrophic cardiomyopathy in which there is excessive thickening of the upper portion of the interventricular septum and distortion of the geometry of the left ventricle.[13] This causes the anterior leaflet of the mitral valve to be drawn toward the septum during left ventricular contraction in systole, producing outflow obstruction.[14] In IHSS, in contrast to valvular aortic stenosis, the degree of left ventricular outflow obstruction is variable and changes in response to interventions that alter left ventricular size and contractility. Vasodilators, which decrease left ventricular size by decreasing both venous return and arterial pressure, augment the obstruction. Similarly, pharmacologic interventions, such as catecholamine stimulation, that enhance myocardial contractility also increase obstruction.

Patients with IHSS should be approached in the same manner as those with valvular aortic stenosis. They are exquisitely sensitive to decreases in preload both because they require adequate diastolic fiber length to maintain normal systolic performance and because reduced ventricular size increases their ventricular outflow obstruction. Consequently, the basic principles of fluid management for patients with aortic stenosis also apply to patients with IHSS.

However, inotropic stimulation should never be used to treat hypotension in patients with IHSS; it aggravates the underlying left ventricular outflow obstruction that may very well be responsible for the hypotension. If hypotension occurs, adequate preload should be insured with volume administration, and afterload should be adjusted to produce sufficient arterial pressure. Frequently, increasing afterload will improve cardiac output by decreasing the severity of left ventricular outflow obstruction.

PROSTHETIC HEART VALVES

Perioperative management of the patient with a heart valve prosthesis depends on the type of prosthesis and its location. Prosthetic valves are of two major types: tissue bioprostheses, which are natural aortic valves from pigs mounted on fabric-covered metal frames, and mechanical prostheses, either of the ball-and-cage type (Starr–Edwards) or of the pivoting-disk design (Bjork–Shiley and St. Jude).

Clinical assessment of prosthetic valve function is quite difficult. Systolic murmurs are present across normally functioning aortic prostheses, and even severely stenotic mitral prostheses do not produce diastolic murmurs. Aortic periprosthetic leaks are typically accompanied by blowing diastolic murmurs; however, the intensity and timing of the murmurs do not correlate with the severity of the leakage. Mitral periprosthetic leaks may be acoustically silent. In general, suspicion of prosthetic dysfunction is warranted only when a patient is doing poorly after what appears to be a technically successful valve replacement and there are no other factors to explain the deterioration.

Valve replacement never completely corrects the underlying heart disease. The chamber(s) that bore the burden of the dysfunctional valve before surgery continue to be variably dysfunctional. Therefore, patients with prosthetic valves cannot be approached as though they have a normal cardiovascular system. The extent of perioperative monitoring employed and the precautions taken should be based on careful clinical and laboratory assessment of overall cardiac function. The role of antibiotic prophylaxis in prosthetic valves is discussed in Chapter 4.

Anticoagulant Therapy

Mechanical prostheses are more prone to thrombosis and embolization than tissue prostheses, and these complications are more common with the valve in the mitral than in the aortic position.[15] Anticoagulation is most critical in patients with mechanical prostheses in the mitral position and least critical in those with bioprostheses in the aortic position.

Anticoagulant management in the perioperative period should be based on the type and position of the prosthesis or prostheses. Patients with bioprostheses in the aortic position frequently are not anticoagulated. Patients with bioprostheses in the mitral position are usually anticoagulated. In those who are anticoagulated, warfarin should be discontinued and anticoagulation maintained with heparin until 12 hr before surgery.[16] Heparin should then be discontinued, restarted only after all danger of bleeding has passed, and maintained until adequate anticoagulation with warfarin is re-established. A similar program of management is appropriate for patients with mechanical prostheses in the aortic position.

The most difficult problem is presented by the patient with a mechanical prosthesis in the mitral position, who is most in need of anticoagulation. The best approach is to discontinue warfarin anticoagulation before surgery and maintain heparinization. In certain types of surgery, it may be possible to maintain heparinization during the procedure and the postoperative period. When this is not possible, heparin can be discontinued at the time of surgery. The effect can be rapidly reversed at any time with protamine sulfate. This approach allows for maintenance of anticoagulation in marginal situations and rapid reversal should bleeding develop.

SUMMARY

1. Noncardiac surgery can be performed safely in virtually every patient with valvular heart disease. It requires recognition of the presence and severity of the valvular defect, assessment of the state of the underlying left ventricular contractile function, and proper control of the hemodynamic and metabolic context in which the heart functions.

2. In high-risk patients, hemodynamic monitoring, including measurement of right-heart pressure and systemic arterial pressure with indwelling catheters, is essential.

3. Patients with aortic and mitral stenosis require careful attention to intravascular volume and cardiac rhythm during and after surgery. Vasodilators are hazardous, and small changes in intravascular volume can produce profound changes in left ventricular filling pressure and cardiac output.

4. Patients with valvular regurgitation are better able to withstand perioperative stresses than are those with stenotic lesions. Their ability to respond to changes in intravascular volume, systolic vascular resistance, and cardiac rhythm is determined principally by left ventricular function.

5. Pronounced fluid shifts in the postoperative period should be anticipated. The hemodynamic monitoring employed during surgery in high-risk patients should be continued postoperatively.

6. Anticoagulation is most critical in patients with a mitral mechanical prosthesis and least critical in patients with an aortic bioprosthesis. Warfarin should be discontinued before surgery and anticoagulation maintained with heparin until 12 hr before the operation. Heparin followed by warfarin should be restarted postoperatively when all danger of bleeding has passed.

7. For specific recommendations regarding antibiotic prophylaxis against bacterial endocarditis in patients with valvular heart disease undergoing surgery, see Chapter 4.

REFERENCES

1. Skinner JF, Pearce ML: Surgical risk in the cardiac patient. J Chron Dis 17:57, 1964
2. Goldman L, Caldera DL, Southwick FS et al: Cardiac risk factors and complications in non-cardiac surgery. Medicine 57:357, 1978
3. Perloff JF: Clinical recognition of aortic stenosis. The physical signs and differential diagnosis of the various signs of obstruction to left ventricular outflow. Prog Cardiovasc Dis 10:323, 1968
4. Eddleman EE, Frommeyer WB, Lyle DP et al: Critical analysis of clinical factors in estimating severity of aortic valve disease. Am J Cardiol 31:687, 1973
5. Gorlin R, Gorlin G: Hydraulic formula for the calculation of area of stenotic mitral valve, other valves and central circulatory shunts. Am Heart J 41:1, 1951
6. Mitchell JH, Shapiro W: Atrial function and the hemodynamic consequences of

atrial fibrillation in man. Am J Cardiol 23:556, 1969

7. Arandi DT, Carleton RA: The deleterious role of tachycardia in mitral stenosis. Circulation 36:511, 1967

8. Goldschlager N, Pfeifer J, Cohn K et al: The natural history of aortic regurgitation. A clinical and hemodynamic study. Am J Med 54:577, 1973

9. Abdulla AM, Frank MJ, Canedo MI et al: Limitations of echocardiography in the assessment of left ventricular size and function in aortic regurgitation. Circulation 61:148, 1980

10. Braunwald E: Mitral regurgitation: Physiological, clinical and surgical considerations. N Engl J Med 281:425, 1969

11. Perloff JK, Roberts WC: The mitral apparatus. Functional anatomy of mitral regurgitation. Circulation 46:227, 1972

12. Yoran C, Yellin EL, Becker RM et al: Mechanism of reduction of mitral regurgitation with vasodilator therapy. Am J Cardiol 43:773, 1979

13. Frank S, Braunwald E: Idiopathic hypertrophic subaortic stenosis. Clinical analysis of 126 patients with emphasis on the natural history. Circulation 37:759, 1968

14. Henry WL, Clark CE, Griffith JM et al: Mechanism of left ventricular outflow obstruction in patients with obstructive asymmetric septal hypertrophy (Idiopathic hypertrophic subaortic stenosis). Am J Cardiol 35:337, 1975

15. Katholi RE, Nolan SP, McGuire LB: Living with prosthetic heart valves. Subsequent noncardiac operations and the risk of thromboembolism or hemorrhage. Am Heart J 92:162, 1976

16. Tinker JH, Tarhan S: Discontinuing anticoagulant therapy in surgical patients with cardiac valve prostheses. JAMA 239:738, 1978

The Surgical Patient on Steroids

DAVID R. GOLDMANN

Ever since Fraser's initial case report of intraoperative cardiovascular collapse in a patient taking exogenous glucocorticoids, the literature has reflected continuing concern for this serious complication.[1-8] The use of steroids for the treatment of a variety of diseases is widespread. However, working through the hypothalamic–pituitary–adrenal (HPA) axis, steroids are the most common cause of unsuspected adrenal suppression, and adrenocortical insufficiency can remain clinically inapparent until the stress of surgery supervenes. In addition, steroids affect both wound healing and host defenses against infection, two important areas of concern in the perioperative period.

Although those who suffer from severe adrenal insufficiency and endogenously or exogenously induced Cushing's syndrome are usually readily recognized, preoperative patients who have taken or are taking steroids can be difficult to identify. Adrenal insufficiency can be subtle in its presentation, with few, if any, clearly defined signs and symptoms to guide the clinician. It can be easily confused with the so-called steroid withdrawal syndrome, which consists of anorexia, weight loss, malaise, myalgias, arthralgias, emotional lability, and even low-grade fever in the patient with normal cortisol levels who has recently discontinued steroids.[9,10] Moreover, endogenous Cushing's syndrome may differ from that produced by exogenous steroids.[11,12] Although obesity, edema, poor wound healing, and psychiatric symptoms are common to both, benign intracranial hypertension, glaucoma, posterior subcapsular cataracts, pancreatitis, panniculitis, and aseptic necrosis of bone are peculiar to persons taking exogenous steroids. Hypertension, acne, menstrual irregularities, hirsutism, striae purpura, and plethora are more commonly seen in cases of endogenous Cushing's syndrome. Equivalent doses of steroids over a given period of time may more readily produce side-effects in some patients than in others. For these reasons, a detailed history of steroid use is often more helpful than physical examination or routine laboratory testing for electrolyte abnormalities.

This chapter reviews the physiology of the HPA axis, the biochemistry and pharmacology of commonly used steroids, and the effects of steroids on three major areas important in the perioperative setting—suppression of the HPA axis, wound healing, and predisposition to infection.

STEROID PHYSIOLOGY, BIOCHEMISTRY, AND PHARMACOLOGY

The production of cortisol by the adrenal cortex is controlled by adrenocorticotropic hormone (ACTH) from the anterior pituitary gland. The secretion of both hormones is episodic and exhibits diurnal variation, with peak secretion in the early morning and a nadir in the evening. The secretion of ACTH is in turn controlled by corticotrophin-releasing hormone (CRH) from the hypothalamus, and neural stimuli from higher centers presumably stimulate the secretion of CRH to work its effect on the rest of the axis. There is a clearly defined negative-feedback mechanism in which cortisol from the adrenal cortex suppresses the secretion of ACTH. This same inhibition of ACTH production and secretion is produced by exogenous steroids.

Pharmacologically active steroids are all variants of cortisol or hydrocortisone with 21 carbon atoms arranged in a characteristic four-ringed compound. Variations in the saturation of the rings and the presence of various side-chains influence the half-lives and potencies of these agents. Table 9-1 lists some of the most commonly used steroids grouped according to their durations of action and relative potencies in suppressing ACTH secretion.[13,14] Equivalent doses of short-acting steroids produce ACTH suppression for 24 hr to 36 hr, intermediate-acting compounds for 26 hr to 48 hr, and long-acting agents for more than 48 hr.

It should be emphasized that duration and potency of action in suppressing ACTH secretion do not correlate strictly with either serum half-life or duration of biologic effect. Though the serum half-life of prednisolone is roughly twice that of

Table 9-1. Commonly Used Glucocorticoids

Steroids	Glucocorticoid Potency *	Equivalent Glucocorticoid Dose (mg)
Short-acting		
Cortisol (hydrocortisone)	1	20
Cortisone	0.8	25
Prednisone	4	5
Prednisolone	4	5
Methylprednisolone	5	4
Intermediate-acting		
Triamcinolone	5	4
Long-acting		
Betamethasone	25	0.60
Dexamethasone	30	0.75

*The values given for glucocorticoid potency are relative. Cortisol is arbitrarily assigned a value of 1.

hydrocortisone, in equivalent doses they are both short-acting in their suppression of ACTH. Since the steroid molecule must enter the cell nucleus and affect the entire post-transcriptional chain of events to exert its biologic effect, neither its serum half-life nor its potency in suppressing ACTH correlates with its duration of action in various other target tissues. Moreover, the duration of one biologic effect exerted by a particular dose of steroid may differ from that of another effect. For example, although several different pulmonary function tests are useful in monitoring the effect of steroids in patients with asthma, the duration of improvement in one parameter may differ from that in another.[15]

The effect of surgical stress on the HPA axis has been well studied. In normal subjects, the plasma concentration of cortisol rises to a peak of 5 to 10 times normal approximately 6 hr after surgery and, unless stress continues, falls to normal levels within 24 hr.[16–18] A similar rise is seen after a dose of exogenous ACTH.[19] Epidural anesthesia delays but does not prevent this response.[20] Cortisol secretion remains episodic during stress, but the number of episodes per unit time and the amount of cortisol secreted during each are greater than under normal conditions.[21] A rise in ACTH occurs before a rise in cortisol and, in one study, was found to first occur 15 to 45 min after skin incision.[22] There are minor, probably clinically unimportant changes in the hepatic conjugation and renal excretion patterns of steroid metabolites after surgery.[23] Though a temporal relationship between the rise in plasma concentration of adenosine $3':5'$-cyclic phosphate (cyclic AMP) and cortisol has been documented, the exact mechanism of HPA activation, whether neural or humoral, remains undefined.[24–27] The adrenal response to the stress of surgery remains essentially intact in the elderly.[28]

Several tests have been used to evaluate the effect of exogenous steroids on one or more components of the HPA axis. Although administration of pyrogen or production of hypoglycemia with insulin provides a simulation of stress, such methods for the evaluation of adrenal response are impractical and potentially dangerous. The two well-standardized and clinically useful tests to measure adrenal reserve and the integrity of the HPA axis are, respectively, the ACTH test and the metyrapone test.[29,30] Adrenal reserve is tested by measurement of the plasma cortisol concentration before and 30 to 60 min after a parenteral dose of 250 μg of synthetic ACTH (cosyntropin).[21–24] From a basal plasma level of 6 μg/dl to 25 μg/dl, a rise to greater than 20 μg/dl or an incremental increase of more than 7 μg/dl in plasma cortisol concentration is considered normal. Although there are several variations of the metyrapone test, all involve inhibition of the final 11-hydroxy-lation step in the biochemical pathway of cortisol production from 11-deoxycortisol (compound S) to cortisol (compound F). After administration of metyrapone, plasma concentration of cortisol falls, ACTH secretion increases, and production of 11-deoxycortisol rises. An increase in plasma 11-deoxycortisol levels to above 10.5 μg/dl with a simultaneous plasma cortisol concentration of 8 μg/dl or less assures the integrity of both the pituitary and the adrenal components of the HPA axis.

SUPPRESSION OF THE HYPOTHALAMIC–PITUITARY–ADRENAL AXIS AND ITS IMPLICATION FOR THE SURGICAL PATIENT

It is generally assumed that adrenal suppression by exogenous glucocorticoids is dangerous during periods of stress because lack of acutely required cortisol leads to hypotension, cardiovascular collapse, and even death. Since the early 1950s, numerous case reports have documented these operative complications in patients taking steroids for a number of inflammatory diseases.[1–8] Some provide histologic evidence of adrenal atrophy at autopsy, but only a few supply biochemical evidence of low plasma concentrations of cortisol or one of its metabolites during the period of these complications.[1–3,31–33]

The many studies of HPA axis suppression by exogenous steroids are summarized elsewhere.[12,14] They fall into two major groups: those that only document suppression by abnormalities in one or more of the above biochemical tests, and those that attempt to correlate suppression with clinical outcome in the surgical setting. Though the latter are more relevant to questions posed in this chapter, both groups suffer from lack of uniform methodology and arrive at different conclusions. They evaluate heterogeneous groups of patients with different underlying diseases on a variety of different steroid regimens and employ different biochemical tests to define suppression. It is important to know what type of steroid given at what dose and frequency produces suppression, what is the best way to define and measure suppression, and how long the suppression lasts and how much time is required for recovery of the HPA axis. Even more important is the question of whether abnormalities in the HPA axis adversely alter surgical outcome. These questions are complex, and available data are limited.

Clinical studies of surgical outcome in patients taking exogenous steroids provide the most relevant data available. Danowski and co-workers studied 117 patients on various steroid regimens approximating replacement doses who went through 80 different stressful episodes, including surgery, pregnancy, diagnostic procedures, and acute illness, without developing signs or symptoms of adrenal insufficiency.[34] Another group of 13 men underwent 15 major or minor surgical procedures 3 to 24 months after interrupting replacement doses of steroid and similarly experienced no mishap. Although no biochemical testing of the HPA axis was performed, this clinical study provides firm evidence that patients taking replacement doses of steroid at the time of surgery or at any time within the preceding 2 years tolerate stress and surgery well and therefore require no perioperative steroid coverage.

Patients taking supraphysiologic doses of steroid greater than the equivalent of about 7.5 mg/day of prednisone present a more difficult problem. The best early study is probably that of Sampson, Brooke, and Winstone.[32] These authors studied 35 patients with ulcerative colitis undergoing elective surgery, 17 of whom had never received steroids and 18 of whom had been on various regimens within 2 years of operation. Two days after steroid was stopped in all patients, ACTH tests were performed, and plasma cortisol concentrations were determined hourly during surgery. In all patients except 3 of those who had taken steroids before surgery, both the ACTH test and intraoperative plasma cortisol determinations were normal. Of the 3 with abnormal ACTH tests, 1 underwent surgery with steroid cover and 2 did so without. Both of the latter had subnormal intraoperative plasma cortisol determinations and suffered unexplained hypotension responsive to intravenous hydrocortisone. Despite the small number of patients studied, the authors concluded not only that exogenous steroid can produce HPA axis suppression and increase the risk of perioperative collapse, but also that a preoperative ACTH test predicts both lack of adrenal response to stress and subsequent surgical complications.

This work has been confirmed and extended by others. Jasani and associates showed that plasma 11-hydroxycorticosteroid responses to synovectomy of the knee were normal in 16 of 21 steroid-treated patients with rheumatoid arthritis who had normal preoperative ACTH stimulation tests.[31] However, they were clearly subnormal in patients with abnormal tests and intermediate in those with a normal response to ACTH but subnormal response to one or more of three other tests of the HPA axis. There was only one case of severe intraoperative hypotension, and this was in a patient on a low-dose steroid who had an abnormal ACTH test. The authors therefore suggested that the results of the ACTH test correlate best with the adrenal response to the stress of surgery and may be useful in predicting intraoperative complications and the need for steroid coverage. The conclusions of this work were reaffirmed by Kehlet and Binder with the caveats that abnormalities in any stimulation test do not always correlate with intraoperative outcome and that intraoperative hypotension may occur for a variety of reasons unrelated to HPA axis function.[19] Coupled with early, isolated reports of intact stress responses in patients with abnormal feedback due to head injury or previous pituitary stalk section, the available data must therefore be viewed critically.

Other studies supply limited information about the time course of suppression and recovery of HPA axis function during and after a course of exogenous steroids. These data are helpful to the physician in deciding what length of steroid course during what period before surgery will most probably produce clinically significant HPA axis suppression, especially when surgery cannot await the results of an ACTH stimulation test. Graber and coworkers studied the recovery of each component of the HPA axis over time after discontinuation of supraphysiologic doses of exogenous steroids given for 1 to 10 years or after surgical removal of an adrenocortical tumor causing Cushing's syndrome.[35] Through measurements of plasma ACTH and basal and ACTH-stimulated 17-hydroxycorticosteroids, these investigators defined four phases of HPA axis recovery. During the first month, ACTH and 17-hydroxycorticosteroid levels were low, and the ACTH stimulation test was abnormal. In the second through the fifth months, ACTH levels rose to normal or supranormal levels while basal and stimulated 17-hydroxycorticosteroids remained low. In the sixth through ninth months, 17-hydroxycorticosteroids returned to normal, but adrenal responsiveness remained abnormal. Only after 9 months did all parameters return to normal. Graber concluded that recovery of adrenocortical function lags behind that of the pituitary and may not occur for up to a year or more after discontinuation of exogenous steroid.

Livanou and colleagues studied the recovery of HPA axis function by measuring plasma levels of 11-hydroxycorticosteroids before and after insulin-induced hypoglycemia in control subjects and patients who were either still on steroids or had discontinued them for periods ranging from 24 hr to more than 1 year.[36] Although basal 11-hydroxycorticosteroid levels returned to normal after about 1 month, normal stimulated levels were not achieved in all patients until after 1 year or more. Patients achieved normal basal levels of 11-hydroxycorticosteroids more quickly if they were taking the equivalent of 7.5 mg/day or less of prednisone, and, in the low-dose group, stimulated levels returned more quickly if the duration of therapy had been less than 18 months. These authors emphasized the importance of considering the variables of dosage and duration of therapy in predicting a person's response to stress.

Data on the steroid dosage and duration of therapy necessary to produce HPA axis suppression are conflicting, but Streck and Lockwood have demonstrated that high-dose short-term steroid therapy twice daily for only 5 days can affect HPA axis function.[37] They measured cortisol responses to both ACTH and insulin-induced hypoglycemia 2 and 5 days after discontinuation of therapy in 10 normal men and found both to be impaired at 2 days and the response to ACTH to be still subnormal at 5 days. Unfortunately, testing was not carried out for more than 5 days after steroids had been stopped.

Steroid regimens involving other routes of administration and dosage frequencies affect HPA axis function differently. Although infrequent, usually mild, and of only minor clinical importance, adrenal suppression has been documented in patients receiving topical or intranasal steroids.[38–41] More important is the effect of dosage frequency on the HPA axis. As early as 1963, Harter and associates documented that alternate-day prednisone therapy not only produced significantly fewer side-effects than daily therapy but also preserved normal adrenal response to ACTH.[42] Ackerman and Nolan found that alternate-day high-dose prednisone lowered basal plasma 17-hydroxycorticosteroid levels but had no effect on response to insulin-induced hypoglycemia.[43] Others have extended this work to other steroids and other intermittent dosage regimens.[44] Alternate-day administration of a long-acting steroid, dexamethasone, produces profound adrenal suppression, and HPA axis dysfunction cannot be avoided by regimens calling for doses on three consecutive days each week.[45–47] There are data to suggest that triamcinolone given once daily in the morning produces less HPA axis suppression than divided or even single doses given later in the day.[48,49] Administration of ACTH does not produce significant HPA axis suppression.[14,50]

In summary, although the available data are far from consistent, it is reasonable to expect HPA axis suppression from supraphysiologic doses of exogenous steroids after as few as 5 days. Full recovery can require up to 1 year and cannot be easily predicted from information on dosage and duration of treatment. Suppression of the HPA axis can be minimized by use of the lowest possible effective quantity in a single daily or, if possible, alternate-day dose, with long-acting potent agents such as dexamethasone being avoided.

A carefully taken history is the most important element in the preparation of the preoperative patient taking steroids. Only precise information regarding the dosage, its duration and frequency, and the interval between the last dose and the operative procedure allows the clinician to predict the possibility of adrenal insufficiency under stress and determine the need for steroid coverage in the perioperative period. When time permits before surgery, especially if an accurate history of steroid use cannot be obtained, an ACTH stimulation test provides the most reliable index of adrenocortical response to stress. In an emergency situation, it is reasonable to provide preoperative steroid coverage when the patient has taken supraphysiologic doses of steroid for more than a week in the year preceding surgery.

There are many available steroid coverage regimens, all of which are empirical.[51–53] In all cases, it is best to avoid intramuscular cortisone acetate because of its uncertain absorption and the need for hepatic reduction to cortisol. For major surgery, hydrocortisone hemisuccinate in a dose of 100 mg can be given intravenously the evening before surgery, at the beginning of the procedure, and every 8 hr until the end of the period of stress. Adequate salt- and glucose-containing fluid should be provided with careful monitoring of serum electrolytes and glucose concentration. If the postoperative course is complicated, steroid coverage should be continued. Unless required for more than a few days or needed in the treatment of an underlying disease, it can be discontinued without tapering. For minor surgical procedures, the same regimen can be used for 24 hr, and, for stressful diagnostic procedures or those involving the use of dye, a simple intravenous dose of 100 mg of hydrocortisone just before the operation should suffice. If a maintenance dose of steroid for an underlying disease is required, it can be resumed when the hydrocortisone is discontinued and the patient is eating.

STEROID THERAPY AND WOUND HEALING

Clinicians have long recognized thinning of skin, easy bruisability, and delayed wound healing in patients with endogenous or exogenous hypercortisolism. However, the literature on surgical wound healing in patients taking steroids is scant. Much must be inferred from series of patients with Cushing's syndrome undergoing adrenalectomy or pituitary surgery, animal work dealing with the physics of wound healing, or in vitro studies of collagen biochemistry. Given the number of patients on long-term steroid therapy going to surgery and those requiring perioperative steroid coverage for suspected HPA axis suppression, it is important that the effect of these agents on the normal process of wound healing be assessed.

Solem and Lund reviewed their experience with 449 steroid-treated patients who underwent surgery under high-dose cortisone cover over a 10-year period.[54] Although the authors do not supply numbers, they documented no tendency for delayed wound healing and stated that steroids rarely interfere with healing, un-less doses are unduly high for long periods of time and protein intake is inadequate. In a later series of 44 patients undergoing bilateral adrenalectomy for Cushing's disease, only 1 patient who could not be easily weaned from replacement cortisone experienced delayed wound healing.[55]

Early animal studies date from the time when steroids were first used widely in clinical practice. Baker and Whitaker inflicted standardized wounds in the skin of rats before and after local application of cortisone and studied the gross and histologic morphology of the healing process.[56] They found that cortisone delayed formation of granulation tissue and wound closure and caused thinning of the dermis, atrophy of collagen fibers, and a decrease in fibroblast and new blood vessel proliferation. This work was supported by that of Howes and co-workers, who found that subcutaneous cortisone affected granulation tissue formation in rabbits and rats in a dose-dependent fashion and significantly decreased the tensile strength of sutured wounds.[57]

Data on the effects of different steroid doses and times of administration in relation to wounding on various parameters of healing is conflicting. Ehrlich and Hunt, as well as Sandberg, found that moderate to large doses of steroids exerted their morphologic effects best within 3 days of injury and postulated that the steroids' inhibition of the early inflammatory process after wounding was responsible for delayed healing.[58,59] Vitamin A was found to be somewhat protective against delayed healing, presumably because of its effect on stabilizing lysosomes. However, other investigators found that small doses of steroid have variable effects.[60,61] Moreover, the effects of different doses of steroid on the proliferation of fibroblasts, production of collagen, and uptake of nucleic and amino acids in tissue culture from humans are far from clear.

The latest work exploits biochemical techniques for measuring many different physical parameters of connective tissue. In one study, rats given long-term moderate-dose cortisol treatment were wounded, and tissue from the wound site and a tendon were tested both biochemically for collagen content and mechanically for tensile strength, stress–strain relationships, failure energy, extensibility, and elastic stiffness.[62] Although the authors found that steroids only slightly impaired the mechanical properties of healing, they documented a systemic effect of wounding itself on skin distant from the wound and independent of steroid treatment; this effect consisted of increased collagen content and decreased stiffness.

These studies are clearly limited in clinical applicability. Not only do most derive their data from animals, but they are also flawed by lack of methodologic uniformity and inability to relate their measured parameters to the overall process of surgical wound healing in humans. However, clinical experience and an overall assessment of the unsatisfactory data suggest that steroid treatment may have a deleterious effect on wound healing. For this reason, it seems appropriate to recommend extra attention to and meticulous care of wounds in patients on glucocorticoids. Although delayed wound healing provides another reason to avoid their indiscriminate use, steroids should not be withheld if underlying adrenal insufficiency is suspected.

STEROID THERAPY AND INFECTION

Increased susceptibility to infection is another generally accepted complication of steroid therapy that is relevant to the surgical setting. Again, however, good data on the basis of which to assess the risk of this complication are difficult to find. Additional information must be derived from studies of infection in steroid-treated nonsurgical patients and from studies that examine the effect of glucocorticoids on the complicated process of host defense *in vitro*.

Winstone and Brooke observed 4 cases of septicemia among 18 surgical patients on steroids given steroid coverage but no similar complication in 17 others also taking steroids but not given coverage.[63] In a controlled retrospective study of 100 patients on steroids undergoing major and minor surgical procedures under appropriate coverage, there were 11 wound infections in the steroid-treated group and only 1 among the controls.[64] Though patients and controls were matched for age and sex, they were not matched for underlying disease. In contrast, Kaalund-Jensen and Elb did not observe an increased incidence of wound or other infections in an uncontrolled series of 419 patients subjected to surgery under steroid cover, and Oh and Patterson found only 1 minor suture abscess among a group of 17 steroid-dependent asthmatics undergoing 21 surgical procedures.[65,66] Four series of patients with Cushing's disease undergoing adrenalectomy gave wound infection rates ranging from 2.3% to 21%.[55,67–69] In one series, urinary tract infection occurred in only 4.5% of the patients. Though these data are conflicting, largely uncontrolled, and drawn from patients with serious underlying diseases, there is some evidence that long-term steroid use and perhaps steroid coverage itself may predispose some surgical patients to postoperative wound infection. It is noteworthy that other infections do not seem to be increased, implying that steroids may affect the local inflammatory response and host defenses at the site of injury only.

Other clinical data to support the contention that steroids may predispose to infection can be drawn from nonsurgical literature already extensively reviewed.[70–72] Soon after their introduction into clinical practice, steroids were found to worsen infection despite their effects in reducing fever and toxicity. Specific attention was soon drawn to the seemingly higher than normal incidence of infection with gram-negative bacteria and other more unusual opportunistic organisms. Despite the fact that the studies carried out to date suffer from small numbers and methodologic problems, there is some evidence to suggest that steroid therapy may predispose patients with systemic lupus erythematosis and patients undergoing renal transplantation to serious complications and death from infection.[73,74] There are also data to suggest that alternate-day steroid therapy may decrease this risk in a variety of chronic diseases.[71,75]

The accumulation of experimental data on the effect of steroids on host defenses and cellular immunity provides a theoretical basis for clinical observation; these data have recently been extensively reviewed.[71] Steroids exert multiple effects on the kinetics, distribution pattern, and function of granulocytes and mononuclear cells. Though glucocorticoids cause a brisk neutrophilic leukocytosis, they suppress accumulation of granulocytes at the inflammatory site, probably by altering their surface and preventing adherence to and egress from the vascular epithelium. Steroid-induced lymphocytopenia is probably due to redistribution of circulating lymphocytes, particularly T lymphocytes, out of the intravascular space through as yet undefined mechanisms. The multiple effects of steroids on the complicated processes of cellular immunity are beyond the scope of this chapter but include antagonism of macrophage interaction with the soluble products of activated lymphocytes. It is ironic that the very mechanisms that allow glucocorticoids to exert their beneficial anti-inflammatory and immunosuppressive effects in so many disease states may be responsible for increasing host susceptibility to infection.

In summary, the incidence of postoperative infection, particularly of the wound, may be increased in steroid-treated patients. For this reason, steroids should be used perioperatively only when required to treat an underlying disease or when adrenal suppression is suspected. Meticulous wound care is essential to prevent infection; however, prophylactic antibiotics are not indicated.

SUMMARY

1. **Decreased adrenal reserve due to suppression of the HPA axis by exogenous steroids should be suspected in any patient who has taken supraphysiologic doses of glucocorticoids (more than the equivalent of 7.5 mg/day of prednisone) for more than a week in the year preceding surgery.**
2. **If the history is unclear, an ACTH stimulation test provides an adequate measure of the ability of the adrenal glands to meet the stress of surgery. When emergency surgery is required and time does not permit testing, steroid coverage should be given.**
3. **Appropriate steroid coverage for major surgery consists of hydrocortisone hemisuccinate, 100 mg intravenously, the evening before surgery, another dose at the beginning of the procedure, and 100 mg every 8 hr thereafter until**

the stress of the postoperative period has passed. The same regimen can be used for 24 hr for minor procedures. One dose of 100 mg of hydrocortisone should be given just before stressful diagnostic procedures. Intramuscular cortisone acetate should be avoided because of its uneven absorption. Adequate glucose- and salt-containing fluid should be given.

4. Tapering of the steroid dose is required only if coverage is required for ongoing postoperative stress for more than a few days. Patients who require maintenance glucocorticoid for their underlying diseases should be continued on parenteral therapy until they start eating, at which time they can restart their usual oral dose.

5. Steroids may delay wound healing and predispose patients to wound infection. They should therefore be used only when indicated in the perioperative period; however, they should not be withheld if adrenal suppression is suspected. Meticulous wound care is essential.

REFERENCES

1. Fraser CG, Preuss FS, Bigford WD: Adrenal atrophy and irreversible shock associated with cortisone therapy. JAMA 149:1542, 1952

2. Lewis L, Robinson RF, Yee J: Fatal adrenal cortical insufficiency precipitated by surgery during prolonged continuous cortisone treatment. Ann Intern Med 39:116, 1953

3. Salassa RM, Bennett WA, Keating FR: Postoperative adrenal cortical insufficiency: Occurrence in a patient previously treated with cortisone. JAMA 152:1509, 1953

4. Slaney G, Brooke BN: Postoperative collapse due to adrenal insufficiency following cortisone therapy. Lancet 1:1167, 1957

5. Hayes MA, Kushlan SD: Influence of hormonal treatment for ulcerative colitis upon the course of surgical treatment. Gastroenterology 30:75, 1956

6. Harmagel EE, Kramer WG: Severe adrenocortical insufficiency following joint manipulation. JAMA 158:1518, 1955

7. Roberts JG: Operative collapse after corticosteroid therapy—A survey. Surg Clin North Am 50:363, 1970

8. Cope CL: The adrenal cortex in internal medicine. Br Med J 2:847, 1966

9. Amatruda TT Jr, Hollingsworth DR, D'Esopo ND et al: A study of the mechanism of the steroid withdrawal syndrome. Evidence for integrity of the hypothalamic–pituitary–adrenal system. J Clin Endocrinol Metab 20:239, 1960

10. Amatruda TT Jr, Hurst MM, D'Esopo ND: Certain endocrine and metabolic facets of the steroid withdrawal syndrome. J Clin Endocrinol Metab 25:1207, 1965

11. Ragan C: Corticotropin, cortisone, and related steroids in clinical medicine: Practical considerations. Bull NY Acad Med 61:1, 1964

12. Christy NP: Iatrogenic Cushing's syndrome in the human adrenal cortex. In Christy NP (ed): The Human Adrenal Cortex, p 395. New York, Harper and Row, 1971

13. Harter JG: Corticosteroids: Their physiologic use in allergic disease. NY State J Med 66:827, 1966

14. Axelrod L: Glucocorticoid therapy. Medicine 55:39, 1976

15. Ellul-Micallef R, Borthuricle RC, McHardy GJR: The time-course of response to prednisolone in chronic bronchial asthma. Clin Sci 47:105, 1974

16. Thoren L: General metabolic response to trauma including pain influence. Acta Anaesthesiol Scand (Suppl) 55:9, 1974

17. Haugen HN, Brinde-Johnsen T: The adrenal response to surgical trauma. Acta Chir Scand (Suppl) 357:100, 1966

18. Plumpton FS, Besser GU: The adrenocortical response to surgery and insulin-induced hypoglycemia in corticosteroid-treated and normal subjects. Br J Surg 55:857, 1968

19. Kehlet H, Binder C: Value of an ACTH test in assessing hypothalamic–pituitary–adrenocortical function in glucocorticoid-treated patients. Br Med J 1:147, 1973

20. Lush D, Thorpe NN, Richardson DJ et al: The effect of epidural analgesia on the adrenocortical response to surgery. Br J Anaesth 44:1169, 1972

21. Wise L, Margraf HW, Ballinger WF: A new concept on the pre- and postoperative regulation of cortisol secretion. Surgery 72:290, 1972

22. Ichikawa Y, Kawagoe M, Nishikai M et al: Plasma corticotropin (ACTH), growth hormone (GH), and 11-OHCS (hydroxycorticosteroid) response to surgery. J Lab Clin Med 78:882, 1971

23. Wise L, Margraf H, Ballinger WF: The effect of surgical trauma on the excretion and conjugation pattern of 17-ketosteroids. Surgery 71:625, 1972

24. Gill GV, Prudhoe K, Cook DB et al: Effect of surgical trauma on plasma concentrations of cyclic AMP and cortisol. Br J Surg 62:441, 1975

25. Hime DH, Bell CC, Barker F: Direct measurement of adrenal secretion during operative trauma and convalescence. Surgery 52:174, 1962

26. Greer MA, Allen CF, Gibbs FB et al: Pathways at the hypothalamic level through which traumatic stress activates ACTH secretion. Endocrinology 86:1404, 1970

27. Witorsch RN, Brodish A: Evidence for acute ACTH release by extrahypothalamic mechanisms. Endocrinology 90:1160, 1972

28. Blichert-Toft M, Hippe E, Kaalund-Jensen H: Adrenal cortical function as reflected by the plasma hydrocortisone and urinary 17-ketogenic steroids in relation to surgery in elderly patients. Acta Chir Scand 133:591, 1967

29. Speckart PF, Nicoloff JT, Bethune JE: Screening for adrenocortical insufficiency with cosyntropin (synthetic ACTH). Arch Intern Med 128:761, 1971

30. Spark RF: Simplified assessment of pituitary–adrenal reserve: Measurement of serum 11-deoxycortisol and cortisol after metapyrone. Ann Intern Med 75:717, 1971

31. Jasani MK, Freeman PA, Boyle JA et al: Studies of the rise in plasma 11-hydroxycorticosteroids (11-OHCS) in corticosteroid-treated patients with rheumatoid arthritis during surgery: Correlations with the functional integrity of the hypothalamo–pituitary–adrenal axis. Q J Med 37:407, 1968

32. Sampson PA, Brooke BN, Winstone NE: Biochemical confirmation of collapse due to adrenal failure. Lancet 1:1377, 1961

33. Sampson PA, Winstone NE, Brooke BN: Adrenal function in surgical patients after steroid therapy. Lancet 2:322, 1962

34. Danowski TS, Bonessi JV, Sabeh A et al: Probabilities of pituitary adrenal responsiveness after steroid therapy. Ann Intern Med 61:11, 1964

35. Graber AL, Ney RI, Nicholson WE et al: Natural history of pituitary–adrenal recovery following long-term suppression with corticosteroids. J Clin Endocrinol Metab 25:11, 1965

36. Livanou T, Ferriman D, James VHT: Recovery of hypothalamo–pituitary–adrenal function after corticosteroid therapy. Lancet 2:856, 1957

37. Streck W, Lockwood DH: Pituitary–adrenal recovery following short-term suppression with corticosteroids. Am J Med 66:910, 1979

38. Munro DD, Feiwel M. James VHT: The influence of topical corticosteroids on hypothalamic–pituitary–adrenal function. In Jadassohn W, Schirren CF (eds): XII Conpressus Internationalis Dermatologiae, p 94. Berlin, Springer Verlag, 1967

39. Scoggins RB, Kliman B: Percutaneous absorption of corticosteroids: Systemic effects. N Engl J Med 273:832, 1965

40. Feiwel M, James VHT, Barnett ES: Effect of potent topical steroids on plasma-cor-

tisol levels of infants and children with eczema. Lancet 2:485, 1969

41. Czarny D, Brostoff J: Effect of intranasal beta-methesone-17-valerate on perennial rhinitis and adrenal function. Lancet 1:189, 1968

42. Harter JG, Reddy WJ, Thorn GW: Studies on an intermittent corticosteroid dosage regimen. N Engl J Med 269:591, 1963

43. Ackerman GL, Nolan CM: Adrenocortical responsiveness after alternate-day corticosteroid therapy. N Engl J Med 278: 405, 1968

44. Jasani MK, Boyle JA, Dick WC et al: Corticosteroid-induced hypothalamo–pituitary–adrenal axis suppression: Prospective study using two regimens of corticosteroid therapy. Ann Rheum Dis 27:352, 1968

45. Rabhan, NB: Pituitary–adrenal suppression and Cushing's syndrome after intermittent dexamethasone therapy. Ann Intern Med 69:1141, 1968

46. Martin MM, Gaboardi F, Podolsky S et al: Intermittent steroid therapy. N Engl J Med 279:273, 1968

47. Malone DN, Brant IWB, Percy-Robb IW: Hypothalamus–pituitary–adrenal function in asthmatic patients receiving long-term corticosteroid therapy. Lancet 1:733, 1970

48. Grant SP, Forsham PH, DiRaimondo VC: Suppression of 17-hydroxycorticosteroids in plasma and urine by single and divided doses of triamcinolone. N Engl J Med 273:1115, 1965

49. Nichols T, Nugent CA, Tyler FH: Diurnal variation in suppression of adrenal function by glucocorticoids. J Clin Endocrinol Metab 25:343, 1965

50. Carter ME, James VHT: Pituitary–adrenal response to surgical stress in patients receiving corticotrophin treatment. Lancet 2:328, 1970

51. Paris J: Pituitary–adrenal suppression after protracted administration of adrenal cortical hormones. Proc Mayo Clin 36:305, 1961

52. Olin R: When should you consider a cortisone prep? Med Times 100:64, 1972

53. Byyny RL: Preventing adrenal insufficiency during surgery. Postgrad Med 67:219, 1980

54. Solem JH, Lund I: Surgery in patients treated with cortisone or cortisone-like steroids: A 10-year study. J Oslo City Hosp 19(1):3, 1969

55. Ernest I, Ekman H: Adrenalectomy in Cushing's disease, a long-term follow-up. Acta Endocrinol (Suppl) (Copenh) 160:3, 1972

56. Baker BL, Whitaker WL: Interference with wound healing by the local action of adrenocortical steroids. Endocrinology 46:544, 1950

57. Howes EL, Plotz CM, Blunt JW et al: Retardation of wound healing by cortisone. Surgery 28:177, 1950

58. Ehrlich HP, Hunt TK: Effects of cortisone and vitamin A on wound healing. Ann Surg 167:324, 1968

59. Sandberg N: Time relationship between administration of cortisone and wound healing in rats. Acta Chir Scand 27:446, 1964

60. Stern SF, Shuman A: The effect of locally administered corticosteroids (soluble and insoluble) on the healing times of surgically induced wounds in guinea pigs. J Am Podiatry Assoc 63:374, 1973

61. Vogel HG: Tensile strength of skin wounds in rats after treatment with corticosteroids. Acta Endocrinol 64:295, 1970

62. Oxlund H, Fogdestam I, Viidik A: The influence of cortisol on wound healing of the skin and distant connective tissue response. Surg Gynecol Obstet 148:876, 1979

63. Winstone NE, Brooke BN: Effects of steroid treatment on patients undergoing operation. Lancet 1:973, 1961

64. Engquist A, Backer OG, Jarnum S: Incidence of postoperative complications in patients subjected to surgery under steroid cover. Acta Chir Scand 140:343, 1974

65. Kaalund-Jensen J, Elb S: Pre-og postoper-

ative komplikationer hos kortikosteroid-behandlede patienter. Nord Med 76:975, 1966

66. Oh SH, Patterson R: Surgery in corticosteroid-dependent asthmatics. J Allergy Clin Immunol 53:345, 1974

67. Walbourn RB, Montgomery DAD, Kennedy TL: The natural history of treated Cushing's syndrome. Br J Surg 58:1, 1971

68. Bennett AH, Cain JP, Dluhy RC et al: Surgical treatment of adrenocortical hypoplasia: 20-year experience. J Urol 109:321, 1973

69. Hradec E: Surgical treatment of hyperadrenocorticism (Cushing's syndrome). J Urol 109:533, 1973

70. David DS, Grieco MH, Cushman P: Adrenal glucocorticoids after twenty years: A review of their clinically relevant consequences. J Chronic Dis 22:637, 1970

71. Fauci AS, Dale DC, Balow JE: Glucocorticoid therapy: Mechanisms of action and clinical considerations. Ann Intern Med 84:304, 1976

72. Dale DC, Petersdorf RG: Corticosteroids and infectious diseases. Med Clin North Am 57:1277, 1973

73. Staples PJ, Gerding DN, Decker JL et al: Incidence of infection in systemic lupus erythematosis. Arthritis Rheum 17:1, 1974

74. Myerowitz RC, Mederios AA, O'Brien TF: Bacterial infection in renal homotransplant recipients: A study of 53 bacteremic episodes. Am J Med 53:3081, 1972

75. Dale DC, Fauci AS, Wolff SM: Alternate-day prednisone: Leukocyte kinetics and susceptibility to infections. N Engl J Med 291:1154, 1974

Perioperative Management of Pituitary Adenoma, Hyperparathyroidism, and Pheochromocytoma

PETER J. SNYDER
MAURICE F. ATTIE
JOSEPH VERBALIS

Endocrinopathies requiring surgery present complex diagnostic and therapeutic problems. This three-part chapter provides an overview of the perioperative management of pituitary adenomas, parathyroid disease, and pheochromocytoma.

PITUITARY ADENOMAS

Treatment of pituitary adenomas is controversial. Both the natural history of the disease and the relative merits of the principal forms of treatment are incompletely understood. Although the indications for transphenoidal surgery, radiotherapy, and drug therapy will not be reviewed here, this section discusses the perioperative management of patients for whom surgical resection is recommended. Medical management of surgically treated patients consists of preoperative neurologic and hormonal evaluation, assistance with immediate postoperative management, re-

peat hormonal evaluation after surgery, and careful long-term follow-up.

Preoperative Evaluation

Patients with pituitary adenomas should undergo detailed neurologic and endocrine evaluation before treatment. Radiologic demonstration of a large and eroded sella turcica by polytomography suggests the presence of a pituitary adenoma but does not exclude that of a primary empty sella or an intrasellar aneurysm.[1] Fluid density within the sella detected by computerized tomography (CT) suggests the presence of an empty sella, and this can be confirmed by CT cisternography using metrizamide. However, if the scan demonstrates increased uptake of contrast material, a pituitary adenoma is likely, though an intrasellar aneurysm cannot be excluded.[2] Extension of an adenoma into the sphenoid sinus can be seen by CT scan. Extension of an adenoma above the sella can be detected by suprasellar enhancement on CT scan and by bitemporal hemianopsia. When surgical treatment of the presumed adenoma is elected, exclusion of an aneurysm by bilateral carotid arteriogram is mandatory before the surgery. Treatment is usually recommended when the adenoma is large and neurologic signs and symptoms are present.

The objectives of preoperative hormonal evaluation are to ensure the safety of the surgical procedure and to provide a baseline by which to judge its efficacy. In this regard, the single most important hormonal requirement is maintenance of the euthyroid state. If the patient is hypothyroid, narcotics and barbiturates administered postoperatively are metabolized more slowly and exert a greater effect than normal. Hypothyroidism should therefore be corrected before surgery. If severe visual field impairment demands immediate decompression, postoperative analgesic medications should be given in minimum doses. Hypocortisolism does not require preoperative correction as long as high doses of glucocorticoids are administered during and after surgery.

Determination of preoperative hormonal status allows assessment of the efficacy of the surgical procedure. Hormonal hypersecretion, which causes obvious clinical changes, such as acromegaly due to growth hormone hypersecretion, is reasonably easy to recognize, but recent developments in pituitary hormone assay techniques provide a means to identify and follow patients with adenomas. It is now recognized that the frequency of prolactin-secreting adenomas is 20% to 65% of all adenomas.[3] Follicle-stimulating hormone (FSH)-secreting adenomas have been documented by immunoassay and found to represent 10% of all untreated adenomas in men.[4] Thyroid-stimulating hormone (TSH)-secreting adenomas have also been described. If the degree of hypersecretion is documented biochemically before surgery, the success of resection can be judged by the fall in serum concentration of the hormone in question.

Immediate Postoperative Management

After surgery, diabetes insipidus often develops. This development is heralded by the excretion of large volumes of dilute urine and is treated by the administration of aqueous vasopressin and sufficient dextrose in water and hypotonic saline to maintain euvolemia. The dose of vasopressin required to maintain urine volume between 2 and 3 liters/day may vary from 5 μg to 20 μg every 8 to 24 hr.[4] Diabetes insipidus is usually transient, perhaps because transphenoidal surgery is likely to damage axons of vasopressin-secreting cells in the posterior pituitary and pituitary stalk rather than cell bodies in the hypothalamus. If symptomatic diabetes insipidus with more than 4 to 5 liters/day of urine volume is still present 5 to 7 days after surgery, treatment with DDAVP or Pitressin Tannate in Oil (vasopressin tannate) may be prescribed.[5] Chlorpropamide is also effective in partial diabetes insipidus but may produce hypoglycemia in patients with growth hormone and adrenocorticotropic hormone (ACTH) deficiencies.

The large doses of glucocorticoid used during surgery should be tapered to a maintenance dose by the time the patient leaves the hospital. Between the time of discharge and readmission for postoperative evaluation 4 to 6 weeks later, the patient should be assumed to be ACTH-deficient and treated with 20 to 30 mg of hydrocortisone or 5.0 to 7.5 mg of prednisone daily until formal testing of ACTH reserve is performed.

Postoperative Hormonal Evaluation

Hormonal evaluation 4 to 6 weeks after surgery allows time for regression of the traumatic effects of the procedure and possible development of hypothyroidism if TSH secretion was impaired by surgery. Determination of the adequacy of TSH secretion requires only measurement of serum thyroxine concentration. In contrast, assessment of the adequacy of ACTH secretion requires testing not only of basal secretion but also of ACTH reserve by measurement of the 11-deoxycortisol response to metyrapone or the cortisol response to insulin-induced hypoglycemia.[6] These tests should be performed 2 to 3 days after discontinuation of maintenance glucocorticoids.

Basal luteinizing hormone (LH) and FSH secretion in women under 50 years of age can be assessed by measurement of serum estradiol concentration. Demonstration of normal cyclical secretion must await the return of regular menses and the increases in basal body temperature and serum progesterone concentration that occur in the luteal phase. Testosterone secretion in men can be evaluated by measurement of serum concentration of the hormone 4 to 6 weeks after surgery, but spermatogenesis is best judged after 3 to 6 months. Screening for vasopressin deficiency can be accomplished by measurement of the 24-hr urine volume 1 or 2 days after DDAVP has been stopped and 2 to 4 days after Pitressin Tannate in Oil has been stopped. If urine volume is less than 2 liters, no further tests or treatment are necessary; if it is 4 to 5 liters or more, a water deprivation test should be performed to document diabetes insipidus.[7] Measurement of the serum concentrations of any hormones that were elevated before surgery should be repeated at this time. Visual field evaluation should also be repeated.

Additional Treatment

Deficiencies in thyroid, adrenocortical, vasopressin, and sex hormone secretion detected at the time of the postoperative evaluation should be treated in the usua. ways. If there is still hormonal secretion, the physician, in conjunction with the neurosurgeon and ophthalmologist, should make a decision regarding the need for further treatment of the adenoma. There is evidence that pituitary adenomas treated by transfrontal surgery alone recur more frequently than those treated by surgery in conjunction with postoperative radiation.[8] Transsphenoidal surgery has not been performed long enough for us to know whether postoperative radiation is necessary after this procedure as well. Residual pituitary hypersecretion after surgery is a relatively clear indication for radiotherapy, whereas correction of hypersecretion may indicate that radiation is not necessary. In the latter case, measurement of the serum concentration of the hormone in question should be repeated every 6 months. If the concentration rises above normal again, radiotherapy can be administered at that time.

If prolactin hypersecretion persists after surgery, the administration of bromocriptine should be considered along with postoperative radiation. Bromocriptine is a potent inhibitor of prolactin secretion, lowering its serum concentration to normal in most patients with prolactin-secreting adenomas.[9] Its effect on tumor size is not yet known. It may be especially helpful when hyperprolactinemia is responsible for hypogonadism. In this regard, other treatment of hypogonadism should be withheld until the effect of bromocriptine has been assessed.

SUMMARY

1. **Preoperative neurologic evaluation of patients who have pituitary adenomas should always include sella polytomography, CT scanning, and visual field assessment.**
2. **Preoperative hormonal evaluation should always include a measurement of serum thyroxine concentration and an evaluation of possible hormonal hypersecretion by the adenoma.**
3. **Immediate postoperative medical management consists of the use of maintenance glucocorticoids and the treatment of diabetes insipidus, should it occur.**
4. **Four to six weeks after surgery, evaluation should include visual field testing, measurement of basal concentrations of any hormones previously hypersecreted, and determination of adequate thyroxine and gonadal steroid levels, ACTH reserve, and vasopressin secretion. On the basis of these results, decisions regarding hormonal replacement therapy and further treatment of the adenoma can be made.**

HYPERPARATHYROIDISM

Widespread use of automated multiphasic chemistry screening has produced a dramatic rise in the apparent incidence of hyperparathyroidism and a large increase in the frequency with which parathyroid surgery is performed. One study estimated that 35,000 to 86,000 new cases of hyperparathyroidism occur yearly in the United States.[10] The success rate of parathyroid surgery in permanently normalizing the serum calcium concentration is usually greater than 80% and, in large series, over 90%.[11-13] Mortality is less than 1%. However, the procedure is beset by unique problems, including a significant failure rate, especially in certain variants of hyperparathyroidism, and, less commonly, hypocalcemia. These problems and some rarer complications of parathyroid surgery will be considered in this section.

Hypercalcemia After Parathyroid Surgery

Persistent or recurrent hypercalcemia after neck exploration for primary hyperparathyroidism can occur for a number of reasons. Hypercalcemia that is persistent or recurs after less than 3 months can be due to the following:

Parathyroid adenoma not found due to its unusual location in the neck
Enlarged gland(s) not excised (parathyroid hyperplasia)
Familial hypocalciuric hypercalcemia
Parathyroid carcinoma with residual disease
Nonparathyroid hypercalcemia

Hypercalcemia that recurs after 3 to 6 months, which usually implies the regrowth of parathyroid tissue, is likely to be caused by one of the following:

Familial forms of hyperparathyroidism, multiple endocrine neoplasia, types I and II, and familial hypocalciuric hypocalcemia
Parathyroid carcinoma
? Recurrent adenoma

In general, early recurrence, within days

or weeks, implies the presence of remaining functional parathyroid tissue. Late recurrence, after several months or years, suggests regrowth. Less frequently, removal of a portion of a large mass of hyperfunctioning parathyroid tissue results in transient remission of hypercalcemia, despite persistently high circulating levels of parathyroid hormone (PTH), indicating a degree of PTH resistance. Surgery alone can produce a transient decrease in or normalization of the serum calcium concentration. Failure of the serum calcium level to fall into the hypocalcemic or low normal range at some point during the postoperative period suggests that surgery may not have been successful.

Approximately 80% of patients with primary hyperparathyroidism have a single enlarged gland representing an adenoma, and failure to find it is the most common cause of unsuccessful surgery.[12] The glands may be in unusual locations in the neck or mediastinum. The finding of four normal glands does not exclude the presence of an adenoma, since a few patients have more than four glands. Fortunately, recurrent disease after removal of an adenoma is distinctly unusual. The distinction between hyperplasia and adenoma cannot reliably be made from the histology of one gland; it must be confirmed by the demonstration that at least one additional gland is normal.

About 15% of patients have enlargement of more than one gland, or parathyroid hyperplasia. In these cases, the surgeon performs a subtotal parathyroidectomy by removing all of the enlarged glands and leaving behind any normal gland(s) or a remnant equal in size to a normal gland. Removing too little tissue will not cure the hypercalcemia, and removing or damaging too much tissue will cause hypoparathyroidism. The surgeon must therefore identify all glands

and use careful judgment in excising them.[14] The risk of hyperparathyroidism after surgery is much higher in patients with hyperplasia than in those with adenoma. A subgroup of patients with hyperplasia, those with familial hyperparathyroidism, have an unusually high risk of recurrence, which can occur years later.

An infrequent cause of recurrent or persistent hypercalcemia is parathyroid cancer, found in less than 5% of patients operated upon for primary hyperparathyroidism. These tumors can spread into local tissues and lymph nodes or metastasize through the blood stream to distant organs. The diagnosis is often made at surgery, when a large hard mass of parathyroid tissue is found to be adherent to local structures, or on histologic examination, in which mitotic figures and capsular or blood vessel invasion are seen. Although some patients have been cured by local excision, parathyroid carcinoma is associated with high mortality. Death is usually due to uncontrollable hypercalcemia.

The management of postoperative hypercalcemia includes several measures. The diagnosis of primary hyperparathyroidism should be reconfirmed by a review and perhaps a refinement of the initial diagnostic evaluation.[15] A careful review of the operative note and surgical specimens sometimes suggests the type of pathology and the possible location of unidentified glands. Adenoma should be suspected if only normal glands were found and hyperplasia if one or more enlarged glands were found. The history should be carefully reviewed for clues to one of the familial forms of hyperparathyroidism.[16] Urinary calcium excretion should be measured to exclude familial hypocalciuric hypercalcemia, in which further surgery would not be indicated.

Finally, if the diagnosis of primary hyperparathyroidism is established, the decision to reoperate must be considered. Repeat exploration is associated with higher risk of complications, failure to find the abnormal gland(s), postoperative hypoparathyroidism, and injury to the recurrent laryngeal nerves. The success of the procedure can be increased by preoperative localization with parathyroid arteriography followed by selective venous sampling for PTH.[17] Although helpful and safe, selective venous sampling is technically difficult and is performed only at a small number of large referral centers. Less invasive methods such as CT, ultrasound, and radioisotope scans have not yet been demonstrated to be useful.

Unfortunately, chronic medical therapy of patients with symptomatic hyperparathyroidism is not entirely satisfactory. Adequate hydration should be ensured in all patients. Oral phosphates can lower both serum and urinary calcium levels and thus may be particularly useful in patients with renal stones. However, they may produce metastatic calcifications, especially if serum phosphorus rises above normal; patients with renal insufficiency are particularly at risk. Moreover, lowering the serum calcium level can theoretically increase the level of PTH secretion and cause more bone osteolysis. Inhibitors of bone osteolysis such as the diphosphonates may become available in the future. Preliminary studies in patients with hyperparathyroidism are encouraging; however, the long-term safety and efficacy of these inhibitors are as yet unknown.[18]

Hypocalcemia After Parathyroid Surgery

After successful surgery for hyperparathyroidism, the serum calcium level usually falls to 8 mg/dl to 9 mg/dl (4.0–4.5 mEq/L) between the second and the seventh postoperative days and then slowly returns to normal. There may be mild symptoms of hypocalcemia such as tingling around the mouth and fingertips. In a minority of cases, hypocalcemia is more profound and can cause tetany. The main causes of hypocalcemia in this setting are hypoparathyroidism, excess calcium uptake by remineralizing bone ("hungry bones"), and pancreatitis.

Hypoparathyroidism or inadequate functional parathyroid tissue results from excision, damage, or atrophy from long-term suppression by hypercalcemia. In the latter two instances, there may be recovery of function. In some patients said to have parathyroid insufficiency, recovery may be partial, and small amounts of calcium supplements will be needed to maintain a normal serum calcium concentration. In other patients said to have latent hypoparathyroidism, hypocalcemia occurs only when calcium homeostasis is stressed during pregnancy or gastrointestinal illness. In general, the risk of postoperative hypoparathyroidism is greatest after subtotal parathyroidectomy or repeat neck exploration.

Although hypomagnesemia is sometimes associated with hyperparathyroidism before surgery, it more often occurs postoperatively as a result of unbalanced uptake of magnesium into healing bone and prior magnesium depletion. Hypomagnesemia may cause functional hypoparathyroidism by impairing both the secretion and the action of PTH.[19,20] Hypomagnesemia renders hypocalcemia more refractory to treatment and aggravates its symptoms.[21]

Excess skeletal uptake of calcium after parathyroidectomy is seen in patients with osteitis fibrosa. The large uptake of mineral into healing bone produces profound hypocalcemia, hypophosphatemia, and hypomagnesemia. Hypocalcemia may persist for 3 months after surgery. Formation of basic bone salts releases hydrogen ions, leading in some patients to metabolic acidosis. The serum alkaline phosphatase concentration usually increases, and, for unknown reasons, renal function may transiently worsen.[22,23]

Patients who develop "hungry bones" typically have severe hyperparathyroidism with increased serum alkaline phosphatase levels, subperiosteal resorption of the phalanges, bone cysts, and brown tumors.[22] Ectopic calcifications including nephrocalcinosis, chondrocalcinosis, and band keratopathy as well as renal insufficiency are common. Patients with chronic renal failure and those with vitamin D deficiency have a higher risk than normal of developing this syndrome.

Severe or persistent hypocalcemia without the clinical findings usually associated with "hungry bones" is most likely due to hypoparathyroidism. In one series, half of the patients who eventually developed permanent hypoparathyroidism had hyperphosphatemia with serum phosphate concentrations in excess of 6 mg/dl during some part of their postoperative course, and no patient who later recovered parathyroid function had a serum phosphate level greater than 5.8 mg/dl.[22]

Measurement of PTH by radioimmunoassay or of urinary adenosine 3':5'-cyclic phosphate (cyclic AMP), an index of circulating PTH activity, can in theory separate "hungry bones" from true hypoparathyroidism, but there is little published data on this matter. In one study comparing a patient with "hungry bones" to one with permanent hypoparathyroidism, both PTH and urinary cyclic AMP were high in the former but low in the latter by the fifth postoperative day.[24] Although these tests may provide prognostic clues, it is important to test for return of normal calcium homeostasis even months after surgery by attempting to wean patients off calcium and vitamin D supplements.

The object of the management of the patient with postoperative hypocalcemia is to minimize discomfort and decrease the risk of more severe manifestations, such as seizures and laryngospasm. Before surgery, the patient should be warned that numbness and tingling may develop postoperatively and told that these are an indication of successful surgery. A useful approach is to ask about symptoms and monitor the Chvostek sign daily. Postoperative laboratory evaluation includes a daily determination of the serum calcium concentration and, in severe hypocalcemia, levels of serum phosphorus, creatinine, and magnesium. If hypocalcemia persists for more than 1 week, an index of PTH concentration, measurement of PTH by radioimmunoassay, or urinary cyclic AMP may be useful.

Mild symptoms of hypocalcemia can be treated by an increase in dietary calcium. Occasionally, oral calcium supplements are required. For most patients, 2 to 3 g/day of elemental calcium in divided doses as often as every 6 hr provides relief, but, occasionally, several times this dose is required. It is best to allow some degree of hypocalcemia, because hypercalcemia or even a normal calcium level may inhibit the recovery of suppressed parathyroid tissue.

Severe hypocalcemia persisting beyond the first few days after surgery calls for the use of a vitamin D preparation with a rapid onset of action and a short enough biologic half-life to allow for quick discontinuation of effect. Vitamin D_2 or ergocalciferol, the most commonly used preparation for chronic hypoparathyroidism, takes several weeks to achieve a therapeutic effect. Calcitriol or 1,25-dihydroxycholecalciferol, the most potent and rapidly effective analogue, begins to work within 1 to 2 days but is presently approved in the United States only for renal osteodystrophy. Dihydrotachysterol requires 1 to 2 weeks to exert adequate effect, but this time can be shortened through a loading dose of 4 mg/day for 2 days, 2 mg/day for 2 days, and then 1 mg/day.

While a patient is on vitamin D therapy, the physician should monitor the serum calcium concentration frequently, aiming for a level high enough to suppress symptoms but enough below the mid-normal range to allow stimulation of any remaining parathyroid tissue and limit hypercalciuria. If therapy is necessary beyond the first few months after surgery, which would suggest the presence of permanent hypoparathyroidism, the serum calcium concentration should be maintained within or close to the lower half of the normal range in order to prevent cataracts. In general, it is preferable to adjust the dose of vitamin D to allow for concurrent administration of at least 1 g/day of oral calcium. This prevents fluctuations in serum calcium resulting from changes in dietary calcium and allows for more rapid restoration of normocalcemia if the serum calcium concentration rises above the desired level. Slow tapering withdrawal of the vitamin D preparation before the calcium should begin as soon after surgery as possible. If this is still not possible after the third month following surgery, it is likely that life-long therapy for hypoparathyroidism will be required.

Hypomagnesemia makes hypocalcemia more difficult to treat.[25] Magnesium can be replaced with parenteral magnesium sulfate in which 1 g of the salt contains 8.12 mEq of magnesium. The dosage and rate of administration are determined by the serum magnesium concentration, which is only a rough index of the deficiency of this primarily intracellular ion as well as the severity of hypocalcemia and level of renal function. In an average-sized adult with moderate to severe hypomagnesemia and normal renal function, 40 to 100 mEq may be given in an intravenous infusion or intramuscularly in divided doses on the first day. Smaller doses may be required on subsequent days to maintain the serum magnesium concentration. Monitoring of serum magnesium level is mandatory in patients receiving vigorous replacement.

Occasionally, severe symptomatic hypocalcemia persists despite vigorous replacement of calcium and magnesium. Since vitamin D preparations do not work quickly enough, treatment with intravenous calcium is indicated. A solution of 10 ml to 30 ml of 10% calcium gluconate containing 180 mg to 450 mg of elemental calcium in 500 ml of normal saline can be administered over 3 to 12 hr while serum calcium concentration and neuromuscular irritability are monitored. If parenteral calcium is still required after 3 to 4 days and oral calcium is insufficient, a vitamin D preparation should be given. Severe full-blown tetany requires prompt intravenous administration of 10 ml to 20 ml of 10% calcium gluconate over 10 to 15 min followed by a continuous infusion as described above. Recently, parathyroid autotransplantation into the forearm has been used in the therapy of postoperative hypoparathyroidism.[26] Although the long-term consequences of grafting abnormal parathyroid tissue are unknown, this technique may be useful in patients with primary hyperplasia undergoing subtotal parathyroidectomy and in patients requiring reoperation for persistent or recurrent hyperparathyroidism.

Miscellaneous Postoperative Problems

Other complications of parathyroid surgery occur less frequently. Pancreatitis, arthritis, and metabolic acidosis usually occur in the subgroup of patients who have severe hyperparathyroidism and osteitis fibrosa. Acute pancreatitis may occur in the early postoperative period and, if severe, can exacerbate postoperative hypocalcemia. Many patients with acute pancreatitis have pancreatic calcifications visible on abdominal roentgenograms. Acute arthritis, including gout and pseudogout, occur with increased frequency in hyperparathyroidism and may be precipitated by parathyroid surgery. The acute arthritis of pseudogout may be a unique complication of parathyroid surgery.[27] Chondrocalcinosis may be seen on radiographs of joints, and the diagnosis can be confirmed by the demonstration of typical crystals in synovial fluid. Hyperchloremic metabolic acidosis in association with a deterioration in renal function can occur transiently after parathyroidectomy. Other cases of postoperative renal insufficiency must be ruled out. Patients in this category usually have a mild acidosis preoperatively as well as some degree of renal insufficiency.

Injury to the recurrent laryngeal nerve is usually unilateral, probably due to edema, and transient, with return of function within 2 to 3 months. The major symptom of unilateral paresis is hoarseness. Bilateral nerve injury is more serious because the cords are usually paralyzed in mid-position and can produce airway obstruction requiring tracheos-

tomy. Return of function may occur over several months; if not, a transoral arytenoidectomy may be necessary to enlarge the airway. Indirect laryngoscopy should be performed routinely after the procedure and preoperatively in any patient who has had previous neck surgery. The finding of clinically inapparent unilateral paresis can serve as a warning of potential danger in the exploration of the contralateral side of the neck.[28]

The Patient with Familial Hyperparathyroidism

Syndromes of familial hyperparathyroidism, outlined in Table 10-1, may be seen in as many as 10% of patients undergoing surgery for primary hyperparathyroidism. The most prevalent syndrome is multiple endocrine neoplasia, type I (MEN I), in which hyperparathyroidism may be the earliest and only manifestation.[29] Familial hypocalciuric hypercalcemia (FHH), although less common, is becoming increasingly apparent, often only in retrospect after parathyroid surgery has failed. MEN II is a rare disorder in which hyperparathyroidism is not a frequent manifestation. Documentation of these traits is important in patients with hyperparathyroidism for a number of reasons. In MEN I and II, other coexisting endocrinopathies may need to be managed before parathyroid surgery is performed. Patients with FHH have enlargement of more than one gland or parathyroid hyperplasia. Unlike patients with adenomas, those with FHH have frequent recurrences, up to 35% in one series, and require periodic monitoring of serum calcium concentration.[11] Furthermore, parathyroidectomy is usually not appropriate therapy for FHH. Patients are usually asymptomatic and have little evidence of clinical disease de-

Table 10-1. Features of the Syndromes of Familial Hypercalcemia

Syndrome	Associated Endocrinopathies	Inheritance	Unique Biochemical Features	Clinical Manifestations	Subtotal Parathyroidectomy
Multiple Endocrine Neoplasia, Type I	Anterior pituitary islet cells	Autosomal dominant	Hyperprolactinemia, hypergastrinemia, hyperinsulinemia, etc.	Similar to nonfamilial hyperparathyroidism	Useful (recurrence rate higher than in nonfamilial hyperparathyroidism)
Multiple Endocrine Neoplasia, Type II	Medullary thyroid cancer or hyperplasia; pheochromocytoma	Autosomal dominant	Hypercalcitonemia	Similar to nonfamilial hyperparathyroidism	Useful (recurrence rate higher than in nonfamilial hyperparathyroidism)
Familial Hypocalciuric Hypercalcemia	None	Autosomal dominant	Low urinary calcium	Usually none	Usually not effective

spite lifelong hypercalcemia. Nephrolithiasis and other renal complications are rare, perhaps because of relative hypocalciuria, and bone involvement has never been described. The biochemical features of FHH are similar to those of typical primary hyperparathyroidism, making confusion between the two frequent.[30]

Screening tests using both hormone assays and radiologic procedures are available for detection of endocrine hyperplasia or neoplasia in the MEN syndromes.[29] These tests should be reserved for patients with suggestive symptoms, signs, or family histories and for patients with recurrent hyperparathyroidism in whom prior surgery has revealed parathyroid hyperplasia. However, FHH should be considered in all candidates for parathyroid surgery except those with obvious bone disease or renal calcifications. Screening can be accomplished with a 24-hr urine collection for calcium. Virtually all patients with FHH but only a minority with typical primary hyperparathyroidism excrete less than 250 mg/day of calcium. The ratio of calcium to creatinine clearance offers even better discrimination; a value below 0.01 is strongly suggestive of FHH.[21] The diagnosis is further substantiated by the finding of hypocalciuric hypercalcemia in first-degree relatives.

SUMMARY

1. Patient education consists of an explanation of the unique, though uncommon, complications associated with neck exploration and parathyroid surgery. These include significant transient or permanent hypocalcemia and recurrent laryngeal nerve injury. Mild symptoms of hypocalcemia are common, and patients should be advised to expect them.

2. Reversible complications of hypercalcemia include dehydration, mental obtundation, and electrolyte disorders. These should be corrected before surgery.

3. Patients with one of the familial forms of hyperparathyroidism have a higher risk than normal of recurrence and may have other endocrinopathies. Familial hypocalciuric hypercalcemia can be detected through urine calcium excretion. Parathyroid surgery in this disorder is usually not indicated and is rarely successful.

4. The serum calcium concentration should be monitored daily during the initial postoperative period. Signs and symptoms of hypocalcemia should be routinely monitored.

5. Hypercalcemia after surgery indicates the presence of excess residual parathyroid tissue or an incorrect diagnosis. If, after re-evaluation, the diagnosis of primary hyperparathyroidism is firmly established, preoperative localization procedures and repeat neck exploration are indicated.

6. Mild postoperative hypocalcemia with mild symptoms is common, usually transient, and can be followed or treated with increased dietary calcium. Severe hypocalcemia requires large amounts of oral calcium supplements, rapidly acting preparations of vitamin D, and, depending on the urgency and severity of the disorder, intravenous calcium. Magnesium deficits can aggravate hypocalcemia and should be corrected. Hypocalcemia is caused by excess mineral uptake by bone or hypoparathyroidism. The latter can be permanent and may require life-long therapy.

PHEOCHROMOCYTOMA

Even with optimal management and anticipation of all potential complications, the surgical resection of pheochromocytomas is often difficult. The surgical mortality rate for pheochromocytoma resection in experienced hands at major medical centers is between 1% and 3%.[31] A complete understanding of the pathophysiology of excess catecholamine secretion, the spectrum of potential complications that may arise during surgery, and the therapeutic options available for treatment of these complications is essential.

Preoperative Preparation

Reliable assays of urinary catecholamines and their metabolites are essential to the establishment of a diagnosis of pheochromocytoma. Before surgery, localization of the tumor should be attempted and unresectable metastatic disease excluded. Two to three percent of pheochromocytomas may present as neck or thoracic masses.[32]

The goal of preoperative medical preparation is to render the patient normotensive and relatively free of the effects of excessive catecholamine secretion for a sufficient period of time to allow the reestablishment of normal vascular tone and intravascular volume. Without such preparation, there is an increased incidence of intraoperative complications, including severe refractory hypotension after removal of the tumor. This refractory hypotension is felt to be secondary to two effects of chronically elevated serum catecholamine levels; decreased intravascular volume due to increased vascular tone, and relative insensitivity of vascular alpha-adrenergic receptors to normal levels of circulating catecholamines after re-

moval of the tumor. Since only a small percentage of patients with pheochromocytomas actually have low plasma volumes, the latter mechanism may be predominant.[33]

Several investigators have challenged the importance of preoperative preparation.[34] Nonetheless, the bulk of clinical evidence remains in favor of preoperative preparation with alpha-adrenergic blockers because of the smooth anesthetic course and the low incidence of intraoperative complications.[35] Therapy might be considered optional in patients without sustained hypertension or frequent paroxysmal attacks. However, even "normal" blood pressure may represent a significant elevation, depending on the baseline level.

Patients are generally prepared with alpha- and beta-adrenergic blocking agents, the exception being those requiring emergency surgery for retroperitoneal or intraabdominal hemorrhage from vascular tumors. Phenoxybenzamine is the drug of choice for long-term alpha-adrenergic blockade. Phentolamine has a shorter half-life and causes wider fluctuations in blood pressure, it is therefore less desirable for preoperative preparation and long-term use. Inhibitors of catecholamine synthesis such as alpha-methylparatyrosine have been used successfully but have relatively serious side-effects; they remain investigational.[36]

The dosage of phenoxybenzamine should be increased slowly over several days until the patient is normotensive and relatively free of paroxysmal symptoms. Occasionally, orthostatic hypotension supervenes before total disappearance of paroxysmal symptoms; in these cases, a compromise between the symptoms of the pheochromocytoma and those of excessive alpha-adrenergic blockade must be accepted. A usual starting dose is 20 mg once or twice daily, and a total dose of 40 to 100 mg/day is sufficient to control most patients. Higher doses of up to 200 mg/day are needed only occasionally. Side-effects, usually minimal, include mild sedation, nasal congestion, gastrointestinal distress, and sometimes postural hypotension with reflex tachycardia. Treatment for 2 weeks after the achievement of normal blood pressure is sufficient for reversal of the major effects of chronic catecholamine hypersecretion. Longer courses may be needed when other medical problems require attention before surgery. A patient with a pheochromocytoma should not undergo any surgery requiring general anesthesia before resection of the pheochromocytoma; even with adequate alpha-adrenergic blockade, the risk of complications is too great to warrant other than essential emergency procedures.

Patients may safely continue the drug through the morning of surgery. If it is given at the appropriate dose level, it will not significantly interfere with attempts at surgery to localize the tumor by intra-abdominal palpation. Even with complete alpha-adrenergic blockade, the beta-adrenergic-mediated tachycardia can still be used as a marker after tumor manipulation. When preoperative localization has been suboptimal and intra-abdominal palpation is important, the last dose of phenoxybenzamine may be given 2 to 3 days before surgery and the shorter-acting agent phentolamine substituted until the time of surgery. The latter is given in doses sufficient to control hypertension, usually 2 mg to 5 mg intramuscularly every 4 to 6 hr. Preoperative alpha-adrenergic blockade also allows invasive preoperative localization procedures such as arteriography to be performed with a low risk of severe hypertensive crisis.

Preoperative preparation with beta-adrenergic blockade is indicated for the control of persistent tachycardia, cardiac arrhythmias, and angina. Some investigators have advocated routine preoperative use of beta-adrenergic blockers such as propranolol, 10 mg to 20 mg every 6 hr for several days, but there is no clear evidence that such therapy alters the intraoperative course. Beta-adrenergic blocking agents should never be started until adequate alpha-adrenergic blockade has been achieved; if they are begun too soon, a paradoxical elevation of blood pressure may result from the unopposed alpha-adrenergic effect of the secreted catecholamines.[36] Consequently, an increased dose of alpha-adrenergic blocking agents may be needed, although sometimes the addition of beta-adrenergic blockers may decrease the dosage of alpha-adrenergic blockers necessary for blood pressure control. The use of enemas in bowel preparations may induce a hypertensive crisis. This effect is minimized with adequate alpha-adrenergic blockade, and the use of a liquid diet in combination with oral cathartics has been recommended.

Intraoperative Management

The three major concerns during surgery are cardiac arrhythmias, hypertensive crises, and maintenance of normal intravascular volume. The patient should have a central venous pressure line, an arterial catheter, and electrocardiographic leads attached before surgery. Intubation can be safely accomplished with standard preanesthetic agents and muscle relaxants. Agents that probably should be avoided because of reported tachycardia and hypotension are atropine, narcotics, and phenothiazines.

After much controversy about the appropriate anesthetic agent, there is now a consensus that the benefits of halogenated hydrocarbons outweigh their drawbacks.[37] The major advantage of these agents is their ability to antagonize the vasopressor effects of catecholamines on peripheral vasculature. As a result, some of the fluctuations in blood pressure that occur during surgery can be controlled by changes in the level of anesthesia given. These anesthetics tend to potentiate the arrhythmogenic effects of catecholamines on myocardial tissue; however, arrhythmias, whether they occur during induction of anesthesia or during surgery, are generally easily controlled with propranolol or lidocaine.

The above-mentioned arrhythmias are frequently ventricular in origin and show a more consistent response to propranolol than to other antiarrhythmic agents. Initial treatment consists of boluses of 1 mg to 2 mg of propranolol given intravenously up to a total dose of 5 mg at any one time. Failure of the patient to respond to initial doses or rapid recurrencce of arrhythmia after 5 mg of propranolol requires the intravenous injection of lidocaine in a bolus of 75 mg to 100 mg followed by appropriate maintenance infusion, if necessary. Lidocaine should be the initial therapy if propranolol is contraindicated because of asthma, chronic obstructive lung disease, or congestive heart failure. Precipitation of congestive heart failure by propranolol in patients with no pre-existing cardiac disease has not been a problem at these doses.

Maintenance of normal blood pressure avoids catastrophic events such as intracerebral hemorrhage and myocardial infarction and helps to preserve hemostasis. The vascular nature of the tumor and alpha-adrenergic blockade makes excessive bleeding a potential problem that can be seriously exacerbated by sudden increases in blood pressure.

Several options are available for control of acute elevations of blood pressure during induction and surgery. The standard accepted approach uses intravenous boluses of the short-acting alpha-adrenergic blocker phentolamine in doses of 1 mg to 5 mg, as needed. The desired effect is achieved within minutes but may be exceedingly short in the presence of extremely high serum catecholamine levels. As much of this agent as necessary, often up to 50 mg/hr, should be used for control of blood pressure. Alternatively, a continuous infusion of phentolamine may be used at levels of 2 to 50 mg/hr titrated to fluctuations in blood pressure.[38] As mentioned above, the level of halogenated hydrocarbon anesthesia can also be varied as an alternative or synergistic measure to control hypertensive episodes. In patients who have been adequately prepared with phenoxybenzamine, fluctuations of blood pressure before manipulation of the tumor can be adequately controlled by an increase in anesthesia. However, even in well-prepared patients, phentolamine is generally required for the large increases in blood pressure that occur with manipulation.

An alternative approach is the infusion of sodium nitroprusside for maintenance of normal blood pressure during induction of anesthesia and surgery.[39] Because this drug is not widely used, and because of reported problems with hypotension in some cases, use of this agent should be limited to physicians with experience. However, sodium nitroprusside is a potentially useful alternative in unusually refractory cases of severe intraoperative hypertension.

Hypotension usually follows removal of a pheochromocytoma or ligation of the last major venous effluent from the tumor even in patients with alpha-adrenergic blocking agents. It often responds poorly to pressor agents but, in most cases, can be reversed or even prevented by the infusion of adequate volumes of intravenous fluid. As discussed earlier, this suggests the presence of either true or functional hypovolemia. Since the volumes required are usually significantly in excess of surgical blood loss, monitoring of central venous pressure is essential as a guide fluid therapy.

Throughout surgery, liberal replacement of estimated surgical blood loss with intravenous saline solutions is indicated. Whole blood or packed red cells should be used only for excessive surgical blood loss of greater than 2 to 3 units, since, postoperatively, some of the infused fluid may have to be removed with diuretics. In addition, an infusion of several units of colloid plasma expander may be started at the beginning of the operation and just before removal of the tumor to decrease the need for rapid infusions of volume. Even with these measures, a precipitous fall in blood pressure should be anticipated at the time of tumor resection and treated with rapid infusion of both saline and colloid as necessary for maintenance of a systolic blood pressure of greater than 100 mm. If these maneuvers fail to restore adequate blood pressure, pressor agents must be used. Direct-acting sympathomimetic amines such as norepinephrine are the most efficacious. Pressor therapy should be necessary only for a short period of time while additional intravenous fluids are infused to expand intravascular volume.

The occurrence of significant hypotension after removal of the tumor is an encouraging sign that all of the pheochro-mocytoma tissue has been resected. However, neither this occurrence nor preoperative localization procedures demonstrating a single mass lesion obviates the need for subsequent thorough abdominal exploration for other tumor foci. Most reported series have found a 10% to 20% incidence of multiple or multicentric pheochromocytomas with a significantly higher incidence in patients with multiple endocrine neoplasia syndrome types II and III. Many of these multiple tumors are too small to be detected by preoperative localization procedures but can be found through a meticulous abdominal exploration. The absence of a significant fall in blood pressure to hypotensive levels should prompt a careful search for multiple tumors or metastases. Because of the need for thorough abdominal exploration, surgeons consider an anterior abdominal approach mandatory for adequate exposure of the entire suprarenal and para-aortic regions, where pheochromocytoma tissue is most likely to be found.

A final issue in the intraoperative management of pheochromocytoma is corticosteroid replacement. If both adrenals contain tumor, they should be removed in their entirety to prevent future local recurrence. When this is done, the patient should receive stress doses of hydrocortisone, a bolus of 100 mg intravenously followed by a continuous infusion of 100 mg every 8 hr. Similar corticosteroid coverage should probably also be started after unilateral adrenalectomy and any significant surgical manipulation other than inspection and palpation of the contralateral adrenal. Such treatment should be continued until the function of the remaining adrenal tissue can be assessed by ACTH stimulation testing.

Postoperative Care

The early postoperative care of patients who have had resection of pheochromocytomas requires the same careful monitoring as during the procedure. New or persistent hypotension requiring large amounts of intravenous fluid or pressors is infrequently seen, and its presence raises the possibility of intra-abdominal or retroperitoneal bleeding. More commonly, within the first 24 hr one sees mild to moderate hypertension, which is due to the volume expansion necessary to maintain blood pressure during surgery. This postoperative hypertension can be explained by re-establishment of normal alpha-adrenergic receptor sensitivity to physiologic levels of serum catecholamines in addition to decreased serum levels of the alpha-adrenergic blocking agents used during the operation. There is thus a reversal of the functional hypovolemia caused by the sudden decrease in catecholamine levels at the time of tumor resection and subsequent increased capacitance of the vascular system. This true hypervolemia is readily treated with small doses of diuretics, or, if the blood pressure elevation is mild, the patient may be allowed to diurese the excess fluid spontaneously. Alpha-and beta-blockers are not indicated for postoperative hypervolemic hypertension.

Markedly elevated blood pressures or failure of the patient to respond to reasonable doses of diuretics should raise the possibility of residual pheochromocytoma tissue. In this case, a trial dose of phentolamine in an intravenous bolus of 5 mg should be given. A prompt fall in blood pressure strongly suggests residual pheochromocytoma. If an appropriately careful exploration of the entire abdomen has been performed, the hypertension should be treated as needed and the presence of residual pheochromocytoma confirmed by measurement of urinary catecholamines and their metabolites 5 to 7 days after surgery. Even when all pheochromocytoma tissue is resected, elevated urinary catecholamine levels may persist for 4 to 5 days.[36] If residual tumor is confirmed biochemically, a repeat search for extra-abdominal tumor in the thorax or neck is indicated before re-exploration of the abdomen should be considered. A rare reported cause of postoperative hypertension is ligation of a renal artery, the presence of which, if suspected, can be ascertained by a radionucleotide renal perfusion scan. However, the most common type of persistent hypertension after resection of a pheochromocytoma is simply essential hypertension of no identifiable origin, occurring in up to 25% in some series. Just as essential hypertension does not protect patients from subsequently developing a pheochromocytoma, patients with a pheochromocytoma have the same incidence of underlying essential hypertension as the rest of the population. Once the presence of residual pheochromocytoma has been ruled out, this hypertension can be treated with the usual antihypertensive agents.

Patients with only mild or transient postoperative hypertension should experience uneventful postoperative recovery, and central venous pressure and intra-arterial catheters may be removed within 24 to 48 hr. Measurement of 24-hr urinary catecholamines and their metabolites should be performed after recovery from surgery; this remains the definitive test for residual tumor. Hydrocortisone can be rapidly tapered over 2 to 3 days to a maintenance dose. If a total adrenalectomy was performed, replacement is needed indefinitely; if some adrenal tissue is felt to be viable, an ACTH stimulation will determine the need for chronic replacement therapy.

Patients found to have metastatic or otherwise unresectable pheochromocytoma tissue should be treated medically with long-acting alpha-adrenergic blockers, as described earlier in the section on Preoperative Preparation. Neither radiotherapy nor chemotherapy has been very successful in controlling progression of the tumor. Since most of the tumors are relatively slow-growing, death is often due to the cardiovascular effects of increasingly elevated levels of serum catecholamines.

SUMMARY

1. **The goal of preoperative medical preparation in pheochromocytoma is to render the patient normotensive. Treatment should be instituted with phenoxybenzamine. Propranolol should be added for persistent tachycardia, arrhythmias, or angina.**
2. **Major intraoperative concerns are cardiac arrhythmias, hypertensive crises, and maintenance of a normal intravascular volume. Arrhythmias are usually controlled with either propranolol or lidocaine. Intravenous boluses of phentolamine should be used for blood pressure control.**
3. Postoperative hypertension is usually due to hypervolemia and responds to diuretics.
4. **If blood pressure does not fall postoperatively, the possibility of unresected pheochromocytoma should be considered. Persistent hypotension may necessitate re-exploration for bleeding.**

REFERENCES

1. Bruneton JN, Drourillard JP, Sabstier, JC et al: Normal variants of the sella turcica. Neuroradiology 131:99, 1979
2. Hatam A, Bergstrom M, Greitz T: Diagnosis of sellar and parasellar lesions by computed tomography. Neuroradiology 18:249, 1979
3. Frantz AC: Prolactin. N Engl J Med 298:201, 1978
4. Snyder PJ, Bigdeli H, Gardner DF et al: Gonadal function in 50 men with untreated pituitary adenomas. J Clin Endocrinol Metab 48:309, 1979
5. Robinson AG: DDAVP in the treatment of pituitary adenomas. N Engl J Med 294:507, 1976
6. Spark RF: Simplified assessment of pituitary–adrenal reserve. Measurement of 11-deoxycortisol and cortisol after metyrapone. Ann Intern Med 75:717, 1971
7. Miller M, Dalakos T, Moses AM et al: Recognition of partial defects in antidiuretic hormone secretion. Ann Intern Med 73:721, 1970
8. Sheline GE: Untreated and recurrent chromophobe adenomas of the pituitary gland. Am J Roentgenol Rad Ther Nucl Med 112:768, 1971
9. Carter JN, Tyson JE, Tolis G et al: Prolactin-secreting tumors and hypogonadism in 22 men. N Engl J Med 299:847, 1978
10. Heath H, Hodgson SF, Kennedy MA: Primary hyperparathyroidism: Incidence, morbidity and potential economic impact in a community. N Engl J Med 302:189, 1980
11. Clark OH, Way LW, Hunt TK: Recurrent hyperparathyroidism. Am Surg 184:391, 1976
12. Wang CA: Parathyroid re-exploration: A clinical and pathological study of 112 cases. Ann Surg 186:140, 1977
13. Attie JN, Wise L, Mir R et al: The rationale against subtotal parathyroidectomy for primary hyperparathyroidism. Am J Surg 136:437, 1978
14. Wang CA: Surgery of the parathyroid glands. Adv Surg 5:109, 1971

15. Mundy GR, Cowe DH, Fiskin R: Primary hyperparathyroidism: Changes in the pattern of clinical presentation. Lancet 1:1317, 1980

16. Marx SJ, Spiegel AM, Brown EM et al: Family studies in patients with primary parathyroid hyperplasia. Am J Med 62:705, 1977

17. Brennan MF, Doppman JL, Marx SJ et al: Preoperative parathyroid surgery for persistent hyperparathyroidism. Surgery 83:669, 1978

18. Douglas DL, Russel RGR, Preston CJ et al: Effect of dichloromethylene disphosphonate in Paget's disease of bone and in hypercalcemia due to primary hyperparathyroidism or malignant disease. Lancet 1:1044, 1980

19. Rude RK, Oldham SB, Sharp CF et al: Parathyroid hormone secretion in magnesium deficiency. J Clin Endocrinol Metab 47:800, 1978

20. Rude RK, Oldham SB, Singer FR: Functional hypoparathyroidism and PTH end organ resistance secondary to human magnesium deficiency. Clin Endocrinol 5:209, 1976

21. Marx SJ, Stock JL, Attie MF et al: Familial hypocalciuric hypercalcemia: Recognition among patients referred after unsuccessful parathyroid exploration. Ann Intern Med 92:351, 1980

22. Mallette LE, Bilezikian JP, Heath DA et al: Primary hyperparathyroidism: Clinical and biochemical features. Medicine 53:127, 1974

23. Purnell DC, Scholz DA, Smith LH et al: Treatment of primary hypoparathyroidism. Am J Med 56:800, 1974

24. Broadus AE: Nephrogenous cyclic AMP as a parathyroid function test. Nephron 23:136, 1979

25. Pösler A, Rabinowitz D: Magnesium-induced reversal of vitamin-D resistance in hypoparathyroidism. Lancet 1:803, 1973

26. Wells SA, Ross AJ, Dale JK et al: Transplantation of the parathyroid glands. Surg Clin North Am 59:167, 1980

27. Bilezikian JP, Aurbach GD, Connor TB et al: Pseudogout following parathyroidectomy. Lancet 1:445, 1973

28. Edis AJ: Prevention and management of complications associated with thyroid and parathyroid surgery. Surg Clin North Am 59:83, 1979

29. Marx SJ, Spiegel AM, Brown EM et al: Family studies in patients with primary parathyroid hyperplasia. Am J Med 62:698, 1977

30. Marx SJ: Familial hypocalciuric hypercalcemia. N Engl J Med 303:810, 1980

31. Manger WM, Gifford RW Jr: Current concepts of pheochromocytoma. Cardiovasc Med 3:289, 1978

32. Stewart BH, Bravo EL, Haaga J et al: Localization of pheochromocytoma by computed tomography. N Engl Med 299:460, 1978

33. Sjoerdsma A, Engelman K, Waldmann TA et al: Pheochromocytoma: Current concepts of diagnosis and treatment. Ann Intern Med 65:1302, 1966

34. Manger WM, Gifford RW Jr: Pheochromocytoma. New York, Springer-Verlag, 1977

35. Loudsberg L, Young JB: Pheochromocytoma. In Bondy PK, Rosenberg LE (eds): Metabolic Control and Disease, p 1663. Philadelphia, WB Saunders, 1980

36. Engelman K: Pheochromocytoma. Clin Endocrinol Metab 6:769, 1977

37. Pratilas V, Pratila MG: Anesthetic management of pheochromocytoma. Can Anaesth Soc J 26:253, 1979

38. Gitlow SE, Pertsemlidis D, Bertani LM: Management of patients with pheochromocytoma. Am Heart J 82:557, 1971

39. Daggett P, Verner I, Carruthers M: Intraoperative management of pheochromocytoma with sodium nitroprusside. Br Med J 2:311, 1978

11

The Surgical Patient with Diabetes

JOHN A. SCARLETT

Despite the advances made in the treatment of diabetes mellitus in the last 50 years, surgery continues to be potentially more dangerous for the diabetic than for the nondiabetic patient. The mortality rate for diabetics undergoing surgical procedures is estimated to be between 3% and 13%, while morbidity may approach 20%.[1,2] The most common causes of this increased risk are cardiovascular complications and postoperative infections.

Even young diabetic patients with no symptoms of ischemic heart disease may have significant coronary artery disease.[3–5] If myocardial infarction occurs, it is more likely to be fatal in diabetics than in nondiabetics.[6] Diabetics frequently suffer from autonomic neuropathy, and painless myocardial infarction or sudden death may result.[7–9]

Over 75% of diabetics undergoing surgery are over the age of 50.[1] The incidence of peripheral vascular disease, obesity, and renal insufficiency is increased in this population, as is the concomitant risk of surgery. Wound healing is delayed in poorly controlled diabetics, probably as a result of atherosclerotic vascular disease and small vessel disease.[10] Infections occur frequently, often in the extremities, and involve an unusual preponderance of

gram-negative organisms.[11–13] Despite these risks, it is possible to successfully manage diabetic patients during surgery with a logical approach that stresses close cooperation among anesthesiologist, surgeon, and internist.[14,15]

CARBOHYDRATE METABOLISM AND SURGERY

The regulation of carbohydrate metabolism is a complex subject.[16,17] Ingested carbohydrate, protein, and fat are stored as glycogen, triglycerides, and protein. Insulin is the predominant anabolic hormone. It stimulates hepatic lipogenesis and glycogenesis, directs glucose into muscle and adipose tissue, and stimulates protein synthesis. Insulin simultaneously inhibits lipolysis and gluconeogenesis, thus avoiding net substrate loss from peripheral tissue. Growth hormone is also anabolic but is quantitatively far less important than insulin.

As a person switches from the fed to the fasting state, insulin levels fall, and catabolic hormones use tissue stores to maintain blood glucose concentrations and provide energy for metabolic needs. Cortisol causes protein breakdown peripherally, sending precursors to the liver, where the hormone also enhances hepatic gluconeogenesis. Glucagon also stimulates hepatic gluconeogenesis and glycogenolysis, and catecholamines promote lipolysis and glycogenolysis. Concurrently, insulin levels fall, and the net effect is a flow of fatty acids and amino acids away from peripheral tissue toward the liver, with an overall loss of peripheral protein and fat. Fatty acids converted by the liver to ketone bodies become an important substrate during starvation.

This sequence is disrupted by the stress of trauma and surgery. Normal nondiabetic individuals frequently become hyperglycemic during surgery and develop associated deficiencies in insulin and C peptide, a response probably related to catecholamine inhibition of the pancreatic beta-cell.[18-25] Insulin resistance also occurs during surgery, most likely owing to increased catecholamine and cortisol levels.[21,23,26,27,28] Although glucagon and growth hormone are elevated after trauma and surgery, their effects in the surgical patient are unclear.[24,29-34] Protein synthesis is impaired, probably owing to a defect in the uptake of precursor amino acids.[35-37] Fatty acid and ketone body levels are paradoxically lowered in normal individuals undergoing surgery. There are no data regarding the effect of surgery on insulin receptor number or affinity in diabetic or nondiabetic patients.

The diabetic patient receiving glucose-free fluids intraoperatively demonstrates only modest hyperglycemia similar to that seen in the nondiabetic patient undergoing surgery.[24,39] However, when glucose is administered to a diabetic patient during surgery, there is often a significant increase in plasma glucose. In some maturity-onset diabetics and in virtually all juvenile-onset diabetics, diabetic keto-acidosis (DKA) or hyperosmolar hyper-glycemic nonketotic coma (HHNK) may result if adequate insulin is not provided.[40-43]

Anesthesia may affect carbohydrate metabolism in both normal and diabetic patients. Ether causes hyperglycemia, suppression of insulin secretion, and fatty acid mobilization by raising catecholamine and cortisol levels.[44] Halothane and other inhalational agents cause similar but less pronounced effects. Extradural and spinal anesthesia have the least effect and in fact may abolish the hyperglycemic response to surgery, even though insulin secretion remains suppressed.[20,45] The effects of anesthesia may be more pronounced in diabetic patients than in normal persons but usually present no significant complications in management.

PREOPERATIVE EVALUATION AND MANAGEMENT

A careful history and physical examination remain the cornerstones of the preoperative evaluation of the diabetic patient. Of particular importance are an in-depth review of the electrocardiogram (ECG) and a complete urinalysis. Before elective surgery, it is acceptable to substitute urine glucose measurements for multiple blood glucose determinations only if a good correlation between renal glucose threshold and blood glucose level has been documented.

Any preoperative evaluation that exposes the diabetic patient to intravenous contrast material should be done only after noninvasive means of evaluation have been exhausted and the patient has been fully hydrated before injection of the dye. Intravenous injection of contrast material has been associated with acute renal failure in diabetics, usually in patients with pre-existing renal disease but also in patients with previously normal serum creatinine levels.[46]

Patients with diabetic cardiac autonomic neuropathy are at risk for intraoperative cardiorespiratory arrest.[9,47] A patient who has evidence of autonomic neuropathy and whose variation in heart rate during deep breathing is very slight or absent should have cardiac monitoring intraoperatively and postoperatively.

Acidemia in the operative diabetic patient may be secondary to ketoacidosis, lactic acidosis, or uremia. Arterial blood gas and electrolyte determinations are imperative for identification of mixed acid–base disturbances and for assessment of the degree of acidemia. Hyperlipidemia, sometimes found in severe DKA, may cause the serum sodium measurement to be artifactually low, in which case the serum should be turbid and the measured plasma osmolality normal. Hyperglycemia may also depress serum sodium, because glucose, like sodium, acts as an osmotic solute in the extracellular fluid. The plasma sodium concentration will decrease by about 1.6 mEq/liter for every elevation of 100 mg/dl of plasma glucose above normal.

Hyperkalemia may be present if the patient is acidemic. A number of diabetic patients with renal insufficiency have been described in whom acute hyperkalemia was found to be induced paradoxically by hyperglycemia. These diabetics, who have been found to have hyporeninemic hypoaldosteronism, may be at great risk for developing hyperkalemia if potassium-sparing diuretics such as spironolactone or triamterene are used.[48,49] Diabetic patients receiving cadaver kidneys at the time of renal transplantation may also be at increased risk for sudden hyperkalemia accompanied by cardiorespiratory arrest.[50]

Metabolic derangements in the acutely ill preoperative diabetic patient may be quite severe. It is suggested that surgery be postponed if possible until blood glucose is under control for 24 to 48 hr, and this recommendation is based on empiric evidence.[51] It is clear that preoperative metabolic abnormalities may be worsened by emergency surgery, but, fortunately, there are usually several hours during which the internist can initiate treatment before the surgery begins. Further complications may be due to the fact that DKA may mimic or mask the symptoms of an acute abdomen.

In large part, treatment of DKA and HHNK is the same in preoperative and medical patients.[52,53] The emphases in both are adequate fluid repletion, prompt correction of severe acid–base abnormalities, institution of insulin therapy, and correction of electrolyte disturbances. If emergency surgery is already underway, intraoperative management should include frequent serum glucose and electrolyte determinations, arterial blood gases, cardiac monitoring, and central venous pressure or Swan–Ganz monitoring. Communication and coordination among the surgeon, anesthesiologist, and consulting internist are essential.

INTRAOPERATIVE MANAGEMENT OF THE INSULIN-DEPENDENT PATIENT

The many methods that exist for managing diabetic patients during surgery all seek to avoid ketosis and hyperglycemia or hypoglycemia. This is customarily accomplished by the subcutaneous administration of one-third to one-half of the patient's usual dose of intermediate-acting insulin on the morning of surgery and the subsequent infusion of intravenous dextrose during and after surgery.[15,52] In practice, plasma glucose is rarely monitored intraoperatively, but several studies in which glucose levels were measured throughout the procedure have shown that few instances of hypoglycemia or hyperglycemia occur with this method.[15,53,54] DKA or HHNK is very unusual without significant intraoperative complications. However, this regimen is cumbersome if the operation is scheduled late in the day, and it may be dangerous if the operation is delayed and the intravenous dextrose infusion has not been started when the insulin is being absorbed. In some brittle patients, such as renal transplant recipients, plasma glucose may then be very hard to control adequately.[54]

An alternative approach, the "no insulin–no glucose" regimen, has gained favor in recent years. When insulin-requiring diabetics are fasted before and during surgery without dextrose infusion, there is minimal deterioration in glucose control.[39] Using a similar protocol, Alberti and Thomas have found increases in ketone body concentration accompanied by negative potassium, phosphate, calcium, and magnesium balance.[15] The clinical significance of these alterations during the short duration of most minor operations remains to be demonstrated.

Continuous intravenous insulin therapy, similar to that used in the treatment of DKA, has been suggested for insulin-requiring diabetics during surgery.[55] The theoretic advantage is achievement of steady-state insulin and dextrose infusion rates and hence near steady-state plasma glucose levels. Such insulin levels throughout the procedure normalize intermediary carbohydrate metabolism, but intraoperative glucose levels must be measured frequently and periodic adjustments made in the insulin and dextrose infusion rates to prevent hypoglycemia. There have been few serious hypoglycemic episodes reported in plasma glucose

control either intraoperatively or postoperatively.[15,53,54]

Several methods for administering insulin and dextrose together have been described. Taitelman and co-workers reported using one infusion line for all parenteral fluids and a separate line for insulin.[53] They recommend 500 ml of 5% dextrose over the first hour followed by 125 ml/hr of dextrose plus 2 units/hr of regular insulin. The dosage of insulin is reduced to 1 unit/hr in patients taking less than 20 units/day of insulin before surgery. Adjustments are made for plasma glucose levels obtained during operation. Alberti and Thomas suggest 5 units of regular insulin (10 units if the plasma glucose level is greater than 108 mg/dl) added to 500 ml of 10% dextrose containing 7.4 mEq of potassium chloride infused at a rate of 100 ml/hr beginning 30 min before the operation.[15] Meyer and associates recommend 50 units of regular insulin mixed in 250 ml of normal saline and a separate line of 5% dextrose running into a common intravenous line.[54] Insulin rate is determined by an algorithm, and dextrose is infused at 50 ml/hr. All other parenteral fluids and medications are administered through a separate line. At Meyer's institution, the medical consultant writes all orders for the insulin-dextrose intravenous line, while the surgeons and anesthesiologists control the other line.

There are no comparative studies of the "no insulin–no glucose," conventional split-dose insulin-and-dextrose infusion, and continuous insulin infusion protocols for insulin-dependent diabetics undergoing surgery. The following recommendations are therefore based on available literature. If the procedure is minor and expected to be short and the patient is not seriously ill, the "no insulin–no glucose" protocol may be used. For the very ill or brittle patient, the continuous infusion protocol is appropriate, and provisions for rapid intraoperative glucose monitoring and infusion rate adjustment are essential. In elective surgery on well-controlled diabetic patients, the conventional split-dose insulin-and-dextrose infusion protocol is reasonable.

INTRAOPERATIVE MANAGEMENT OF THE INSULIN-INDEPENDENT PATIENT

The protocols discussed above are also useful in the management of patients controlled by diet or oral hypoglycemic agents. No special treatment is necessary if the surgery is minor and the patient is well controlled with diet. Treatment of patients on oral hypoglycemic agents is more controversial. Recognition that significant hyperglycemia and insulin resistance may accompany even minor procedures has led to the proposal that patients receiving oral agents be switched to insulin and dextrose infusion while they are not eating. Several authors have suggested that less antigenic pure pork insulin rather than standard beef and pork insulin be used for patients who will return to diet or oral agents.[57] If these patients need another course of insulin treatment in the future, their chance of developing insulin allergy may be decreased. However, if the procedure is minor and the patient is in good control, the oral agent can be discontinued the day before surgery and the "no insulin–no glucose" protocol followed perioperatively. The oral agent is reinstituted when the patient begins to eat. Supplemental regular pork insulin can be used if control deteriorates in the perioperative period.

Long-acting sulfonylureas such as chlorpropamide have long half-lives and may cause severe, unremitting hypoglycemia if carbohydrate intake is diminished. Such agents should be stopped 3 days before surgery, the patient should be allowed normal carbohydrate intake until the evening before surgery, and preoperative plasma glucose should be measured before induction of anesthesia. Regardless of which oral agent has been used, it is always wise to check the plasma glucose intraoperatively during a lengthy procedure. Phenformin, which has been removed from the market in the United States because of its association with lactic acidosis, has no place in the management of diabetic surgical patients.

FLUID AND ELECTROLYTE MANAGEMENT DURING SURGERY

The dextrose infusion rate should remain constant throughout surgery unless plasma glucose concentrations dictate otherwise.[24] Intravascular volume should be maintained with saline. Hartman's and Ringer's lactate solutions should not be used in the diabetic surgical patient because the lactate may worsen a metabolic acidosis already present or serve as a substrate for conversion into glucose, which will contribute to the deterioration of diabetic control.[56] If the plasma glucose level undergoes significant changes over a short period of time, potassium levels should be closely monitored and appropriately treated.

POSTOPERATIVE MANAGEMENT AND COMPLICATIONS OF SURGERY

Postoperative care of the diabetic patient requires careful attention to fluid and electrolyte management, cardiovascular and pulmonary status, and metabolic stability. Plasma glucose and electrolyte levels should be measured for all but the most routine cases. It is not safe to rely on urinary glucose measurements (fractionals) to determine appropriate postoperative carbohydrate and insulin orders. The level of glucose in the urine lags several hours behind that in the plasma and may not accurately reflect current plasma glucose. Fractional orders are frequently written so that no insulin is given if the patient spills little or no glucose into the urine. However, postoperative patients need some insulin even if the urine fractional is negative. They are usually still receiving a dextrose drip, and actions of counterregulatory hormones affected by surgery peak 12 to 24 hr postoperatively. Severe hyperglycemia or DKA may therefore occur if no insulin is given. Thus, frequent plasma glucose levels should guide postoperative insulin management.

If circumstances require urine fractional coverage, several steps should be taken to minimize its potential danger. Double-voided urines reduce the differential in plasma and urine glucose levels over time; fixed doses of insulin at regular intervals prevent wide swings in plasma glucose. Five units of regular insulin can be given subcutaneously every 6 hr with additional insulin for positive urine fractionals. The rate of dextrose infusion can be increased if hypoglycemia occurs. Alternatively, one-half of the patient's usual intermediate-acting insulin can be given before surgery and one-half after surgery with supplemental regular insulin for positive urine fractionals.

Insulin requirements may be altered dramatically by the stress of surgery, tissue infection, or necrosis. Drugs given intraoperatively or postoperatively, such as thiazides, propranolol, and steroids may also alter insulin requirements. For the severely ill patient requiring an intensive care unit, it may be feasible to give a continuous insulin infusion and vary the insulin and dextrose infusion rates to correct the urine fractionals. Careful monitoring by the physician is mandatory, no matter which method is used.

Perhaps the most common postoperative complication for diabetics is infection. Over 13% of a large series of diabetic patients followed by Galloway and Shuman developed postoperative infections.[1] It has been speculated that abnormalities of phagocytic function, as well as disorders of cell-mediated immune function, underlie this propensity of diabetics for infection.[12,58] Wound healing is also delayed in diabetics, owing to poor vascular supply to the affected tissue and possibly to impaired protein synthesis and collagen synthesis in diabetic skin fibroblasts.[59,60]

Cardiovascular complications, often associated with tissue ischemia and necrosis, account for many of the observed postoperative complications in diabetics. Myocardial infarction, stroke, and gangrene after systemic emboli are not infrequent. Unexplained hypotension or tachycardia may mean silent myocardial infarction or sepsis with subsequent rapid development of DKA or profound lactic acidosis. Postoperative DKA and HHNK are uncommon if not present preoperatively and usually reflect an intraoperative metabolic catastrophe. Poor control of plasma glucose with subsequent urinary loss of free water coupled with hypertonic fluid replacement and inadequate insulin treatment may predispose the patient to the development of HHNK, although this is an infrequent postoperative complication.[41,42]

SUMMARY

1. **The management of the diabetic patient during surgery demands careful**

attention to detail and a rational approach to treatment on the part of the consulting internist.

2. Essential preoperative evaluation includes plasma glucose, electrolytes, blood urea nitrogen (BUN), creatinine, complete blood count, chest x-ray, ECG, and urinalysis.

3. Elective surgery should be postponed in the patient with severe hyperglycemia, DKA, or HHNK.

4. Insulin-requiring diabetics undergoing short procedures may usually be managed with the "no insulin–no glucose" protocol.

5. Well-controlled insulin-requiring diabetic patients undergoing major surgery are often most conveniently managed with the split insulin–dextrose infusion protocol.

6. Insulin-requiring diabetic patients who are poorly controlled, extremely ill, or undergoing long procedures should be managed with a continuous infusion of insulin, provided that intraoperative glucose monitoring is available.

7. Diabetic patients controlled with diet or short-acting oral hypoglycemics who are undergoing minor surgery require no special treatment. The oral agents should be stopped 1 day before surgery.

8. Long-acting sulfonylureas should be stopped 3 days before surgery. Dextrose infusion and insulin may be necessary if the patient is not eating postoperatively.

9. Plasma glucose rather than urine fractionals should guide postoperative management of the diabetic patient.

10. Close cooperation and communication among surgeon, anesthesiologist, and internist are essential.

REFERENCES

1. Galloway JA, Shuman CR: Diabetes and surgery. A study of 667 cases. Am J Med 34:177, 1963

2. Alieff A: Das Risiko chirurgischer Eingriffe beim Diabetiker. Zentralbl Chir 941:857, 1969

3. Kannel WB, McGee DL: Diabetes and cardiovascular risk factors: The Framingham study. Circulation 59:8, 1979

4. Weinrauch LA, D'Elia JA, Healy RW et al: Asymptomatic coronary artery disease—Angiography in diabetic patients before renal transplantation. Ann Intern Med 88:346, 1978

5. Bennett WM, Kloster F, Rosch J et al: Natural history of asymptomatic coronary arteriographic lesions in diabetic patients with end-stage renal disease. Am J Med 65: 779, 1978

6. Solar NG, Pentecost BL, Bennett MA et al: Coronary care for myocardial infarction in diabetics. Lancet 1:475, 1974

7. Clarke BF, Ewing DJ, Campbell IW: Diabetic autonomic neuropathy. Diabetologia 17:195, 1979

8. Faerman I, Faccio E, Milei J et al: Autonomic neuropathy and painless myocardial infarction in diabetic patients. Histologic evidence of their relationship. Diabetes 26:1147, 1977

9. Page MB, Watkins PJ: Cardiorespiratory arrest and diabetic autonomic neuropathy. Lancet 1:14, 1978

10. Goodson WH, Hunt TK: Wound healing and the diabetic patient. Surg Gynecol Obstet 149:600, 1979

11. Louis TJ, Bartlett JG, Tally FP et al: Aerobic and anaerobic bacteria in diabetic foot ulcers. Ann Intern Med 85: 461, 1976

12. Bagdade JD, Nielson KL, Bulger RJ: Reversible abnormalities in phagocytic function in poorly controlled diabetic patients. Am J Med Sci 263:451, 1972

13. Mowat AG, Baum J: Chemotaxis of polymorphonuclear leukocytes from patients with diabetes mellitus. N Engl J Med 284: 621, 1971

14. Molitch ME, Reichlin S: The care of the diabetic patient during emergency surgery and postoperatively. Orthop Clin North Am 9:811, 1978

15. Alberti KGMM, Thomas DJB: The management of diabetes during surgery. Br J Anaesthes 51:693, 1979

16. Cahill GF: Starvation in man. Clin Endocrinol Metab 5:397, 1976

17. Newsholme EA: Carbohydrate metabolism in vivo: Regulation of the blood glucose level. Clin Endocrinol Metab 5:543, 1976

18. Allison SP, Tomlin PJ, Chamberlain MJ: Some effects of anaesthesia and surgery on carbohydrate and fat metabolism. Br J Anaesth 41: 588, 1969

19. Brandt MR, Kehlet H, Binder C et al: Effect of epidural anesthesia on the glycoregulatory endocrine response to surgery. Clin Endocrinol (Oxf) 5:107, 1976

20. Brandt MR, Kehlet H, Faber O et al: C-peptide and insulin during blockade of the hyperglycaemic response to surgery by epidural anesthesia. Clin Endocrinol (Oxf) 6:167, 1977

21. Clarke RSJ, Johnston H, Sheridan B: The influence of anaesthesia and surgery on plasma cortisol, insulin and free fatty acids. Br J Anaesth 42:295, 1970

22. Aarimaa M, Slatis P, Haapaniemi L et al: Glucose tolerance and insulin response during and after elective surgery. Ann Surg 179:926, 1974

23. Wright PD, Henderson K, Johnson IDA: Glucose utilization and insulin secretion during surgery in man. Br J Surg 61:5, 1974

24. Schwartz SS, Horwitz DL, Zehfus B et al: Use of a glucose-controlled insulin infusion system (artificial beta cell) to control diabetes during surgery. Diabetologia 16:157, 1979

25. Port D, Graber AL, Kuzuya T et al: The effect of epinephrine on immunoreactive insulin levels in man. J Clin Invest 45:228, 1966

26. Giddings AEB: The control of plasma glucose in the surgical patient. Br J Surg 61:787, 1974

27. Bromage PR, Shibata HR, Willoughby HW: Influence of prolonged sugar and cortisol responses to operations upon the upper part of the abdomen and thorax. Surg Gynecol Obstet 132:1051, 1971

28. Nistrup-Madsen S, Engquist A, Badawi et al: Cyclic AMP, glucose, and cortisol in plasma during surgery. Horm Metab Res 8:483, 1976

29. Wilmore DW, Lindsey CA, Moylan JA: Hyperglucagonemia after burns. Lancet 1:73, 1974

30. Russell RCG, Walker CJ, Bloom SR: Hyperglucagonemia in the surgical patient. Br Med J 1:10, 1975

31. Wright PD, Johnston IDA: The effect of surgical operation on growth hormone levels in plasma. Surgery 77:479, 1975

32. Giddings AEB, O'Conner KJ, Rowlands BJ et al: The relationship of plasma glucagon to the hyperglycemia and hyperinsulinemia of surgical operations. Br J Surg 63:612, 1976

33. Lindsay A, Santensanio F, Braaten J et al: Pancreatic alpha cell function in trauma. J Am Med Assoc 227:757, 1974

34. Miyata M, Yamamoto T, Nakao K: Suppression of glucagon secretion during surgery. Horm Metab Res 8:239, 1976

35. O'Keefe SJD, Sender PM, James WPT: Catabolic loss of body nitrogen in response to surgery. Lancet 2:1035, 1974

36. Crane CW, Picor D, Smith R: Protein turnover in patients before and after elective orthopaedic operations. Br J Surg 64:129, 1977

37. Elia M, Smith R, Williamson DII: Oral protein and blood branched-chain amino acids. Lancet 1:448, 1979

38. Foster KJ, Alberti KGMM, Binder C: Lipid metabolites and nitrogen balance after abdominal surgery in man. Br J Surg 66:242, 1979

39. Fletcher J, Langman MJS, Kellock TD: Effect of surgery on blood sugar levels in diabetes mellitus. Lancet 2:52, 1965

40. Flanigan WJ, Thompson BW, Casali RE et al: The surgical significance of hyperosmolar coma. Am J Surg 120:652, 1970

41. Greenstein AJ, Dreiling DA: Nonketotic hyperosmolar coma in the postoperative patient. Am J Surg 121:698, 1971

42. Bedford RF: Hyperosmolar hyperglycemic non-ketotic coma following general anesthesia. Report of a case. Anesthesiology 35:652, 1971

43. Brenner WI, Lansky Z, Engelman RM et al: Hyperosmolar coma in surgical patients. Ann Surg 178:651, 1972

44. Schweizer O, Howland WS: Some metabolic changes associated with anesthesia and operation. Surg Clin North Am 49:223, 1969

45. Nistrup-Madsen S, Brandt MR, Engquist E: Inhibition of plasma cyclic AMP, glucose and cortisol response to surgery by epidural analgesia. Br J Surg 64:669, 1977

46. Vesely DL, Mintz DH: Acute renal failure in insulin-dependent diabetics. Arch Intern Med 138:1858, 1978

47. Page MM, Watkins PJ: The heart in diabetes. Autonomic neuropathy and cardiomyopathy. Clin Endocrinol Metab 6:377, 1977

48. Goldfarb S, Cox M, Singer I et al: Acute hyperkalemia induced by hyperglycemia. Hormonal mechanisms. Ann Intern Med 84:426, 1976

49. Cox M, Sterns RH, Singer I: The defense against hyperkalemia. The roles of insulin and aldosterone. N Engl J Med 299:525, 1978

50. Hirshman CA, Edelstein G: Intraoperative hyperkalemia and cardiac arrests during renal transplantation in an insulin-dependent diabetic patient. Anesthesiology 51:161, 1979

51. Steinke J: Management of diabetes mellitus and surgery. N Engl J Med 282:1472, 1970

52. Rossini AA, Hare JW: How to control the blood glucose level in the surgical diabetic patient. Arch Surg 111:945, 1976

53. Taitelman U, Reece EA, Bessman AN: Insulin in the management of the diabetic surgical patient. Continuous intravenous infusion vs. subcutaneous administration. J Am Med Assoc 237:658, 1977

54. Meyer EJ, Lorenzi M, Bohannon NV et al: Diabetic management by insulin infusion during major surgery. Am J Surg 137:323, 1979

55. Page MM, Alberti KGMM, Greenblood R et al: Treatment of diabetic coma with continuous low-dose infusion of insulin. Br Med J 2:687, 1974

56. Thomas DJB, Alberti KGMM: The hyperglycemic effects of Hartmann's solution in maturity-onset diabetics during surgery. Br J Anaesth 50:185, 1978

57. Asplin CM, Hartog M, Goldie DJ: Change of insulin dosage, circulating free and bound insulin, and insulin antibodies on transferring diabetics from conventional to highly purified porcine insulin. Diabetologia 14:99, 1978

58. Kolterman OG, Olefsky JM, Kurahara C et al: A defect in cell-mediated immune function in insulin-resistant diabetic and obese subjects. J Lab Clin Med 96:535, 1980

59. Rowe DW, Starman BJ, Fujimoto WY et al: Abnormalities in proliferation and protein synthesis in skin fibroblast cultures from patients with diabetes mellitus. Diabetes 26:284, 1977

60. Tenni R, Tavella D, Donnelly P et al: Cultured fibroblasts of juvenile diabetics have excessively soluble pericellular collagen. Biochem Biophys Res Commun 92:1071, 1980

12

The Surgical Patient with Thyroid Disease

GAIL B. SLAP

Anatomic or functional abnormalities of the thyroid gland are common in surgical patients. The discovery of nonendemic goiter on physical examination is reported in 4% to 7% of the population, and autopsy surveys report nodular thyroid glands in 8% to 50% of all patients.[1–4] The annual incidence of Graves' disease and thyroiditis is 0.2 to 0.8 per 1000.[5–7] Spontaneous myxedema is rare, occurring in only 0.01% to 0.08% of all persons admitted to the hospital, but the incidence of [131]I- and drug-induced hypothyroidism is rising.[7]

The thyroid physiology of the euthyroid surgical patient is discussed in the first section. Particular attention is given to assessment of the functional status of the thyroid; such assessment may be difficult in the chronically ill or malnourished patient. The second section explores the surgical risks, presentation, diagnosis, and treatment of thyrotoxicosis. Thyroid storm and thyroid surgery require detailed management and are discussed separately. The final sections deal with hypothyroidism and myxedema coma.

THYROID PHYSIOLOGY IN THE SURGICAL PATIENT

Thyroxine (T_4) and 3,5,3'-triiodothyronine (T_3) are the principal biologically active thyroid hormones. T_4 is produced by the thyroid and T_3 by both the thyroid (20%) and peripheral tissues (80%). In the euthyroid patient, T_3 is produced in extrathyroidal tissues by deiodination of T_4 to T_3, which occurs most actively in the liver and kidney. Another route of T_4 metabolism is monodeiodination to 3,3',5'-triiodothyronine, or reverse T_3 (rT_3). This inactive hormone is produced largely (95%) in peripheral tissues.[8] The serum concentrations of total T_4, free T_4, thyroxine-binding globulin, as estimated by the T_3-resin uptake (T_3RU), and T_3 provide biochemical estimates of thyroid status.

Thyroid physiology is altered by anesthesia, surgery, chronic illness, infection, and fasting. Certain types of anesthesia may alter serum T_4 concentration. Fore and co-workers found that serum T_4 increases during ether anesthesia.[9] Oyama and associates confirmed this finding in

153

a study of the distribution of ^{131}I-labeled thyroxine during and after diethyl–ether and thiopental–nitrous oxide anesthesia without surgery. The authors speculated that the ether stimulates the hepatic release of T_4 and suggested that it be avoided in thyrotoxic patients.[10] Other explanations for the change in serum T_4 concentration include decreased hepatic uptake of the hormone or inhibition of the hepatic enzyme responsible for conversion of T_4 to T_3.[11] Although ether is rarely used because of its flammability, changes in the serum concentration of thyroid hormone (TH) after anesthesia with any agent should be considered in the evaluation of a postoperative patient for thyroid disease.

Surgery is not associated with a change in serum T_4, but it does induce a fall in T_3 and a rise in rT_3.[9] Burr and co-workers measured the concentration of TH in seven euthyroid patients before and after elective nonthyroidal procedures. Serum T_3 fell significantly to values in the hypothyroid range within 24 hr and persisted at this level for at least 6 days postoperatively. Serum rT_3 increased significantly for 3 days and then returned to baseline values. Despite these changes, the patients remained clinically euthyroid and required no treatment.[12]

Acute illness may be associated with a slight increase in serum T_4 and T_3 resin uptake (RU) and a decrease in serum T_3 owing to lowered production.[11] The serum thyroid-stimulating hormone (TSH) and thyrotropin-releasing hormone (TRH)-stimulation tests remain normal. As the illness continues, T_4 and T_3RU fall to normal, T_3 may decrease to 25% of normal, and rT_3 rises.[11,14] An increase in the absolute free T_4, a common occurrence, is probably due to the interaction of thyroxine-binding globulin (TBG) with plasma proteins, which decrease the binding of T_4 to TBG.[16,17] In severe chronic illness, serum T_4, T_3RU, and T_3 may all be low, and rT_3 may be normal. Lack of response to TRH is common in severe chronic illness, consistent with depressed pituitary function.

Chronic liver disease may cause marked changes in TH concentrations. Although the values obtained from them suggest hypothyroidism, patients with chronic liver disease are clinically euthyroid.[17–19] Total T_4 is normal or only minimally decreased, TBG is decreased, free T_4 is increased, and absolute free T_4 is normal.[18–21] T_3 is decreased, and rT_3 is increased.[18,22,23] In acute hepatitis, unlike chronic liver disease, serum T_4 may be very high, T_3RU is normal, and free T_4 is slightly increased.

Total T_4, free T_4, and T_3 may all be decreased in severe chronic renal failure.[17,24] The rT_3 usually remains normal.[22] Patients with this disorder are clinically euthyroid and do not require exogenous TH.[24,25]

Infection or fever may increase T_4 and T_3 turnover as much as fourfold by activating hepatic enzymes. T_4 usually remains normal, T_3 falls, and rT_3 rises. The increase in T_4 turnover may explain the precipitation of myxedema coma by infection that occurs in hypothyroid patients.[26]

The effects of chronic starvation or malnutrition on the TH are usually similar to those seen in chronic illness. T_3 falls, rT_3 rises, T_4 and TSH are unchanged, and free T_4 is elevated.[27,28] A 36-hr fast in adults of normal weight, unlike those in a state of chronic starvation, results in a 50% fall in TSH and a diminished response to TRH.[29]

The many changes in thyroid physiology that accompany surgery and its complications may confuse assessment of thyroid function in the perioperative period. Laboratory values alone do not necessarily indicate a hypothyroid or hyperthyroid state. Serum T_3 concentration is an especially poor measure of thyroid status in this setting and should never be used to diagnose suspected hypothyroidism, since many nonthyroidal diseases cause a fall in T_3 and many hypothyroid patients have normal T_3 values. Although T_3 concentration is usually a reliable indicator of hyperthyroidism, coexisting nonthyroidal illness may depress T_3 in a truly thyrotoxic patient.[11] Management decisions must be based on clinical evaluation along with laboratory data.

THYROTOXICOSIS

Risk of Surgery

The greatest risk confronting surgical patients with untreated thyrotoxicosis is thyroid storm. Of 2033 thyrotoxic patients admitted to the Massachusetts General Hospital over a 25-year period, 36 (1.8%) developed thyroid storm. Of the 36 episodes, 25 followed surgery; 64% of the patients died. In all cases, preoperative thyrotoxicosis was severe. Of the 25, 19 had received no effective treatment before hospitalization, and 6 had received iodine alone.[30] The use of antithyroid medication and adrenergic antagonists over the last 40 years has decreased the risk of thyroid storm.[31] However, for those patients who develop thyroid storm, the mortality rate is 20% to 40%.[32-34]

Any thyrotoxic patient facing surgery has a higher than normal risk of developing thyroid storm and requires close attention. Case reports of cardiac arrest or storm after minor procedures in patients with unrecognized thyrotoxicosis stress the importance of preoperative clinical recognition and treatment.[35,36] Reports of storm in surgical patients on seemingly adequate regimens emphasize the need for close perioperative monitoring.[37]

Clinical Manifestations

Separation of the signs and symptoms of hyperthyroidism into adrenergic and metabolic categories is artificial but clinically useful. Recognition of metabolic effects separate from adrenergic effects permits the diagnosis of apathetic hyperthyroidism. The catecholamine-related effects are the most easily corrected. Metabolic effects due to excess TH develop over weeks or months and take longer to reverse. If hyperthyroidism is due to Graves' disease, some of the manifestations are autoimmune.

Adrenergic Effects

Adrenergic effects place the surgical patient at greatest risk. Palpitations, tremors, increased sweating, heat intolerance, and anxiety are common. Resting cardiac output is increased, and peripheral vascular resistance is decreased because of increased beta- and decreased alpha-adrenergic effects.[38] Atrial fibrillation occurs in 10% of thyrotoxic patients; arrhythmias are difficult to control until a euthyroid state is achieved.[39] During surgery or stress, the basal increase in cardiac output due to hyperthyroidism significantly limits reserve.[40-42]

Protein-Turnover Effects

Although both synthesis and catabolism of protein are increased in thyrotoxicosis, breakdown is greater with resultant negative nitrogen balance. Evidence that propranolol dimishes this turnover suggests that the adrenergic effects of TH also play a role.[43] Increased basal oxygen consumption, atrial fibrillation, underlying heart disease, or vitamin-B_6 deficiency due to increased coenzyme requirements may contribute to cardiac decompensation. Response to digoxin is often inadequate and may reflect increased drug metabolism.[44]

Dyspnea without congestive heart failure, a common occurrence, is probably due to weakened respiratory muscles. Vital capacity and pulmonary compliance are decreased, and basal minute ventilation is increased.[45] Bulbar involvement, present in 16.4% of patients in one study, may complicate postoperative respiratory management in the untreated thyrotoxic patient.[46]

Most thyrotoxic patients are malnourished, despite increased food intake. Preparation for surgery may therefore require sufficient time for nutritional supplementation. Hypoalbuminemia reflects generalized protein wasting. Insulin metabolism is increased, glucose tolerance may be abnormal, and net lipid degradation may produce ketosis, especially when the patient is fasting.[47,48]

Intestinal hypermotility and mucosal edema, common in thyrotoxicosis, may complicate the evaluation of a patient with abdominal pain.[49] Hepatomegaly and splenomegaly accompanied by lymphadenopathy may be present.[39,50–52] Anorexia occurs in as many as 30% and constipation is seen in 25% of elderly hyperthyroid patients.[51] The insidious onset of hyperthyroidism in patients over the age of 60 and its often nonspecific symptoms place elderly patients at greatest risk for misdiagnosis before surgery.

Laboratory abnormalities in hyperthyroidism include an elevated alkaline phosphatase level and a prolonged prothrombin time.[52] Neutropenia with relative lymphocytosis is not unusual. Thrombocytopenia may be critical in the surgical patient. Several patients with presumed idiopathic thrombocytopenic purpura (ITP) have been found to be thyrotoxic.[54,55] Serum T_4 and T_3RU should be checked in all patients with ITP before splenectomy. Platelet counts return to normal with re-establishment of the euthyroid state.

Aspects Unique to Graves' Disease

The third group of signs and symptoms of hyperthyroidism are unique to Graves' disease and appear unrelated to TH or catecholamines. Thyroid-stimulating immunoglobulins (TSIG) are a group of antibodies found in the serum of patients with Graves' disease. Patients with infiltrative ophthalmopathy and pretibial myxedema usually have detectable levels of TSIG.[56,57] Autoimmune diseases such as myasthenia gravis and pernicious anemia are associated with both Graves' disease and Hashimoto's thyroiditis and may complicate perioperative management.[58–62]

Diagnosis

The differential diagnosis of hyperthyroidism is aided by a careful neck examination. This is especially important in patients undergoing general anesthesia and intubation. Tracheal displacement or recurrent laryngeal nerve compression by a thyroid neoplasm or goiter increases the risk of respiratory compromise. The hyperfunctioning gland of Graves' disease is usually soft and large, whereas that of Hashimoto's thyroiditis is firmer. The gland in acute thyroiditis is enlarged and tender. A toxic multinodular goiter usually arises spontaneously in a nontoxic multinodular gland but may be precipitated by exposure to a large dose of iodine.[63] Other less common causes of hyperthyroidism include ingestion of TH, pituitary or hypothalamic thyrotoxicosis, ectopic TH production, and ectopic thyroid stimulator production.

When hyperthyroidism is suspected, measurement of serum T_4 and T_3RU is usually sufficient for diagnosis. Serum T_4 alone may be misleading, because increased serum protein binding may cause elevation of T_4 in euthyroid patients, and decreased binding may cause a normal or low T_4 level in hyperthyroid patients. Occasionally, a patient with early hyperthyroidism has a normal free thyroxine index as estimated by from T_4 and T_3RU. An elevated serum T_3 level measured by radioimmunoassay (RIA) usually confirms the diagnosis.

Serum TSH is rarely helpful, since secondary hyperthyroidism is exceedingly uncommon and most RIAs cannot distinguish a low from a normal value. Radioactive iodine uptake (RAIU) may be misleading in the diagnosis of hyperthyroidism. A hyperthyroid patient exposed to iodine by way of food, intravenous catheters, or angiographic dye may have a normal or low uptake, and a euthyroid patient from an iodine-deficient environment may have a high uptake.

The TRH-stimulation test allows diagnosis of all types of primary hyperthyroidism. In this test, serum TSH is measured before and after a single intravenous dose of TRH of 400 µg. The normal TSH surge in response to TRH is blocked in the hyperthyroid patient.

Once the diagnosis of hyperthyroidism is made, the treatment of choice may vary, depending on the etiology of the disease. If surgery can be postponed, optimal treatment should be carried out. If surgery is emergent, the goal in all thyrotoxic patients, regardless of etiology, is prevention of thyroid storm.

Perioperative Management

Medical management of hyperthyroid patients before and during an extrathyroidal procedure is similar to that before and during thyroidectomy.

Preoperative Screening

Preoperative screening for cardiopulmonary disease is essential in all hyperthyroid patients. Measurement of arterial blood gases, forced expiratory volume, minute ventilation, and maximum breathing capacity are recommended. Congestive heart failure should be treated before surgery, and all patients should be monitored continuously for arrhythmias. If cardiopulmonary disease is present, an arterial line and Swan–Ganz catheter should be inserted preoperatively. All hyperthyroid patients should be placed on a cooling blanket, which can be started during the operation if hyperthermia develops.[64]

Antithyroid Agents

If surgery can be delayed for several months, hyperthyroid patients should be prepared with an antithyroid agent of the thionamide class. Propylthiouracil (PTU) and methimazole are the agents most commonly used in the United States. Both act by inhibiting the oxidation and organification of iodide and the coupling of iodotyrosines. In high doses, PTU also inhibits the peripheral conversion of T_4 to T_3.[65] Because synthesis but not release of TH is impaired, the hyperthyroid state persists until TH stores are depleted. Clinical improvement begins after about 2 weeks, and the euthyroid state is usually re-established within 6 weeks. However, if the patient has received large quantities of iodine before treatment, it may take months for the stores of hormone within the thyroid gland to be depleted. Larger doses of antithyroid agent may help shorten the latency period.

Dosage must be titrated to the patient's clinical status. The minimum initial dose of PTU is 100 mg orally every 6 hr. Patients with severe thyrotoxicosis or large goiters may require much higher doses. It is often helpful to both increase the daily dosage and shorten the dosing interval to every 4 hr. Once the patient is euthyroid, the dose can usually be decreased by as much as one-third.[39]

Patients undergoing emergency surgery should be given 1000 mg of PTU orally to block organification of iodide and peripheral conversion of T_4 to T_3. Propranolol is begun immediately if there are no contraindications to block catecholamine effects, if they are present, and sodium iodide is given 1 hr after the PTU (see below). PTU and methimazole must be administered orally; there are no parenteral preparations.

Adverse reactions to PTU or methimazole are reported in 3% to 12% of patients.[66] Most are mild hypersensitivity reactions such as skin rash or drug fever that tend to occur early in treatment with high doses and resolve with discontinuation of the drug. The alternate drug may be tried in patients who have such reactions. Much more serious are reactions similar to serum sickness and agranulocytosis, which are reported in less than 0.5% of patients. Although these may occur at any time, they are also more common early than late in treatment. Patients should be told to discontinue the drug immediately should fever, sore throat, stomatitis, or proctitis develop. Because as many as 10% of hyperthyroid patients have a baseline white blood-cell count below 4000 with neutropenia, the diagnosis may be a difficult one.[66] Recovery of the marrow occurs in virtually all patients after discontinuation of the drug.

Iodine

Iodine is rarely used alone in the treatment of hyperthyroidism. It is used with an antithyroid agent in patients due to undergo subtotal thyroidectomy, in patients facing emergency surgery, and in

patients with thyroid storm. Iodine acutely inhibits the release of T_4, thus avoiding the latency of the antithyroid agents.[67] Iodine also acutely but transiently inhibits organification (Wolff–Chaikoff effect).[68,69] However, because exacerbation of thyrotoxicosis may occur when the iodine is stopped, and because some patients escape from the initial effectiveness of the iodine, the agent is unsafe when used alone. Should iodine fail, radioiodine ablation and antithyroid agents are ineffective for several weeks or months, because they are not taken up by the iodine-replenished gland.

The recommended dose of iodine is 2 drops of saturated solution of potassium iodide (SSKI) orally 3 times daily for 1 week before surgery. When emergency surgery is necessary, 5 drops 3 times daily are used along with an antithyroid agent, propranolol, and corticosteroids. The first dose of iodine should be given 1 hr after the loading dose of PTU to allow time for the PTU to block organification. Iodine should be discontinued after 7 to 14 days. Adverse reactions are uncommon when the recommended dosages are used. At large doses, iodism may occur. Headache, mucosal edema, skin rash, fever, and sialadenitis are characteristic of iodism; they resolve with discontinuation of iodine.

Sodium iodide is available intravenously and can be given in doses of 1 gr every 8 to 12 hr to acutely ill patients who cannot take SSKI orally or by nasogastric tube. It is in these patients that iodine must be administered without an antithyroid agent, since none of the thionamides is available for parenteral use.

Adrenergic Antagonists

Propranolol, reserpine, and guanethidine are useful adjuncts in severe thyrotoxicosis. Propranolol acts by blocking beta-adrenergic receptor sites. Reserpine and guanethidine act by depleting catecholamine stores. None of the drugs alters serum TH concentration.

Propranolol is the drug of choice for patients with symptomatic thyrotoxicosis and impending or actual thyroid storm and for intraoperative management of thyrotoxicosis.[70,71] Doses of 10 mg to 40 mg orally every 6 hr usually control the symptoms of catecholamine excess while antithyroid medication of ^{131}I takes effect.[72] Occasionally, much larger doses may be required. Propranolol is contraindicated in patients with asthma and should be avoided in patients with congestive heart failure or brittle insulin-dependent diabetes. In patients with cardiac dysfunction due to thyroid disease, iodine and antithyroid drugs are preferred over propranolol in the acute management of thyrotoxicosis, since TH exerts direct inotropic and chronotropic effects on the myocardium that are unaffected by propranolol. Intraoperatively, intravenous propranolol in small doses of 1 mg/min is used to control tachycardia, hypertension, fever, and arrhythmias.

Corticosteroids

If time or patient tolerance does not allow adequate preoperative preparation with antithyroid agents, corticosteroids are usually added to the propranolol–iodine regimen. This both protects against adrenal insufficiency and decreases serum levels of T_4 and TSH.[73] Thyrotoxicosis may be associated with increased degradation of corticosteroids and compensatory hyperplasia of the adrenal cortex. Although the adrenal response to acute stress is usually normal in thyrotoxicosis, adrenal reserve as measured after a 2-day course of ACTH is often subnormal.[39]

Anesthesia

Heavy preoperative sedation is not adequate prophylaxis against thyroid storm. The anesthesiologist often avoids the use of atropine and morphine, which may stimulate adrenergic activity. Short-acting barbiturates or diazepam may be used as premedications.[51] Thiopental is used for induction because it suppresses the sympathetic nervous system and effects direct antithyroid activity.[64,74] Nitrous oxide and halothane or enflurane are the anesthetic agents of choice. Diethyl ether and cyclopropane stimulate the sympathoadrenal axis and are therefore contraindicated in the thyrotoxic patient.[51]

Thyroid Storm

The thyrotoxic patient faces as great a risk of thyrotoxic crisis during the first 18 hr after surgery as during the procedure. Because elective surgery is usually postponed until good control of thyrotoxicosis is achieved, it is usually the patient undergoing emergency surgery who develops thyroid storm. However, crises precipitated by medical complications are even more common than those due to surgical complications.[33–35,75,96]

Regardless of the precipitating factor, thyroid storm is nearly always abrupt in onset. In one series, all 22 patients studied had fever, diaphoresis, and tachycardia. Fourteen patients (63.6%) had sinus tachycardia, and eight (36.4%) had arrhythmias. Twelve patients (54.5%) were hyperkinetic, ten (45.4%) were somnolent, two (9.1%) were psychotic, and four (18.2%) were comatose. Eleven patients (50%) experienced diarrhea or hyperdefecation. Eleven developed congestive heart failure, and two became hypotensive. Also reported, but less common, were jaundice, tender hepatomegaly, and abdominal pain.[34]

Laboratory studies in patients with thyroid storm give non-specific results. Thyroid function studies do not differ from those seen in stable thyrotoxicosis.[34,77,78] Hyperglycemia occurs in 50% of patients because TH causes impaired insulin secretion, insulin resistance, and increased glycogenolysis.[34,79,80] Plasma cortisol levels measured in 3 patients were below 12 μg/dl, suggesting decreased adrenal reserve. Leukocytosis of 10,000 to 20,000 is present in about half of the patients.[34]

Thyroid storm is fatal if untreated. Stupor or coma develops within 24 hr, rapidly followed by pulmonary edema, circulatory collapse, and death.[79] With treatment, improvement begins within 12 hr and the crisis resolves in an average of 3 days.[33,51]

Treatment must begin as soon as the diagnosis is considered, even before laboratory documentation. PTU in a dose of 1000 mg is immediately given orally to block organification of iodide; it is followed by 200 mg every 6 hr until the patient is euthyroid. PTU is preferred over methimazole because, in addition to blocking thyroid synthesis of hormone, it inhibits the peripheral conversion of T_4 to T_3.[65] Hydrocortisone should be given immediately in a dose of 300 mg followed by 100 mg daily until the crisis resolves.

Propranolol is given intravenously at a rate of 1 mg/min to a maximum of 10 mg; this may be repeated as necessary every 3 hr.[79,82] Oral propranolol in a dose of 20 mg to 80 mg every 6 hr has a slower onset of action than intravenous propranolol (1 hr vs. 2–10 min) but a longer duration (4–8 hr vs. 3–4 hr). The benefit of propranolol to the patient with congestive heart failure and thyroid storm probably outweighs the risk.[71,79,83] However, digoxin should be given before propranolol in these patients to compensate for depression of myocardial contractility.[79]

Propranolol should not be used in patients with asthma.

Reserpine in a dose of 5 mg intramuscularly followed by 2.5 mg every 6 hr, or guanethidine in doses of 50 mg to 150 mg orally, may be used in patients in whom propranolol is contraindicated. However, both agents have important disadvantages. Reserpine may cause hypotension, flushing, diarrhea, and depression. Guanethidine has a delayed onset of action of 12 hr to 24 hr, does not achieve peak efficacy for 3 days, and may also cause hypotension and diarrhea.[79]

Iodine should be given 1 hr after the first dose of PTU to ensure that organification is blocked. SSKI, 5 drops orally every 4 hr, or sodium iodide, 1 g intravenously every 8 hr to 12 hr, may be used.

Aggressive supportive care with cooling blankets, intravenous fluids, glucose, and oxygen is essential. Aspirin may displace T_4 from its carrier protein and should not be used to lower temperature.[81] Serum electrolytes, glucose, calcium, and arterial blood gases must be followed closely. Congestive heart failure should be treated as usual with diuretics and digoxin. Vitamin supplementation, especially of B complex, is often recommended.[66,79] Precipitating factors causing thyroid storm must be identified and treated promptly. Antibiotics should not be used prophylactically.

Plasmapheresis and peritoneal dialysis have been used during thyroid storm to remove TH but are not necessary if medical care is aggressively pursued.[79,84]

Thyroid Surgery

Risk

The major risk of thyroid surgery is thyroid storm in the thyrotoxic patient who has been inadequately prepared preoperatively. However, the most common post-operative complication is hypothyroid-ism, which is reported in 4% to 43% of patients, depending on the length of fol-low-up.[100,102] Recurrent hyperthyroidism occurs in 0.6% to 25% of patients.[100,103] It occurs within 5 years in 57% of patients, after 10 years in 37%, and after 20 years in 16%.[104] The incidence of early hypo-thyroidism in post-thyroidectomy pa-tients treated with ^{131}I is higher than in those not treated with [131]I.[104]

Permanent hypoparathyroidism has been reported in up to 3.6% of patients.[100] After long follow-up, Davis and co-work-ers reported hypoparathyroidism in as many as 24% of patients.[105] Postoperative hypocalcemia usually appears within a week of surgery and may be transient. Suggested etiologies include transient is-chemia of the parathyroid glands and bone retention of calcium in the thyro-toxic patient after surgery.[106] Hypocal-cemia appearing months or years postop-eratively may be due to atrophy of the parathyroid glands after ischemic injury. The risk of permanent hypocalcemia has decreased as subtotal has replaced total thyroidectomy as the procedure of choice.

Vocal-cord paralysis is reported in up to 4% of patients after thyroid surgery.[100] Many of the symptoms that are attributed to recurrent laryngeal nerve injury may actually be due to laryngeal edema. Lar-yngeal edema after thyroid surgery is more commonly due to surgical trauma than to difficult intubation, appears within 3 days, and resolves within 5 days of operation.[107] Tracheostomy is rarely necessary. Postoperative bleeding is a sur-gical emergency requiring evacuation to prevent airway obstruction. Because of the risk of both bleeding and laryngeal edema, patients should be observed in an intensive care unit for at least 24 hr post-operatively.

Preoperative Preparation

PTU in doses of 400 to 1200 mg daily is given for several weeks preoperatively un-til the patient is euthyroid according to clinical and laboratory criteria. SSKI, 2 drops orally 3 times daily, is added to the PTU for 7 to 14 days before the procedure. Surgery is performed during the second week, when the iodine effect reaches its peak.[66] In addition to ensuring control of hyperthyroidism, iodine reduces the vas-cularity of the thyroid gland, making the surgery technically easier.

Although an antithyroid agent and io-dine constitute the traditional preparation for partial thyroidectomy, several inves-tigators have established the safety of preparation with propranolol and iodine or propranolol alone.[83,108–114] This is es-pecially significant for patients who can-not tolerate antithyroid agents. The dos-age of propranolol is 40 mg orally every 6 hr for 3 to 4 days before surgery, and it is continued for 1 week postoperatively.[115]

Bewsher and colleagues compared 49 thyrotoxic patients prepared with pro-pranolol and iodine with 42 patients pre-pared with the antithyroid agent carbi-mazole and iodine. Preparation required less time, pulse rates were lower before and after operation, and surgery was tech-nically easier in the group treated with propranolol and iodine.[109] Feek and as-sociates prepared 10 patients for subtotal thyroidectomy with propranolol at a dos-age of 80 mg orally 3 times daily for a mean of 40 days through the fifth post-operative day and potassium iodide at a dosage of 60 mg orally 3 times daily for 10 days until surgery. No significant changes in serum concentration of T_4 or T_3 were found between the starting of pro-pranolol and the starting of potassium io-dide. Both T_4 and T_3 fell to normal in all patients after 10 days of potassium iodide.

Because not all of the effects of TH are mediated by beta-adrenergic receptors, the authors argue against preparation with propranolol alone.[110]

Although the propranolol and iodine regimen appears promising, the regimen of PTU and iodine should remain standard until further study is completed.

HYPOTHYROIDISM

Risk of Surgery

The hypothyroid patient clearly has a higher than normal risk of complications and death when subjected to anesthesia, surgery, trauma, and infection. Extreme sensitivity to central nervous system depressants increases the risk of postoperative respiratory depression. Decreased cardiac reserve limits tolerance of intravenous fluids, transfusions, and depressant effects of anesthesia. If hypotension develops, the response to pressor amines is poor.

The greatest risk faced by the hypothyroid surgical patient is myxedema coma. Although rare, it carries a mortality rate as high as 80%.[116,117] Urbanic and Mazzaferri report the incidence of myxedema coma among hospitalized patients with hypothyroidism to be 0.1% over a 10-year period.[79] Over 50% of all reported cases of myxedema coma occur after hospital admission, often in patients with unrecognized hypothyroidism.[118]

Prompt diagnosis and treatment of hypothyroidism are essential in the surgical patient. Elective surgery should be postponed to allow time for gradual TH replacement. Once the euthyroid state has been re-established, the risk of surgery decreases to that of the patient without hypothyroidism. The hypothyroid patient facing emergency surgery must be treated aggressively and monitored closely for signs of myxedema coma.

Clinical Manifestations

The symptoms of early hypothyroidism due to glandular hypofunction may be insidious and nonspecific.[120] However, development of the full clinical picture is rapid in patients who either discontinue their exogenous hormone or from whom replacement is withheld after thyroidectomy. Symptoms appear within 3 weeks and are flagrant within 3 months.[39]

The term myxedema is derived from the puffy edematous appearance of patients with severe hypothyroidism. Hyaluronic acid accumulates in all tissues, binds water, and produces mucinous edema. The skin becomes pale, cool, and dry. Bruising is common because of capillary fragility. Surgical wounds heal slowly owing to the slow growth rate of all tissues in hypothyroidism.[39]

Hemodynamic Abnormalities

The term "myxedema heart" refers to the cardiomegaly, electrocardiographic (ECG), hemodynamic, and enzymatic changes of hypothyroidism. Blood volume, stroke volume, heart rate, and cardiac output are decreased.[121-123] Peripheral vascular resistance is increased, and pulse pressure is narrowed. The untreated patient facing anesthesia and emergency surgery is prone to congestive heart failure and hypotension, which are usually refractory until TH is replaced. Ventricular fibrillation has been reported when exogenous TH and vasopressors are given together.[124] Blood loss is poorly tolerated, often requiring rapid replacement, but transfusion may precipitate congestive heart failure because of decreased myocardial contractility. Fluid replacement must begin preoperatively and proceed cautiously during the procedure with monitoring of blood pressure and central venous pressure.[125] If there is evidence of congestive heart failure or blood pressure instability preoperatively, an arterial line and Swan–Ganz catheter should be inserted.

Pericardial effusion is common but rarely causes tamponade.[39] ECG changes include sinus bradycardia, PR prolongation, decreased amplitude, and flattened T waves. Angina in the patient with coronary artery disease is usually not a problem while the patient is hypothyroid but may develop with thyroid replacement, especially if replacement is rapid or if the patient is stressed.[126] The serum concentration of cardiac enzymes in hypothyroidism may be very high without apparent heart disease, making the diagnosis of myocardial infarction difficult.[127] Hypothyroid patients who do have angina before TH replacement usually have severe coronary artery disease. Paine and coworkers described four patients who underwent successful cardiac catheterization and revascularization with minimal thyroid replacement. Full replacement was successfully achieved postoperatively.[128]

Pulmonary Abnormalities

The pulmonary abnormalities that occur in myxedema include pleural effusion, myxedematous infiltration of respiratory muscles, and depression of the respiratory center. Patients with myxedema alone usually have normal lung volumes, minute ventilation, PO_2, and P_{CO_2}. However, maximal breathing capacity (MBC), ventilatory response to CO_2, and diffusing capacity (D_{CO}) are lower than normal. Reduced D_{CO} is believed to be due to thickened capillary membranes or a decreased pulmonary capillary bed and is

reversible with treatment. Alveolar hypoventilation is probably due to central nervous system or chest muscle dysfunction.[129] Responsiveness of the respiratory center to hypoxia and hypercapnea is lower than normal.[130,131]

Gastrointestinal Abnormalities

Decreased peristalsis with distention and constipation is common in myxedema and may complicate diagnosis in the surgical patient. Hypomotility may progress to atony and, if accompanied by pain and vomiting, resembles mechanical obstruction. Myxedematous ascites is high in protein and mucopolysaccharides and resembles effusions in other organ systems. Autoimmune diseases involving the gastrointestinal tract are associated with hypothyroidism, although malabsorption is uncommon. Among patients with primary hypothyroidism, half have achlorhydria, one-third have circulating parietal cell antibodies, and 12% have pernicious anemia.[132,133]

Hematologic Abnormalities

Hemostatic abnormalities in hypothyroidism have been recognized since the first descriptions over 30 years ago of easy bruising and menorrhagia. Case reports of serious bleeding tendencies and factor deficiencies have appeared since 1962.[134,135] Edson and associates studied the hemostatic profiles of 16 hypothyroid patients. Twelve of the sixteen, or 75%, exhibited decreased platelet adhesiveness. Six of eight patients without intercurrent illness, or 75%, had decreased levels of at least one of factors VII, VIII, IX, and XI. These abnormalities disappeared after replacement with TH.[136]

Close monitoring for bleeding is essential in the hypothyroid surgical patient. If there are no known clotting abnormalities, special preoperative testing or preparation is not necessary. Should bleeding develop postoperatively with a prolonged protime or partial thromboplastin time, fresh frozen plasma should be used.

Anemia, usually normocytic normochromic anemia, is common in the hypothyroid patient.

Fluid and Electrolytes

Hyponatremia associated with myxedema is a well-recognized entity of unclear etiology.[137–142] Abnormal free water excretion is reported in 75% of hypothyroid patients and can be corrected with replacement of TH.[141,143] In the hypothyroid patient, the additive effects of the baseline defect and the superimposed secretion of antidiuretic hormone precipitated by postoperative pain or analgesics may lead to life-threatening hyponatremia. Serum electrolytes and intravenous fluid replacement should be followed closely.

Adrenal Function

Patients with primary hypothyroidism due to Hashimoto's thyroiditis have a higher incidence than normal of Addison's disease.[144] Patients with secondary hypothyroidism due to pituitary disease often have associated adrenal insufficiency.[66] Any hypothyroid patient may have decreased adrenal reserve when stressed or when undergoing rapid replacement of TH. Therefore, the hypothyroid patient should receive supplemental glucocorticoid during the operative period.

Central Nervous System Abnormalities

Cerebral blood flow is reduced in hypothyroidism without a concomitant decrease in cerebral oxygen consumption.[39] Therefore, during anesthesia, the patient is prone to cerebral hypoxia. The patient's extreme sensitivity to central nervous system depressants makes minimal use of tranquilizers, narcotics, and hypnotics important.[119]

Diagnosis

Total serum T_4, free T_4, and the free thyroxine index as estimated through T_4 and T_3RU are decreased in hypothyroidism of all etiologies. Serum T_3 may be normal or decreased and therefore is not helpful in making the diagnosis. Radioactive iodine uptake may be normal, increased, or decreased, depending on the etiology of the disorder, and is valuable for diagnosis only as part of the TSH-stimulation test. Direct measurement of serum TSH by RIA usually differentiates primary from secondary hypothyroidism, thus making both the TSH- and TRH-stimulation tests unnecessary. If a patient has been on TH, 4 to 6 weeks off replacement should be allowed before the diagnosis of hypothyroidism is confirmed and therapy reinstituted.[145]

The causes of hypothyroidism are divided into those of thyroid and those of suprathyroid origin. Of note among the thyroidal causes is drug-induced hypothyroidism. Defective TH synthesis secondary to lithium carbonate has become a common reversible cause of hypothyroidism.

Perioperative Management

When the diagnosis of hypothyroidism has been established, replacement with L-thyroxine should be instituted. Although young patients usually tolerate rapid replacement, gradual therapy is recommended in adults to avoid cardiac stress.

Elective surgery should be postponed until the patient is euthyroid. An initial oral dose of 25 μg of L-thyroxine daily can be increased by 25 μg every 2 weeks. During the first 6 months of replacement, serum T_4 and T_3 do not reflect the final optimal dose. In six myxedematous patients, serum T_4 and T_3 concentrations were 35% to 120% greater than values obtained 4 to 8 months later. Clinical status rather than laboratory values should therefore dictate early dose adjustments in myxedematous patients.[146]

Hypothyroid patients with angina may not tolerate TH replacement. However, pretreatment angina is not a contraindication to replacement if the patient has symptoms of hypothyroidism. In some patients, angina improves with replacement. The initial dose of L-thyroxine should be 15 μg daily, with increases of 15 μg every 2 weeks. If angina worsens, replacement should be discontinued or decreased.

Emergency surgery and trauma are poorly tolerated by the hypothyroid patient and require aggressive replacement. For the severely hypothyroid patient, an intravenous dose of 300 μg to 500 μg of L-thyroxine increases the basal metabolic rate and corrects electrocardiographic abnormalities within 6 hr.[124] Hydrocortisone in a dose of 300 mg should also be administered preoperatively and continued in a dose of 100 mg daily for several days, since the acute increase in basal metabolic rate may exhaust limited adrenal reserve. The effect of a single large dose of intravenous L-thyroxine persists for several days; therefore, the dose need not be repeated. Oral L-thyroxine in smaller daily doses as described above should be instituted as soon as possible. There is no clinical indication for the use of T_3.

Intravenous fluids should be administered cautiously because of the underlying difficulty with free water excretion. Serum electrolyte concentrations should be checked daily in the hypothyroid patient receiving intravenous fluids postoperatively.

Myxedema Coma

Myxedema coma is a medical emergency that, even with aggressive treatment, carries a mortality rate of 50%.[118,147,148] It is the end-stage of untreated hypothyroidism and is usually precipitated by infection, cold exposure, central nervous system depressants, or trauma. Causes of coma in myxedema include hypothermia, hypercarbia, and hyponatremia.

Hypothermia is present in over 80% of patients with myxedema coma.[79] Heat loss should be prevented and intravenous fluids warmed to body temperature, but external warming, which may worsen hypotension, is contraindicated. Although hypotension is present at presentation in 50% of patients, hypertension has also been reported.[116] Grand mal seizures occur in 25%, cerebellar signs are common, and frank psychosis may precede coma.[147,149] The electroencephalogram is usually markedly abnormal but correlates poorly with prognosis.[79] Recovery has been reported in patients with flat electroencephalograms.[149]

Hypoventilation and CO_2 retention may contribute to the development of coma. Airway obstruction is common and may precipitate acute respiratory failure. If the severely myxedematous patient is breathing spontaneously, an oral airway should be inserted to prevent obstruction by the tongue. Respirations should be monitored continuously and arterial blood gases checked every few hours. Oxygen therapy should be carefully controlled to prevent further CO_2 retention. The patient should be intubated and placed on a respirator for increasing hypercarbia.

Hyponatremia occurs in 50% of patients and may also contribute to coma.[116,150] Free water restriction is generally sufficient treatment. However, if hyponatremia is severe, with serum sodium concentrations of less than 115 mEq/liter, hypertonic saline may be given cautiously. If the patient is hypotensive, fluids should be given before pressors. Response to pressors is poor in hypothyroidism, and simultaneous administration of TH and pressors may precipitate life-threatening arrhythmias.[151]

In one study, hypoglycemia was reported in 4 (17.4%) of 23 severely myxedematous patients; 3 of the 4, or 75%, died.[150] Glucose-containing solutions should therefore be given along with corticosteroids to prevent adrenocortical insufficiency as the basal metabolic rate increases.

Administration of TH is critical in the treatment of myxedema coma. Because of severe hypometabolism and variable gastrointestinal absorption, intravenous L-thyroxine is recommended. A single dose of 500 µg replaces the extrathyroidal pool and need not be repeated for several days.[152] When the patient is conscious, oral L-thyroxine should be administered daily.

SUMMARY

1. The serum concentrations of T_4, T_3, and T_3RU change with surgery, anesthesia, chronic illness, and fasting. These laboratory changes alone may not indicate hypo- or hyperthyroidism.

2. The thyrotoxic patient has a higher risk than normal of complications and death during surgery and anesthesia. If surgery can be delayed, PTU in oral doses of 300 to 1200 mg should be administered daily for several weeks. Surgery can be performed with no increased risk when the patient is euthyroid according to clinical and laboratory criteria.

3. If surgery in the thyrotoxic patient cannot be delayed, PTU in an oral dose of 1000 mg and hydrocortisone in a dose of 300 mg are followed by SSKI, 5 drops orally 3 times daily, or sodium iodide, 1 g intravenously 3 times daily. Propranolol in an intravenous dose of 1 mg/min intravenously is used to control tachycardia, fever, hypertension, and arrhythmias.

4. Thyroid storm is a medical emergency that demands immediate treatment before laboratory documentation of thyrotoxicosis can be made. PTU, hydrocortisone, iodine, and propranolol should be given as described in (3) above.

5. Thyrotoxicosis after emergency surgery or after control of thyroid storm is managed with PTU, approximately 200 mg 4 times daily, and propranolol, 20 mg to 80 mg orally 4 times daily. SSKI, 2 drops orally 3 times daily, and hydrocortisone, 100 mg daily, are continued for 1 week.

6. The risks of subtotal thyroidectomy include hypothyroidism, recurrent hyperthyroidism, hypoparathyroidism, vocal-cord paralysis, laryngeal edema, and hemorrhage. Preparation of the thyrotoxic patient for subtotal thyroidectomy includes administration of PTU, as outlined in (2) above, with the addition of SSKI, 2 drops 3 times daily for 1 week before surgery.

7. A regimen of propranolol and iodine is an effective alternative preparation for the thyrotoxic patient facing subtotal thyroidectomy.

8. The hypothyroid patient also has a higher than normal risk of complications and death during surgery and anesthesia. If surgery can be delayed, L-thyroxine in an oral dose of 25 μg should be administered daily with increases of 25 μg every 2 weeks. Surgery can be performed with no increased risk when the patient is euthyroid according to clinical and laboratory criteria.

9. Slower replacement (15 μg daily with increments of 15 μg every 2 weeks) is suggested for elderly patients or patients with angina.

10. If surgery in the hypothyroid patient cannot be delayed, L-thyroxine in intravenous doses of 300 μg to 500 μg and hydrocortisone in a dose of 300 mg should be administered preoperatively. Hydrocortisone, 100 mg daily, should be continued for 1 week. L-thyroxine in a daily oral dose of 25 μg can be instituted several days postoperatively.

11. Myxedema coma is a medical emergency requiring immediate treatment. L-thyroxine and hydrocortisone should be given as described in (10) above.

REFERENCES

1. Vander JB, Gaston, EA, Dawber TR: Significance of solitary nontoxic thyroid nodules. N Engl J Med 251:970, 1954
2. Stagger, RP, Welch JW, Hellwig CA et al: Nodular goiter. Arch Intern Med 106:10, 1960
3. Schlesinger MG, Gargill JL, Saxe IH: Studies in nodular goiter. I. Incidence of thyroid nodules in routine necropsies in non-goitrous region. JAMA 110:1638, 1938
4. Mortensen JD, Woolner LB, Bennett WA: Gross and microscopic findings in clinically normal thyroid glands. J Clin Endocrinol Metab 15: 1270, 1955
5. Furszyfer JL, Kurland LT, McConahey WM et al: Graves' disease in Olmstead County, Minnesota, 1935–1967. Mayo Clin Proc 45:636, 1970
6. Iversen, K: Temporary Rise in the Frequency of Thyrotoxicosis in Denmark, 1941–1945. Copenhagen, Rosenkilde & Bagger, 1948
7. Degroot LJ, Stanbury JB: The Thyroid and its Diseases, pp 263, 411, 638. New York, John Wiley & Sons, 1975
8. Schimmel M, Utiger RD: Thyroid and peripheral production of thyroid hormones: Review of recent findings and their clinical implications. Ann Intern Med 87:760, 1977
9. Fore W, Kohler P, Wynn J: Rapid redistribution of serum thyroxine during ether anesthesia. J Clin Endocrinol Metab 26:821, 1966
10. Oyama T, Shibata S, Matsuki A: Thyroxine distribution during ether and thiopental anesthesia in man. Anesth Analg (Cleve) 48:1, 1969
11. Utiger RD: Decreased extrathyroidal triiodothyronine production in nonthyroidal illness: Benefit or harm? Am J Med 69:807, 1980
12. Burr WA, Black EG, Griffiths RS et al: Serum triiodothyronine and reverse triiodothyronine concentration after surgical operations. Lancet 2:1277, 1975
13. Cavalieri RR, Rapoport B: Impaired peripheral conversion of thyroxine to triiodothyronine. Annu Rev Med 28:57, 1977
16. Chopra IJ: An assessment of daily production and significance of thyroidal secretion of 3, 3', 5'-triiodothyronine (reverse T₃) in man. J Clin Invest 58:32, 1976
15. Bellabarba D, Inada M, Varsanoaharan N et al: Thyroxine transport and turnover in major non-thyroidal illness. J Clin Endocrinol Metab 28:1023, 1968

16. Brown-Grant K, Brennan RD, Yates FE: Simulation of the thyroid hormone-binding protein interactions in human plasma. J Clin Endocrinol Metab 30:733, 1970

17. Gregerman RI, Davis PJ: Effects of intrinsic and extrinsic variables on thyroid hormone economy. In Werner SC, Ingbar SH (eds): The Thyroid, 4th ed, p 235. Hagerstown, Harper & Row, 1978

18. Chopra IJ, Solomon DH, Chopra U et al: Alterations in circulating thyroid hormones and thyrotropin in hepatic cirrhosis: Evidence for euthyroidism despite subnormal serum triiodothyronine. J Clin Endocrinol Metab 39:501, 1974

19. Cuttelod S, Lenarchand-Béraud T, Magnenat P et al: Effect of age and role of kidneys and liver on thyrotropin turnover in man. Metabolism 23:101, 1974

20. Inada M, Sterling K: Thyroxine turnover and transport in Laennec's cirrhosis of the liver. J Clin Invest 46:1275, 1967

21. McConnon J, Row VV, Volpe R: The influence of liver damage in man on the distribution and disposal rates of thyroxine and triiodothyronine. J Clin Endocrinol Metab 34:144, 1972

22. Chopra IJ, Chopra U, Smith SR et al: Reciprocal changes in serum concentrations of 3, 3′, 5′-triiodothyronine (reverse T_3) and 3, 3′, 5-triiodothyronine (T_3) in systemic illness. J Clin Endocrinol Metab 41:1043, 1975

23. Nomura S, Pittman CS, Chambers JB et al: Reduced peripheral conversion of thyroxine to triiodothyronine in patients with hepatic cirrhosis. J Clin Invest 56:643, 1975

24. Spector D, Helderman H, David P et al: Low serum triiodothyronine (T_3) with euthyroidism in chronic renal failure (abstr). Presented at the Eighth Annual Meeting of the American Society of Nephrology, Washington, DC, November 25–26, 1975. Kidney Int 8:420, 1975

25. Pokroy N, Epstein S, Hendricks S et al: Thyrotrophin response to intravenous thyrotrophin-releasing hormone in patients with hepatic and renal disease. Horm Metab Res 6:132, 1974

26. Gregerman RI, Solomon N: Acceleration of thyroxine and triiodothyronine turnover during bacterial pulmonary infections and fever: Implications for the functional state of the thyroid during stress and in senescence. J Clin Endocrinol Metab 27:93, 1967

27. Portnay GI, O'Brian JT, Bush J et al: The effect of starvation on the concentration and binding of thyroxine and triiodothyronine in serum and on the response to TRH. J Clin Endocrinol Metab 39: 191, 1974

28. Chopra IJ, Smith SR: Circulating thyroid hormones and thyrotropin in adult patients with protein-calorie malnutrition. J Clin Endocrinol Metab 40:221, 1975

29. Vinik AI, Kalk WJ, McLaren H et al: Fasting blunts the TSH response to synthetic thyrotropin releasing hormone (TRH). J Clin Endocrinol Metab 40:509, 1975

30. McArthur JW, Rawson RW, Means JH et al: Thyrotoxic crisis. JAMA 134:868, 1947

31. Nelson NC, Becker WF: Thyroid crisis: Diagnosis and treatment. Ann Surg 170:263, 1969

32. Rives JD, Shepard RM: Thyroid crisis. Am Surg 17:406, 1951

33. Waldstein SS, Slodki SJ, Kaganiec I et al: A clinical study of thyroid storm. Ann Intern Med 52:626, 1960

34. Mazzaferri EL, Skillman TG: Thyroid storm: A review of 22 episodes with special emphasis on the use of guanethidine. Arch Intern Med 124:684, 1969

35. Blum M, Kranjac T, Park CM et al: Thyroid storm after cardiac angiography with iodinated contrast medium. JAMA 235:2324, 1976

36. Wolfson B, Smith K: Cardiac arrest following minor surgery in unrecognized thyrotoxicosis: A case report. Anesth Analg (Cleve) 47:672, 1968

37. Eriksson M, Rubenfeld S, Garber AJ et al: Propranolol does not prevent thyroid storm. N Engl J Med 296:263, 1977

38. Grossman W, Robin NI, Johnson LW et

al: The enhanced myocardial contractility of thyrotoxicosis: Role of the beta adrenergic receptor. Ann Intern Med 74:869, 1971

39. Ingbar SH, Woeber KA: The thyroid gland. In Williams RH (ed): Textbook of Endocrinology, 5th ed, p 95. Philadelphia, W B Saunders, 1974

40. Buccino RA, Spann JF Jr, Pool PE et al: Influence of thyroid state on the intrinsic contractile properties and energy stores of the myocardium. J Clin Invest 46:1669, 1967

41. Grossman W, Robin NI, Johnson LW et al: The enhanced myocardial contractility of thyrotoxicosis: Role of the beta adrenergic receptor. Ann Intern Med 74:869, 1971

42. Shafer RB, Bianco JA: Assessment of cardiac reserve in patients with hyperthyroidism. Chest 78:269, 1980

43. Dratman MB: The mechanism of thyroxine action. In Lie CH (ed): Hormonal Proteins and Peptides, Vol 6, p 205. New York, Academic Press, 1978

44. Doherty JE, Perkins WH: Digoxin metabolism in hypo and hyperthyroidism. Ann Intern Med 64:489, 1966

45. Stein M, Kimbel P, Johnson RL et al: Pulmonary function in hyperthyroidism. J Clin Invest 40:348, 1961

46. Ramsay ID: Muscle dysfunction in hyperthyroidism. Lancet 2:931, 1966

47. Doar JWH, Stamp TCB, Wynn V et al: Effects of oral and intravenous glucose loading in thyrotoxicosis: Studies of plasma glucose, free fatty acids, plasma insulin and blood pyruvate levels. Diabetes 18:663, 1969

48. Nikkilä EA, Kekki M: Plasma triglyceride metabolism in thyroid disease. J Clin Invest 51:2103, 1972

49. Hellerson C, Friis T, Larsen E et al: Small intestinal histology, radiology and absorption in hyperthyroidism. Scand J Gastroenterol 4:169, 1969

50. Sterling LC: Anaesthetic management of the patient with hyperthyroidism. Anesthesiology 41:585, 1974

51. Klion FM, Segal R, Schaffner F et al: The effect of altered thyroid function on the ultrastructure of the human liver. Am J Med 50:317, 1971

52. Dooner HP, Parada J, Aliaga C et al: The liver in thyrotoxicosis. Arch Intern Med 120:25, 1967

53. David PJ, Davis FB: Hyperthyroidism in patients over the age of 60 years. Medicine 53:161, 1974

54. Herman J, Resnitzky P, Fink A: Association between thyrotoxicosis and thrombocytopenia: A case report and review of the literature. Isr J Med Sci 14:469, 1978

55. Herman J: Thrombocytopenic purpura and thyroid disease. Ann Intern Med 93:934, 1980

56. Hetzel BS, Mason EK, Wang HK: Studies of long-acting thyroid stimulator in relation to exophthalmos after therapy for thyrotoxicosis. Aust Ann Med 17:307, 1968

57. Hetzel BS, Wall JR: Pretibial myxedema. Aust J Derm 10:18, 1969

58. Pinals RS, Tomar RH, Haas DC et al: Graves' disease, myasthenia gravis and purpura. Ann Intern Med 87:250, 1977

59. Segal BM, Weintraub M: Hashimoto's thyroiditis, myasthenia gravis, idiopathic thrombocytopenic purpura. Ann Intern Med 85:761, 1976

60. Sahay BM, Blendis LM, Greene R: Relation between myasthenia gravis and thyroid disease. Br Med J 1:762, 1965

61. Durston JH: Myasthenia gravis, Hashimoto's thyroiditis and pernicious anemia. Postgrad Med J 45:290, 1969

62. Krol TC: Myasthenia gravis, pernicious anemia and Hashimoto's thyroiditis. Arch Neurol 36:594, 1979

63. Vagenakis AG, Wang C, Burger A et al: Iodine-induced thyrotoxicosis in Boston. N Engl J Med 287:523, 1972

64. Bendixen HH, Ngai SH: Anesthesia in thyroid surgery. In Werner SC, Ingbar SH (eds): The Thyroid, 4th ed, p 584. Hagerstown, Harper & Row, 1978

65. Oppenheimer JH, Schwartz HJ, Surks MI: Propylthiouracil inhibits the conversion of L-thyroxine to L-triiodothyronine. J Clin Invest 51:2493, 1972

66. Mills LC: Drug treatment in thyroid disease. Semin Drug Treat 3:377, 1974

67. Wartofsky L, Ransil BJ, Ingbar SH: Inhibition by iodine of the release of thyroxine from the thyroid glands of patients with thyrotoxicosis. J Clin Invest 49:78, 1970

68. Wolff J, Chaikoff IL: Plasma inorganic iodide as homeostatic regulator of thyroid function. J Biol Chem 174:555, 1948

69. Wolff J, Chaikoff IL, Goldberg RC et al: The temporary nature of the inhibitory action of excess iodide on inorganic iodine synthesis in the normal thyroid. Endocrinology 45:504, 1949

70. Shanks RG, Lowe DC, Hadden DR et al: Controlled trial of propranolol in thyrotoxicosis. Lancet 1:993, 1969

71. Das G, Krieger M: Treatment of thyrotoxic storm with intravenous propranolol. Ann Intern Med 70:985, 1969

72. Hadden DR, Montgomery DAD, Shanks RG et al: Propranolol and iodine-131 in the management of thyrotoxicosis. Lancet 2:852, 1968

73. Wilber JF, Utiger RD: The effects of glucocorticoids on thyrotropin secretion. J Clin Invest 48:2096, 1969

74. Wase AW, Foster WC: Thiopental and thyroid metabolism. Proc Soc Exp Biol Med 91:89, 1956

75. Hanscom D, Ryan RJ: Thyroid crisis and diabetic ketoacidosis. N Engl J Med 257:697, 1957

76. Roizen M, Becker C: Thyroid storm: A review of cases at University of California, San Francisco. Cal Med 115:5, 1971

77. Brooks M, Waldstein S, Bronsky D et al: Serum triiodothyronine concentration in thyroid storm. J Clin Endocrinol Metab 40:339, 1975

78. Jacobs H, Eastman C, Ekins R et al: Total and free triiodothyronine and thyroxine levels in thyroid storm and recurrent hyperthyroidism. Lancet 2:236, 1973

79. Urbanic RC, Mazzaferri EL: Thyrotoxic crisis and myxedema coma. Heart Lung 7:435, 1978

80. Holdsworth CD, Besser GM: Influence of gastric emptying rate and insulin response on oral glucose tolerance in thyroid disease. Lancet 2:700, 1968

81. Larsen P: Salicylate-induced increase in free triiodothyronine in human serum. J Clin Invest 51:1125, 1972

82. Mackin JF, Canary JJ, Pittman CS: Current concepts of thyroid storm and its management. N Engl J Med 291:1396, 1977

83. Lee TC, Coffee RJ, Mackin J et al: The use of propranolol in the surgical treatment of thyrotoxic patients. Ann Surg 177:643, 1973

84. Ashkar FS, Katims RB, Smock WM et al: Thyroid storm treatment with blood exchange and plasmapheresis. JAMA 214:1275, 1970

85. Dobyns BM, Sheline GE, Workman JB et al: Malignant and benign neoplasms of the thyroid in patients treated for hyperthyroidism: A report of the cooperative thyrotoxicosis therapy follow-up study. J Clin Endocrinol Metab 38:976, 1974

86. Saenger EL, Thoma GE, Tompkins EA: Incidence of leukemia following treatment of hyperthyroidism. JAMA 205:855, 1968

87. Safa AM, Schumacher OP, Rodriguez-Antunez A: Long-term follow-up results in children and adolescents treated with radioactive iodine (^{131}I) for hyperthyroidism. N Engl J Med 292:167, 1975

88. Hung W, Wilkins L, Blizzard R: Medical therapy of thyrotoxicosis in children. Pediatrics 30:17, 1962

89. Reeve TS, Hales IB, White B et al: Thyroidectomy in the management of thyrotoxicosis in the adolescent. Surgery 65:694, 1969

90. Werner SC: Radioiodine. In Werner SC (ed): The Thyroid, 4th ed, p 827. Hagerstown, Harper & Row, 1978

91. Starr P, Jaffe HL, Oettinger L: Later results of ^{131}I treatment of hyperthyroidism in 73 children and adolescents. J Nucl Med 10:586, 1969

92. Hayek A, Chapman EM, Crawford JD: Long-term results of treatment of thyrotoxicosis in children and adolescents

with radioactive iodine. N Engl J Med 283:949, 1970

93. Black BM: Surgery for Graves' disease. Mayo Clin Proc 47:966, 1972

94. Burrow GN: Hyperthyroidism during pregnancy. N Engl J Med 298:150, 1978

95. Colcock BP: Modern indications for thyroidectomy. Am J Surg 122:296, 1971

96. Colcock BP, Pena O: Diagnosis and treatment of thyroiditis. Postgrad Med 44:83, 1968

97. Lindem MC, Clark JH: Indications for surgery in thyroiditis. Am J Surg 118:829, 1969

98. Gershengorn MC, McClung MR, Chu EW et al: Fine needle aspiration cytology in the preoperative diagnosis of thyroid nodules. Ann Intern Med 87:265, 1977

99. Walfish PG, Hazani E, Strawbridge HTG et al: Combined ultrasound and needle aspiration cytology in the management of hypofunctioning thyroid nodules. Ann Intern Med 87:270, 1977

100. Hershman JM: The treatment of hyperthyroidism. Ann Intern Med 64:1306, 1966

101. Nofal MM, Beierwaltes WH: Treatment of hyperthyroidism with sodium iodide¹³¹I. JAMA 197:605, 1966

102. Welsum, MV, Feltkamp TEW, DeVries MJ et al: Hypothyroidism after thyroidectomy for Graves' disease: A search for an explanation. Br Med J 4:755, 1974

103. Hedley AJ, Flemming CJ, Marian CI et al: Surgical treatment of thyrotoxicosis. Br Med J 1:519, 1970

104. Kalk WJ, Durbach D, Kantor S et al: Postthyroidectomy thyrotoxicosis. Lancet 1:291, 1978

105. Davis RH, Fourman P, Smith JW et al: Prevalence of parathyroid insufficiency after thyroidectomy. Lancet 2:1432, 1961

106. Michie W, Duncan T, Hamer-Hodges DW et al: Mechanism of hypocalcemia after thyroidectomy for thyrotoxicosis. Lancet 1:508, 1971

107. Martis C, Athanassiades S: Post-thyroidectomy laryngeal edema. Am J Surg 122:58, 1971

108. Pimstone B, Joffee B: The use and abuse of beta-adrenergic blockade in the surgery of hyperthyroidism. S Afr Med J 44:1059, 1970

109. Bewsher PD, Pegg CAS, Stewart DJ et al: Propranolol in the surgical management of thyrotoxicosis. Ann Surg 180:787, 1974

110. Feek CM, Sawers SA, Irvine WJ: Combination of potassium iodide and propranolol in preparation of patients with Graves' disease for thyroid surgery. New Engl J Med 302:883, 1980

111. Michie W, Pegg CAS, Hamer-Hodges DW et al: Beta-blockade and partial thyroidectomy for thyrotoxicosis. Lancet 1:1009, 1974

112. Zonszein J, Santangelo RP, Mackin JF et al: Propranolol therapy in thyrotoxicosis: A review of 84 patients undergoing surgery. Am J Med 66:411, 1979

113. Caswell HT, Marks AD, Channick BJ: Propranolol for the preoperative preparation of patients with thyrotoxicosis. Surg Gynecol Obstet 146:908, 1978

114. El-Khodary AZ, Thiffault C, Deschenes L et al: Preparation for the surgical treatment of hyperthyroidism using propranolol. Can J Surg 17:304, 1974

115. Toft AD, Irvine WJ, Campbell RWF: Assessment by continuous cardiac monitoring of minimum duration of preoperative propranolol treatment in thyrotoxic patients. Clin Endocrinol 5:195, 1976

116. Forrester CF: Coma in myxedema. Arch Intern Med 111:734, 1963

117. Blum M: Myxedema Coma. Am J Med Sci 264:432, 1972

118. Senior RM, Birge SJ, Wessler S et al: The recognition and management of myxedema coma. JAMA 217:61, 1971

119. Kim JM, Hackman L: Anesthesia for untreated hypothyroidism: Report of three cases. Anesth Analg (Cleve) 56:299, 1977

120. Means JH: The Thyroid and its Diseases, 2nd ed. Philadelphia, JB Lippincott, 1968

121. Bough EW, Crowley WF, Ridgway EC et al: Myocardial function in hypothyroidism: Relation to disease severity and re-

sponse to treatment. Arch Intern Med 138:1476, 1978

122. Crowley WF, Ridgway EC, Bough EW et al: Non-invasive evaluation of cardiac function in hypothyroidism: Response to gradual thyroxine replacement. N Engl J Med 296:1, 1977

123. Hillis WS, Bremner WF, Lawrie TDV et al: Systolic time intervals in thyroid disease. Clin Endocrinol 4:617, 1975

124. Holvey DN, Goodner CJ, Nicoloff JT et al: Treatment of myxedema coma with intravenous thyroxine. Arch Intern Med 113:89, 1964

125. Abbott TR: Anesthesia in untreated myxedema. Br J Anaesth 39:510, 1967

126. Steinberg AD: Myxedema and coronary artery disease—A comparative autopsy study. Ann Intern Med 68:338, 1968

127. Aber CP, Noble RL, Thompson GS et al: Serum lactic dehydrogenase isoenzymes in "myxoedema heart disease." Br Heart J 28:663, 1966

128. Paine, TD, Rogers WJ, Baxley WA et al: Coronary arterial surgery in patients with incapacitating angina pectoris and myxedema. Am J Cardiol 40:226, 1977

129. Wilson WR, Bedell GN: The pulmonary abnormalities in myxedema. J Clin Invest 39:42, 1960

130. Massumi RA, Winnacker JL: Severe depression of the respiratory center in myxedema. Am J Med 36:876, 1964

131. Zwillich CW, Pierson DJ, Hofeldt FD et al: Ventilatory control in myxedema and hypothyroidism. N Engl J Med 292:662, 1975

132. Ardeman S, Chanarin I, Krafchik B et al: Addisonian pernicious anemia and intrinsic factor antibodies in thyroid disorders. Q J Med 35:421, 1966

133. Tudhope GR, Wilson GM: Deficiency of vitamin B12 in hypothyroidism. Lancet 1:703, 1962

134. Orr FR: Hemorrhage in myxedema coma. Lancet 2:1012, 1962

135. Simone JV, Abildgaard CF, Schulman I: Blood coagulation in thyroid dysfunction. N Engl J Med 273:1057, 1965

136. Edson JR, Fecher DR, Doe RP: Low platelet adhesiveness and other hemostatic abnormalities in hypothyroidism. Ann Intern Med 82:342, 1975

137. Crispell KR, Parson W, Sprinkle P: A cortisone-resistant abnormality in diuretic response to ingested water in primary myxedema. J Clin Endocrinol 14:640, 1954

138. Vogt JH: Impaired water excretion capacity in primary myxedema improved by corticosteroids, corticotrophin and thyroid substitution. Acta Endocrinol (Coph) 35:277, 1960

139. Bleifer RH, Belsky JL, Saxon L et al: The diuretic response to administered water in patients with primary myxedema. Clin Res 7:245, 1959

140. Aikawa JK: The nature of myxedema: Alterations in the serum electrolyte concentrations and in the exchangeable sodium and potassium contents. Ann Intern Med 44:30, 1956

141. Goldberg M, Reivich M: Studies on the mechanism of hyponatremia and impaired water excretion in myxedema. Ann Intern Med 56:120, 1962

142. DeRubertis FR, Michelis MF, Bloom ME et al: Impaired water excretion in myxedema. Am J Med 51:41, 1971

143. Showsky WR, Kikuchi TA: The role of vasopressin in the impaired water excretion of myxedema. Am J Med 64:613, 1978

144. Carpenter CCJ, Solomon N, Silverberg SG et al: Schmidt's syndrome (thyroid and adrenal insufficiency): A review of the literature and a report of 15 new cases including 10 instances of coexistent diabetes mellitus. Medicine 43:153, 1964

145. Vagenakis AG, Braverman LE, Azizi E et al: Recovery of pituitary thyrotropic function after withdrawal of prolonged thyroid-suppression therapy. N Engl J Med 293:681, 1975

146. Brown ME, Refetoff S: Transient elevation of serum hormone concentration after initiation of replacement therapy in myxedema. Ann Intern Med 92:491, 1980

147. Catz B, Russell S: Myxedema, shock and coma. Arch Intern Med 108:407, 1961

148. Rosenberg IN: Hypothyroidism and coma. Surg Clin North Am 48:353, 1968

149. Jellinek EH: Fits, faints, coma and dementia in myxedema. Lancet 2:1010, 1962

150. Nickerson JF, Hill SR Jr, McNeill JH et al: Fatal myxedema, with and without coma. Ann Intern Med 53:475, 1960

151. Winawer SJ, Rosen SM, Cohn H: Myxedema coma with ventricular tachycardia. Arch Intern Med 111:647, 1963

152. Green WL: Guidelines for the treatment of myxedema. Med Clin North Am 52:431, 1968

13

Perioperative Management of the Overweight Patient

SANKEY V. WILLIAMS

In the United States, 30% of men and 20% of women between the ages of 30 and 60 are 20% or more above ideal weight; 15% of men and 20% of women in this age group are 35% or more above ideal weight. This chapter begins with a definition of obesity and a review of its natural history. The numerous medical consequences of being overweight and their particular relevance to the surgical patient are presented next. The chapter concludes with a discussion of surgical complications that are common in the overweight patient.

DEFINITION OF OBESITY

Understanding what is known about the health of overweight persons is complicated, because different investigators have used different measures of body size. Simple body weight in pounds or kilograms does not take into account the subject's height. In most cases in which weight is associated with health, it is not known whether body size or body composition is the more important measure.

The predominant opinion is that amount of body fat is usually more important than size alone. Because of this, different indexes have been developed that combine height and weight to provide an indirect measure of body fat. In white adult females, the preferred index is probably weight divided by height.[1] In white adult males, the preferred index is weight divided by the square of height (the Quetelet or body-mass index).[1-3] Some investigators have used a mathematically equivalent technique that divides the person's weight by the average weight of a standard population (relative weight) or by the weight at which mortality is lowest (the desirable or ideal weight).[4] It is convenient that these measures are all closely correlated and that few, if any, of the important conclusions drawn from the literature would be different if an alternative index were used.[5]

Whatever measure of body size is used, there is still the problem of distinguishing normal people from people who are larger or smaller than normal. There is no completely satisfactory solution to this problem, and thus no simple estimate can be made of the proportion of the population that is overweight enough to be considered abnormal.

The natural history of obesity reveals that weight may vary over short periods of time but is relatively stable over long periods of time. When 5209 residents of the town of Framingham, Massachusetts, were weighed every other year for 18 years, the mean difference between the highest and lowest weights for each person was 21 lb.[6] This represented short-term fluctuation, however, and persistent changes occurred very slowly. For most people, weight at one age was closely related to weight later in life. There was a high correlation between weight at entry and final weight 18 years later. Although complicated by changes over time, average weight increased to age 54, plateaued to age 62, and then declined.

MEDICAL COMPLICATIONS OF OBESITY

Longevity

Between 1903 and 1979, five large investigations based on pooled life insurance records examined the relationship between weight and longevity, and all found increased weight to be associated with decreased longevity.[6] Five additional studies not restricted to holders of life insurance policies support this conclusion.[8-13] As weight increases, mortality increases even faster. Persons who are 30% to 40% heavier than average have a mortality rate 50% higher than that of persons of average weight. Persons who are 40% or more heavier than average have a mortality rate 90% higher than that of persons of average weight.[10] Being overweight at a younger age may be worse than being overweight at an older age.[11] Deaths attributed especially to coronary artery disease and diabetes mellitus but also to digestive diseases, cerebrovascular disease, and cancer account for much of the excess mortality.[10]

However, there is some disagreement about the weight at which mortality is lowest.[14] In the 1959 life insurance study, the lowest mortality was found in those who were most underweight.[5,12] In the 1979 life insurance study, the lowest mortality rate was found among those who were 10% under the average weight; those who were 20% underweight had a higher mortality.[5] A prospective study of 750,000 men and women drawn from the general population and followed from 1959 to 1972 found the lowest mortality among both those of average weight and those 10% to 20% below average weight. Men who were 20% or more below average weight had a 25% higher mortality rate than those of average weight.[10] The Framingham study found the lowest mortality among those of average weight, with increased mortality for those below average weight.[12]

A single study suggests that weight loss decreases mortality.[15] Death rates are described in 2300 people who were charged an extra premium for life insurance because they were overweight but who subsequently reduced their weight enough to be charged lower rates. For both men and women, the death rate was higher than normal but lower in the group who lost weight than in a similar group who were initially charged the extra premium and did not lose weight.

Hypertension

The association between hypertension and obesity is supported by convincing epidemiologic information.[16-18] The relationship is strongest in persons with a family history of obesity and hypertension, in the extremely obese, and in young age groups. Between one-fifth and one-third of adult hypertensives are overweight. In the Framingham study, there was a moderately strong correlation between blood pressure and body weight.[6,17] Correlations were stronger for diastolic than for systolic blood pressure and were slightly more pronounced in women and in young age groups. Depending on age and sex, between 17% and 47% of the most overweight patients were hypertensive.

Universal acceptance of the relationship between hypertension and body weight has been delayed by conflicting answers to two questions: (1) In obese patients, are the same blood pressure measurements obtained with a blood pressure cuff as with intra-arterial recordings? (2) Does weight loss without salt restriction decrease blood pressure? Several studies demonstrate that mean blood pressure measurements in groups are approximately the same whether one uses the auscultatory method with an adequate cuff or the intra-arterial method.[16,19,20] However, in individual patients, there are unpredictable differences between the two methods. Although several studies have documented that weight loss produces a drop in blood pressure, only two have measured sodium balance. The first failed but the second succeeded in showing a decrease in blood pressure when weight was lost without salt restriction. A weight loss of approximately 10 lb produced decreases in mean blood pressure of approximately 20 torr.

Lipid Abnormalities

Body weight is correlated with blood lipid levels, and changes in weight produce changes in these levels. In the Framingham study, relative weight was positively correlated with triglycerides, total cholesterol, low-density lipoprotein (LDL)-cholesterol, and very low-density lipoprotein (VLDL)-cholesterol.[23,24] The strongest association was the inverse correlation between relative weight and high-density lipoprotein (HDL)-cholesterol. The associations were strongest in men and young persons, except in the case of HDL-cholesterol, for which there were no age or sex differences.

A large study conducted by the Lipid Research Clinics confirmed the inverse correlation between weight and HDL-cholesterol.[25,26] The difference in mean HDL-cholesterol between the 10th and 90th percentiles for body weight was 6 to 7 mg/dl, enough to alter cardiovascular mortality. These relationships persisted when the effects of other factors that affect lipid levels were removed. When all variables were considered simultaneously, body weight, cigarette smoking, and alcohol use were the factors most strongly and consistently associated with HDL-cholesterol.[26]

A stronger relationship was found between changes in body weight and changes in lipid levels than between the simple level of body weight and the simple level of blood lipid. For each 10% change in relative weight for men, there was a change of 11.3 mg/dl in total cholesterol. In women, the corresponding change was 6.3 mg/dl.[24] Five other studies describe similar changes in cholesterol levels with weight loss and gain, and four additional studies document comparable changes for HDL-cholesterol.[24,26]

Atherosclerotic Cardiovascular Disease

Through its effects on other risk factors, obesity is indirectly associated with a higher incidence than normal of coronary artery disease and congestive heart failure. In the Framingham cohort, persons who weighed 35% more than their ideal weight had a relative risk of congestive heart failure of 1.7 for men and 2.1 for women and a relative risk of coronary heart disease of 1.6 for men and 1.4 for women.[6,27,28] The risk factors known to be associated simultaneously with body weight and atherosclerotic cardiovascular disease include the components of serum cholesterol and blood pressure. When the effects of these risk factors are removed, body weight is no longer correlated with congestive heart failure or coronary artery disease.[6,29–31] Obesity therefore should be thought of as a cause of other cardiovascular risk factors and thus as a marker of their presence rather than as a risk factor itself.

The relationship between body weight and stroke is similar to the relationship between body weight and atherosclerotic heart disease.[6,28,32] Obesity is associated with elevated blood pressure, the risk factor most highly correlated with stroke, and obesity probably exerts its apparent effect on stroke through this risk factor.

Since obesity exerts such a powerful, if indirect, effect on atherosclerotic heart disease and stroke, it is surprising that increasing body weight is inversely correlated with peripheral vascular disease, the third major category of atherosclerotic cardiovascular disease.[6,28] The negative effect of obesity on peripheral vascular disease is as strong and significant as its positive effect on atherosclerotic heart disease and stroke, especially for men. One suggested explanation is that increased weight limits exercise and that the obese person thus avoids the stress that would otherwise lead to symptoms.[28]

Other Cardiopulmonary Abnormalities

As body weight increases, the cardiovascular system responds with comparable increases in blood volume, resting cardiac output, and heart size.[33] Increased heart size results from myocardial hypertrophy and not from fatty infiltration as was once thought. The increase in cardiac output with exercise is normal, but pulmonary artery pressure and left ventricular end-diastolic filling pressure rise above normal with exercise in most obese subjects. With increasing obesity, there is an increase in cardiac work that can be disproportionate to the level of obesity.

The pulmonary system responds to moderate increases in body weight with increased minute ventilation resulting in normal arterial oxygen levels and normal or reduced levels of arterial carbon dioxide, despite increased resting oxygen consumption and carbon dioxide production.[34] Increased resting oxygen consumption and carbon dioxide production implies an increased work of breathing, which is explained by two mechanisms. First, respiratory muscles must work against an abnormal compliance caused largely by the chest wall with its heavy load of fat but also by the lung, which is probably made stiffer by an expanded pulmonary blood volume. Second, the respiratory muscles are inefficient in the overweight patient. Fatty infiltration of the diaphragm may explain part of the inefficiency, but abnormal neuromuscular coupling and an unfavorable configuration of the chest wall with upward displacement of the diaphragm by abdominal fat also play a role.

These abnormalities are responsible for the overweight subject's abnormal pulmonary function tests. There is a reduced volume that can be expired from the resting volume of the lung (expiratory reserve volume, ERV), and there is a reduction in the resting volume itself (functional residual capacity, FRC). As a consequence, the overweight patient breathes shallowly, exhibiting a reduction in vital capacity (VC), but rapidly to maintain minute ventilation. This breathing pattern is useful at rest, because the oxygen cost of breathing is lower than it would be with other combinations of volume and rate. With effort, however, an increasing rate causes a disproportionate increase in oxygen consumption that is worsened by an increase in relative dead space. The result is a decrease in maximum voluntary ventilation (MVV).

Shallow breathing also produces relative overventilation of the upper lungs and underventilation of the lower lungs, where perfusion is greater. The resulting ventilation–perfusion inequality is worsened if the ERV is reduced below the closing volume (CV) of the alveoli, which collapse but continue to be perfused. Hypoxemia in the obese patient is caused by these ventilation–perfusion inequalities, and it is worsened when the patient is in the supine position because of further reductions in ERV.

Diabetes Mellitus

The association between obesity and diabetes mellitus is supported by good epidemiologic information.[23,35-37] The prevalence of diabetes increases in all age groups as relative weight increases, but the effect appears at lower relative weights in older age groups.[19] When 3751 men were followed for 10 years, a rapidly accelerating increase in the risk of diabetes was found as initial weight increased from normal to more than 45% overweight.[8] The Framingham study found that, for each 10% change in relative weight, there was a change in blood glucose of 2.5 mg/dl in men and 1.3 mg/dl in women.[24]

The association between obesity and diabetes is also supported by a growing understanding of the mechanism through which obesity exerts its effects. Independent of other factors known to influence insulin resistance and insulin secretion, obesity interferes with the ability of muscle and fatty tissues to take up glucose and promotes higher circulating insulin levels in response to oral glucose. The primary effect is probably an increase in insulin resistance that requires the obese person to secrete larger than normal amounts of insulin for normal glucose homeostasis.[38] These effects are partly explained by a decrease in the number of insulin receptors on cell surfaces, but there are also postreceptor abnormalities involving glucose transport, glucose phosphorylation, and other cellular systems.[39,40]

Gallstones

Several studies have demonstrated an association between increasing weight and increasing prevalence of gallstones, independent of age, sex, or parity.[41-44] The abnormal cholesterol metabolism found in obese people may be responsible for this association, acting through elevated biliary cholesterol secretion and gallbladder bile that is supersaturated with cholesterol.[45,46]

Abnormalities in Sex Hormones and Reproductive Function

In both women and men, there are changes in the levels of sex hormones with obesity, but only in women have clinically important disorders been documented. In one study, women who reported irregular menstrual cycles lasting more than 36 days were more than 30 lb heavier than women who reported no menstrual abnormalities, with height and age adjusted for.[47] The polycystic ovary, or Stein–Leventhal, syndrome is associated with obesity. Multiple, small ovarian cysts and irregular menstrual cycles progress to amenorrhea. Women who had surgery for polycystic ovaries reported more teenage obesity than women who had ovarian surgery for other causes.[47] Morbidly obese women who do not have polycystic ovaries have other pathologic changes in their ovaries that are not present in control patients of normal weight and that suggest a predisposition to premature ovarian failure.[48]

Hyperuricemia and Gout

Increasing weight is the single most important variable associated with elevated serum uric acid levels, and one study suggests that weight loss causes a decrease in uric acid levels.[6,49,50] In the Framingham study, the prevalence of gout was also correlated with relative weight.[6]

Cancer

Prevalence studies suggest an association between obesity and death from a variety of cancers.[10] A number of case-control studies have demonstrated correlation between obesity and endometrial cancer.[51–54] Obesity has been suggested as a risk factor for breast cancer, but many studies show weak correlations that are not significant, and some of the results are conflicting.[55,56]

Psychiatric and Emotional Disorders

As a group, people with mild or moderate obesity do not score differently on psychologic tests or have consistently different indices of anxiety and depression from control groups, and people with morbid obesity have no more psychopathology than control groups when specific criteria for psychiatric disease are used.[57–63] Nevertheless, there are two emotional disturbances related to obesity that have been found in subgroups of obese persons.[64] First, almost half of juvenile-onset obese persons have a disturbed body image; they perceive themselves as grotesque and loathsome and think others view them with hostility and contempt. Second, young upper-class women are subject to two eating disorders that are precipitated by stress. In one, there is morning anorexia and evening hyperphagia with insomnia. In the other (bulimia), there is compulsive ingestion of a large amount of food in a short period of time, usually followed by agitation and self-condemnation.

Although overweight persons are no more subject to psychopathology than normal-weight persons, they experience more worry and pain because of their weight. Nearly 8000 persons in 2756 families from six geographic areas in the United States have been enrolled in the Rand Health Insurance Study. A comprehensive, initial assessment of the participants found that, of those who were most overweight, 79% worried about their weight, 32% experienced pain due to their weight, and 29% restricted their activities because of their weight. Comparable values for normal-weight and moderately overweight persons were substantially lower.[65]

SURGICAL COMPLICATIONS IN THE OVERWEIGHT PATIENT

Although surgeons and anesthesiologists generally agree that overweight patients have an increased risk of perioperative complications and death, relatively few studies adequately document these beliefs.[66,67]

Surgical Mortality

There have been only two well-controlled studies of surgical mortality. In the first, each of 300 consecutive women weighing over 200 lb and undergoing abdominal hysterectomy was matched with the next consecutive nonobese patient undergoing the same procedure.[68] Obese patients weighed an average of 60 lb more than their controls. There were 3 deaths among the obese patients and none among the controls. Although not statistically significant, the difference may be clinically important, given the difficulty of establishing statistical significance in a study of this size and the very low death rates expected with this operation. In a cooperative study of surgical therapy for duodenal ulcer conducted in Veterans Administration hospitals, patients were classified as obese if they weighed more than 35 lb over their ideal weight.[69] Of 116 obese patients, 8, or 7%, died postoperatively; in contrast, only 72 of 2649 nonobese patients, or 2.7%, died postoperatively. Other authors reach conflicting conclusions about relative death rates in obese and nonobese patients after inadequately controlled studies of cholecystectomy, surgery for endometrial carcinoma, cesarean section, and other operations.[70–74]

Large numbers of morbidly obese patients have undergone major surgical procedures designed to promote weight loss. The surgical mortality rate of jejunoileal bypass procedures is approximately 1.8% to 3% in the majority of published studies from experienced centers, but one study described no deaths among 130 patients.[75–78] The surgical mortality rate of gastric bypass procedures is probably lower than that of jejunoileal procedures.[79–82]

There are no studies that describe the effect of weight loss before surgery on surgical mortality or complications in the obese patient.

Pulmonary Complications

During surgery, morbidly obese patients experience a decrease in arterial oxygen concentration that may reach unacceptably low levels despite inspiration of 40% oxygen.[83] Intraoperative hypoxemia is worsened when the patient is in the head-down position or when subdiaphragmatic packs are used, and it is not corrected by use of positive end-expiratory pressure (PEEP).[83,84] Morbidly obese patients also experience postoperative hypoxemia that can persist for as long as 5 days after surgery.[85] Early postoperative hypoxemia can be improved by placement of the patient in the semirecumbent position and is probably greater in patients undergoing abdominal surgery with a transverse than with a vertical incision.[86,87]

Postoperative atelectasis may be more frequent in the obese than in the normal patient. Although criteria for diagnosis of atelectasis were not described, 11 of 124 obese patients, or 8.9%, and 127 of 2695 nonobese patients, or 4.7%, developed atelectasis in one series of patients undergoing surgery for duodenal ulcer.[69] In contrast, a second study, which also omitted criteria for diagnosis of atelectasis, reported the disorder to be less frequent in obese (2 of 48, or 4.2%) than in nonobese (14 of 236, or 5.9%) female patients undergoing cholecystectomy.[70] A higher than normal frequency of macroatelectasis in obese patients has been described for 46 patients undergoing elective upper abdominal surgery and for 40 patients having elective cholecystectomy.[88,89]

Postoperative pneumonia is not more frequent in obese patients. In one controlled study that did not define the criteria for diagnosis of pneumonia, there were fewer postoperative pneumonias in obese patients (4 of 120, or 3.3%) than in nonobese subjects (163 of 2532, or 6.4%).[69] A second study with carefully defined criteria found no significant relationship between weight and incidence of postoperative chest infections.[90] Obese patients do have a greater volume of gastric contents with a lower pH than nonobese patients, and special preoperative care has been recommended to prevent aspiration pneumonitis.[91]

Wound Complications

All five studies of the relationship between obesity and postoperative wound infection report a statistically significant association between the two. This association is strengthened by the diverse nature of the studies and is probably not compromised by the widely varying infection rates that were found. In a case-control study of women undergoing abdominal hysterectomy, 17 of 300 obese women, or 5.7%, and 2 of 300 nonobese women, or 0.8%, developed wound infections.[68] In a study of patients undergoing surgery for duodenal ulcer, 19 of 125 obese patients, or 15.3%, and 221 of 2695 nonobese patients, or 8.2%, suffered wound infections.[69] In a study of the value of topical antiseptic for preventing wound infection, 6 of 29 obese patients, or 20.7%, and 6 of 115 nonobese patients in the control group, or 5.1%, developed such infections. Intraoperative application of povidine–iodine to the wound reduced the incidence of wound infection in the obese

patients.[92] In a study of the value of wound drains in 250 patients with abdominal incisions, 11 of 23, or 47.8%, and 3 of 26, or 11.5%, obese and nonobese patients with obviously contaminated wounds developed wound infection, respectively. Wound drains were thought to be helpful in obese but not in nonobese patients. However, there were no significant differences between obese and nonobese patients if the wounds were either clean or only potentially contaminated.[93] In a study of patients who underwent cesarean section, 33 of 61 obese patients, or 54.1%, and 21 of 68 nonobese patients, or 30.9%, developed postoperative fever; the fever was probably caused by bacterial infection, since it was found to be preventable with antibiotics.[94]

Few of the studies reported are adequately controlled, but the evidence clearly implicates obesity as an important risk factor for wound dehiscence, probably because of mechanical factors and because wound infection is an important precursor of dehiscence.[95–99]

Postoperative Thromboembolism

Although there is contradictory evidence about the association of obesity with pulmonary embolism, there is uniform evidence about its association with venous thrombosis.[100,101] In a study of patients undergoing surgery for duodenal ulcer, 5 of 124 obese patients, or 4%, and 19 of 2676 nonobese patients, or 0.7%, developed clinically manifest thrombophlebitis.[69] Two studies have used radioactively labeled fibrinogen to show a higher incidence of postoperative thrombosis in the calf of obese than nonobese patients.[102,103]

The evidence that obesity may be an important risk factor for the development of pulmonary embolus comes from autopsy studies of hospitalized patients and from prospective clinical studies. An autopsy study published in 1927 reported that 40 of 156 obese patients, or 25.6%, and 130 of 1942 nonobese patients, or 7.9%, died from postoperative pulmonary embolism and that the rate of fatal embolism increased with increasing weight.[104] Coon's widely quoted autopsy study found pulmonary emboli in 119 of 544 obese patients, or 21.9%, and 584 of 4056 nonobese patients, or 14.4%, but the figures for postoperative pulmonary embolism were not correlated with actual body weight.[105] A recent study of 508 autopsies reported 280 pulmonary emboli, but there was no correlation between body weight and occurrence of emboli.[106]

Prospective clinical trials are no more conclusive. Clinical features of patients with pulmonary emboli who were treated with urokinase and streptokinase have been described.[107] Of 167 patients who had submassive or massive pulmonary emboli demonstrated by pulmonary angiography, 40, or 30%, were obese; however, there was no control group. In a prospective study of admissions to the medical and surgical services of three Philadelphia hospitals, 322 of 6527 patients or 4.9%, had pulmonary emboli confirmed by pulmonary angiograms, autopsies, and pulmonary scans for diagnosis. Relative weight was not associated with pulmonary embolism.[108] Of 57 morbidly obese patients who underwent gastric bypass surgery and were followed postoperatively with serial Doppler studies of the common femoral vein, 7 developed clinical evidence of either deep venous thrombosis or pulmonary embolus; however, again, there was no comparison group of nonobese patients.[109]

Problems with Anesthesia

Anesthesia in overweight patients is complicated by a variety of technical and, to a lesser extent, metabolic and physiologic problems.[67,74] It is difficult to establish and maintain intravenous routes for drugs and fluids. Laryngoscopy and endotracheal intubation are complicated by distorted anatomy. With a face mask, the high pressures required for ventilation may promote gastric aspiration by rendering the gastroesophageal sphincter incompetent. A reduced FRC may allow unexpectedly rapid increases in the alveolar tension of insoluble anesthetic gases. It is difficult to identify the anatomic landmarks needed for regional and spinal anesthesia. Spinal anesthesia is further complicated by the possibility of reductions in ventilation and by unpredictable requirements for anesthetic that may result from unpredictable spinal canal volumes.[110] Maintaining fluid balance is difficult because of difficulty in evaluating dehydration and hypovolemia. Obese patients probably metabolize methoxyflurane and halothane differently from normal patients, and, unless anesthesia time is limited, the elevated serum fluoride levels that result from this biotransformation could cause renal and perhaps hepatic damage.[111]

SUMMARY

1. The more overweight the patient, the more likely and severe are the problems that have been described in this chapter and the more often practice should deviate from the usual pattern.
2. Extra care should be taken with the history and physical examination of

the obese patient to elicit information about the medical consequences of being overweight. These include hypertension, lipid disorders, atherosclerotic cardiovascular disease, the obesity-hypoventilation syndrome, diabetes mellitus, gallstones, gout, abnormalities of reproductive function in women, and endometrial cancer.

3. Few of the recommendations for preoperative testing given in Chapter 2 need be altered for the overweight patient. Special attention must be given to preventing pulmonary complications.

4. Medical and surgical problems should be managed no differently in the overweight than in the normal-weight patient.

5. Surgical complications are more common in the obese than in the normal patient. These include hypoxemia, wound infection, wound dehiscence, atelectasis, and, perhaps, thromboembolic disease.

6. A calorie-restricted diet should not be instituted for the obese patient admitted to the hospital for surgery. It will not lead to weight loss after discharge and may interfere with postoperative recovery.

REFERENCES

1. Florey C dV: The use and interpretation of ponderal index and other weight–height ratios in epidemiological studies. J Chronic Dis 23:93, 1970
2. Keys A, Fidanzia F, Karvonen MJ et al: Indices of relative weight and obesity. J Chronic Dis 25:329, 1972
3. Goldburt U, Medalie JH: Weight–height indices. Br J Prevent Soc Med 28:116, 1974
4. Benn RT: Some mathematical properties of weight-for-height indices used as measures of adiposity. Br J Prevent Soc Med 25:42, 1971
5. Stewart AL, Brook RH, Kane RL: Conceptualization and Measurement of Health Habits for Adults in the Health Insurance Study, Vol 2: Overweight, p14. R-2374/2-HEW, Santa Monica, The Rand Corporation, 1980
6. Kannel WB, Gordon T: Physiological and medical concomitants of obesity: The Framingham study. In Bray GA (ed): Obesity in America. Publ No 79-359, Washington DC, National Institutes of Health, 1979
7. Stunkard AJ: Introduction and overview. In Stunkard AJ (ed): Obesity. Philadelphia, WB Saunders, 1980
8. Westlund K, Nicolaysen R: Ten-year mortality and morbidity related to serum cholesterol. Scand J Clin Lab Invest (Suppl) 30:1, 1972
9. Sorensen TIA, Sonne-Holm S: Mortality in extremely overweight young men. J Chronic Dis 30:359, 1977
10. Lew EA, Garfinkel L: Variations in mortality by weight among 750,000 men and women. J Chronic Dis 32:563, 1979
11. Drenick EJ, Bale GS, Seltzer F et al: Excessive mortality and causes of death in morbidly obese men. JAMA 243:443, 1980
12. Sorlie P, Gordon T, Kannel WB: Body build and mortality in the Framingham study. JAMA 243:1828, 1980
13. Comstock GW, Kendrick MA, Livesay V: Subcutaneous fatness and mortality. Am J Epidemiol 83:548, 1966
14. Andres R: Effect of obesity on total mortality. Int J Obes 4:381, 1980
15. Dublin LI: Relation of obesity to longevity. N Engl J Med 248:971, 1953
16. Chiang BN, Perlman LV, Epstein FH: Overweight and hypertension. Circulation 39:403, 1969
17. Kannel WB, Brand N, Skinner JJ Jr et al: Relation of adiposity to blood pressure

and development of hypertension: Framingham study. Ann Intern Med 67:48, 1967

18. Rimm AA, Werner LH, Yserloo BV et al: Relationship of obesity and disease in 73,532 weight-conscious women. Public Health Rep 90:44, 1975

19. Nielson PE, Janniche H: The accuracy of auscultatory measurement of arm blood pressure in very obese subjects. Acta Med Scand 195:403, 1974

20. Bray GA: The risks and disadvantages of obesity. In Bray GA: Major Problems in Internal Medicine, Vol 9: The Obese Patient. Philadelphia, WB Saunders, 1976

21. Dahl LK, Silver L, Christie RW: The role of salt in the fall of blood pressure accompanying reduction in obesity. N Engl J Med 258:1186, 1958

22. Reisin E, Abel R, Modan M et al: Effect of weight loss without salt restriction on the reduction of blood pressure in overweight hypertensive patients. N Engl J Med 298:1, 1978

23. Kannel WB, Gordon T, Castelli WP: Obesity, lipids and glucose intolerance in the Framingham study. Am J Clin Nutr 32:1238, 1979

24. Ashley FW, Kannel WB: Relation of weight change to changes in atherogenic traits in the Framingham study. J Chronic Dis 27:103, 1974

25. Glueck CJ, Taylor HL, Jacobs D et al: Plasma high-density lipoprotein cholesterol: Association with measurements of body mass. Circulation (Suppl) 62:IV62, 1980

26. Heiss G, Johnson NJ, Reiland S et al: The epidemiology of plasma high-density lipoprotein cholesterol levels. Circulation (Suppl) 62:IV116, 1980

27. Truett J, Cornfield J, Kannel W: A multivariate analysis of the risk of coronary heart disease in Framingham. J Chronic Dis 20:511, 1967

28. Gordon T, Kannel WB: The effects of overweight on cardiovascular diseases. Geriatrics 28(8):80, 1973

29. Gordon T, Castelli WP, Hjortland C et al: Diabetes, blood lipids, and the role of obesity in coronary heart disease for women: The Framingham study. Ann Intern Med 87:393, 1977

30. Keys A, Aravanis C, Blackburn H et al: Seven Countries: A Multivariate Analysis of Death and Coronary Heart Disease. Cambridge MA, Harvard University Press, 1980

31. The Pooling Research Group: The relationship of blood pressure, serum cholesterol, smoking habit, relative weight and ECG abnormalities to incidence of major coronary events: Final report of the pooling project. J Chronic Dis 31:201, 1978

32. Ostfeld AM: A review of stroke epidemiology. Epidemiol Rev 2:136, 1980

33. Sharp JT, Barrocas M, Choksoverty S: The cardiorespiratory effects of obesity. Clin Chest Med 1:103, 1980

34. Luce JM: Respiratory complications of obesity. Chest 78:626, 1980

35. Berger M, Muller WA, Renold AE: Relationship of obesity to diabetes: Some facts, many questions. In Katzen HM, Mahler RJ (eds): Diabetes, Obesity and Vascular Disease, Part I. Washington DC, Hemisphere Publishing Corporation, 1978

36. West KM, Kalbfleisch JM: Influence of nutritional factors on prevalence of diabetes. Diabetes 20:99, 1971

37. Hundley JM: Diabetes—overweight: U.S. problems. J Am Diet Assoc 32:417, 1956

38. Reaven GM: Insulin-dependent diabetes mellitus: Metabolic characteristics. Metabolism 29:445, 1980

39. Kolterman OG, Insel J, Saekow M et al: Mechanism of insulin resistance in human obesity: Evidence for receptor and postreceptor defects. J Clin Invest 65:1272, 1980

40. Crettaz M, Jeanrenaud B: Postreceptor alterations in the states of insulin resistance. Metabolism 29:467, 1980

41. Friedman GD, Kannel WB, Dawber TR:

The epidemiology of gallbladder disease: Observations in the Framingham study. J Chronic Dis 19:273, 1966

42. Wheeler M, Hills LL, Laby B: Cholelithiasis: A clinical and dietary survey. Gut 11:430, 1970

43. Sturdevant RAL, Pearce ML, Payton S: Increased prevalence of cholelithiasis in men ingesting a serum-cholesterol-lowering diet. N Engl J Med 288:24, 1973

44. Bernstein RA, Werner LH, Rimm AA: Relationship of gallbladder disease to parity, obesity, and age. Health Serv Rep 88:925, 1973

45. Bennion LJ, Grundy SM: Effects of obesity and caloric intake on biliary lipid metabolism in man. J Clin Invest 56:996, 1975

46. Shaffer EA, Small DM: Biliary lipid secretion in cholesterol gallstone disease. The effect of cholecystectomy and obesity. J Clin Invest 59:828, 1977

47. Hartz AJ, Barboriak PN, Wong A et al: The association of obesity with infertility and related menstrual abnormalities in women. Int J Obes 3:57, 1979

48. Fisher ER, Gregorio R, Stephan T et al: Ovarian changes in women with morbid obesity. Obstet Gynecol 44:839, 1974

49. Goldbourt U, Medalie JH, Herman JB et al: Serum uric acid: Correlation with biochemical, anthropomorphic, clinical and behavioral parameters in 10,000 Israeli men. J Chronic Dis 33:435, 1980

50. Nichols A, Scott JT: Effect of weight loss on plasma and urinary levels of uric acid. Lancet 2:1223, 1972

51. David JL, Rosenshein NB, Antunes CMF et al: A review of the risk factors for endometrial carcinoma. Obstet Gynecolog Surv, in press.

52. MacMahon B: Risk factors for endometrial cancer. Gynecol Oncol 2:122, 1974

53. Elwood JM, Cole P, Rothman KJ et al: Epidemiology of endometrial cancer. J Nat Cancer Inst 59:1055, 1977

54. Blitzer PH, Blitzer EC, Rimm AA: Association between teen-age obesity and cancer in 56,111 women: All cancers and endometrial carcinoma. Prev Med 5:20, 1976

55. Kelsey JL: A review of the epidemiology of breast cancer. Epidemiol Rev 1:74, 1979

56. Thomas DB: Epidemiologic and related studies of breast cancer etiology. Rev Cancer Epidemiol 1:154, 1980

57. Friedman J: Weight problems and psychological factors. J Consult Clin Psychol 23:524, 1959

58. Weinberg N, Mendelson M, Stunkard AJ: A failure to find distinctive personality features in a group of obese men. Am J Psychiatry 117:1035, 1961

59. Silverstone JT: Psychosocial aspects of obesity. Proc R Soc Med 61:371, 1968

60. Crisp AH, McGuiness B: Jolly fat: Relation between obesity and psychoneurosis in a general population. Br Med J 1:7, 1976

61. Moore ME, Stunkard AJ, Strole L: Obesity, social class, and mental illness. JAMA 118:962, 1962

62. Holland J, Masling L, Copley D: Mental illness in lower class normal, obese, and hyperobese women. Psychosom Med 32:351, 1970

63. Halmi KA, Long M, Stunkard AJ et al: Psychiatric diagnosis of morbidly obese gastric bypass patients. Am J Psychiatry 137:470, 1980

64. Stunkard AJ: Obesity. In Kaplan HI, Freedman AM, Sadock BJ (eds): Comprehensive Textbook of Psychiatry, 3rd ed. Baltimore, Williams & Wilkins, 1980

65. Stewart AL, Brook RH, Kane RL: Conceptualization and Measurement of Health Habits for Adults in the Health Insurance Study, Vol 2: Overweight, p 98. R-2374/2-HEW, Santa Monica, The Rand Corporation, 1980

66. Strauss RJ, Wise L: Operative risks of obesity. Surg Gynecol Obstet 146:286, 1978

67. Fisher A, Waterhouse TD, Adams AP:

Obesity: Its relation to anesthesia. Anaesthesia 30:633, 1975

68. Pitkin RM: Abdominal hysterectomy in obese women. Surg Gynecol Obstet 142:532, 1976

69. Postlethwait RW, Johnson WD: Complications following surgery for duodenal ulcer in obese patients. Arch Surg 105:438, 1972

70. Pemberton LB, Manax WG: Relationship of obesity to postoperative complications after cholecystectomy. Am J Surg 121:87, 1971

71. Prem KA, Mensheha NM, McKelvey JL: Operative treatment of adenocarcinoma of the endometrium in obese women. Am J Obstet Gynecol 92:16, 1965

72. Stevenson CS, Behney CA, Miller NF: Maternal death from puerperal sepsis following cesarean section. Obstet Gynecol 29:181, 1967

73. Sicuranza BJ, Tisdall LH: Cesarean section in the massively obese. J Reprod Med 14:10, 1975

74. Putnam L, Jenicek JA, Allen CR et al: Anesthesia in the morbidly obese patient. South Med J 67:1411, 1974

75. Iber FL, Cooper M: Jejunoileal bypass for the treatment of massive obesity. Prevalence, morbidity, and short-term and long-term consequences. Am J Clin Nutr 30:4, 1977

76. Bray GA, Greenway FL, Barry RE et al: Surgical treatment of obesity: A review of our experience and an analysis of published reports. Int J Obes 1:331, 1977

77. Nachlas MM, Crawford DT, Pearl JM: Current status of jejunoileal bypass in the treatment of morbid obesity. Surg Gynecol Obstet 150:256, 1980

78. The Danish Obesity Project. Randomised trial of jejunoileal bypass versus medical treatment in morbid obesity. Lancet 2:1255, 1979

79. Hermreck AS, Jewell WR, Hardin CA: Gastric bypass for morbid obesity: Results and complications. Surgery 80:498, 1976

80. Mason EE, Printen KJ, Blommers TJ et al: Gastric bypass for obesity after ten years experience. Int J Obes 2:197, 1978

81. Griffen WO: Gastric bypass for morbid obesity. Surg Clin North Am 59(6):1103, 1979

82. Pace WG, Martin EW Jr, Tetirick T et al: Gastric partitioning for morbid obesity. Ann Surg 190:392, 1979

83. Vaughan RW, Wise L: Intraoperative arterial oxygenation in obese patients. Ann Surg 184:35, 1976

84. Salem MR, Dalal FY, Zygmunt MP et al: Does PEEP improve intraoperative arterial oxygenation in grossly obese patients? Anesthesiology 48:280, 1978

85. Vaughan RW, Engelhardt RC, Wise L: Postoperative hypoxemia in obese patients. Ann Surg 180:877, 1974

86. Vaughan RW, Wise L: Postoperative arterial blood gas measurement in obese patients: Effect of position on gas exchange. Ann Surg 182:705, 1975

87. Vaughan RW, Wise L: Choice of abdominal operative incision in the obese patient: A study using blood gas measurements. Ann Surg 181:829, 1975

88. Latimer RG, Dickman M, Day WC et al: Ventilatory patterns and pulmonary complications after upper abdominal surgery determined by preoperative and postoperative computerized spirometry and blood gas analysis. Am J Surg 122:622, 1971

89. Hansen G, Prablos PA, Steinert R: Pulmonary complications, ventilation and blood gases after upper abdominal surgery. Acta Anaesth Scand 21:211, 1977

90. Presley AP, Alexander-Williams J: Postoperative chest infection. Br J Surg 61:448, 1974

91. Vaughan RW, Bauer S, Wise L: Volume and pH of gastric juice in obese patients. Anesthesiology 43:686, 1975

92. Gilmore OJA, Sanderson PJ: Prophylactic interparietal povidone-iodine in abdominal surgery. Br J Surg 62:792, 1975

93. Higson RH, Kettlewell MGW: Parietal wound drainage in abdominal surgery. Br J Surg 65:326, 1978

94. Green SL, Sarubbi FA Jr: Risk factors associated with post cesarean section febrile morbidity. Obstet Gynecol 49:686, 1977

95. Schmitz HE, Beaton JH: Wound disruption and its management. Am J Obstet Gynecol 43:806, 1942

96. Efron G: Abdominal wound disruption. Lancet 1:1287, 1965

97. Reitamo J, Moller C: Abdominal wound dehiscence. Acta Chir Scand 138:170, 1972

98. Keill RH, Keitzer WF, Nichols WK et al: Abdominal wound dehiscence. Arch Surg 106:573, 1973

99. Helmkamp BF: Abdominal wound dehiscence. Am J Obstet Gynecol 128:803, 1977

100. Tibutt DA, Chesterman CN: Pulmonary embolism: Current therapeutic concepts. Drugs 11:151, 1976

101. Moser KM: Pulmonary embolism. Am Rev Resp Dis 115:829, 1977

102. Kakkar VV, Howe CT, Nicholaides AN et al: Deep vein thrombosis of the leg. Is there a "high risk" group? Am J Surg 120:527, 1970

103. Clayton JK, Anderson JA, McNicol GP: Preoperative prediction of postoperative deep vein thrombosis. Br Med J 4:910, 1976

104. Snell AM: The relation of obesity to fatal post-operative pulmonary embolism. Arch Surg 15:237, 1927

105. Coon WW: Risk factors in pulmonary embolism. Surg Gynecol Obstet 143:385, 1976

106. Havig O: Pulmonary thromboembolism: Clinicopathological correlations and multiple regression analysis of possible risk factors. Acta Chir Scand Suppl 478:48, 1977

107. Bell WR, Simon TL, DeMets DL: The clinical features of submassive and massive pulmonary emboli. Am J Med 62:355, 1977

108. Sigel B, Justin JR, Gibson RJ et al: Risk assessment of pulmonary embolism by multivariate analysis. Arch Surg 114:188, 1979

109. Printon KJ, Miller EV, Mason EE et al: Venous thromboembolism in the morbidly obese. Surg Gynecol Obstet 147:63, 1978

110. Vaughan RW: Anesthetic considerations in jejunoileal small bowel bypass for morbid obesity. Anesth Analg (Cleve) 53:421, 1974

111. Young SR, Stoelting RK, Peterson C et al: Anesthetic biotransformation and renal function in obese patients during and after methoxyflurane or halothane anesthesia. Anesthesiology 42:451, 1975

Nutrition and the Surgical Patient

GORDON P. BUZBY
JAMES L. MULLEN

Malnutrition contributes substantially to increased morbidity and mortality in surgical patients. The demonstration by Dudrick, Vars, and Rhoads in 1966 that total intravenous nutrition could support normal growth introduced the modern era of surgical nutrition.[1–3] Total parenteral nutrition (TPN) was initially reserved for patients in whom starvation was assured. However, as evidence accumulated that wound healing, infection, and response to stress could be improved by perioperative nutritional support, the use of TPN expanded.

No definitive study has been done on the efficacy of TPN. One randomized, controlled trial of 70 patients who had undergone surgery for gastric cancer found significantly fewer wound infections in patients who had received 7 to 10 days of preoperative nutritional support than in patients who had not. There was no significant difference in the occurrence of other complications or in mortality.[4] Holter and co-workers found no significant differences between nutritionally supported patients and others when TPN was initiated 48 hr preoperatively.[5] A nonrandomized study at the University of Pennsylvania surveyed identical groups of TPN and non-TPN patients. Although age, sex, diagnosis, and overall nutritional status were equivalent in both groups, preoperative TPN in high-risk patients reduced the incidence of all complications by 60% ($p < 0.01$), major septic complications by 85% ($p < 0.05$), and mortality by 81% ($p < 0.01$).[6]

Many hospitalized patients are malnourished. The incidence of malnutrition approaches 50% in most series and is independent of the type of hospital studied, the socioeconomic background of the patient population, or the medical service surveyed (pediatric, general medicine, general surgical, oncologic, or geriatric).[7–12] The diagnosis of malnutrition no longer rests on obvious cachexia or chronic inanition. Acute stress may result in adverse nutritional alterations within days. Many patients with potentially curable disease succumb to complications related to their underlying nutritional or metabolic status. The internist must recognize nutritional needs and work with the surgeon in developing a nutritional regimen.

Optimal nutritional support is a four-phase procedure. First is nutritional assessment, in which the nutritional status of the patient is determined and nutritional deficiencies that may predispose the patient to postoperative complications are identified. As a preoperative consultant, the internist may play a major role in this regard by making a nutritional assessment screen an integral part of the routine preoperative evaluation of patients who are to be "cleared" for surgery. The second phase is determination of the nutrients required for maintenance of the well-nourished patient or repletion of the malnourished patient. A regimen of support must be tailored to provide nutrients in a manner that is consistent with the patient's condition and that does not aggravate underlying disorders. The consulting internist plays a major role in patients who have diseases that render administration of fluids and electrolytes critical or in patients who demonstrate intolerance to some nutrient substrate. The third phase of nutritional support is delivery of the regimen to the patient by an oral, enteral, or parenteral route. Traditionally, delivery of nutritional support, particularly parenteral administration, has been the responsibility of the surgeon. The fourth phase is monitoring of the patient receiving nutritional support to determine therapeutic efficacy and to avoid metabolic complications. This chapter reviews the state of the art of nutritional assessment requirements and regimens.

NUTRITIONAL ASSESSMENT

The purpose of nutritional assessment, the first phase of nutritional support, is identification of the malnourished patient. Traditionally, physicians have relied on a patient's weight or a history of weight loss to identify patients with significant nutritional deficits. As early as 1936, Studley reported a 33% mortality rate in ulcer surgery patients who had lost more than 20% of their usual body weight compared to a 3.5% operative mortality rate in patients with no weight loss.[13] However, several studies have demonstrated that weight loss is frequently an insensitive indicator of major nutritional deficits, particularly in the acutely stressed or septic patient.[10,14] Recognizing that malnutrition is common in surgical patients and that weight loss is not a sensitive predictor, investigators have sought to define objective measures with which to detect and quantitate nutritional deficits.

In recent years, many nutritional measures have appeared in the literature. These measures fall into one of three broad categories: anthropometric, biochemical, or immunologic. Anthropometric measurements are physical measures of various body compartments, usually skinfolds or muscle circumferences, which provide a crude estimate of fat and muscle stores, respectively. Measures exceeding 90% of predicted values are considered normal. Biochemical nutritional measures include levels of circulating proteins with relatively short half-lives, such as albumin, prealbumin, retinal binding protein, complement, and transferrin. The levels of these proteins may reflect acute changes in the relative rates of protein synthesis and degradation. Urinary constitutents such as creatinine and 3-methylhistidine may also be measured. They are by-products of muscle metabolism and may reflect muscle mass.

Numerous measures of immunologic function appear to be sensitive to nutritional status. In 1973, Law, Dudrick, and Abdou described abnormalities of both T-cell and B-cell function in malnourished patients.[15] This immune dysfunction is easily assessed by determination of delayed hypersensitivity skin-test reactivity to recall antigens. Numerous studies have documented the complex multifactorial relationship between malnutrition and anergy.[10,16] Abnormalities in serum immunoglobulin G (IgG), complement, lymphocyte count, lymphocyte response to phytohemagglutinin, and neutrophil chemotaxis have been described by Dionigi and colleagues in malnourished dogs.[17] These deficiencies are corrected with nutritional repletion. Meakins and his associates studied the immune response in seriously ill malnourished patients and demonstrated abnormalities of neutrophil chemotaxis, T-lymphocyte rosette formation, and lymphocyte chemotaxis in anergic patients.[18,19] The cause of anergy in patients who are both malnourished and seriously ill is not clear. Shizgal and co-workers and Spanier and associates have demonstrated a close correlation between skin test anergy and an erosion of the body cell mass.[20,21] Reconstitution of the body cell mass by TPN is frequently followed by restoration of skin-test reactivity. Failure of restoration of the body cell mass despite adequate nutrition is associated with persistent skin-test anergy and poor prognosis.

Although numerous biochemical, anthropometric, and immunologic measures of malnutrition are available to the clinician, interpretation of these measures to assess a patient's operative risk is difficult. Most patients exhibit one or more abnormalities when multiple nutritional markers are screened.[10] Studies have identified those nutritional measures that, when abnormal, are associated with increased operative morbidity and mortality. Serum albumin, serum transferrin (derived from total iron-binding capacity (TIBC): transferrin = 0.8 TIBC − 43), and cutaneous delayed hypersensitivity are the most important. Mullen and colleagues demonstrated a 2.5-fold increase in complications in patients whose serum

albumin was less than 3 mg/dl before surgery. Serum transferrin levels less than 220 mg/dl were associated with a fivefold increase in morbidity and cutaneous anergy with a twofold increase in surgical complications. Kaminski demonstrated a 2.5-fold increase in mortality with serum transferrin less than 170 mg/dl.[22] Seltzer reported a fourfold increase in complications and a sixfold increase in deaths among patients with serum albumin levels less than 3.5 mg/dl.[23] Hypoalbuminemia and lymphocytopenia (a lymphocyte count less than 500/mm^3) increased mortality 20-fold. Meakens and co-workers reported a surgical mortality rate of 74% in anergic patients relative to 5% in reactive patients.[18] Harvey and colleagues demonstrated a similar correlation between mortality and serum transferrin, albumin, and delayed hypersensitivity.[16] Buzby and associates found that nutritional repletion produced a significant increase in serum transferrin in 4 to 10 days.[24] Failure to achieve a response after 14 days was associated with a fivefold increase in mortality (from 8% to 39%).

Researchers at the University of Pennsylvania have developed a Prognostic Nutritional Index (PNI) that relates operative risk to the patient's nutritional status on admission.[14,25] Components of the index are serum albumin (ALB, expressed in g/dl), serum transferrin (TFN, expressed in mg/dl), triceps skinfold (TSF, expressed in mm) and cutaneous reactivity to mumps, candida, or streptokinase–streptodornase (SKSD) (expressed as DH grade 0 = nonreactive, grade 1 = 5 mm reactivity, grade 2 = >5 mm reactivity). The equation is as follows.

Prognostic Nutritional Index (%) = 158 − 16.6(ALB) − 0.78(TSF) − 0.2 (TFN) − 5.8 (DH), where the PNI is the risk of operative complications in an individual patient.

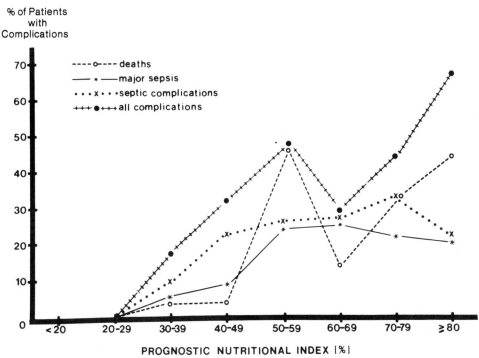

Fig. 14-1. *Actual* postoperative complications observed in patients undergoing major gastrointestinal procedures as a function of risk (%) as *predicted* by an index of nutritional status. This index (termed the Prognostic Nutritional Index) uses four measures of preoperative nutritional status (serum albumin, serum transferrin, cutaneous skin test reactivity, and triceps skinfold) to quantitatively assess operative risk. All classes of complications, including death, increase with increasing predicted risk. (Buzby GP, Mullen JL, Hobbs CL et al: Am J Surg 139:160–167, 1980)

The PNI has been validated prospectively in several studies.[14,26] In one, patients with a predicted risk of less than 30% demonstrated a complication rate of 11.7% and a mortality rate of 2%; patients with a predicted risk of 60% or greater had a complication rate of 81% and mortality rate of 59%. The incidence of complications as a function of risk as predicted by this index in patients undergoing gastrointestinal surgery are shown in Figure 14-1. A subsequent study has demonstrated that 5 to 7 days of adequate preoperative nutritional support is effective in reducing morbidity in high-risk patients to a level approximating that in well-nourished patients.[27] Studies such as these provide an objective means of identifying high-risk patients. They offer a readily available method for screening for clinically significant nutritional deficits. Determination of at least serum albumin and serum transferrin should be included in the routine battery of preoperative studies.

More than 90% of malnourished patients are identified simply by a serum albumin level of less than 3 gm/dl and a transferrin level of less than 200 mg/dl. These patients must be considered can-

Table 14-1. Guidelines for Initiation of Nutritional Support

Baseline Nutritional Status	Severity of Actual or Anticipated Clinical Stress	Duration of Actual or Anticipated Starvation Before Initiation of Nutritional Support (Days)
Well nourished (ALB > 3.5, TFN > 220, DH reactive)	Moderate *	7–10
Well nourished	Severe †	5–7
Moderate malnutrition (ALB 3.0–3.5, TFN 180–220, DH reactive)	Moderate	3–5
Moderate malnutrition	Severe	2–3
Severe malnutrition (ALB < 3, TFN < 180, DH nonreactive)	Moderate or severe	<2

* For example, elective colon resection, biliary procedure, or thoracotomy.
† For example, combined thoracoabdominal procedure, hepatic resection, massive bowel resection, or intra-abdominal abscess.
Approximate guidelines for initiation of adjuvant nutritional support in surgical patients when there are no *specific* primary indications (e.g., inflammatory bowel disease, enteric fistula, etc.). The decision to initiate support is based on the patient's baseline nutritional status, severity of clinical stress, and period of actual or anticipated starvation. ALB = Serum albumin (gm/dl); TFN = Serum transferrin (mg/dl); DH = Skin-test reactivity.

didates for preoperative nutritional repletion. Similarly, patients who demonstrate reduction in these measures 1 week postoperatively must also be considered candidates, unless adequate oral intake is imminent. Guidelines followed at the University of Pennsylvania for initiation of nutritional support are shown in Table 14-1. These guidelines apply to all surgical patients who have no specific indications for nutritional support such as bowel fistula or inflammatory bowel disease. Such indications are discussed in comprehensive texts devoted to nutritional support.[28–30]

DETERMINATION OF NUTRIENT REQUIREMENTS/EFFECT OF SURGICAL STRESS

The goals of nutritional therapy are maintenance of the well-nourished patient or repletion of the malnourished patient. The first step is determination of protein and calorie requirements. Deficiencies of specific vitamins, minerals, or trace elements are unusual except for folate, vitamin B$_{12}$, and vitamin K. This determination requires an understanding of the normal metabolic adaptation to starvation and the alterations that occur when a surgical stress is superimposed. Grant's description of the metabolic alterations of surgical stress is discussed below.[29]

When the supply of exogenous nutrients is abruptly discontinued, the body immediately turns to utilization of endogenous substrates to provide energy for essential functions. The central nervous system metabolizes 100 to 150 g/day of glucose to carbon dioxide and water. The renal medulla, bone marrow, red blood cells, and peripheral nervous system require an additional 30 to 40 g/day of glucose, which is metabolized to lactate and pyruvate. This mandatory glucose requirement rapidly depletes hepatic glycogen stores. Hepatic and renal gluconeogenesis from alanine and glutamine must then supply the glucose-dependent tissues with energy substrates. The nitrogenous by-products, ammonia and urea, are either excreted in the urine or reutilized in protein synthesis.

During early starvation, 75 g of protein and 160 g of lipid are metabolized daily to supply 1800 kcal. It appears that all body proteins are catabolized, including plasma and liver proteins and enzymes.[31-33] Serum albumin is utilized in a ratio of approximately 1 g of albumin for each 30 g of tissue protein.[34] All tissues except the heart and red blood cells use the fatty acids produced by lipolysis. Although glycerol is readily converted to glucose, it provides only about 18 g/day of glucose.[35] The metabolism of triglycerides to serum ketones gives rise to starvation ketosis.

As dietary deprivation continues, metabolic rate and total body energy expenditure decrease. There is a gradual shift to the use of lipid as energy substrate with a decrease in the mandatory requirement for glucose.[29] Hence, gluconeogenesis from protein decreases, and protein catabolism falls from 75 g/day to 20 g/day with a marked decrease in urinary nitrogen excretion. Even the central nervous system gradually adapts to the metabolism of ketones for energy. After 3 weeks of unstressed starvation, mandatory glucose utilization is so minimal that protein catabolism provides only 5% of the total daily caloric requirements. Of the total caloric requirement, 60% is derived from metabolism of fat to carbon dioxide, 10% from the conversion of free fatty acids to ketone bodies, and 25% from the direct metabolism of ketone bodies in peripheral tissues.[36] This adaptation permits remarkable tolerance of relatively prolonged periods of unstressed starvation in persons with adequate fat stores. Muscle protein and circulating proteins are well maintained until very late in starvation.

Two important alterations occur when a major stress is added to simple starvation. Energy requirements increase as much as twofold, and this is reflected by increased oxygen consumption. Protein is no longer conserved, and, as a consequence, urinary nitrogen excretion is increased. As much as 40 g/day of nitrogen

may be excreted in the urine; this represents the catabolism of approximately 1 kg of wet muscle.[37] Peripheral catabolism may be necessary not only for gluconeogenesis but also for synthesis of acutephase globulins, protein mediators of the immune system, white blood cells, and wound healing. Nutritional support does not prevent occurrence of the normal response to stress and starvation. Rather, it provides exogenous substrates to meet the metabolic needs of the patient and obviates the need to catabolize endogenous stores. This is particularly true for endogenous proteins serving crucial structural or enzymatic functions.

DETERMINATION OF NUTRIENT REQUIREMENTS AND REGIMENS

There is apparently little difference between the enteral and parenteral routes in the supplying of nutrients to the cell. Nutrient requirements are influenced primarily by the age, height, weight, activity, and metabolic milieu of the patient. The recommended dietary allowance sets the protein requirement for an average 22-year-old at approximately 0.8 g/kg of body weight per day for maintenance of nitrogen balance. This requirement is increased substantially in the hypermetabolic, stressed patient and must be increased further if the goal of therapy is protein repletion. Surprisingly, slightly more protein must be supplied by the parenteral route than by the enteral route. Positive nitrogen balance is achieved by provision of 1.3 g/kg/day of protein by the enteral route or 1.5 g/kg/day by the parenteral route. A severely stressed patient may require up to 2.5 g/kg/day.

The recommended dietary allowance for a 150-lb man engaged in moderate physical activity is 2700 cal daily. This energy requirement decreases progressively with age and is markedly dependent on body weight. A convenient estimate of caloric requirements based solely on weight is 30 to 35 cal/kg/day for the well-nourished unstressed adult patient. If there is a severe catabolic stress or baseline nutritional deficiency, as much as 55 cal/kg/day may be necessary to maintain nitrogen homeostasis.

An alternative method for calculating caloric requirements is based on the basal energy expenditure (BEE), which is the predicted caloric expenditure for a patient in the resting, unstressed state. The equation for a BEE is as follows:[38]

In men: BEE (kcal/day) = 66 + (13.7 ×
  W) + (5 × H) − (6.8 × A)
In women: BEE = 655 + (9.6 × W) +
  (1.7 × H) − (4.7 × A), where
  W = weight (kg); H = height (cm); A
  = age (years).

To determine the actual caloric requirement for a patient, one must multiply this basal expenditure by some factor that reflects the degree of activity, stress, and baseline nutritional depletion involved. The normally active unstressed patient requires approximately 1.5 × BEE and the moderately stressed catabolic patient as much as 2.5 × BEE.

In addition to calorie and protein requirements, water, electrolytes, vitamins, minerals, and trace elements must also be considered. These requirements are similar for patients receiving and patients not receiving nutritional support. An abrupt shift from the catabolic to the anabolic state may alter requirements; serum levels of these constituents must therefore be monitored closely.

After nutrient requirements are defined, the route of administration must be determined. Oral or enteral feedings are preferred if the patient's gastrointestinal tract is functional. Several recent advances in enteral formulations and techniques of delivery have substantially improved therapeutic efficacy and patient satisfaction with tube feedings even in the immediate postoperative period.[39–41] Nutrients must be supplied by the parenteral route when the gastrointestinal tract is nonfunctional.

The composition of a representative solution for TPN is shown in Table 14-2. This solution provides 1000 non-nitrogenous calories and 40 g of protein per 1000 ml of water. Solutions such as this are appropriate for 80% to 90% of patients requiring TPN. Patients with renal or hepatic disorders may require specifically designed solutions. The reader is referred to several excellent monographs for a detailed discussion of nutritional support in these disorders.[28,29,42]

Most patients require 2 to 3 liters/day of intravenous hyperalimentation (IVH) solution. This volume supplies enough water, minerals, and electrolytes so that, if there are no abnormal losses, supplemental fluids are rarely required. All nonnitrogenous calories in this regimen are

Table 14-2. Representative Composition of IVH Solution

Component	Quantity
Water	1000 ml
Dextrose	250 g
Crystalline amino acids	35–50 g
Sodium (as chloride or acetate)	0–40 mEq
Potassium (as chloride)	0–20 mEq
Phosphate (as potassium acid salt)	20 mEq
Calcium (as gluconate)	4.8 mEq
Magnesium (as sulfate)	8 mEq
Multivitamin concentrate	1 unit
Folate	5 mg

Specific diseases may necessitate modification of the water/or electrolyte content (e.g., congestive heart failure), glucose content (e.g., uncontrolled diabetes mellitus), or amino acid content or profile (e.g., renal or hepatic failure).

supplied as dextrose. An alternative form of high-density calories is now available as a lipid emulsion. Most patients develop chemical evidence of essential fatty acid deficiency within 2 weeks of the institution of routine lipid-free IVH solutions. Clinical evidence, manifested by scaling skin and hair loss, is usually not apparent for at least a month. Although the importance of the chemical deficiency is unknown, lipid emulsion should be administered weekly beginning on day 15 of TPN. Other indications for lipid administration include extreme uncontrolled glucose intolerance and necessity for peripheral administration, since lipid solutions are nearly isotonic and obviate the need for central venous administration. Some investigators favor routine provision of a portion of the daily caloric load as fat.

COMPLICATIONS OF TOTAL PARENTERAL NUTRITION

A major concern of physicians unaccustomed to caring for patients receiving TPN is fear of complications. This fear is based on well-publicized complications prevalent during early experience and a continued disproportionate emphasis on rare complications in the surgical literature. With currently available solutions, hardware, and techniques, most complications are readily avoidable. Those that do occur usually represent a break in technique or improper monitoring and are easily treated with no long-term sequelae.

Three categories of complications occur during TPN: mechanical complications related to catheter insertion and maintenance, septic complications, and metabolic complications. Insertion of central catheters and management of associated

Table 14-3. Mechanical Complications Associated with Central Venous Catheterization

Great Vessel Injury
  Subclavian artery (including false aneuryms)
  Subclavian vein (with or without hemothorax)
  Carotid artery
  Arteriovenous fistula
Pleural Injury
  Pneumothorax (including tension pneumothorax)
  Hemothorax
  Hydrothorax (catheter tip in pleural space)
Mediastinal Injury
  Hemomediastinum
  Hydromediastinum (catheter tip in mediastinum)
Superior vena caval syndrome
Nerve Injury
  Brachial plexus
  Phrenic nerve
  Vagus nerve
  Recurrent laryngeal nerve
Lymphatic Injury
  Chylothorax (thoracic duct injury)
Tracheal/Bronchial Injury
Myocardial Injury
  Hydropericardium
  Tamponade
Embolic Phenomena
  Air embolism
  Catheter embolism
Thrombotic Phenomena
  Subclavian vein
  Superior vena cava
  Hepatic vein
  Septic thrombophlebitis
Catheter Occlusion

complications are generally the responsibility of the surgeon. The internist's familiarity with potential pitfalls in catheter insertion and maintenance is essential for prompt recognition of complications. Mechanical complications are summarized in Table 14-3. Grant found a 4.2% complication rate in a survey of 10,130 subclavian vein catheterizations reported in the English language between 1956 and 1978.[29] Improved techniques and meticulous care, including dressing change and use of the line for TPN only, have decreased major complications in most series to approximately 1%.[43]

Sepsis associated with hypertonic dextrose solutions and indwelling central venous catheters is a major concern in patients receiving TPN. The frequency of septic complications reported during parenteral nutrition ranges from 2% to 33%. Candida sepsis predominated in early re-

ports. Gram-negative and gram-positive bacteria are now more common.[29] The incidence of catheter-related sepsis varies inversely with the quality of the aseptic technique employed in solution preparation and delivery and in catheter insertion and care. Centers with rigid protocols for catheter care report infection rates of approximately 3%.[44,45] Even in immunocompromised patients, catheter sepsis is rare if meticulous care is provided.[46] If there

Table 14-4. Metabolic Complications Associated with Total Parenteral Nutrition

Complications	Selected References
Glucose Metabolism	
Hyperglycemia (nonketotic hyperosmolar coma)	28,47,48,53,68
	28,47,53,68
Hypoglycemia (postinfusion)	
Amino Acid Metabolism	
Prerenal azotemia	53,68
Hyperammonemia	28,53,54,68
Hyperchloremic metabolic acidosis	28,53,54,68
Plasma amino acid imbalance	53
Electrolyte and Water Balance	
Hypo/hypernatremia	68
Hypo/hyperkalemia	28,68
Fluid overload	28
Calcium and Phosphate Metabolism	
Hypo/hyperphosphatemia	28,42,49–51,53,68
Hypo/hypercalcemia	28,53,68
Lipid Metabolism	
Essential fatty acid deficiency	53,58–62,64
Hepatic Dysfunction	
Hepatomegaly	64
Elevated liver function tests	52,55–57
Cholestasis	28,52,55,56
Anemia	
Vitamin B_{12} deficiency	28
Folate deficiency	28,63
Trace Metal Deficiencies	
Zinc	63–66
Copper	63–65
Chromium	69
Miscellaneous	
Hyper/hypomagnesemia	28,42
Hypoprothrombinemia	28
Hypervitaminosis A, D	28,63

is documented bacteremia, secondary seeding of central catheters occurs in 5% to 7% of patients.[29]

A frequent issue in the patient with an indwelling central venous catheter who develops fever is whether the catheter should be removed. In general, if the fever is accompanied by systemic signs of sepsis, the catheter should be removed and cultured after blood cultures are drawn both through the catheter and by peripheral venipuncture. The solution should also be cultured. If there is no apparent source for the fever and the patient defervesces within 8 hr to 12 hr, antibiotics should be withheld, and TPN can be resumed through a new line. If the patient does not defervesce, broad-spectrum antibiotics should be instituted. If fever is not accompanied by signs of sepsis, the catheter may be evaluated as a potential source without being removed or TPN being discontinued. Blood cultures should be drawn through the catheter, the catheter changed over a guidewire, and the tip cultured. Positive cultures necessitate removal of the catheter. This technique is useful in patients in whom central access is difficult and the catheter is considered an unlikely source of the fever.

Numerous metabolic complications described in patients receiving TPN are summarized in Table 14-4. In general, the clinical manifestations of these metabolic complications are identical in patients receiving and patients not receiving TPN, and virtually all are avoidable with proper monitoring. A protocol for monitoring to prevent these complications appears in Table 14-5.

Table 14-5. Variables Monitored During Total Parenteral Nutrition with Suggested Frequency of Monitoring

Variables Monitored	Suggested Frequency
Nutritional	
Body weight	daily
Serum albumin	weekly
Serum transferrin (from TIBC)	weekly
Anthropometrics (if available)	biweekly
Skin tests (if available)	biweekly
Metabolic	
Urine glucose and specific gravity	2–4 × daily
Fluid intake and output	daily
Serum electrolytes (Na, K, Cl, CO_2)	3 × weekly
Blood glucose and urea nitrogen	3 × weekly
Serum total calcium and inorganic phosphorus	weekly
Serum magnesium	weekly
Liver function tests (SGOT, SGPT, alkaline phosphatase, bilirubin)	weekly
Prothrombin time	weekly
Hemoglobin/white blood count	weekly
Serum triglycerides	weekly
Clinical	
Vital signs	every 4 hr
Level of activity and mentation	every 4 hr
Total (IV & PO) calorie and protein intake	daily

SUMMARY

1. Optimal nutritional care may substantially improve survival and decrease morbidity associated with major surgical procedures.
2. A nutritional assessment including measurement of least serum albumin and transferrin should be part of the routine preoperative evaluation.
3. A determination of nutrient requirements involves an estimate of protein and caloric needs, which are dependent on sex, age, size, activity, and level of stress.
4. Oral or enteral administration is preferred but depends upon gastrointestinal integrity and function.
5. Familiarity of the physician with potential mechanical, septic, and metabolic complications associated with parenteral feeding is essential.

REFERENCES

1. Dudrick SJ, Vars HM, Rhoads JE: Growth of puppies receiving all nutritional requirements by vein. Symp Int Soc Parent Nutr 2:16, 1967
2. Dudrick SJ, Wilmore DW, Vars HM et al: Longterm total parenteral nutrition with growth development and positive nitrogen balances. Surgery 64:134, 1968
3. Dudrick SJ, Wilmore DW, Vars HM et al: Can intravenous feeding as the sole means of nutrition support growth in the child and restore weight loss in the adult? Ann Surg 169:974, 1969
4. Williams RH, Heatley RV, Lewis MH et al: A randomized controlled trial of preoperative intravenous nutrition in patients with stomach cancer. Br J Surg 63:667, 1976
5. Holter AR, Rosen HM, Fincher JE: The effects of hyperalimentation on major surgery in patients with malignant disease: A prospective study. Acta Chir Scand (Suppl) 466:86, 1976
6. Mullen JL, Buzby GP, Matthews DC et al: Reduction of operative morbidity and mortality by combined preoperative and postoperative nutritional support. Ann Surg 192:604 1980
7. Shaw S, Cooper A, Roth K et al: Nutritional status and neuroblastoma—Correlation with survival. J Parent Ent Nutr 3:506, 1979
8. Bistrian BR, Blackburn GL, Vitale J et al: Prevalence of malnutrition in general medical patients. JAMA 235:1567, 1976
9. Bistrian BR, Blackburn GL, Hallowell E et al: Protein status of general surgical patients. JAMA 230:858, 1974
10. Mullen JL, Gertner MH, Buzby GP et al: Implications of malnutrition in the surgical patient. Arch Surg 114:121, 1979
11. Lundvick JL: Evaluation of a nutritional screen when used on oncology patients. J Parent Ent Nutr 3:521, 1979
12. Shaver HJ, Loper JA, Lutes R: Nutritional status of a nursing home population. J Parent Ent Nutr 3:523, 1979
13. Studley HO: Percentage of weight loss: A basic indicator of surgical risk in patients with chronic peptic ulcer. JAMA 106:458, 1936
14. Buzby GP, Mullen JL, Hobbs CL et al: Prognostic Nutritional Index in gastrointestinal surgery. Am J Surg 139:160, 1980
15. Law DK, Dudrick SJ, Abdou NI: Immunocompetence of patients with protein–calorie malnutrition. Ann Intern Med 79:545, 1973
16. Harvey KB, Ruggiero JA, Regan CS et al: Hospital morbidity–mortality risk factors using nutritional assessment. J Clin Res 26:581A, 1978
17. Dionigi R, Zonta A, Dominioni L et al: The effects of total parenteral nutrition on immunodepression due to malnutrition. Ann Surg 185:467, 1977
18. Meakins JL, Pietsch JB, Bubenick O et al: Delayed hypersensitivity: Indicator of acquired failure of host defenses in sepsis and trauma. Ann Surg 186:241, 1977
19. Christou NV, Meakins JL: Delayed hyper-

sensitivity: A mechanism for anergy in surgical patients. Surgery (in press)

20. Shizgal HM, Spanier AH, Kurtz RS: The effect of parenteral nutrition on body composition in the critically ill patient. Am J Surg 131:156, 1976

21. Spanier AH, Pietsch JB, Meakins JL et al: The relationship between immune competence and nutrition. Surg Forum 27:332, 1976

22. Kaminski MV, Fitzgerald MJ, Murphy RJ et al: Correlation of mortality with serum transferrin and anergy. J Parent Ent Nutr 1:27, 1977

23. Seltzer MH, Bastidas JA, Cooper DM: Instant nutritional assessment. J Parent Ent Nutr 3:157, 1979

24. Buzby GP, Forster J, Rosato EF: Transferrin dynamics in total parenteral nutrition. J Parent Ent Nutr 3:34, 1979

25. Mullen JL, Buzby GP, Waldman MT et al: Prediction of operative morbidity and mortality by preoperative nutritional assessment. Surgical Forum 30:80, 1979

26. Smale BF, Buzby GP, Rosato EF: Prognostic nutritional index in cancer surgery. Proc Am Soc Clin Oncol 20:336, 1979

27. Mullen JL, Buzby GP, Matthews DC: Reduction of operative morbidity and mortality by combined preoperative and postoperative nutritional support. Ann Surg (in press)

28. Fischer JE: Total Parenteral Nutrition. Boston, Little, Brown & Co, 1976

29. Grant JP: Total Parenteral Nutrition. Philadelphia, W B Saunders, 1980

30. Schneider, HA: Nutritional Support of Medical Practice. Hagerstown MD, Harper & Row, 1977

31. Dudrick SJ, Rhoads JE: Metabolism in surgical patients. In Sabiston, DC (ed): Davis–Christopher Textbook of Surgery, 11th ed. Philadelphia W B Saunders, 1977

32. Whipple GH: The dynamic equilibrium of body proteins. Springfield IL, Charles C Thomas, 1956

33. Filkins, JP: Lysosomes and hepatic regression during fasting. Am J Physiol 219: 923, 1970

34. Elman, R: Parenteral Alimentation in Surgery. New York, Hoeber Medical Books, 1947

35. Cahill GF, Herrera MG, Morgan AP et al: Hormone—Fuel interrelationships during fasting. J Clin Invest 45:1751, 1966

36. Owen OE, Felig P, Morgan AP et al: Liver and kidney metabolism during prolonged starvation. J Clin Invest 48:574, 1969

37. Cahill GF, Felig P, Marliss EP: Some physiological principles of parenteral nutrition. In Nahas G, Fox C (eds): Body Fluid Replacement in the Surgical Patient, Part IV. New York, Grune & Stratton, 1969

38. Ruflen P, Blackburn GL, Flatt JP et al: Determination of optimal hyperalimentation infusion rate. J Surg Res 18: 477, 1975

39. Kaminski MV: Enteral hyperalimentation. Surg Gynecol Obstet 143:12, 1976

40. Heymsfield SB, Bethel RA, Ansley JD et al: Enteral hyperalimentation: An alternative to central venous hyperalimentation. Ann Intern Med 90:63, 1979

41. Page CP, Ryan JA, Haff RC: Continual catheter administration of an elemental diet. Surg Gynecol Obstet 142:184, 1976

42. Ballinger WF: Manual of Surgical Nutrition. Philadelphia, W B Saunders, 1975

43. Vogel CM, Kinsbury RJ, Bave AE: Intravenous hyperalimentation. A review of two and one half years experience. Arch Surg 105:414, 1972

44. Sanderson I, Deitel M: Intravenous hyperalimentation without sepsis. Surg Gynecol Obstet 136:577, 1973

45. Ryan JA, Abel RM, Abbott WM et al: Catheter complications in total parenteral nutrition. A prospective study of 200 consecutive patients. N Engl J Med 290: 757, 1974

46. Copeland EM, MacFadyen BV, McGown C et al: The use of hyperalimentation in patients with potential sepsis. Surg Gynecol Obstet 138:377, 1974

47. Sanderson I, Deitel M: Insulin response in patients receiving concentrated infusions of glucose and casein hydrolysate for complete parenteral nutrition. Ann Surg 179:387, 1974

48. Doromal NM, Canter JW: Hyperosmolar hyperglycemic non-ketotic coma compli-

cating intravenous hyperalimentation. Surg Gynecol Obstet 136:729, 1973

49. Sand DW, Pastore RA: Paresthesias and hypophosphatemia occurring with parenteral alimentation. Am J Dig Dis 18:709, 1973

50. Sheldon GF, Grzyb S: Phosphate depletion and repletion: Relation to parenteral nutrition and oxygen transport. Ann Surg 182:683, 1975

51. Silvis SE, Paragas PD: Paresthesias, weakness, seizures, and hypophosphatemia in patients receiving hyperalimentation. Gastroenterology 62:513, 1972

52. Rodgers BM, Hollenbeck JI, Donnelly WH et al: Intrahepatic cholestasis with parenteral alimentation. Am J Surg 131:149, 1976

53. Dudrick SJ, MacFadyen BV, VanBuren CT et al: Parenteral hyperalimentation: Metabolic patterns and solutions. Ann Surg 176:259, 1972

54 Johnson JD, Albritton WL, Sunshine P: Hyperammonemia accompanying parenteral nutrition in newborn infants. J Pediatr 81:154, 1972

55. Peden VH, Witgleben CL, Skelton MA: Letter: Total parenteral nutrition. J Pediatr 78:180, 1971

56. Touloukian RJ, Downing SE: Cholestasis associated with long-term parenteral alimentation. Arch Surg 106:58, 1973

57. Grant JP, Kleinman LM, Maher MM et al: Serum hepatic enzyme and bilirubin elevations during parenteral nutrition. Surg Gynecol Obstet 145:573, 1977

58. Faulkner WJ, Flint LM: Essential fatty acid deficiency associated with total parenteral nutrition. Surg Gynecol Obstet 144:665, 1977

59. Riella MC, Broviac JW, Wells M: Essential fatty acid deficiency in human adults during total parenteral nutrition. Ann Intern Med 83:786, 1975

60. Goodgame JT, Lowry SF, Brennan MF: Essential fatty acid deficiency in total parenteral nutrition: Time course of development and suggestions for therapy. Surgery 84:271, 1978

61. Conner WE: Pathogenesis and frequency of essential fatty acid deficiency during total parenteral nutrition. Ann Intern Med 83:895, 1975

62. Press M, Kikuchi H, Shimoyama T et al: Diagnosis and treatment of essential fatty acid deficiency in man. Med J 2:247, 1974

63. Editorial: Deficiencies in parenteral nutrition. Br Med J 2:913, Editorial: 1978

64. McCarthy DM, May RJ, Maher M et al: Trace metal and essential fatty acid deficiency during total parenteral nutrition. Am J Dig Dis 23:1009, 1978

65. Lowry SF, Goodgame JT, Smith JC et al: Abnormalities of zinc and copper during total parenteral nutrition. Ann Surg 189:120, 1979

66. Kay RG, Tasman–Jones C, Pybus J: A syndrome of acute zinc deficiency during total parenteral alimentation in man. Ann Surg 183:331, 1976

67. Ballard HS, Lindenbaum J: Megaloblastic anemia complicating hyperalimentation therapy. Am J Med 56:740, 1974

68. Myers RN, Smink RD, Goldstein F: Parenteral hyperalimentation—Five years' clinical experience. Am J Gastroenterol 62:313, 1974

69. Jeejeebhoy KN, Chu RC, Marliss EB et al: Chromium deficiency, glucose intolerance and neuropathy reversed by chromium supplementation in a patient receiving longterm total parenteral nutrition. Am J Clin Nutr 30:531, 1977

Postoperative Acute Renal Failure

LAURENCE H. BECK

Postoperative acute renal failure remains an ominous complication with a mortality of 40% to 80%, depending on the setting. Although little has been accomplished in the last 20 years to improve the survival rate, an understanding of the factors that contribute to the development of acute renal failure can help to prevent this feared complication. In this chapter, the term "acute renal failure" (ARF) will be used inclusively, indicating any abrupt reduction in excretion of nitrogenous wastes with subsequent azotemia and, usually, oliguria. This definition is operationally sound because it forces the clinician to refine and clarify the diagnosis further and to determine whether the ARF is due to prerenal, postrenal, or intrinsic renal factors. The method involved in making this important differentiation will be fully discussed below. The traditional term "acute tubular necrosis" (ATN) will not be used because it defines a histologic lesion, which may or may not be present; instead, the somewhat awkward but more precise term "acute reversible intrinsic renal failure" (ARIRF) will be employed.[1,2] Other authors have chosen to use terms like "acute ischemic failure" or "nephrotoxic renal failure," emphasizing the common etiologies of ARIRF.

Bywaters described the clinical picture of ARIRF in traumatized and surgical patients in 1944 during the bombing of London.[4] At that time, mortality was in excess of 90%. Mortality was similar during World War II, but, with the advent of hemodialysis, the mortality of patients with ARIRF in the Korean conflict fell to 53%.[5,6] Mortality among patients in the Vietnam conflict requiring hemodialysis rose slightly to 64%, but, owing to more rapid evacuation of the injured the overall incidence of ARIRF had fallen from 1 in 200 injuries during World War II to 1 in 600 in Vietnam.[5] Recent reviews of ARIRF in surgical patients yield mortality figures between 56% and 70%, similar to those from battlefield casualties.[7–10]

Certain factors make for a better or worse prognosis in patients with postoperative ARIRF. Those associated with a worse prognosis include the patient's age, the extent of extrarenal disease, past occurrence of myocardial infarction, and the development of peritonitis.[5,10] Those tending to improve prognosis are the occurrence of nonoliguric rather than oliguric renal failure and the use of total parenteral nutrition (TPN).[8,10–12]

RENAL RESPONSE TO SURGERY

In the evaluation of renal function in post-operative patiens, it is important to recognize the physiologic effects of general anesthesia and surgery per se in normal persons. Although anesthetics like halothane increase renal blood flow in the isolated kidney, numerous studies have reported that major changes in renal hemodynamics occur in humans undergoing general anesthesia, with decreases in renal blood flow and glomerular filtration rate and increases in renal vascular resistance and filtration fraction.[13] These renal hemodynamic changes are secondary to the depression of myocardial function that occurs with all inhalational anesthetics. Preoperative or intraoperative volume losses would be expected to produce additional changes in the same direction.

Urinary concentration as measured by osmolality increases during surgery, while urine flow and osmolar clearance decrease. Although it was thought that an-esthetic-induced vasopressin release was the cause of this oliguria and increase in urinary concentration, recent studies indicate that anesthesia by itself does not cause vasopressin release but that surgery during anesthesia results in large increases in plasma vasopressin concentration.[14] Postoperative pain and some narcotics that stimulate vasopressin release independently continue the antidiuretic stimulus. Therefore, one would expect that most patients emerging from surgery and general anesthesia would be relatively oliguric with concentrated urine.[15] As discussed below, it is not oliguria per se but a decrease in normal urinary concentrating ability that can serve as a key to the diagnosis of ARIRF in the early postoperative period.

EVALUATION OF ACUTE RENAL FAILURE

One of the major determinations to be made in the initial evaluation of the patient with oliguria and a rising blood urea nitrogen (BUN) level is whether acute renal insufficiency is due to prerenal, postrenal, or intrinsic renal factors. Postrenal failure, or obstructive uropathy, although uncommonly acute in hospitalized patients, occurs often enough to be considered a possibility in every patient. Bladder outlet obstruction induced by drugs, bed rest, or urinary tract infection is easily diagnosed by physical examination and straight catheterization of the bladder. Obstruction higher in the urinary tract can occur in the surgical patient for a number of reasons but is usually due to extrinsic ureteral compression by hematoma, abscess, or inadvertent suturing. Obstructive uropathy need not be manifested by anuria or persistent oliguria, and a high index of suspicion of its presence must be maintained. Although an intravenous urogram has been the traditional method for making the diagnosis of upper tract obstruction, renal ultrasound is currently the method of choice. A normal renal sonogram virtually excludes obstructive uropathy as the cause of acute renal insufficiency.[16]

A more difficult task, and one that is critical for determination of the prognosis, is differentiation between the patient with failure due to renal hypoperfusion and the patient with ARIRF. Numerous methods have been advocated in the literature, and one that is widely recommended and practiced involves the use of a "test dose" of a potent "loop" diuretic like furosemide or ethacrynic acid.[17-19] Induced diuresis is thought to indicate that the kidney tubules are intact and that prerenal factors underlie the oliguria; the absence of diuresis indicates established ARIRF. This hypothesis is based primarily on experimental studies in dogs and has not been tested critically in humans in a prospective manner.[20-22] Experience indicates that the test is poorly predictive, since false-positive and negative results occur. Patients who are markedly hypovolemic may not respond to potent diuretics because of enhanced reabsorption of glomerular filtrate in the proximal nephron; in this test, such patients would be mislabeled as having ARIRF. Conversely, some patients with established ARIRF may have a diuretic response to a diuretic-like furosemide (see below), and this test would lead in their case to an erroneous diagnosis of prerenal azotemia. The use of potent diuretics in critically ill patients can even contribute to the development of ARIRF by inducing further volume losses.[23]

An alternative approach to the oliguric patient has been the use of urine and serum electrolyte and osmolality measurements in the assessment of tubular salt and water reabsorptive function in the kidney. The underperfused but otherwise normal kidney should conserve sodium and water, whereas the kidney in ARIRF loses its ability to do so, as well as its ability to concentrate the urine maximally.[24] It is generally taught that urine sodium concentration and osmolality can be used to differentiate the patient with prerenal azotemia from that with established ARIRF. Prerenal azotemia is usually characterized by a urinary sodium concentration (U_{Na}) of less than 20 mEq/liter and a urine osmolality (U_{osm}) of more than 500 milliosmoles (mOsm)/liter, whereas ARIRF usually has a U_{Na} of more than 40 mEq/ liter and a U_{osm} of less than 350 mOsm/ liter. However, some patients with ARIRF exhibit a low U_{Na}, and there is a gray zone in which individual values may not serve to separate the two conditions.

Schrier and his colleagues have recently developed refined criteria for the differentiation of prerenal states from ARIRF.[26] Since the kidney with ARIRF has a failure of both urinary concentration and sodium reabsorption, an index combining measurements of both functions could be more precise in separating the two. In his prospective series of 102 patients with acute renal failure, Schrier found that U_{Na} and U_{osm} provided only fair discrimination, with considerable overlap between the two groups for U_{osm} from 350 to 500 and for U_{Na} from 20 to 40. He derived two functions, the fractional excretion of sodium (FE_{Na}) and the Renal Failure Index, which are easily calculated with values obtained from plasma and spot urine measurements:

$$FE_{Na} = \frac{U_{Na}/P_{Na}}{U_{creat}/P_{creat}}$$

$$\text{Renal Failure Index} = \frac{U_{Na}}{U_{creat}/P_{creat}}$$

An index of less than 1 was found in 84% of patients with prerenal azotemia but in no patients with ARIRF. An FE_{Na} of less than 1 was obtained for 90% of prerenal cases but for only 1 of 25 patients with ARIRF. These indices also proved useful, although not as specific, in nonoliguric ARIRF, in which 2 and 3 of 31 patients had values of less than 1 for the Renal Failure Index and FE_{Na}, respectively.

These indices can aid in the categorization of patients with ARF and help in the planning of therapeutic strategy; however, two important provisos must be stated. First, the Schrier study excluded patients who had received a diuretic or mannitol within 24 h before initial evaluation. Since mannitol and diuretics block tubular sodium reabsorption even in prerenal patients, these diagnostic indices are useless after such agents have been given. The "automatic" urge to administer a potent diuretic to the oliguric patient must be resisted until after urine and serum samples have been taken if the FE_{Na} and Renal Failure Index results are to prove predictive. Secondly, the classification of ARIRF or prerenal azotemia does not obviate the necessity of attempting to improve renal perfusion in *every* patient with ARF. Although prerenal indices indicate that azotemia and oliguria can be reversed if renal perfusion is improved (e.g., by volume repletion or treatment of heart failure), the same hemodynamic factors may be operating in patients with ARIRF and, in fact, may have caused the ARIRF. Failure to recognize and correct these factors may prolong the course of renal failure or complicate it in other ways.

ETIOLOGIES OF ACUTE REVERSIBLE INTRINSIC RENAL FAILURE

In establishing the diagnosis of ARIRF, one must consider likely causes in each patient so that contributing factors can be altered or removed. There are often multiple potential etiologies in ARIRF in surgical patients, and the clinician may be unable to determine which one(s) provoked renal failure. Although early studies separated nephrotoxic from ischemic causes of ARIRF on a histologic basis, the clinical presentation is sufficiently similar in all categories of ARIRF to enable

etiologic differentiation to be made only by careful review of the history, medication regimen, and operative record of each patient.[27] In this section, two general types of ARIRF, hemodynamic and nephrotoxic, are reviewed, and several specific causes of ARIRF seen most commonly in the surgical patient are discussed. In each case, distinctive clinical features, predisposing factors, and methods of prevention are highlighted.

Ischemic (Hemodynamic)

The most dramatic and easily recognized cause of ARIRF is sustained hypotension secondary to blood loss, anesthesia, drugs, heart failure, or other causes. The end result, decreased blood flow to the kidney, is the same. In most of these situations, active renal vasoconstriction in response to systemic hypotension further compromises renal blood flow and the glomerular filtration rate (GFR). The resultant oliguria is appropriate, preventing more extracellular fluid loss. With rapid correction of hypotension or volume loss, this prerenal state is reversible without damage to the kidney. However, depending on the duration of hypotension and the previous level of renal function, the patient may rapidly develop ARIRF with progressive elevation in BUN and creatinine despite treatment.

The patient with ischemic ARIRF is usually oliguric from the time of the hypotensive episode on and remains so during the course of the renal failure until diuresis ensues. Occasionally, a brief period of several hours of continued urine flow ensues between the causative event and the onset of oliguria. The hypotensive event may seem trivial. In some patients, it lasts only minutes; others may be hypotensive for hours without subsequently developing ARIRF. Although it is difficult to predict who will develop ARIRF, it is generally held that persons who are old, have underlying renal insufficiency, or are volume-contracted at the time of the hemodynamic insult are at greatest risk. Ischemic ARIRF usually results in 7 to 10 days of oliguria followed by diuresis.[28] As discussed below, treatment with dialysis obviously alters that time course, commonly blunting the diuresis that would be seen during the recovery phase.

Septicemia, often due to gram-negative organisms, is a common cause of "ischemic" ARIRF in surgical patients.[10,29,30] Although frank hypotension can often be identified as the initiating event in ARIRF, septicemia alone, without systemic hypotension, can cause oliguric ARIRF, apparently mediated through intense splanchnic and renal vasoconstriction.[31]

Nephrotoxic

The most recently published series of patients with ARIRF identify nephrotoxins as common etiologic agents even in surgical patients.[10,12] Although the number of drugs and chemicals capable of causing ARIRF is vast, aminoglycoside antibiotics, most commonly gentamicin, account for the majority of cases.[32] The clinical course of gentamicin-induced renal failure is sufficiently uniform to be characteristically described in detail.[33] The aminoglycoside has been administered for a minimum of 2 to 3 days, generally in combination with other antibiotics, when the BUN and creatinine levels begin to rise, usually without oliguria. The rate of rise may not be as rapid as in ischemic ARIRF, in which serum creatinine usually rises 1.0 to 1.5 mg/dl/day, and the total duration of renal failure is variable. Some patients recover in a few days, after the drug is stopped; others experience prolonged azotemia with renal function slowly improving over several weeks.

Predisposing factors for the development of aminoglycoside nephrotoxicity include pre-existent renal insufficiency, advanced age, and a dose of aminoglycoside that is excessive on the basis of weight and renal function nomograms.[33] If serum gentamicin levels are measured, elevated peak or trough levels are usually demonstrated in patients with nephrotoxicity.[34] Unfortunately, elevated serum levels probably occur as a result of renal failure, obviating their successful use for prediction or prevention of ARIRF.[35] Newer methods that assess early tubular toxicity, such as urinary excretion of lysozyme or other markers, appear promising but have not yet proved clinically useful.[36,37]

It has been suggested that the combination of gentamicin and a cephalosporin is more nephrotoxic than an aminoglycoside alone. Clinical reports are anecdotal, and experimental models and an epidemiologic survey suggest no additive deleterious or protective effect of cephalosporins.[38-43] Since most patients who require an aminoglycoside receive other antibiotics as well, the question is not easily answered. Furthermore, the relative toxicities of new aminoglycosides have not been established. Although some studies show no major difference in nephrotoxicity between gentamicin and tobramycin, a recent prospective study indicates that tobramycin may be less nephrotoxic.[45,46]

Renal Failure After Cardiac Bypass Surgery

The patient undergoing cardiac surgery is at unusual risk for postoperative ARIRF, a complication that carries a particularly serious prognosis. Cardiopulmonary bypass has been described as "a form of controlled clinical shock."[47] In addition to the variable period of low flow during the initial stages of bypass, hemolysis, intravascular hemagglutination, and redistribution of circulating blood volume may occur. Nonpulsatile blood flow is thought to be particularly deleterious to renal function.[48]

Four retrospective studies and one prospective study have been published on the incidence and course of acute renal failure after cardiac surgery.[49–53] Despite the 15-year spread of the publication dates and the variety of institutions reporting, the combined results represent 3000 patients and are remarkably uniform. The incidence of postoperative renal dysfunction indicated by a creatinine level of 1.6 mg/dl or higher is 25% to 30%. Within this large group of patients, there appear to be three distinct categories of increasing severity. In the report of 490 patients from New York University, the largest group, 14% of the total, developed nonoliguric mild renal failure with creatinine never exceeding 2 mg/dl.[52] Renal function returned to normal by the fourth day after surgery. A second group, 12% of the total, developed more severe renal failure, with peak creatinine reaching 2 to 5 mg/dl. These patients did not experience oliguria, and none required dialysis. Recovery of renal function occurred after a mean of 7 days. Mortality in these first two groups was low at 7% and 8%, respectively; however, in the group of patients who did not develop postoperative renal failure mortality was only 0.5%. The worst prognosis was seen in the smallest group, representing 4% of the total, in whom oliguric renal failure developed with creatinine rising above 5 mg/dl. Most of these patients required dialysis, and

mortality in this group was 66%. These data were similar to those reported from the Massachusetts General Hospital, which showed a mortality rate of 89% among the 4% of patients who developed severe renal failure with creatinine over 5 mg/dl. All those who required dialysis died.[53]

Preoperative factors that were predictive of postoperative renal failure in the above studies were old age and pre-existing renal dysfunction. Operative risk factors included prolonged bypass time, hypotension, low output syndrome, aortic cross-clamping, and hemoglobinemia. None of the studies demonstrated a protective effect of preoperative or intraoperative mannitol or furosemide administration. In fact, the study of Abel and colleagues cautions strongly against the routine use of furosemide in the oliguric patient.

Dye-Induced

As recently as ten years ago, iodinated radiocontrast materials were thought to carry little or no risk of producing renal failure.[54] Over the last several years, however, numerous reports have documented ARIRF following radiocontrast studies, and some predisposing factors have been identified.[55–61] Within 12 hr to 24 hr of a dye study, such as an intravenous urogram or a coronary arteriogram, oliguria is noted. The oliguria is brief, lasting only 2 to 4 days, but the serum creatinine level usually continues to rise, peaking approximately 7 days after exposure. The majority of patients fully recover renal function, although a small proportion with pre-existing renal disease may progress immediately to irreversible chronic renal failure.[60,62] A mortality rate of 5% to 10% in dye-induced ARIRF is reported from most centers. Dialysis is not commonly required, and since oliguria is brief, hyperkalemia does not usually occur.

Oral cholecystographic dyes rarely cause ARIRF; however, the incidence of ARIRF after intravenous or intra-arterial administration of radiocontrast material is high in some groups of patients.[63–67] Risk factors include previous renal insufficiency, diabetes mellitus, advanced age, dehydration, and multiple myeloma.[61] The major risk factor is probably pre-existing renal insufficiency with or without diabetes mellitus.[58] The combination of diabetes and renal insufficiency is a contraindication to a dye study. Harkonan and Kjellstrand reported that, although only 1 of 23 diabetics with a creatinine level less than 2 mg/dl developed ARIRF after intravenous pyelography, 22 of 29 (76%) with a creatinine level above 2 mg/dl did.[62] The incidence was 93% in those in whom the serum creatinine was greater than 5 mg/dl. An incidence of 92% was reported by Weinrauch and co-workers in 13 diabetics with nephropathy and a mean serum creatinine level of 6.8 mg/dl in whom coronary arteriograms were performed.[56]

Although other reports suggest that the incidence of dye-induced ARIRF is low or nonexistent, the consensus of published reports suggests that this complication occurs commonly in the high-risk groups identified above.[55,68] Since many surgical patients have dye studies performed before operation, and since the oliguric period is often brief, dye-induced ARIRF may not be recognized unless serial creatinine values are obtained.

Dye-induced ARIRF can be prevented if alternative imaging techniques such as radioisotopic scans, ultrasound, computerized tomographic (CT) scans without contrast are used instead of dye studies in high-risk patients. If dye studies must be performed, use of the smallest possible dose of contrast agent and avoidance of dehydration should be recommended.

Acute Interstitial Nephritis

Acute (allergic) interstitial nephritis (AIN) is a condition that has been recognized only in the last few years as a common cause of ARF. In one renal biopsy series, AIN accounted for about 11% of the cases with ARIRF.[69] Because the course of AIN mimics that of ARIRF in many ways, it often goes unrecognized clinically. The histologic hallmark of AIN is an intense diffuse inflammatory infiltrate in the interstitium of the kidney, usually with mononuclear and plasma cells. In some cases, polymorphonuclear leukocytes and eosinophils predominate.[70]

AIN is usually caused by drugs or infection. Although numerous drugs have been implicated, penicillins, sulfas, and methicillin are the most common offenders.[71,72] The clinical picture is not distinctive and can vary from transient renal insufficiency to acute oliguric renal failure.[73] Clinical features that may distinguish AIN from ARIRF are unilateral or bilateral kidney pain with flank tenderness and frequent systemic "allergic" signs including fever, skin rash, and eosinophilia. The urinary sediment usually shows pyuria, and some authors suggest that eosinophiluria be looked for on a Wright's stained preparation of the sediment.[72] Urinary indices are usually indistinguishable from those of ARIRF.[70]

The clinical course is generally that of ARF with oliguria in about 50%. Renal insufficiency varies in severity and occasionally requires dialysis. Discontinuation of the responsible drug is followed by recovery of renal function in days or weeks. There is some evidence that the administration of steroids may hasten the recovery of renal function, but the prognosis for complete recovery is excellent without steroids.[70,72]

Other

Although the causes discussed above account for most cases of ARIRF in the surgical patient, three other factors—hemoglobinuria, myoglobinuria, and methoxyflurane—can cause ARIRF, each having unique features that distinguish it from other types. The heme pigments hemoglobin and myoglobin are capable of producing ARIRF in the surgical patient in certain clinical circumstances, generally those of volume depletion, acidosis, or serious illness.[3] In the surgical patient, hemoglobinuria usually results from a serious blood transfusion reaction, and myoglobinuria follows crushing muscle injuries. A clue to the presence of these pigments is a positive urine dip-stick test for blood or benzidine reaction when there are no red blood cells in the urinary sediment. When the pigments are present in significant amounts, they color the urine red. Because myoglobin is rapidly cleared from the serum, patients with myoglobinuria almost never have red serum, but those with hemoglobinuria usually do. In either case, the presence of orange red granular casts in the urine sediment is typical.

Although hemoglobinuric ARIRF follows the usual course of ARF, certain features of myoglobinuric renal failure are distinctive.[74,75] Serum creatinine phosphokinase levels are usually elevated, and, because of the release of muscle cell contents into the extracellular fluid, there is often a particularly rapid rise in serum potassium and creatinine concentration. In most types of ARIRF, serum creatinine rises about 1.0 to 1.5 mg/dl/day, but, in myoglobinuric renal failure, creatinine may rise by as much as 3 to 5 mg/dl/day.

Both experimental and clinical evidence suggest that mannitol diuresis can abort acute pigment nephropathy if it is administered before ARIRF has fully developed.[76–78] Therefore, the patient with acute hemolysis or muscle injury should be given 12.5 g to 25 g of 25% mannitol to initiate a diuresis of 2 to 3 liters/day. This urine volume should be maintained until there is clinical evidence that the pigment load has been reduced.

The inhalational anesthetic methoxyflurane has been associated with a unique type of renal injury that manifests itself as polyuric ARF. Although numerous case reports have appeared, the most definitive work is found in two controlled prospective studies comparing methoxyflurane with halothane.[79,80] The study by Mazze and co-workers showed that patients receiving methoxyflurane developed a syndrome characterized by polyuria unresponsive to the administration of vasopressin and increased serum BUN and creatinine levels.[79] Similar although less severe changes were reported by Merkle and associates.[80] In each case, halothane produced none of the above changes.

Although oliguric ARF can occur after methoxyflurane anesthesia, polyuria of 2 to 4 liters accompanied by azotemia on the first postoperative day is more common.[81,82] The polyuria is due to a concentrating defect that cannot be corrected by vasopressin.[83] The severity of the renal failure is variable but, in several cases, has been irreversible despite prolonged periods of dialysis.[81,82] Cousins and Mazze have related the acute nephrotoxicity to the level of blood fluoride, one of the metabolites of methoxyflurane.[84] Crystallized oxalate, the other major metabolite, has been found in the interstitium in most kidney biopsies and is thought to lead to interstitial fibrosis and persistent renal failure.[82,85–87] Prolonged exposure time correlates with incidence of methoxyflurane-induced renal failure. Recent reports of another fluorinated inhalational anesthetic, enflurane, suggest that, in high doses, this agent may cause renal toxicity similar to that caused by methoxyflurane.[88,89]

TREATMENT OF ACUTE REVERSIBLE INTRINSIC RENAL FAILURE

The management of ARIRF is similar in surgical and nonsurgical patients and will not be discussed in detail. The major concerns are salt and water balance, potassium homeostasis, acid–base problems, and uremic manifestations. Infection and progression of the underlying primary disease are the major threats to survival even in the well-managed patient with ARIRF.

As for any patient with renal failure, all medications must be reviewed. Potentially nephrotoxic drugs must be totally avoided if possible; others that are cleared predominantly by the kidney should be given in appropriately adjusted dosage. Excellent tables of revised drug dosages in renal failure are published regularly in the literature.[90] In the setting of ARIRF with a rising serum creatinine level, one can assume that the GFR is close to zero and use dosage modifications for anephric patients. During the patient's recovery from ARIRF, the serum creatinine can be used to estimate GFR; however, for some drugs, particularly those with potential nephrotoxicity, serum drug levels are necessary.

Certain characteristics of ARF may be exaggerated and require a more aggressive approach in the surgical patient than in the medical patient. Because of trauma and accelerated catabolism, serum creatinine and, in particular, serum BUN may rise rapidly with the early development of uremic signs and symptoms. Large endogenous potassium loads make hyperkalemia common. "Third-space" accumulation of extracellular fluid (e.g., in the lumen of the bowel or at operative sites) and extrarenal fluid losses, coupled with the frequent need for large quantities of intravenous fluids, make assessment of intravascular volume difficult. Swan–Ganz catheter placement is therefore useful and often necessary in the critically ill patient.

Two subjects of special interest in regard to the surgical patient are early or "prophylactic" dialysis and the use of parenteral hyperalimentation. Most nephrologists institute dialysis in nonsurgical patients with ARIRF only when clinical indications such as hyperkalemia, uremic symptoms, or volume overload are present. However, several authors recommend prophylactic dialysis in ARIRF and suggest that it improves survival.[91–93] These studies are difficult to interpret, because they use historical controls. In view of the continuing improvement in intensive care of critically ill patients over the last two decades, it may not be justifiable to attribute improvement in survival to early dialysis. However, there has been a single prospective controlled study comparing intensive prophylactic dialysis to conventional dialysis in post-traumatic patients matched for severity and type of injury.[94] In the conventional group, hemodialysis was carried out only when the creatinine level reached 10 mg/dl and the BUN level 150 mg/dl or when the patient developed a clinical sign indicating earlier intervention. The intensive group received hemodialysis early and frequently enough to maintain the serum creatinine level below 5 mg/dl and the BUN level under 70 mg/dl. Among the 18 patients in the study, 5 of 8 (64%) in the prophylactic dialysis group survived, compared to 2 of

10 (20%) in the routine group. Gram-negative septicemia was less frequent in the intensive group (50%) than among controls (80%). Although neither comparison proved statistically significant (p < 0.05), the results suggest that early dialysis is beneficial.

The choice between peritoneal dialysis and hemodialysis depends upon the type of surgery being performed and the availability of capable personnel. Although peritoneal dialysis is technically easier, requires fewer personnel, and avoids the risk of anticoagulation, hemodialysis is often preferred in the surgical setting because of risks posed by peritoneal dialysis in patients who have undergone recent abdominal surgery, have prosthetic vascular grafts, or suffer from pulmonary insufficiency. Moreover, the rate of catabolism in surgical patients is often so high that peritoneal dialysis cannot keep pace with the production of nitrogenous wastes.

Malnutrition probably underlies much of the morbidity and mortality in ARF, particularly in postoperative patients in whom rates of catabolism are inordinately high. The traditional approach to nutrition in ARF has been to severely restrict protein intake in order to minimize azotemia while attempting to provide "protein-sparing" carbohydrate calories.[28] The work of Giordano provides evidence that dietary essential amino acids (EAA) given in the proper ratio allow for reutilization of urea for synthesis of non-EAA and underlies current recommendations for oral nutrition in patients with renal failure.[95] However, surgical patients, many of whom experience enormous nitrogen wasting and cannot eat, require another approach. Dudrick and colleagues demonstrated that a positive nitrogen balance could be achieved in surgical patients receiving TPN with solutions of balanced EAA, hypertonic glucose, and other nutrients.[96]

Whether TPN with EAA improves morbidity and mortality in ARIRF is less certain. The most definitive study is that of Abel and his colleagues, who carried out a prospective randomized double-blind study comparing the use of "renal failure fluid" (EAA with hypertonic glucose) with the use of hypertonic glucose alone in patients with ARIRF.[97] The two groups were matched for etiology of renal failure, age, and other characteristics. Of those receiving renal failure fluid (RFF), 75% survived; of those receiving glucose alone, 44% survived. The duration of renal failure, number of required dialyses, and incidence of fatal and nonfatal sepsis were all decreased in those given RFF.

Although another clinical trial supporting these findings has been reported, others have not shown improved morbidity or mortality rates.[98,99] Current commercial renal failure solutions, Freamine-E and Nephramine, are similar to the RFF used in Abel's study. However, studies by Blackburn and Blumenkrantz and their associates suggest that different ratios of amino acids, especially those involving important branched-chain ketogenic amino acids, and some non-EAA may be necessary to influence survival with TPN.[100,101]

PREVENTION OF ACUTE REVERSIBLE INTRINSIC RENAL FAILURE AND "CONVERSION" TO THE NONOLIGURIC STATE

Meticulous attention to intraoperative fluid balance and hemodynamics, avoidance of radiocontrast dyes and nephrotoxic drugs in the high-risk patient, and rapid treatment of systemic infections will certainly prevent some cases of ARIRF. Recent interest in the renal effects of nonsteroidal anti-inflammatory drugs suggests that these agents may contribute to the development of ARF in some patients.[102,103] In experimental animals, indomethacin enhances renal ischemia during hemorrhagic hypovolemia through its effect on renal prostaglandin synthesis.[104,105] Because ARIRF has been reported in a patient with congestive heart failure receiving indomethacin, it seems prudent to avoid these agents in preoperative patients.[103]

Preoperative mannitol administration, stressed recently in an animal study by Abbott and Austin, has been recommended for prevention of ARF in high-risk procedures such as abdominal aortic surgery.[106-108] On the other hand, similar protection can be provided by preoperative administration of saline, and most nephrologists recommend careful volume repletion with saline in preoperative patients who have a high risk of developing ARIRF.[109,110]

The use of mannitol or potent loop diuretics in incipient or established ARIRF is more controversial. Since ARIRF is associated with decreased total renal blood flow and redistribution of flow away from the renal cortex, these agents, which cause increases in cortical blood flow in normal persons, have become widely used for reversal of early ARIRF or at least for establishment of a diuresis.[111,112] The evidence that mannitol can reverse oliguria and alter the clinical course of ARIRF is scanty. The best study, that of Luke and associates, although not randomized, suggests that some patients with established ARIRF respond to mannitol with diuresis and a shortened period of azotemia and that this favorable response can be predicted by a urine-to-plasma osmolality ratio of greater than 1.05.[113] Although these authors state that careful volume repletion was accomplished be-fore administration of mannitol, it is possible that the "responders" were still in a prerenal state.

Because mannitol causes marked intravascular volume expansion, it cannot be recommended routinely in oliguric patients, especially if the patients have already been volume-repleted. Intravenous furosemide and the more ototoxic diuretic ethacrynic acid have been widely recommended for the oliguric patient.[114,115] Although furosemide has been shown to have protective effect in certain animal models, it has no significant effect in man.[116-118] Some authors have suggested that furosemide may cause renal failure in patients who otherwise would not have developed it.[23,53]

Furosemide may not reverse already established ARIRF; nevertheless, many nephrologists feel that it is useful in early ARF, when the clinical course may occasionally be changed from oliguria to nonoliguria.[119] The value of such a response, should it occur, is undeniable, because nonoliguric patients are generally more easily managed than oliguric patients, with less hyperkalemia, fewer dialyses, and a better survival rate.[12] The standard approach is to infuse about 200 mg of furosemide intravenously over 20 to 30 min. The dose may be doubled if there is no diuresis. Lack of response to 400 mg to 500 mg of furosemide suggests that further efforts at diuresis are probably futile. If diuresis does ensue, the dose should be repeated every 6 to 12 hr for maintenance of high urine output.

An alternative approach has recently been suggested by Shin and co-workers.[120] Using pulmonary artery catheters in 18 consecutive trauma patients with ARIRF, they found that, when necessary, cardiac output could be maximized by an increase in preload with plasma protein fractions and by a reduction in afterload with nitroprusside. They attempted to increase preload despite an elevated pulmonary capillary wedge pressure as long as cardiac output increased and pulmonary edema did not develop. This aggressive approach to fluid therapy resulted in maintenance of a nonoliguric state with a mean urine output of 100 ml/hr in all 18 patients for the duration of ARIRF. These results contrast sharply with those obtained for the 17 preceding ARIRF patients, in whom less aggressive fluid management was employed. Of those 17, 14 were oliguric throughout the course of ARIRF. The impressive results of Shin and his colleagues deserve confirmation in a prospective controlled trial. The ability to "convert" a sizable fraction of patients with postoperative ARIRF into a nonoliguric state may have an important beneficial effect on survival.

SUMMARY

1. Prevention of ARF
   a. Avoid nephrotoxic drugs if possible. If they are necessary, pay close attention to recommended doses, especially in the patient about to undergo surgery.
   b. Consider alternatives to radiocontrast dye studies for diabetic patients and for patients with renal impairment. If dye studies are necessary, avoid dehydration, and consider saline infusion for 24 hr before the study. Check daily serum creatinine in the high-risk patient after a dye study to avoid sending him to surgery while he is already in the course of undetected ARIRF.
   c. Always volume-replete the patient before surgery. The volume-depleted patient is more susceptible to ARF than normal.
   d. Do not use methoxyflurane anesthesia.
   e. Replace intraoperative fluid losses rapidly to avoid prolonged hypotension.
   f. If a hemolytic transfusion reaction occurs, administer mannitol to protect kidneys from ARF.
2. Diagnosis in the acutely azotemic or oliguric patient
   a. Before administering diuretics or fluids, send a spot urine sample for measurement of sodium and creatinine concentrations and osmolality as well as a serum sample for measurement of creatinine concentration. Calculate the Renal Failure Index (RFI):

$$RFI = \frac{U_{Na}}{U_{creat}/P_{creat}}$$

   If RFI is <1, azotemia is probably prerenal; if RFI is >1, azotemia is probably due to ARIRF.
   b. Immediately assess the patient's volume status. If there is evidence of volume depletion, administer a fluid challenge until hemodynamics are normal. Look for manifestations of congestive heart failure, and, if it is present, attempt to improve cardiac output.
   c. Always consider postrenal (obstructive) failure. Straight bladder catheterization and renal ultrasound study can rule out obstruction. The obstructed patient need not be anuric or even oliguric.
   d. Discontinue drugs known to cause acute interstitial nephritis (e.g., semisynthetic penicillins and sulfas). These may also cause accompanying fever, rash, and eosinophilia. Urinalysis shows pyuria and sometimes eosinophiluria on Wright's stain.

e. If azotemia persists after volume repletion and exclusion of obstruction and interstitial nephritis, treat the patient for ARIRF.

3. Management of ARIRF

a. Attempt to determine from the history, physical examination, anesthesia record, and medication list the most likely cause of ARIRF. Attempt to correct any possible causes that remain (*e.g.*, hypovolemia, nephrotoxic drugs, sepsis).

b. If the patient has oliguric ARIRF, a trial of up to 500 mg of intravenous furosemide in the first 24 to 48 hr is occasionally useful in "converting" the dysfunction to a nonoliguric ARIRF.

c. Principles of management are generally the same as in the non-surgical patient. Because of high catabolic rates, rapid rises in serum BUN, creatinine, and potassium levels may occur.

d. Early "prophylactic" dialysis is recommended. Attempt to keep the BUN level below 100 to 120 mg/dl and the creatinine level below 10 mg/dl.

e. Parenteral nutrition with EAA and hypertonic glucose should be administered unless the course of ARIRF is expected to be brief or the patient can obtain an adequate number of calories and EAA by oral feeding.

f. Adjust all drug dosages appropriately. Consider the patient with ARIRF to be anephric until serum creatinine has peaked. Serum drug levels may be necessary.

REFERENCES

1. Finckh ES, Jeremy D, Whyte HM: Structural renal damage and its relation to clinical features in acute oliguric renal failure. Q J Med 31:429, 1962

2. Bohle A, Jahnecke J, Meyer D et al: Morphology of acute renal failure: Comparative data from biopsy and autopsy. Kidney Int 10:S9, 1976

3. Finn WF: Acute renal failure. In Earley LE, Gottschalk CW (eds): Diseases of the Kidney, p. 167. Boston, Little, Brown & Co, 1979

4. Bywaters EGL: Ischemic muscle necrosis. JAMA 124:1103, 1944

5. Griffith GL, Maull KI, Coleman CC et al: Acute reversible intrinsic renal failure. Surg Gynecol Obstet 146:631, 1978

6. Smith LH, Post RS, Teschan PE et al: Post-traumatic renal insufficiency in military casualties. Am J Med 18:187, 1955

7. Kennedy AC, Burton JA, Luke RG et al: Factors affecting the prognosis in acute renal failure. Q J Med 42 (165):73, 1973

8. Baek SM, Makabali GG, Shoemaker WC: Clinical determinants of survival from postoperative renal failure. Surg Gynecol Obstet 140:685, 1975

9. Merino GE, Buselmeier TJ, Kjellstrand CM: Postoperative chronic renal failure: A new syndrome? Ann Surg 182:37, 1975

10. McMurray SD, Luft FC, Maxwell DR et al: Prevailing patterns and predictor variables in patients with acute tubular necrosis. Arch Intern Med 138:950, 1978

11. Brooks HB, Schulhoff JW: Acute nonoliguric renal failure in the postoperative patient. Crit Care Med 4:193, 1976

12. Anderson RJ, Linas SL, Berns AS et al: Nonoliguric acute renal failure. N Engl J Med 296:1134, 1977

13. Ngai SH: Current concepts in anesthesiology: Effects of anesthetics on various organs. N Engl J Med 302:564, 1980

14. Philbin DM, Coggins CH: Plasma antidiuretic hormone levels in cardiac surgical patients during morphine and halothane anesthesia. Anesthesiology 49:95, 1978

15. Moore FD: Metabolic Care of the Surgical Patient, p 289. Philadelphia, WB Saunders, 1959

16. Ellenbogen PH, Scheible FW, Talner LB et al: Sensitivity of gray scale ultrasound

in detecting urinary tract obstruction. Am J Roentgenol 130:731, 1978

17. Hardy JD: Surgical complications. In Sabiston DC (ed): Textbook of Surgery, 11th ed, p 428. Philadelphia, WB Saunders, 1977

18. Frank IN, McDonald DF: Urology. In Schwartz SI (ed): Principles of Surgery, 3rd ed, p 1687. New York, McGraw-Hill, 1979

19. Whelton A: Post-traumatic acute renal failure. Bull NY Acad Med 55:150, 1979

20. Stone AM, Stahl WM: Effect of ethacrynic acid and furosemide on renal function in hypovolemia. Ann Surg 174:1, 1971

21. Eng K, Stahl WM: Correction of the renal hemodynamic changes produced by surgical trauma. Ann Surg 174:19, 1971

22. Baek SM, Brown RS, Shoemaker WC: Early prediction of acute renal failure and recovery. II. Renal function response to furosemide. Ann Surg 178:605, 1973

23. Lucas CE, Zito JG, Carter KM et al: Questionable value of furosemide in preventing renal failure. Surgery 82:314, 1977

24. Schrier RW: Acute renal failure. Kidney Int 15:205, 1979

25. Coe FL: Proteinuria, hematuria, azotemia and oliguria. In Isselbacher KJ, Adams RD, Braunwald E et al (eds): Principles of Internal Medicine, 9th ed, p 218. New York, McGraw-Hill, 1980

26. Miller TR, Anderson RJ, Linas SL et al: Urinary diagnostic indices in acute renal failure. Ann Intern Med 89:47, 1978

27. Oliver J, MacDowell M, Tracy A: The pathogenesis of acute renal failure associated with traumatic and toxic injury. Renal ischemia, nephrotoxic damage and the ischemic episode. J Clin Invest 30:1305, 1951

28. Franklin SS, Merrill JP: Acute renal failure. N Engl J Med 262:711, 761, 1960

29. Elmgren DT, Cheung LY, Bloomer A et al: Acute renal failure after abdominal surgery. Am J Surg 128:743, 1974

30. Fischer RP, Polk HC: Changing etiologic patterns of renal insufficiency in surgical patients. Surg Gynecol Obstet 140:85, 1975

31. Levinsky N: Pathophysiology of acute renal failure. N Engl J Med 296:1453, 1977

32. Maher JF: Toxic nephropathy. In Brenner BM, Rector FC (eds): The Kidney, p 1355. Philadelphia, WB Saunders, 1976

33. Appel GB, Neu HC: Gentamicin in 1978. Ann Intern Med 89:528, 1978

34. Bennett WM, Plamp C, Porter GA: Drug-related syndromes in clinical nephrology. Ann Intern Med 87:582, 1977

35. Bennett WM, Gilbert DN, Houghton D et al: Gentamicin nephrotoxicity—Morphologic and pharmacologic features. West J Med 126:65, 1977

36. Wellwood JM, Lovell D, Thompson AE et al: Renal damage caused by gentamicin: A study of the effects on renal morphology and urinary enzyme excretion. J Pathol 118:171, 1976

37. Luft FC, Patel V, Yum MN et al: Experimental aminoglycoside nephrotoxicity. J Lab Clin Med 86:213, 1975

38. Bobrow SN, Jaffe E, Young RC: Anuria and acute tubular necrosis associated with gentamicin and cephalothin. JAMA 222:1546, 1972

39. Kleinknecht D, Ganeval D, Droz D: Acute renal failure after high doses of gentamicin and cephalothin. Lancet 1:1129, 1973

40. Harrison WO, Silverblatt FJ, Turck M: Gentamicin nephrotoxicity: Failure of three cephalosporins to potentiate injury in rats. Antimicrob Agents Chemother 8:209, 1975

41. Dellinger P, Murphy T, Pinn V et al: Protective effect of cephalothin against gentamicin-induced nephrotoxicity in rats. Antimicrob Agents Chemother 9:172, 1976

42. Luft FC, Patel V, Yum MN et al: Nephrotoxicity of cephalosporin–gentamicin combinations in rats. Antimicrob Agents Chemother 9:831, 1976

43. Fanning WL, Gump D, Jick H: Gentamicin- and cephalothin-associated rises in blood urea nitrogen. Antimicrob Agents Chemother 10:80, 1976

44. Klastersky J, Hensgens C, Henri A et al: Comparative clinical study of tobramycin

and gentamicin. Antimicrob Agents Chemother 5:133, 1974

45. Modsen PO, Kjaer TB, Mosegaard A: Comparison of tobramycin and gentamicin in the treatment of complicated urinary tract infections. J Infect Dis (Suppl) 134:S150, 1976

46. Smith CR, Lipsky JJ, Laskin OL et al: Double-blind comparison of the nephrotoxicity and auditory toxicity of gentamicin and tobramycin. N Engl J Med 302:1106, 1980

47. Norman JC: Renal complications of cardiopulmonary bypass. Dis Chest 54:50, 1968

48. Wilkens H, Regelson W, Hoffmeister FS: The physiologic importance of pulsatile blood flow. N Engl J Med 267:443, 1962

49. Doberneck RC, Reiser MP, Lillebei CW: Acute renal failure after open-heart surgery utilizing extracorporeal circulation and total body perfusion. J Thorac Cardiovasc Surg 43:441, 1962

50. Yeboah ED, Petrie A, Pead JL: Acute renal failure and open heart surgery. Br Med J 1:415, 1972

51. Abel RM, Wick J, Beck CH et al: Renal dysfunction following open-heart operations. Arch Surg 108:175, 1974

52. Bhat JG, Gluck MC, Lowenstein J et al: Renal failure after open heart surgery. Ann Intern Med 84:677, 1976

53. Abel RM, Buckley MJ, Austen WG et al: Etiology, incidence, and prognosis of renal failure following cardiac operations. J Thorac Cardiovasc Surg 71:323, 1976

54. Ansell G: Adverse reactions to contrast agents. Invest Radiol 5:374, 1970

55. Diaz-Buxo JA, Wagoner RD, Hattery RR et al: Acute renal failure after excretory urography in diabetic patients. Ann Intern Med 83:155, 1975

56. Weinrauch LA, Healy RW, Leland OS et al: Coronary angiography and acute renal failure in diabetic azotemic nephropathy. Ann Intern Med 86:56, 1977

57. Alexander RD, Berkes SL, Abuelo JG: Contrast media-induced oliguric renal failure. Arch Intern Med 138:381, 1978

58. Carvallo A, Rakowski TA, Argy WP et al: Acute renal failure following drip infusion pyelography. Am J Med 65:38, 1978

59. Swartz RD, Rubin JE, Leeming BW et al: Renal failure following major angiography. Am J Med 65:31, 1978

60. VanZee BE, Hoy WE, Talley TE et al: Renal injury associated with intravenous pyelography in nondiabetic and diabetic patients. Ann Intern Med 89:51, 1978

61. Byrd L, Sherman RL: Radiocontrast-induced acute renal failure: A clinical and pathophysiologic review. Medicine 58:270, 1979

62. Harkonen S, Kjellstrand CM: Exacerbation of diabetic renal failure following intravenous pyelography. Am J Med 63:939, 1977

63. Rene RM, Mellinkoff SM: Renal insufficiency after oral administration of a double dose of a cholecystographic medium. N Engl J Med 261:589, 1959

64. Blythe WB, Woods JW: Acute renal insufficiency after ingestion of a gall-bladder dye. N Engl J Med 264:1045, 1961

65. Gottlieb A, Spiera H, Gordis E: Fatal renal insufficiency after oral cholecystography. N Engl J Med 267:389, 1962

66. Seaman WB, Cosgriff S, Wells J: Renal insufficiency following cholecystography. Am J Roentgenol 90:859, 1963

67. Canales CO, Smith GH, Robinson JC et al: Acute renal failure after the administration of iopanoic acid as a cholecystographic agent. N Engl J Med 281:89, 1969

68. Eisenberg RL, Bank WO, Hedgcock MW: Renal failure after major angiography. Am J Med 68:43, 1980

69. Wilson DM, Turner DR, Cameron JS et al: Value of renal biopsy in acute intrinsic renal failure. Br Med J 2:459, 1976

70. Van Ypersele de Strihou C: Acute oliguric interstitial nephritis. Kidney Int 16:751, 1979

71. Ditlove J, Weidmann P, Bernstein M et al: Methicillin nephritis. Medicine 56:483, 1977

72. Galpin JE, Shinaberger JH, Stanley TM et al: Acute interstitial nephritis due to methicillin. Am. J Med 65:756, 1978

73. Ooi BS, Jao W, First MR et al: Acute interstitial nephritis: A clinical and path-

ologic study based on renal biopsies. Am J Med 59:614, 1975

74. Grossman RA, Hamilton RW, Morse BM et al: Nontraumatic rhabdomyolysis and acute renal failure. N Engl J Med 291:807, 1974

75. Koffler A, Friedler RM, Massry SG: Acute renal failure due to nontraumatic rhabdomyolysis. Ann Intern Med 85:23, 1976

76. Teschan PE, Lawson NL: Studies in acute renal failure. Nephron 3:1, 1966

77. Wilson DR, Thiel G, Arce ML et al: Glycerol-induced hemoglobinuric acute renal failure in the rat. Nephron 4:337, 1967

78. Levinsky BG, Alexander EA: Acute renal failure. In Brenner BM, Rector FC (eds): The Kidney, p 806. Philadelphia, WB Saunders, 1976

79. Mazze RI, Shue GL, Jackson SH: Renal dysfunction associated with methoxyflurane anesthesia. JAMA 216:278, 1971

80. Merkle RB, McDonald FD, Waldman J et al: Human renal function following methoxyflurane anesthesia. JAMA 218:841, 1971

81. Hollenberg NK, McDonald FD, Cotran R et al: Irreversible acute oliguric renal failure. N Engl J Med 286:877, 1972

82. Churchill D, Knaack J, Chirito E et al: Persisting renal insufficiency after methoxyflurane anesthesia. Am J Med 56:575, 1974

83. Singer I, Forrest JN: Drug-induced states of nephrogenic diabetes insipidus. Kidney Int 10:82, 1976

84. Cousins MJ, Mazze RI: Methoxyflurane nephrotoxicity: A study of dose response in man. JAMA 225:1611, 1973

85. Vandam LD: Editorial: The crystal ball. N Engl J Med 283:705, 1970

86. Frascino JA, Vanamee P, Rosen PP: Renal oxalosis and azotemia after methoxyflurane anesthesia. N Engl J Med 283:676, 1970

87. Halpren BA, Kempson RL, Coplon NS: Interstitial fibrosis and chronic renal failure following methoxyflurane anesthesia. JAMA 223:1239, 1973

88. Mazze RI, Calverley RK, Smith NT: Inorganic fluoride nephrotoxicity. Anesthesiology 46:265, 1977

89. Cousins MJ, Fulton A, Haynes WDG et al: Enflurane nephrotoxicity and pre-existing renal dysfunction. Anaesth Intensive Care 6:277, 1978

90. Bennett WM, Muther RS, Parker RA et al: Drug therapy in renal failure: Dosing guidelines for adults. Ann Intern Med 93 (I): 62, 1980

91. Kleinknecht D, Jungers P, Chanard J et al: Uremic and nonuremic complications in acute renal failure: Evaluation of early and frequent dialysis on prognosis. Kidney Int 1:190, 1972

92. Teschan PE, Bacter CR, O'Brien TF et al: Prophylactic hemodialysis in the treatment of acute renal failure. Ann Intern Med 53:992, 1960

93. Fischer RP, Griffen WO, Clark DS: Early dialysis in the treatment of acute renal failure. Surg Gynecol Obstet 123:1019, 1966

94. Conger JD: A controlled evaluation of prophylactic dialysis in post-traumatic acute renal failure. J Trauma 15:1056, 1975

95. Giordano C: Use of exogenous and endogenous urea for protein synthesis in normal and uremic subjects. J Lab Clin Med 62:231, 1963

96. Dudrick SJ, Steiger E, Long JM: Renal failure in surgical patients. Treatment with intravenous essential amino acids and hypertonic glucose. Surgery 68:180, 1970

97. Abel RM, Beck CH, Abbott WM et al: Improved survival from acute renal failure after treatment with intravenous essential L-amino acids and glucose. N Engl J Med 288:695, 1973

98. Baek SM, Makabali GG, Bryan-Brown CW et al: The influence of parenteral nutrition on the course of acute renal failure. Surg Gynecol Obstet 141:405, 1975

99. Leonard DC, Luke RG, Siegel RR: Parenteral essential amino acids in acute renal failure. Urology 6:154, 1975

100. Blackburn GL, Etter G, Mackenzie T: Criteria for choosing amino acid therapy in acute renal failure. Am J Clin Nutr 31:1841, 1978

101. Blumenkrantz MJ, Kopple JD, Koffler A et al: Total parenteral nutrition in the management of acute renal failure. Am J Clin Nutr 31:1831, 1978

102. Kimberly RP, Bowden RE, Keiser HR et al: Reduction of renal function by newer nonsteroidal anti-inflammatory drugs. Am J Med 64:804, 1978

103. Walshe JJ, Venuto RC: Acute oliguric renal failure induced by indomethacin: Possible mechanism. Ann Intern Med 91:47, 1979

104. Henrich WL, Berl T, McDonald KM et al: Angiotensin II, renal nerves, and prostaglandins in renal hemodynamics during hemorrhage. Am J Physiol 235:F46, 1978

105. Henrich WL, Anderson RJ, Berns AS et al: The role of renal nerves and prostaglandins in control of renal hemodynamics and plasma. Renin activity during hypotensive hemorrhage in the dog. J Clin Invest 61:744, 1978

106. Barry KG, Cohen A, Knochel JP et al: Mannitol infusion. II. The prevention of acute functional renal failure during resection of an aneurysm of the abdominal aorta. N Engl J Med 264:967, 1961

107. Seitzman DM, Mazze RI, Schwartz FD et al: Mannitol diuresis: A method of renal protection during surgery. J Urol 90:139, 1963

108. Abbott WM, Austen WG: The reversal of renal cortical ischemia during aortic occlusion by mannitol. J Surg Res 16:482, 1974

109. Barry KG, Mazze RI, Schwartz FD: Prevention of surgical oliguria and renal–hemodynamic suppression by sustained hydration. N Engl J Med 270:1371, 1964

110. Blythe WB: The management of intercurrent medical and surgical problems in the patient with chronic renal failure. In Earley LE, Gottschalk CW (eds): Diseases of the Kidney, p 517. Boston, Little, Brown & Co, 1979

111. Hollenberg NK, Epstein M, Rosen SM et al: Acute oliguric renal failure in man: Evidence for preferential renal cortical ischemia. Medicine 47:455, 1968

112. Mudge GH: Diuretics and other agents employed in the mobilization of edema fluid. In Goodman LS, Gilman A (eds): The Pharmacological Basis of Therapeutics, p 817. New York, Macmillan, 1975

113. Luke RG, Briggs JD, Allison MEM et al: Factors determining response to mannitol in acute renal failure. Am J Med Sci 259:168, 1970

114. Stahl WM, Stone AM: Prophylactic diuresis with ethacrynic acid for prevention of postoperative renal failure. Ann Surg 172:361, 1970

115. Cantarovich F, Galli C, Benedetti L et al: High dose furosemide in established acute renal failure. Br Med J 4:449, 1973

116. Bailey RR, Natale R, Turnbull DI et al: Protective effect of furosemide in acute tubular necrosis and acute renal failure. Clin Sci 45:1, 1973

117. Kramer HJ, Schürmann J, Wassermann C et al: Prostaglandin-independent protection by furosemide from oliguric ischemic renal failure in conscious rats. Kidney Int 17:455, 1980

118. Kleinknecht D, Ganeval D, Gonzalez-Duque LA et al: Furosemide in acute oliguric renal failure: A controlled trial. Nephron 17:51, 1976

119. Minuth AN, Terrell JB, Suki WN: Acute renal failure: A study of the course and prognosis of 104 patients and of the role of furosemide. Am J Med Sci 271:317, 1976

120. Shin B, Mackenzie CF, McAslan TC et al: Postoperative renal failure in trauma patients. Anesthesiology 51:218, 1979

16

The Surgical Patient with Chronic Renal Failure

THOMAS G. MURRAY

More than 45,000 patients with end-stage renal disease (ESRD) are currently maintained on dialysis in the United States, and many times this number of people have milder degrees of renal insufficiency.[1] Most surgical conditions develop at least as frequently in patients with chronic renal failure (CRF) as in those with normal renal function, and some surgical procedures are required more commonly (e.g., parathyroidectomy) or exclusively (e.g., vascular access surgery, renal transplantation) in patients with CRF.

Pre-existing renal insufficiency increases the risk of complications in the perioperative period.[2] Surgery can be performed in patients with CRF with an acceptably low rate of complications; achieving this, however, requires careful preoperative evaluation and treatment.[3,4]

SURGICAL RISK OF CHRONIC RENAL FAILURE

The kidneys play an important role in compensating for the stresses of surgery. Excretion of intracellular constituents released into the extracellular fluid (ECF) during surgery and changes in sodium excretion occur in response to surgically induced shifts in the volume of ECF are essential to homeostasis. In patients with CRF, the capacity of the kidneys to respond to these stresses is compromised. As renal function decreases, much of the adaptive ability of the remaining viable kidney is used to maintain ECF homeostasis in the steady state; therefore, very little is available to defend against the acute stresses of the perioperative period. In addition, CRF is often complicated by systemic abnormalities like hypertension, anemia, and coagulopathy, which further decrease the patient's ability to tolerate the stresses of surgery. Finally, dysfunction of other organs caused by CRF or by diseases responsible for the renal failure may further increase the risk of surgery.

The chance that systemic complications will occur in the perioperative period in a patient with CRF increases with the severity of the renal failure. If the glomerular filtration rate (GFR) is above 50 ml/min, surgery is usually well tolerated, and, in most patients, no specific precautions are necessary. If the GFR is below 20 ml/min, complications are likely to occur unless specific preventive steps are taken. The type of underlying renal disease may influence the risk of perioperative complications, but this factor is less important than the level of azotemia. For example, patients with chronic interstitial renal disease are more likely than normal to develop complications secondary to abnormal tubular function, like hyperkalemia and metabolic acidosis, but complications can occur in patients with any type of renal disease.

COMPLICATIONS OF DECREASED RENAL FUNCTION

Extracellular Fluid Volume

CRF limits the ability of the kidney to respond to situations requiring either maximum sodium excretion or maximum sodium conservation.[5] ECF volume expansion does not occur until severe azotemia has developed, usually with a GFR of less than about 10 ml/min. In patients with mild or moderately advanced renal failure, normal dietary or intravenous sodium intake can be excreted by the kidneys. Volume overload does not supervene unless underlying conditions that independently inhibit sodium excretion (congestive heart failure, cirrhosis, or the nephrotic syndrome) are also present. Maximum sodium excretion is nonetheless decreased even in patients with only moderately advanced azotemia, and extremely large sodium loads given in the perioperative period can cause significant volume expansion.

The consequences of volume overload in the perioperative period are the same in patients with CRF as in persons with normal renal function. If ECF volume expansion is present preoperatively, it should be treated with sodium restriction and either diuretics or, for the patient with ESRD, dialysis.[6] Potent diuretics like furosemide or ethacrynic acid are usually required in patients with CRF, often in large doses. The addition of a modest dose of metalozone to a large dose of either furosemide or ethacrynic acid will significantly increase the diuresis.

ECF volume depletion is a common complication of CRF, and, in patients with mild or moderately advanced renal failure, volume depletion is probably more common than expansion. The presence of CRF necessarily results in a urinary sodium loss. Decreased sodium intake or increased loss from an extrarenal source, as in fever, diarrhea, or vomiting, can cause further ECF volume depletion in patients with CRF. The assessment, risks, and treatment of volume depletion are the same in patients with CRF as in normals. It is important to remember that volume depletion in patients with CRF commonly goes unrecognized until serious complications develop.

Careful monitoring of the ECF volume is necessary in patients with CRF during and after surgery. In many patients, this requires the use of central venous pressure monitoring, although, in patients with relatively normal cardiovascular function, physical assessment should be sufficiently sensitive for accurate measurement of volume status.

Tonicity/Serum Sodium Concentration

In CRF, the ability to conserve or excrete free water is limited.[5] Despite these abnormalities, ECF tonicity is usually normal because water intake is adjusted by the thirst mechanism. However, if enough free water is given in the perioperative period, the ability of the kidneys to excrete it is exceeded, and hyponatremia can develop. This is particularly likely to occur if levels of antidiuretic hormone are acutely elevated, which can be the case owing to any number of factors in the perioperative period. Conversely, if free water intake is inappropriately restricted in the perioperative period, hypernatremia may develop. The clinical consequences and the treatment of these ECF abnormalities are the same for patients with CRF as for patients with normal renal function (see Chap. 17).

Acidosis

Chronic metabolic acidosis is usually present in patients with moderately advanced CRF.[7] The serum bicarbonate concentration begins to decrease when the GFR falls below 20 to 30 ml/min. The acidosis of CRF is usually well compensated by secondary respiratory hyperventilation, and blood pH is maintained at a level only slightly below normal.

Despite the presence of only modest acidemia in the steady state, patients with CRF can develop severe acidemia if there is a sudden increase in the rate of introduction of hydrogen ions into the ECF. This may occur because most of the compensatory mechanisms that allow persons with normal renal function to tolerate an increased hydrogen ion load are already being used in patients with CRF to maintain a steady-state bicarbonate concentration and a pH as close to normal as possible. The serum bicarbonate concentration should be 18 mEq/liter or higher before surgery.[6] In most patients with CRF, the untreated bicarbonate concentration is above this level. In those in whom the bicarbonate concentration is below 18 mEq/liter, enough oral or intravenous bicarbonate should be given postoperatively to increase the concentration to that level. The sodium load given with the bicarbonate is tolerated in the majority of these patients. In patients on chronic dialysis, the bicarbonate concentration is generally above 18 mEq/liter in the periods between dialysis, making supplemental bicarbonate unnecessary.

It is important to obtain preoperative blood gases for patients with CRF who have a bicarbonate concentration of less than 20 mEq/liter. Blood gas measurements should also be obtained for patients with a serum creatinine significantly elevated to levels greater than 6 mg/dl regardless of serum bicarbonate concentration, because a normal serum bicarbonate may be the consequence of a mixed acid–base disorder. If the blood gases reveal through Winter's formula ($p_{CO_2} = 1.5$ [HCO_3] $+ 8 \pm 1$) that the degree of respiratory compensation is inadequate for the serum bicarbonate concentration, evaluation of pulmonary function before surgery is crucial.

During and after surgery, hydrogen ions are released from ischemic cells into the ECF. Cellular ischemia occurs at the operative site and in other areas of the body secondary to changes in blood pressure, regional blood flow, or systemic oxygenation. This release of hydrogen ions causes an added acid load that requires buffering. The patient with CRF is already hyperventilating to compensate for the chronic metabolic acidosis. If the same level of hyperventilation is not maintained throughout the perioperative period, the lowered p_{CO_2} will rise and the pH will fall.[8] Even an increase in p_{CO_2} to normal will result in a significant fall in pH. The clinical consequences and the treatment of acute acidemia are the same in patients with CRF as in normals (see Chap. 18).

Hyperkalemia

Hyperkalemia does not appear in most patients with CRF until end-stage disease develops.[5] Though they can usually maintain a normal steady-state serum potassium concentration, patients with CRF do not tolerate sudden shifts of potassium ions into the ECF.[6] Hyperkalemia is therefore a common complication of surgery in patients with CRF.[9,10] The risk of hyperkalemia increases with the severity of renal failure. In addition, intraoperative hyperkalemia is more likely to occur at any given level of renal insufficiency in patients with chronic interstitial disease than in patients with other types of renal failure.

The risk of hyperkalemia during surgery correlates with the preoperative serum potassium concentration and, in patients on chronic dialysis, with the predialysis potassium concentration. Therefore, in the case of two dialysis patients with the same preoperative potassium concentration, the chances that intraoperative hyperkalemia will occur are greater in the patient with the higher potassium concentration before the last dialysis. For the risk of intraoperative hyperkalemia to be minimized, the serum potassium level should be below 5 mEq/liter immediately before surgery.

The assessment and treatment of an elevated preoperative serum potassium concentration should proceed in an orderly manner. Any reversible factor that may be interfering with potassium excretion should be ameliorated or eliminated. Volume depletion and increased sodium reabsorption secondary to heart failure, cirrhosis, and the nephrotic syndrome can all interfere with potassium excretion. Under these conditions, there is increased sodium reabsorption in the proximal tubule with decreased delivery of sodium to distal tubular sites, where sodium reabsorption is necessary for potassium secretion. Volume expansion in patients who are volume-depleted or on diuretics should be used to increase the delivery of sodium to the distal tubule. If more than 50 to 60 mEq/day of sodium are excreted in the urine, distal sodium delivery can be assumed to be adequate to permit potassium secretion.

Various drugs can interfere with potassium excretion. Drugs that inhibit the action of aldosterone, such as aldactone and triamterene, should be discontinued. A number of other drugs have been reported to cause hyperkalemia in a small number of patients, usually in persons with decreased renal function. Nonsteroidal anti-inflammatory agents can cause hyperkalemia by inhibiting prostaglandin production and should be discontinued before surgery if hyperkalemia is present.[11] Heparin inhibits the production of aldosterone and may rarely contribute to hyperkalemia.[12] Beta-adrenergic blocking drugs may predispose the patient to the development of intraoperative hyperkalemia.[13] Tolerance of a potassium load is decreased in the patient receiving beta-blocking drugs, apparently as a result of a decreased cellular uptake of potassium. Since patients with CRF may be particularly dependent on cellular buffering relative to renal excretion for defense against the development of acute hyperkalemia, they may be adversely affected by these agents.

If preoperative hyperkalemia cannot be attributed to a reversible process, the serum potassium level must be lowered by other means that are not dependent on kidney function. Kayexalate (sodium polystyrene sulfonate) is the treatment of choice in this circumstance. If it is appropriately used (30 g to 50 g every 2 to 3 hr in sufficient sorbitol to promote its elimination), Kayexalate is as or more effective than dialysis in removing potassium. If Kayexalate proves ineffective or cannot be used because of gastrointestinal disease, dialysis should be employed preoperatively to lower the serum potassium concentration.

During and after surgery, the load of potassium introduced into the ECF increases significantly. This is potentially dangerous in the patient with CRF. Causes of this increase include acidemia, cellular ischemia, the release of potassium ions from muscle cells in response to the use of succinylcholine, and the introduction of potassium ions in transfused blood or as the cation in various drugs like antibiotics. The principle risk of hyperkalemia is cardiac irritability.[14] In one large series of patients with ESRD undergoing renal transplantation, the incidence of intraoperative cardiac arrhythmias was approximately 10%, with a 3% incidence of serious rhythm disturbances. Postoperative hyperkalemia in patients with CRF is the major indication for emergency dialysis in the first 24 hr after surgery, a time when dialysis is likely to be complicated by postoperative bleeding. Efforts to control the serum potassium concentration in the pre- and intraoperative periods are therefore also important to reduce the need for emergency dialysis.

Calcium and Phosphate

Though disorders of calcium and phosphate homeostasis are common in patients with CRF, they are not exacerbated by surgery and do not generally cause postoperative complications. Severe hypocalcemia increases the cardiovascular risk of general anesthesia and should be treated preoperatively, but hypocalcemia is seldom severe enough in patients with CRF to constitute a risk factor. The treatment of severe hypocalcemia should begin with control of the serum phosphate level. If hyperphosphatemia at a level of greater than 6 mg/dl is present in a patient with severe hypocalcemia, oral phosphate binders or, in an emergency situation, dialysis should be used to lower the phosphate level. Lowering the serum phosphate to 5.5 mg/dl or less may itself cause the serum calcium to increase slightly, but it will also allow the serum calcium concentration to be increased safely. If time permits (a period of several days is needed), the hypocalcemia can then be treated with oral calcium supplements in doses of at least 1 g/day of elemental calcium and vitamin D derivatives, which have a rapid onset of action. 1,25-Dihydroxycholecalciferol is the drug of choice for this purpose. If the serum calcium level must be increased more rapidly, intravenous calcium can be given.

Symptomatic hypocalcemia may also develop again in the postoperative period. If a large amount of intracellular phosphate is released into the ECF during surgery, the serum phosphate level may rise dramatically. Because renal phosphate excretion is limited in the patient with CRF, the serum calcium level may fall. Serum phosphate should be controlled as above before direct efforts to increase serum calcium are made. Only if definite signs and symptoms of hypocalcemia are present should intravenous calcium be considered.

SYSTEMIC COMPLICATIONS OF CHRONIC RENAL FAILURE

Hypertension

Hypertension is seen commonly in patients with CRF, particularly in those with advanced azotemia. The operative risks of inadequately treated hypertension are the same for patients with CRF as for normals. Although treatment generally proceeds in the same way for patients with CRF as for normals, there are a few differences. First, in patients with renal failure, hypertension is often due to ECF volume expansion, so efforts should be made to reduce the ECF volume to normal.[15] Potent diuretics or, in the case of ESRD, dialysis will accomplish this and thereby reduce the blood pressure. However, not all hypertension is volume-dependent, even in patients with ESRD; when it is not, depletion of the ECF volume is not likely to be effective in controlling the blood pressure and may produce complications independently. Second, the use of nitroprusside to control malignant hypertension in patients with CRF increases the risk of side-effects due to the accumulation of thiocyanate, the elimination of which is largely dependent on glomerular filtration.[16] Even in patients with CRF, however, complications generally occur only if the infusion of nitroprusside is continued for more than a few days. Finally, beta-adrenergic blocking drugs should—if possible—be discontinued before surgery in patients with CRF. These patients are particularly sensitive to shifts in volume and run the risk of intraoperative hypotension.

Anemia

Anemia is an almost universal feature of advanced CRF. The presence of anemia theoretically increases the risk of perioperative complications; however, most patients with CRF do not develop complications due to anemia.[6] Because their anemia is chronic and compensatory changes have occurred, it is remarkably well tolerated. Even patients with ESRD who have hematocrits between 20% and 24% tolerate major surgery without prior transfusion in most instances.

The risks associated with transfusion in CRF patients include hepatitis, iron overload, transfusion reactions, and volume overload. Transfusions should not be given preoperatively to all patients with CRF and anemia but should be reserved for cases in which they are specifically indicated. Patients with hematocrits above 25% generally do not require transfusions before surgery, whereas those below 20% probably should be transfused. Decreased postoperative wound healing, a feared consequence of anemia, does not seem to be a major factor in patients with CRF, although it is in those with acute renal failure. If transfusions are required, frozen or washed red cells should be used to decrease the chance of sensitizing the patient to future renal transplants and to decrease the risk of hepatitis.

Coagulation Defects

Patients with moderately severe or advanced azotemia have defective platelet aggregation. A circulating factor retained in the serum as a result of the decreased GFR affects otherwise normal platelets, producing a defect in platelet aggregation that can be demonstrated experimentally. The bleeding time is usually prolonged to $1\frac{1}{2}$ or 2 times normal. In patients with renal failure not requiring dialysis and in patients with ESRD who are adequately dialyzed, this defect has no major clinical consequence.[17] There is usually no increased bleeding, even when major surgery is done.[2]

The major risk factor for intraoperative and postoperative bleeding is dialysis and not CRF itself. If dialysis is performed less than 6 hr before surgery or in the first 24 hr after surgery, the risk of bleeding is increased.[18] Therefore, it is best to avoid dialysis during these intervals.

Nutritional Status

Many patients with severe renal failure, especially those maintained on dialysis, are malnourished.[5] As a result of decreased protein intake and uremia itself, many patients develop both somatic and visceral protein depletion. Postoperatively, malnutrition may contribute to poor wound healing and infectious complications. In patients who are maintained on dialysis and in the majority of patients with severe renal failure, hyperalimentation with essential amino acids and hypertonic glucose (renal failure fluid) given either orally or intravenously should be considered after major surgery.[19] Patients with mild or moderate renal failure are usually not significantly malnourished and do not require routine hyperalimentation unless it is indicated for other reasons.

Infections

Infectious complications do not occur more frequently than normal in the perioperative period in patients with CRF or ESRD, nor do they present more difficulty in treatment. Except for necessary changes in antibiotic dosage due to a decreased GFR, the indications for prophylactic antibiotics and the treatment of established infections are the same for patients with renal failure as for patients with normal renal function.

Atherosclerotic Cardiovascular Disease

Atherosclerotic vascular disease is commonly present in patients with renal failure, often a consequence of underlying conditions other than renal failure.[20] The risks associated with atherosclerotic vascular disease and its treatment are the same for patients with CRF as for normals.

PERIOPERATIVE PRESERVATION OF RENAL FUNCTION

The preservation of renal function in the perioperative period is crucial in patients with CRF who have not progressed to ESRD. Pre-existing renal insufficiency is one of the most important risk factors for the development of postoperative acute renal failure, and a substantial number of patients with CRF suffer an acute decrease in renal function with surgery. Moreover, a postoperative decrement in renal function in a patient with CRF is seldom fully reversible. It is therefore imperative that risk factors for the development of acute renal failure be avoided or minimized.

The causes and treatment of acute renal failure are presented in detail in Chapter 15. Volume depletion, common in patients with CRF in the perioperative period, is of particular concern in this regard. Its high frequency is a consequence of a defect in renal sodium conservation, which complicates CRF. The use of nonsteroidal anti-inflammatory drugs in the immediate preoperative period constitutes another possible, although unproved, risk factor for the development of acute renal failure in these patients.[21] Patients with CRF may be particularly dependent on renal prostaglandin production for maintenance of maximum renal function. In the face of prostaglandin synthesis inhibition by nonsteroidal anti-inflammatory agents, the stresses of surgery on the kidney may be poorly tolerated and the likelihood of acute renal failure increased.

Concern for the preservation of renal function also influences the choice of general anesthetic agents to be used in patients with CRF. Methoxyflurane is a potential nephrotoxin that probably works through the metabolic production of either oxalate or fluoride.[22] The incidence of renal failure after methoxyflurane anesthesia is low in patients with normal renal function, but this agent should not be used in patients with pre-existing renal failure who are not on dialysis. Enflurane, which is also metabolized to fluoride, has been associated with acute renal failure in a number of patients with pre-existing renal failure.[23] Fluoride levels are elevated only after prolonged exposure to enflurane; short exposures may be safe, even for patients with CRF. Enflurane should not be used for prolonged surgical procedures in patients with significant renal failure.

ANESTHETIC CONCERNS

Preoperative sedation with almost any of the commonly used agents is safe for patients with CRF. Although the metabolism of some of these drugs is altered owing to a decreased GFR, one or two doses will not cause complications.

Muscle relaxants should be carefully chosen for patients with CRF. Succinylcholine is generally well tolerated. It causes a rise in serum potassium level in both patients with CRF and normals. Although this increase is similar in the two groups of patients (approximately 0.5 mEq/liter after a dose of 1 mg/kg), it may cause complications in patients with CRF who have previously been hyperkalemic or in those who require repeated doses of the drug. Gallamine should be avoided in patients with decreased renal function. It depends primarily on glomerular filtration for its elimination, and prolonged paralysis commonly follows its use in patients with CRF.[24] Although the half-life of D-tubocurarine is increased in patients with CRF by 30 to 70 min, it can be used

safely. Cases of prolonged or recurrent paralysis after successful reversal by neostigmine have been reported in patients with renal failure; however, such cases are uncommon and, if accurately diagnosed, can be easily managed.[25] Pancuronium is handled primarily by the liver, and, consequently, its metabolism and elimination are not significantly altered by CRF.[26] When its use is possible, it is the muscle relaxant of choice for patients with CRF. Local and spinal anesthesia can be used in patients with CRF without modification of dosage or route of administration.

MODIFICATION OF DRUG DOSES

Alterations in the dosages of some drugs are necessary in cases of CRF because the drugs themselves or their active or toxic metabolites are eliminated by the kidneys. The dosage of such agents must be decreased in the patient with decreased renal function in order for safe concentrations of the drug or its metabolites to be maintained in the body. Changes in dosages of other drugs are necessary because of changes in protein binding or volume of distribution that are induced by azotemia. A detailed discussion of dosage modifications for individual drugs is contained in a review by Bennett and co-workers.[27]

DIALYSIS AND SURGERY

Most patients with CRF who are not already on chronic dialysis do not require dialysis immediately before surgery. As discussed above, electrolyte and volume disturbances generally can be corrected without dialysis. Patients occasionally require both their first dialysis and surgery at the same time. The presence of one or more complications of uremia is the indication for dialysis in these patients.

If possible, surgery should be postponed until a minimum of 4 or 5 hemodialyses or at least 48 hr to 72 hr of peritoneal dialysis have been carried out. If surgery must be performed immediately, 3 or 4 hemodialyses should be performed with an anticoagulation protocol designed to minimize postdialysis bleeding. Between the completion of dialysis and the beginning of surgery, 2 hr to 3 hr should be allowed to elapse. If absolutely necessary, dialysis can be continued throughout the operative procedure; fortunately, this is rarely called for.

In the patient on a regular dialysis program, the last dialysis should be completed between 4 and 30 hr before surgery. If it is performed more than 30 hr before, the chance of intraoperative hyperkalemia is greatly increased. If it is performed less than 4 hr before, the possibility of intraoperative bleeding is increased. If surgery must be performed less than 4 hr after dialysis is completed, the anticoagulation protocol should be designed to minimize the chance of bleeding.[18]

Dialysis should be delayed for as many hours after surgery as possible; in order for bleeding complications to be kept minimal, at least 24 hr and ideally 48 hr should elapse before elective dialysis is performed. For 5 to 7 days after surgery, a special anticoagulation protocol designed to minimize bleeding should again be used.

Chronic hemodialysis access sites are commonly lost in the perioperative period as a result of thrombosis.[2] Hypotension is one cause of this loss. Pressure on the access site during surgery, another cause of thrombosis, can be prevented. Proper at-tention to positioning of the limb, protection of the site during surgery, and frequent observation of the access site in the postoperative period for detection of decreased function should all serve to minimize the loss of access routes. Alterations in function should immediately be brought to the attention of the vascular surgeons.

SUMMARY

1. **The presence of CRF increases the incidence of perioperative systemic complications and of postoperative acute renal failure. Despite this risk, surgery can be performed safely even in patients with ESRD if appropriate attention is given to preventing or treating expected complications.**
2. **The patient should be euvolemic at the time of surgery. Volume overload is usually easy to detect and should be treated with large doses of potent diuretics or, in patients with ESRD, with dialysis. Volume depletion is common, especially in mild or moderately advanced renal failure, but it is often not appreciated clinically.**
3. **Serum electrolyte concentrations should be measured preoperatively in all patients. Hyponatremia or hypernatremia may develop postoperatively because of defective water handling by the kidney. If either of these complications develops, free water intake should be appropriately altered, the serum sodium concentration being maintained between 125 and 150 mEq/liter.**
4. **If the serum bicarbonate concentration is less than 20 mEq/liter or the serum creatinine level greater than 6 mg/dl, blood gas measurements should be obtained preoperatively.**

The serum bicarbonate concentration should be kept above 18 mEq/liter throughout the perioperative period. Hyperventilation should be maintained intraoperatively to prevent a rise in p_{CO_2} and a resultant fall in pH.

5. The preoperative serum potassium concentration should be below 5 mg/dl. However, even if it is normal, intraoperative hyperkalemia may still occur. The serum potassium level should be monitored and treated aggressively if elevated. Kayexalate is as effective as dialysis in removing potassium from the body.

6. Disorders of calcium and phosphate do not generally create problems in the perioperative period. If severe hypocalcemia (less than 7.5 mEq/liter) is present, it should be corrected preoperatively, but only after the serum phosphate concentration has been adjusted to normal.

7. The treatment of hypertension for patients with CRF is the same as for patients with normal renal function. In severe renal failure, hypertension is often volume-dependent. Nitroprusside toxicity due to thiocyanate accumulation is common in CRF if the drug is continued for more than a few days.

8. The anemia of CRF is remarkably well tolerated despite its severity; intra- or postoperative complications are rare. If the hematocrit is above 25%, preoperative transfusion is not required; it is less than 20%, transfusion should be carried out for all but minor procedures. Washed or frozen red blood cells should be used.

9. Except in patients with ESRD who should be but are not on dialysis,

clinical bleeding is usually not a problem. Patients with CRF and patients with ESRD on dialysis tolerate surgery without developing bleeding complications. Anticoagulation required for hemodialysis is more of a risk during surgery. Dialysis should be completed at least 4 hr before or 24 hr to 48 hr after surgery. Preoperative dialysis within 4 hr of surgery and postoperative dialysis during the first 7 days should be performed with an anticoagulation regimen that minimizes the degree of systemic anticoagulation.

10. Many patients with severe renal failure and those on dialysis are protein-malnourished. Since adequate nutrition is essential for optimum wound healing and resistance to infection, these patients should be considered for oral or intravenous hyperalimentation with essential amino acids (renal failure fluids) in the postoperative period.

11. Postoperative infections do not occur with greater incidence or severity than normal in patients with CRF, including those with ESRD on dialysis. The indications for antibiotics are the same as in normals, although the dose may have to be adjusted.

12. The presence of CRF greatly increases the risk for acute renal failure in the postoperative period. Volume depletion, the preoperative use of nonsteroid anti-inflammatory agents, and certain anesthetics like methoxyflurane should be avoided because of their likely contribution to postoperative deterioration of renal function.

13. The presence of CRF influences the choice of muscle relaxants and general anesthetics to be used. Doses of

many drugs must be modified for patients with CRF, and dosage modification is not limited to drugs excreted by the kidneys.

14. Correct positioning of the limb containing an access route, avoidance of pressure during surgery, and frequent postoperative monitoring are crucial for maintenance of the functional integrity of the access site.

REFERENCES

1. Burton BT, Hirschman GH: Demographic analysis: End-stage renal disease and its treatment in the United States. Clin Nephrol 11:47, 1979
2. Brenowitz JB, Williams CD, Edwards WS: Major surgery in patients with chronic renal failure. Am J Surg 134:765, 1977
3. Hampers CL, Bailey GL, Hager EB et al: Major surgery in patients on maintainence hemodialysis. Am J Surg 115:747, 1968
4. Lissos I, Goldberg B, Van Blerk PJP et al: Surgical procedures on patients in end-stage renal failure. Br J Urol 45:359, 1973
5. Depner TA, Gulyassy PF: Chronic renal failure. In Earley LE, Gottshalk CW (eds): Straus and Welts Diseases of the Kidney, p 211. Boston, Little, Brown & Co, 1979
6. Blythe WB: The management of intercurrent medical and surgical problems in the patient with chronic renal failure. In Earley LE, Gottshalk CW (eds): Straus and Welts Diseases of the Kidney, p 517. Boston, Little, Brown & Co, 1979
7. Sebastian A, McSherry E, Morns RC: Metabolic acidosis with special reference to the renal acidosis. In Brenner BM, Rector FC (eds): The Kidney, p 165. Philadelphia, W B Saunders, 1976
8. Goggin MJ, Joeskes AM: Gas exchange in renal failure. I. Dangers of hyperkalemia during anesthesia. Br Med J 2:244, 1971
9. Takacs FJ: Surgery with impaired renal function. Surg Clin North Am 50:719, 1970
10. Aldrete JA, O'Higgins JW, Starzl TE: Changes in serum potassium during renal homotransplantation. Arch Surg 101:82, 1970
11. Tan SY, Shapiro R, Franco R et al: Indomethacin-induced prostaglandin inhibition with hyperkalemia. A reversible cause of hyporeninemic hypoaldosteronism. Ann Intern Med 90:783, 1979
12. Phelps KR, Oh MS, Carroll HJ: Heparin-induced hyperkalemia: Report of a case. Nephron 25:209, 1980
13. Rosa RM, Silva P, Young JB et al: Adrenergic modulation of extrarenal potassium disposal. N Engl J Med 302:401, 1980
14. Korde M, Ward BE: Serum potassium concentrations after succinylcholine in patients with renal failure. Anesthesiology 36:142, 1972
15. Davidson RC, Scribner BIJ: Cardiovascular manifestations of renal failure. In Earley LE, Gottshalk CW (eds): Straus and Welts Diseases of the Kidney, p 263. Boston, Little, Brown & Co, 1979
16. Cohn JN, Burke LP: Nitroprusside. Ann Intern Med 91:752, 1979
17. Rabiner SF: Bleeding abnormalities. In Massry SG, Sellers AL (eds): Clinical Aspects of Uremia and Dialysis, p 179. Springfield, Charles C Thomas, 1976
18. Kjellstrand CM, Buselmeier TJ: A simple method of anticoagulation during pre- and postoperative hemodialysis avoiding rebound phenomenon. Surgery 72:630, 1972
19. Dudrick SJ, Steiger E, Long JM: Renal failure in surgical patients. Treatment with intravenous essential amino acids and hypertonic glucose. Surgery 68:180, 1970
20. Rostan SG, Greles JC, Kirk KA et al: Ischemic heart disease in patients with uremia undergoing maintainence hemodialysis. Kidney Int 16:600, 1979
21. Torres VE, Strong CG, Romero JC: Indomethacin enhancement of glycerol-induced acute renal failure in rabbits. Kidney Int 7:170, 1975
22. Churchill D, Knaack J, Chirito E et al: Persisting renal insufficiency after methoxyflurane anesthesia. Report of two cases and review of literature. Am J Med 56:575, 1974

23. Cousins MS, Fulton A, Haynes WD et al: Enflurane nephrotoxicity and pre-existing renal dysfunction. Anaesth Intensive Care 6:277, 1972

24. Slawson KB: Anesthesia for the patient in renal failure. Br J Anaesth 44:277, 1972

25. Miller RD, Cullen DJ: Renal failure and postoperative respiratory failure: Recurarization. Br J Anaesth 48:253, 1976

26. Miller RD, Stevens WC, Way WL: The effect of renal failure and hyperkalemia on the duration of pancuranium neuromuscular blockade in man. Anesth Analg (Cleve) 52:661, 1973

27. Bennett WM, Muthers, Parker RA et al: Drug therapy in renal failure. Dosage guidelines for adults. Ann Intern Med 93:62, 1980

Disorders of Volume, Tonicity, and Potassium in the Surgical Patient

MICHAEL A. GEHEB
MALCOLM COX

Surgical patients commonly develop problems with volume, tonicity, or potassium homeostasis. Even healthy patients may retain sodium and water and release potassium into the extracellular fluid during the postoperative period. In patients with underlying systemic disease, the ability to maintain normal volume and electrolyte balance may be significantly impaired. The three sections of this chapter review disorders of volume, tonicity, and potassium homeostasis and present an ordered approach to their complex management.

DISORDERS OF VOLUME HOMEOSTASIS

Fundamental Principles

Several fundamental principles help to unravel the most clinically important abnormalities of volume homeostasis:

1. Extracellular fluid (ECF) volume is determined by total body sodium content.

2. The distribution of ECF between the intravascular and interstitial fluid compartments is determined by the balance between plasma and interstitial oncotic and hydrostatic pressures acting at the level of the microcirculation.

3. The effective arterial blood volume (EABV) is a function of tissue perfusion that is determined by cardiac output and peripheral vascular resistance. Under normal circumstances, changes in EABV are concordant with changes in intravascular and ECF volumes.

4. Renal sodium excretion does not respond directly to changes in either ECF or intravascular volume but is a function of EABV.

5. Contraction of the ECF compartment or sodium depletion is always associated with contraction of the intravascular compartment; however, intravascular volume depletion may coexist with increased or decreased ECF volume (Table 17-1).

6. Although expansion of the ECF compartment or sodium excess is always

associated with expansion of the interstitial fluid compartment, it is not necessarily associated with expansion of the intravascular compartment.[1]

The renal response to surgery or trauma is retention of sodium and water. The factors responsible for sodium retention have not been completely delineated, but "third-space" sequestration of fluid, by producing intravascular volume depletion and a decrement in EABV, probably plays a role in many patients.[2-4] In addition, aldosterone secretion generally increases during surgery and undoubtedly contributes to antinatriuresis. Hyperaldosteronism is due both to an EABV-mediated increase in the renin–angiotensin system and to a stress-related increase in adrenocorticotropic hormone (ACTH) secretion.[5] However, since the ACTH-mediated increase in aldosterone secretion is generally short-lived, EABV remains the dominant influence controlling aldosterone secretion in surgical patients.

Intravascular Volume Depletion with Decreased Extracellular Fluid Volume

Intravascular volume depletion is generally characterized by tachycardia and hypotension, and the associated decrease in EABV leads to enhanced reabsorption of sodium and water by the kidney. This is manifested by oliguria with a urine volume of less than 20 ml/hr, a low urine sodium concentration of less than 20 mEq/liter, a high urine osmolality of greater than 500 mOsm/kg, and the same elevated blood urea nitrogen (BUN): plasma creatinine ratio that is seen in prerenal azotemia.[6] Intravascular volume depletion can coexist either with decreased ECF volume, as in acute blood loss, third-space fluid sequestration, and sodium depletion, or with increased ECF, as in hypoalbuminemia (Table 17-1).[1,7]

The presence of hypotension, the principal clinical sign of significant intravascular volume depletion, in a patient without edema provides good evidence for the

Table 17-1. Disorders of Volume Homeostasis

	IVF	IF	ECF	EABV
Intravascular Volume Depletion				
With Decreased ECF Volume				
Acute blood loss	↓↓	⇔	↓	↓
Third-space sequestration*	↓↓	↓	↓	↓
Sodium depletion	↓	↓	↓	↓
With Increased ECF Volume				
Hypoalbuminemia				
Chronic	⇔	↑↑	↑↑	↓
Acute	↓↓	↑	↑	↓
Intravascular Volume Expansion				
With Increased ECF Volume				
Isotonic saline infusion	↑	↑	↑	↑
Renal failure	↑	↑	↑	↑
Congestive heart failure	↑	↑↑	↑↑	↓
Hepatic cirrhosis	↑	↑↑	↑↑	↓

*Under normal circumstances, the IVF makes up one-fourth and the IF three-fourths of the ECF volume (Fig. 17-1). In the case of third-space sequestration, that portion of the ECF volume "trapped" in the third space behaves as if it had been lost externally. Consequently, patients with this dysfunction present with symptoms and signs of intravascular and ECF volume depletion.
IVF = intravascular fluid; IF = interstitial fluid; ECF = extracellular fluid; EABV = effective arterial blood volume.

coexistence of intravascular volume depletion and true ECF volume depletion rather than ECF maldistribution. ECF volume depletion can be due to a relatively selective contraction of the intravascular compartment, as in acute blood loss, to sequestration of fluid in a so-called third space, or to a more generalized proportional contraction of both the intravascular and the interstitial fluid compartments, as in sodium depletion.[4]

Large volumes of fluid rich in albumin can be lost in third spaces. Accumulations can be especially voluminous in patients with gastrointestinal tract obstruction and sequestration of fluid in the bowel wall and lumen and in patients with extensive burns in which fluid is trapped in cutaneous vesicles and bullae.[4,8] After resolution of the primary process, the sequestered fluid is reabsorbed and re-enters the functional ECF compartment. Since fluid sequestration during the initial injury and fluid reabsorption during recovery from the injury can markedly influence intravascular volume, these fluid shifts must be carefully considered in the management of surgical patients.

Sodium Depletion

Sodium depletion can result from renal or extrarenal losses of sodium-containing fluid, as shown below.

Renal sodium losses
    Diuretics
    Osmotic diuresis (glucose, mannitol, urea)
    Postobstructive diuresis
    Diuretic phase of acute tubular necrosis
    Chronic interstitial nephritis
    Polycystic kidney disease
    Medullary cystic disease
    Addison's disease
    Vomiting, nasogastric suction

Gastrointestinal sodium losses
    Vomiting, nasogastric suction
    Diarrhea
    Fistulas
Cutaneous sodium losses
    Sensible perspiration
    Serous drainage (burns, open wounds)

Excessive renal losses of sodium are most commonly caused by diuretics. Patients with renal sodium loss may not have the classic laboratory findings of intravascular volume depletion, oliguria, and low sodium urine concentration. They do have accompanying hypokalemia, increased urinary chloride concentration, and metabolic alkalosis.[9] Osmotic diuresis of any etiology also produces obligate urinary sodium losses.[10] Renal sodium depletion is also common in patients with uncontrolled diabetes mellitus, cerebral edema treated with mannitol, postobstructive diuresis, and the diuresis associated with recovery from acute tubular necrosis.[11–14]

Patients with chronic interstitial nephritis, polycystic kidney disease, and medullary cystic disease have large obligate sodium losses and are particularly susceptible to sodium depletion, especially during periods of sodium restriction.[15] Particular attention must be paid to volume status in these patients during the perioperative period. Since the patients may have associated defects in urinary concentration and in potassium and hydrogen ion secretion, they may also manifest hypertonicity, hyperkalemia, and hyperchloremic metabolic acidosis.

Primary adrenal insufficiency (Addison's disease) may lead to profound sodium depletion, hypercalcemia, and hypotension. Immediate therapy includes ECF volume expansion and glucocorticoid administration. Chronic therapy should include both mineralo- and glu-

Table 17-2. Gastrointestinal Secretions: Normal Volume and Composition

	Volume (liters/day)	Concentration (mEq/liter)			
		Na^+	K^+	Cl^-	HCO_3^-
Saliva	~ 1	20–80	10–20	20–40	20–160
Gastric juice	1–2	20–100	5–10	120–160	—
Bile	~ 1	150–250	5–10	40–60	20–60
Pancreatic juice	1–2	120	5–10	10–60	80–120
Succus entericus	1–2	140	5	Variable	Variable

(After Phillips SF: In Maxwell MH, Kleeman CR (eds): Clinical Disorders of Fluid and Electrolyte Metabolism, 3rd ed. New York, McGraw Hill, 1980)

cocorticoid replacement. Selective hypoaldosteronism does not usually cause sodium depletion of clinical significance.

The gastrointestinal tract is a common source of excessive sodium losses in surgical patients. Under normal circumstances, the daily volume of all gastrointestinal secretions is about 8 liters to 10 liters. However, the volume and electrolyte compositions of different gastrointestinal secretions vary widely (Table 17-2).[16,17] Gastric fluid contains relatively small amounts of sodium and potassium and large amounts of hydrochloric acid. Patients with gastric fluid losses can become markedly sodium-and potassium-depleted, not only because of direct electrolyte losses in the gastric fluid, but also because the resulting hypochloremic metabolic alkalosis is associated with renal sodium and potassium wasting.[18] Pancreatic fluid contains large amounts of sodium bicarbonate with a sodium concentration approaching that of plasma, and large volume losses produce both sodium depletion and hyperchloremic acidosis. Diarrhea varies markedly in composition, depending on its underlying cause, but generally contains appreciable amounts of sodium and potassium and large quantities of alkali-equivalent. Consequently, patients with severe diarrhea usually present with sodium and potassium depletion and hyperchloremic acidosis.

Since insensible perspiration is virtually sodium-free, such losses, unless large, are not associated with clinically significant reductions in ECF volume. In the surgical patient, the loss of sodium in serous drainage from burns or open wounds may also lead to sodium depletion.[8]

Intravascular Volume Depletion with Increased Extracellular Fluid

The presence of edema, the principle clinical sign of ECF volume expansion, in a patient with hypotension provides good evidence for the coexistence of intravascular volume depletion and ECF volume expansion. The edema indicates maldistribution of fluid between the intravascular and interstitial fluid compartments rather than ECF volume depletion.[7]

Since albumin is normally restricted to the intravascular fluid compartment, plasma oncotic pressure is a major determinant of the distribution of fluid between the intravascular and interstitial fluid compartments. Hypoalbuminemia is associated with a shift of fluid from the intravascular to the interstitial fluid compartment. This leads to a decrement in intravascular volume and EABV, an increase in interstitial fluid volume, manifested as edema, and renal sodium and water retention. However, because of the hypoalbuminemia, most of the retained fluid accumulates in the interstitial fluid compartment, and relatively little remains in the intravascular space.[5]

Hypoalbuminemia has many causes and is best classified on the basis of the underlying defect in albumin turnover.[19] Three etiologic categories exist: (1) defects in hepatic albumin synthesis (starvation, malnutrition, debilitating chronic diseases, hepatic cirrhosis); (2) substantial external losses that exceed hepatic synthetic capacity (nephrotic syndrome, protein-losing gastroenteropathy, radiation ileitis, thoracic duct fistulas, chronic peritoneal dialysis, burns); and (3) redistribution of albumin from the intravascular space to either the interstitial fluid compartment (diffuse capillary leak syndrome) or to a third space such as the peritoneal cavity (peritonitis, pancreatitis, hepatic cirrhosis), bowel wall or lumen (bowel obstruction), or cutaneous bullae (burns).

Chronic Hypoalbuminemia

When hypoalbuminemia develops gradually over a period of weeks or months, a new steady state is reached in which intravascular volume is maintained at a near normal level at the expense of increases in the volume of the interstitial and ECF compartments. Consequently, the presentation of patients with chronic hypoalbuminemia is dominated by edema. Significant hypotension ascribable to hypoalbuminemia *per se* is unusual.

Acute Hypoalbuminemia

When hypoalbuminemia develops rapidly over hours or days, renal sodium and water retention cannot match the loss of intravascular fluid, and hypotension is common. One cause is the so-called diffuse capillary leak syndrome, which is usually associated with sepsis in which bacterial toxemia leads to increased capillary permeability.

Hypoalbuminemia can also develop rapidly when patients sequestering fluid rich in albumin in a third space are treated with large volumes of crystalloid. Under these circumstances, hypotension reflects both transudation of fluid from the intravascular to the interstitial fluid compartment due to hypoalbuminemia and the loss of intravascular fluid into the third space.

Intravascular Volume Depletion: Fluid Therapy

The therapy of intravascular volume depletion should be determined by the patient's circulatory status and the nature of the fluid lost. Acute hemorrhage is best treated with blood. Other colloid solutions like plasmanate or albumin, which remain in the intravascular space, can be substituted if blood is unavailable. Isotonic crystalloid solutions like 0.9% saline or Ringer's lactate, which distribute throughout the ECF compartment, can be used in an emergency, but only until colloid is available. Since isotonic saline distributes throughout the ECF compartment, only one-fourth of each liter infused remains in the intravascular compartment. Similarly, since 5% dextrose in water distributes throughout total body water (TBW), only one-twelfth of each liter infused remains in the intravascular compartment. It is for this reason that 5% dextrose in water is not a useful intravascular volume expander. Similar principles apply to patients with third-space sequestration of fluid; however, blood transfusion is not required in such cases.[4,20-22]

Infusions of albumin can be life-saving in disorders associated with acute hypoalbuminemia and in the emergency therapy of hypovolemic shock of any etiology. The continued infusion of large quantities of albumin is generally unnecessary once blood pressure has been stabilized and may lead to intravascular volume expansion and pulmonary edema, especially in patients with underlying heart disease. Hypertonic albumin infusions can also sometimes be helpful in initiating diuresis in patients with chronic hypoalbuminemia and diuretic-resistant edema, such as those with nephrotic syndrome. Once again, however, care must be taken to avoid pulmonary congestion.[23]

There is no rationale for long-term albumin therapy in patients with hypoalbuminemia and edema due to excessive external losses of albumin. Albumin infusions only transiently reduce hypoalbuminemia in patients with nephrotic syndrome, given that the exogenous albumin is rapidly excreted in the urine. Similarly, such therapy is not indicated in patients with hypoalbuminemia and edema due to decreased albumin synthesis. In patients with hepatic cirrhosis, the infused albumin is rapidly sequestered in the peritoneal cavity and contributes to the ascites. Under these circumstances, therapy should be directed at the underlying disorder, if possible. In addition, adequate protein intake is an important prerequisite for normal albumin synthesis. In the case of chronic albumin therapy, as employed for patients with extensive burns or malnourished patients who require prolonged nutritional support before surgery, the raising of plasma albumin levels above normal is of questionable value, since hyperalbuminemia may decrease the synthesis of hepatic albumin and other serum proteins.[19,24]

Four considerations should guide the therapy of the sodium-depleted patient: (1) the nature and magnitude of the deficit already incurred; (2) the nature and magnitude of ongoing losses; (3) the presence of associated disturbances in acid-base and potassium homeostasis; and (4) the availability of therapy for the underlying disorder.[1,4,17]

The magnitude of the initial sodium deficit is often difficult to estimate clinically, but hypotension due to sodium depletion usually indicates a loss of more than 15% of ECF volume or more than 2 liters in a person weighing 70 g. Irrespective of such estimates, sufficient fluid should be provided to stabilize blood pressure. Repletion of intravascular volume is the most immediate concern, and colloid solutions should be used. Thereafter, correction of the sodium deficit should be achieved with crystalloids. Whenever feasible, the replacement solution should reflect the characteristics of the fluid lost.

When hypotension is less severe, replacement therapy with crystalloids can be initiated from the outset, and isotonic saline is the solution of choice. Although rapid infusion of isotonic saline may produce metabolic acidosis, this is generally trivial unless the patient is already acidemic.[25] In patients with shock and associated lactic acidosis, the infusion of half-isotonic saline (0.45% NaCl) made approximately isotonic by the addition of 1 to 2 ampules of bicarbonate (50 mEq Na^+/ ampule) can be used.

Ringer's lactate is a widely used alternative to isotonic saline but has several potential disadvantages. Organic anions like lactate are normally rapidly converted to bicarbonate by the liver, but this process may be compromised by hepatic dysfunction due to severe hypotension. It is therefore advisable to administer bicarbonate directly to any patient with shock and acidemia as outlined above. Additionally, Ringer's lactate contains small amounts of potassium and calcium, which the patient may not require. It is preferable to tailor fluid replacement therapy to the specific situation.

Once existing deficits have been repleted, ongoing losses need to be considered. In any but the simplest situation, it is advisable to estimate losses directly by calculating the electrolyte composition and volume of all fluids being lost. This is particularly important in seriously ill patients, surgical patients expected to experience long-term ongoing fluid and electrolyte losses, and patients with compromised renal function.

Despite such measurements, however, the adequacy of intravascular volume in such patients is often difficult to assess, especially in surgical patients with third-space sequestration of fluid. Intravascular volume status must finally be judged by such parameters as blood pressure, pulse, and urine output. When there is no renal disease, a urine output of greater than 20 ml/hr and a urine sodium concentration of greater than 20 mEq/liter are considered good markers of adequate intravascular volume.

Intravascular Volume Expansion with Increased Extracellular Fluid Volume

The hallmark of intravascular volume expansion is pulmonary vascular congestion manifested clinically by the presence of dyspnea. Although intravascular volume expansion is always clinically associated with expansion of the entire ECF compartment, pulmonary function may be markedly compromised well before sufficient sodium has accumulated in the interstitial fluid compartment to cause edema. The coexistence of intravascular and ECF volume expansion can result from symmetric increases in the intravascular and the interstitial fluid compart-

ments, as in renal failure, or from a maldistribution of fluid between these two compartments, as in congestive heart failure or hepatic cirrhosis.

Renal Failure

Mild degrees of renal insufficiency are not generally associated with sodium retention unless the patient's diet is high in sodium. In advanced acute or chronic renal insufficiency, intravascular and ECF volume expansion are common. Both subdivisions of the ECF compartment are expanded proportionally by retained sodium and water in a fashion identical to that seen during the infusion of isotonic saline (Table 17-1).[26]

Congestive Heart Failure

Two events account for maldistribution of ECF in cardiac failure. First, as cardiac output decreases, venous hydrostatic pressure increases, and fluid shifts from the intravascular to the interstitial fluid compartment. Second, the decrease in tissue perfusion that is associated with significant reductions in cardiac output leads to an EABV-mediated increase in renal sodium and water retention.[27,28] Progressive retention of salt and water increases intravascular volume, but most of the retained fluid accumulates in the interstitial compartment as edema. For any given degree of myocardial dysfunction, therefore, a new steady state is reached in which tissue perfusion and EABV are maintained at nearly normal levels at the expense of increases in intravascular, interstitial, and ECF volumes (Table 17-1).[1,7]

Patients with underlying heart disease are particularly prone to the development of iatrogenic congestive heart failure when they are stressed with excessive sodium or colloid loads. Increasing weight, oliguria, pulmonary congestion, and the appearance of edema may all portend worsening cardiac failure. Consequently, dietary and parenteral fluid management during the perioperative period should be closely scrutinized in such patients. The therapy of iatrogenic fluid overload should be aimed at the relatively rapid removal of excess sodium and water with a potent loop diuretic such as furosemide.

Hepatic Cirrhosis

Multiple factors produce cirrhotic ascites and edema.[29,30] The disruption of hepatic architecture results in hepatic venous obstruction and increased hepatic lymph formation. When formation exceeds removal by the thoracic duct, exudation into the peritoneal cavity occurs. Cirrhosis also produces portal venous hypertension, which, in conjunction with chronic hypoalbuminemia, leads to the transudation of fluid across the splanchnic capillaries and to worsening ascites. Portal venous hypertension is also associated with the formation of an extensive portacaval venous collateral network, resulting in expanded capacitance in the splanchnic circulation.

These factors reduce intravascular volume and lead to the retention of renal sodium and water. Progressive retention of sodium and water restores intravascular volume relative to vascular capacitance and simultaneously increases absolute intravascular volume. Ultimately, for any given degree of liver dysfunction, as for myocardial dysfunction (see above), a new steady state is reached in which tissue perfusion and EABV are maintained at nearly normal levels at the expense of increases in intravascular, interstitial, and ECF volumes.

Most patients with decompensated hepatic cirrhosis do not exhibit pulmonary vascular congestion despite the fact that their intravascular volumes are increased. The absence of pulmonary vascular congestion is easily explained. Although absolute intravascular volume is increased, intravascular volume in relation to vascular capacitance is decreased. However, patients with hepatic cirrhosis may develop iatrogenic congestive heart failure when they are stressed with excessive sodium loads. Therefore, dietary and parenteral fluid management in such patients should be carefully monitored during the perioperative period.

Small volumes of ascitic fluid can be removed safely for diagnostic purposes. However, since ascitic fluid is in equilibrium with intravascular fluid, paracentesis should always be approached with caution. The removal of more than 1 to 2 liters of fluid may lead to hypovolemic shock as ascites reaccumulates at the expense of intravascular volume. If hypotension does occur, the infusion of 25% albumin will temporarily restore intravascular volume but may also increase portal venous pressure and precipitate esophageal variceal bleeding. In general, unless tense ascites severely compromises respiratory status, it is best not to attempt to remove it directly.

Diuretic Therapy of Edematous Disorders

The presence of edema alone does not necessitate the administration of diuretics. Three factors in particular should always be considered: (1) intravascular volume status; (2) the presence of pulmonary vascular congestion; and (3) whether the edema is adversely affecting some vital function such as respiration, cutaneous integrity, or wound healing.

Diuretics decrease intravascular volume and venous return to the heart but do not necessarily improve myocardial performance. They reduce the expanded intravascular volume and pulmonary vascular congestion that are characteristically present in patients with congestive heart failure. The resultant improvement in oxygenation of the blood may benefit myocardial function.[31,32] However, caution should be observed, since rigorous diuresis can reduce venous return to such an extent that stroke volume may be markedly compromised. Furthermore, diuresis can lead to potassium depletion and hypokalemia with resultant digitalis toxicity.

Diuretics should be employed with caution in patients with nephrotic edema. The intravascular volume in patients with nephrotic syndrome is decreased, and pulmonary vascular congestion does not occur. Overvigorous diuresis may further diminish intravascular volume and lead to the worsening of prerenal azotemia, hypotension, and even shock. In general, it is best to restrict diuretic therapy to patients in whom marked peripheral edema restricts normal activities. Diuretics should be used if edema compromises the integrity of the skin of the lower extremities or interferes with wound healing. Intermittent administration of diuretics is best, allowing time for re-equilibration of the intravascular and interstitial fluid compartments.[9,33,34]

Diuretics should be used with caution in patients with hepatic cirrhosis. Overvigorous diuresis can result in marked intravascular volume depletion, particularly in the patient who has ascites without peripheral edema. Peripheral edema can be mobilized relatively rapidly, but a reduction in ascites is limited to about 1 liter/day. In general, a diuretics-induced weight loss of about 0.5 kg/day is more than adequate in cirrhotic patients. Slow diuresis allows time for re-equilibration among intravascular, interstitial, and peritoneal spaces.

Any regimen that leads to potassium depletion in the patient with cirrhosis can precipitate hepatic coma. Hepatic coma has been attributed to the increased production of renal ammonia that is characteristically associated with potassium depletion. Acetazolamide is particularly dangerous in this regard, since it not only causes potassium depletion but also alkalinizes the urine, thereby decreasing the amount of ammonia trapped as ammonium and excreted in the urine. Therefore, a potassium-sparing diuretic such as spironolactone or triamterene should be used in conjunction with other diuretics in the treatment of cirrhotic edema. However, since spironolactone inhibits hydrogen ion secretion in the distal nephron and causes some patients with cirrhosis to develop distal renal tubular acidosis, acid–base status should be carefully monitored when this drug is employed.[35]

In patients with edema due to renal insufficiency, therapy depends on the severity of the disease. When the glomerular filtration rate is only mildly decreased, restriction of sodium intake is often sufficient. As renal insufficiency progresses, diuretics can be added to the regimen. In the severely oliguric or anuric patient, dialysis is necessary. The indiscriminate use of potent diuretics in patients with renal insufficiency should be avoided, since intravascular volume depletion, prerenal azotemia, and hypotension may ensue. In addition, potent diuretics may produce a variety of electrolyte and acid–base disturbances that are then superimposed on disturbances related to the renal insufficiency per se.

Although many edematous patients can be controlled for long periods of time with a given dose of a single diuretic of medium potency such as a thiazide, some may become refractory and begin to develop more edema. Three factors may contribute to this: (1) surreptitious increases in dietary sodium intake; (2) worsening renal function; and (3) progression of the basic disease process underlying the edema-forming state.

In patients with decreased renal function, failure of delivery of an adequate amount of a drug to its tubular site of action is generally responsible for diminished diuretic response. In contrast, in patients not responding because of progression of underlying disease, there is more avid tubular sodium reabsorption at progressively more proximal tubular sites. Less sodium is therefore delivered to the site of thiazide action in the distal nephron, and natriuresis decreases despite therapy.

In patients truly refractory to thiazides, a more potent diuretic such as furosemide or ethacrynic acid should be used, and the thiazide should be discontinued. In patients refractory to loop diuretics, the dosage can be increased progressively up to several hundred milligrams per day. In patients with severe congestive heart failure, acetazolamide, which inhibits sodium reabsorption in the proximal tubule, can be combined with a loop diuretic. Such diuretics act proximally but are usually ineffective when used alone. The combination of relatively low doses of metalazone, an agent that blocks sodium reabsorption in the proximal convoluted tubule and at the cortical diluting site, and a loop diuretic can also be effective in restoring natriuresis in otherwise refractory cases, whether they are due to renal insufficiency or to worsening of the underlying edema-forming process. Frequent monitoring of the serum electro-lytes, especially potassium levels, is mandatory when any regimen of multiple diuretics is used.[9,33,34]

DISORDERS OF TONICITY HOMEOSTASIS

Fundamental Principles

An understanding of five fundamental principles is essential to the analysis of disorders of body-fluid tonicity.

1. Since cell membranes are freely permeable by water, the osmolality of the two major body-fluid compartments at equilibrium must be equal. Water moves rapidly between the intracellular fluid (ICF) and the extracellular fluid (ECF) compartments to equalize any induced osmolal gradient.

2. Total body water (TBW) is 60% of body weight, and its distribution between the ICF and ECF depends on the distribution of osmotically active solute. The ICF and ECF compartments contain two-thirds and one-third of total body solute and therefore two-thirds and one-third of TBW, respectively. Therefore, in a 70-kg person, whose TBW is 42 liters, 28 liters are in the ICF, and 14 liters are in the ECF.

3. Body-fluid osmolality is determined by the ratio of total body solute to TBW. If there is a fixed amount of total body solute, TBW determines the body-fluid osmolality. Therefore, tonicity homeostasis can generally be accounted for by abnormalities in water balance.

4. Disorders of tonicity homeostasis are associated with characteristic alterations in cellular volumes. Hypotonicity is associated with expansion, and hypertonicity with contraction, of the ICF compartment.

5. Disorders of tonicity homeostasis are generally detected clinically by the presence of an abnormal serum sodium concentration. However, since symptoms relate to the abnormal tonicity and not to abnormalities in the serum sodium concentration *per se*, it is important to realize that, although hypernatremia always implies hypertonicity, hyponatremia cannot always be equated with hypotonicity.[2]

Plasma osmolality is commonly used to assess body-fluid osmolality. It can be measured directly in an osmometer or, under normal circumstances, can be calculated as follows:

$$2[Na^+] + \frac{Glucose}{18} + \frac{BUN}{2.8}$$

$$= (2 \times 140) + \frac{90}{18} + \frac{14}{2.8}$$

$$= 290 \text{ mOsm/KgH}_2\text{O}$$

Osmolality is not the same as effective osmolality, that is, tonicity. The latter expresses the concentration only of those solutes that are relatively restricted to a particular compartment and thereby exert an osmotic force affecting the distribution of water between ICF and ECF compartments. Plasma tonicity is calculated as follows:

$$2(Na^+) + \frac{glucose}{18} = (2 \times 140) + \frac{90}{18}$$

$$= 285 \text{ mOsm/KgH}_2\text{O}$$

The BUN is excluded from this calculation, since urea distributes freely across cell membranes and therefore does not alter the distribution of water between the two body-fluid compartments. Other clinically relevant solutes that contribute to osmolality but not to tonicity are ethanol and methanol, both of which distribute rapidly throughout TBW. In contrast, mannitol, sorbitol, and glycerol are relatively restricted to the ECF compartment and, consequently, contribute both to osmolality and to tonicity.

The two major body-fluid compartments differ markedly in composition. The major intracellular solute is potassium with its associated anions; the major extracellular solute is sodium with its associated anions. Intracellular and extracellular solute contents are largely determined by systems that are independent of those that determine water balance. In this sense, total body solute content or $2([K^+]_{ICF} + [Na^+]_{ECF})$ is fixed, and body-fluid tonicity can be considered to be determined by water balance alone. However, body-fluid tonicity is in reality a function of the ratio of total body solute to TBW, or $\frac{2([K^+]_{ICF} + [Na^+]_{ECF})}{TBW}$; therefore, under certain circumstances, hypotonicity can result directly from potassium or sodium depletion *per se*. For example, the hypotonicity that is sometimes associated with severe potassium depletion may reflect in part, the direct effect of potassium losses on this ratio. In addition, although the hypotonicity that is characteristically associated with the syndrome of inappropriate antidiuretic hormone secretion (SIADH) is largely due to an increase in TBW, it may also reflect some degree of sodium depletion.

There are two clinically important circumstances in which hyponatremia can exist without hypotonicity. First, if the ECF contains a large amount of an effective osmotic solute other than sodium, such as glucose or mannitol, water moves from the ICF to the ECF to maintain osmotic equilibrium between the two body-fluid compartments. The result is ICF volume depletion, hyponatremia, and hypertonicity. Second, since lipids and proteins distort the normal relationship between plasma volume and plasma water content but have negligible effects on osmolality, excessive amounts of lipid or protein in the plasma can produce apparent hyponatremia in the face of normal plasma tonicity, or so-called pseudohyponatremia. Pseudohyponatremia should be suspected in any asymptomatic patient with severe hyponatremia, especially if the serum is creamy, as in hypertriglyceridemia, or viscous, as in the presence of a paraprotein. The presence of pseudohyponatremia can be confirmed by measurement of plasma osmolality and the finding that it normal. Once pseudohyponatremia and the presence of an osmotically active solute other than sodium in the ECF have been excluded, hyponatremia can safely be equated with hypotonicity.

Control of Water Balance

For body-fluid tonicity to remain constant, the amount of water lost each day must be replenished. The usual rate of insensible water loss through skin and lungs is approximately 0.6 ml/kg/hr.[36] However, insensible losses are markedly influenced by a wide variety of factors, including body and ambient temperature, humidity, and body hydration. For example, insensible losses increase by approximately 10% for each increase of 1°F in body temperature above normal. When body solute content is fixed, positive water balance produces hyponatremia and dilution of all body fluids, and negative water balance produces hypernatremia and concentration of all body fluids.

Oral ingestion and renal excretion regulate water balance, as shown in Figure 17-1. The hypothalamus serves as the osmostat for sensing body tonicity. The normal range for plasma osmolality is 280 to 295 mOsm/kg, although it varies no more than 1 to 2% over an extended period of time in any given person.[37,38]

Since abnormalities in body-fluid tonicity are generally due to derangements in water balance, abnormalities in thirst, antidiuretic hormone (ADH) synthesis or release, and renal water excretion account for most disorders of body-fluid tonicity homeostasis. Consequently, a thorough understanding of these processes is a pre-

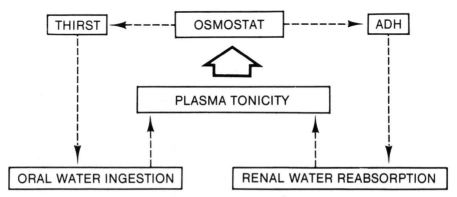

Fig. 17-1. Homeostatic control of body fluid tonicity. Geheb M, Singer I, Cox M: In McDonald FD (ed): Progress in Clinical Kidney Disease and Hypertension. Thieme-Stratton, New York, 1980)

requisite to the clinical evaluation of disorders of tonicity homeostasis.

Water Ingestion and Thirst

The importance of thirst in osmoregulation is immediately apparent in patients with central diabetes insipidus. Provided that their thirst sensation is intact and they have free access to water, such patients do not develop significant hypernatremia despite the complete absence of ADH. Many surgical patients do not have free access to water and consequently cannot respond appropriately to changes in tonicity by altering water intake.[39,40]

Antidiuretic Hormone Synthesis and Release

Most stimuli that increase thirst increase ADH release. ADH is synthesized in the supraoptic and paraventricular nuclei of the hypothalamus, stored in the posterior pituitary, and released directly from the hypothalamus as well as from the posterior pituitary.[41] The primary physiologic stimulus for ADH release is a rise in body-fluid tonicity; as little as a 1% change in plasma osmolality will alter the rate of ADH release. Changes in body-fluid tonicity, not osmolality, modulate ADH release. Thus, whereas increases in osmolality resulting from infusions of hypertonic saline or mannitol are associated with rises in plasma ADH levels, infusions of equimolar amounts of urea have no effect on ADH release.[42] The behavior of glucose is anomalous. Although glucose infusions are associated with decreases in ADH release, hyperglycemia associated with uncontrolled diabetes mellitus is associated with increased ADH levels. Volume stimuli in diabetic patients may override the tendency for hyperglycemia to reduce ADH secretion.[43]

Although tonicity normally controls ADH release, changes in central blood volume sensed by volume receptors in the atria and great veins and those in arterial blood pressure sensed in baroreceptors in the aortic arch and carotid sinus also influence the hypothalamic osmostat. Small decreases in central blood volume or arterial blood pressure have relatively little effect on ADH secretion. However, larger changes of 10% to 15% are associated with dramatic increases in circulating ADH levels. Decreased central blood volume and arterial hypotension enhance ADH release by altering the threshold and possibly the sensitivity of the osmostat rather than by directly affecting ADH release *per se*. These changes are important in the surgical patient in whom volume depletion and hypotension occur frequently. It may be impossible to normalize body-fluid tonicity and water excretion unless ECF volume deficits and hypotension are corrected first.[42]

Other factors that have special relevance to surgical patients and are associated with alterations in ADH release include the following.

Stress
Nausea, with or without emesis
Intestinal traction
Central nervous system disorders
    Trauma
    Tumors
    Vascular disease
    Meningitis
    Encephalitis
    Subarachnoid hemorrhage
    Abscesses
    Psychiatric disorders
Pulmonary diseases
    Tuberculosis
    Pneumonia
    Asthma
Positive pressure ventilation

Drugs
    Oxytocin
    Chlorpropamide
    Vincristine, vinblastine
    Cytoxan
    Clofibrate
    Carbamazepine
    Nicotine
    Narcotics
    General anesthetics
    Indomethacin
    Aspirin
    Acetominophen
    Tricyclic antidepressants
    Phenothiazides
Tumors
    Carcinoma of the lung
    Carcinoma of the duodenum
    Carcinoma of the pancreas
    Carcinoma of the bladder or ureter
    Carcinoma of the prostate
    Lymphoma, Hodgkin's disease
    Thymoma

The renal response to trauma, surgically or otherwise induced, is water retention. Circumstantial evidence suggests that increased ADH secretion, not decreased EABV, has the major role in intra- and postoperative renal water retention. For example, when patients are volume-expanded postoperatively, their urine often remains concentrated as their plasma osmolality falls; thus, antidiuresis persists when EABV is presumably increased.[44] Patients may become severely hypotonic if large water loads are administered indiscriminately.

Dramatic increases in plasma ADH levels occur in response to nausea or vomiting even when blood pressure is stable. Stimulation of the hypothalamic emesis center activates the osmostat and is associated with ADH release irrespective of prevailing body-fluid tonicity.[45] In addition, traction on the intestine in anesthetized humans results in large increases in plasma ADH levels, which are probably mediated through vagal afferents to the emesis center. Pain, anxiety, and stress have all been reported to increase ADH secretion, but whether these factors act directly or indirectly through unrecognized hemodynamic effects is unknown.[45,46] General anesthetics have been thought for many years to directly increase ADH release, but the data are not convincing. For example, ether increases plasma ADH levels only if it induces hypotension.[45] Acute administration of narcotics also appears to increase ADH release, but several narcotic antagonists have the opposite effect. Whether these effects are independent of narcotics-induced hemodynamic changes is uncertain. Finally, many patients receiving positive-pressure ventilation behave as if they have elevated circulating ADH levels.[47] It has been suggested that ADH release under these circumstances is the result of stimulation of volume receptors by the associated decrease in central blood volume.

Renal Water Excretion

Three basic processes control renal water excretion: (1) delivery of adequate amounts of electrolyte-containing fluid from the proximal tubule to the ascending limb of Henle's loop and early distal convoluted tubule, the diluting segments of the nephron; (2) separation of electrolyte from water in the diluting segments of the nephron to generate electrolyte-free water; and (3) variable recombination of water and electrolyte by more distal portions of the nephron (Figure 17-2).[1,37,48]

The first two processes are independent of prevailing body-fluid tonicity and occur irrespective of final urine osmolality. The third process, by virtue of its depen-

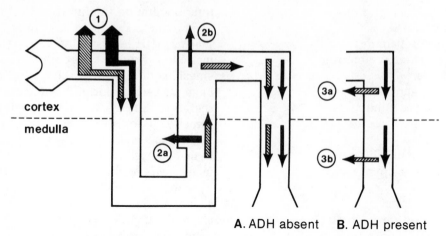

A. ADH absent **B.** ADH present

Fig. 17-2. Renal handling of water. *Solid arrows* represent electrolyte, and *hatched arrows* represent water. Physiologic processes are indicated by circled numbers. In the proximal tubule *(1)*, fluid is reabsorbed isotonically. The remaining fluid is delivered to the medullary *(2a)* and cortical *(2b)* diluting sites, where electrolyte and water are separated, producing dilute (hypotonic) tubular fluid. When ADH is absent *(A)*, the distal convoluted tubule, the cortical collecting tubule, and the collecting duct remain relatively water-impermeable, and dilute tubular fluid is excreted in the urine. When ADH is present *(B)*, the water-permeability of the ADH-responsive portions of the nephron is increased, net water reabsorption occurs *(3a* and *3b)*, and concentrated tubular fluid is excreted in the urine. (Geheb M, Singer I, Cox M: *In* McDonald FD (ed): Progress in Clinical Kidney Disease and Hypertension. Thieme-Stratton, New York, 1980)

dence on ADH, is sensitive to changes in body-fluid tonicity. Small changes in plasma osmolality are translated into large changes in urine osmolality and consequently into large changes in water excretion. A change in plasma osmolality from 280 to 295 mOsm/kg, an increase of 5%, is associated with a change in urine osmolality from 100 to 1000 mOsm/g and a tenfold decrease in urine volume. At the lowest level of plasma osmolality, around 280 mOsm/kg, circulating ADH levels are low, and urine osmolality is minimal at less than 100 mOsm/kg. At the highest level of plasma osmolality, around 295 mOsm/kg, ADH levels are high, and urine osmolality is maximal at 800 to 1200 mOsm/kg.

Normally, 60% to 70% of the glomerular filtrate is isosmotically reabsorbed in the proximal tubule (site 1 in Fig. 17-2). EABV is of major importance in the determination of proximal tubular fluid reabsorption. As EABV decreases, proximal tubular fluid reabsorption increases.

A variety of factors can interfere with the diluting segments of the nephron in the ascending limb of Henle's loop and early distal convoluted tubule. Any pathologic process that disrupts the renal interstitium, such as chronic interstitial nephritis or papillary necrosis, irreversibly interferes with gradient formation and maintenance. There are also a number of contexts in which reversible defects in diluting segment function occur. These include osmotic diuresis of any etiology, the use of potent diuretics such as furosemide and ethacrynic acid, and hypercalcemia, all of which are associated with inhibition of sodium and chloride reabsorption in the ascending limb of Henle's loop. Malnutrition results in decreased urea production and subsequently lower concentrations of urea in the renal medulla, and this also leads to defective diluting segment function.

The more distal portions of the nephron constitute an optional volume-reduction system that uses the concentration gradient established by the loop of Henle (countercurrent multiplication) and maintained by the vasa recti (countercurrent exchange) to reabsorb water from tubular fluid previously rendered hypotonic by the diluting segments. The amount of water reabsorbed varies as a continuous function of the circulating level of ADH. Maximal urinary concentration is dependent on the integrity of all these processes.

Hypotonic States

The clinical evaluation of the hypotonic patient should begin with an assessment of the patient's state of sodium balance. Hypotonicity can occur in association with decreased, increased, or normal total body sodium content (ECF volume) (Table 17-3).[1]

Hypotonicity with Decreased Total Body Sodium

Patients who are hypotonic and have lower than normal total body sodium present with both sodium and water de-
pletion; however, since they are hypotonic and hyponatremic, the sodium deficit is greater than the water deficit. Negative sodium balance results from excessive renal, gastrointestinal, or cutaneous sodium losses for reasons already listed and is associated with a fall in EABV.

There are two reasons why the fall in EABV resulting from sodium depletion may lead to hypotonicity. First, sodium and water reabsorption in the proximal tubule is enhanced by a reduction in EABV, thereby decreasing fluid delivery to the diluting sites and impairing electrolyte-free water generation. Second, if of sufficient magnitude, decreased EABV results in increased ADH secretion and thereby increases water reabsorption in the distal nephron. Consequently, water ingested by or administered to the sodium-depleted patient cannot be excreted in sufficient quantities for normal water balance to be maintained. Progressive hypotonicity will ensue if water intake continues to exceed the impaired renal water excretory capacity.

Re-establishment of adequate circulating blood volume and hence EABV will restore water excretion to normal. Since the hypotonicity associated with sodium depletion is usually mild, volume expansion with isotonic saline or by the provision of a high-sodium diet is generally all that is needed to produce a water diuresis and to restore plasma tonicity and serum sodium concentration to normal.

Hypotonicity with Increased Total Body Sodium

Patients who have hypotonicity with higher than normal total body sodium present with both sodium and water excess; however, since they are hypotonic and hyponatremic, the increase in TBW

Table 17-3. Evaluation of Hypotonic States

Total Body Sodium	Pathophysiology		Edema	$U_{Na} + V$	Condition
↓	Na⁺ deficit > H₂O deficit	Renal fluid loss	−	↑	See text
		GI fluid loss Cutaneous fluid loss	− ↓		See text
↑	H₂O excess > Na⁺ excess	Renal Na⁺ and H₂O retention	+	↓	Renal failure Hypoalbuminemia Congestive heart failure Hepatic cirrhosis
Normal*	Pure H₂O excess	↑ Intake	−	↕	Psychogenic polydipsia
		Renal H₂O retention	−	↕	SIADH

*See text.
$U_{Na} + V$ = urinary sodium excretion; GI = gastrointestinal; SIADH = syndrome of inappropriate ADH section.
(After Geheb M, Singer I, Cox M: In McDonald FC (ed): Progress in Clinical Kidney Disease and Hypertension. New York, Thieme-Stratton, 1980)

is greater than that in total body sodium. Positive sodium balance is the consequence of diminished renal sodium excretory capacity secondary either to a reduction in glomerular filtration rate, as in renal insufficiency, or to a fall in EABV, as in any pathologic edema-forming state.

In patients with renal insufficiency, the ability of the kidney to adjust sodium and water excretion to match intake is limited. If both water balance and sodium balance are positive but more water is ingested or retained than sodium, hypotonicity will coexist with increased total body sodium. In contrast, if both water balance and sodium balance are negative but more water is ingested or retained than sodium, hypotonicity will coexist with decreased total body sodium. The degree of renal insufficiency, the nature of the underlying renal disease, the concomitant use of diuretics, and dietary or parenteral intake of sodium will determine whether total body sodium is increased, decreased, or normal in such patients. Whatever the case, however, it is the continued intake of water in amounts greater than those that can be excreted that leads to hypotonicity. Parenteral fluid management of patients with renal insufficiency can therefore be complex; careful monitoring of such patients is mandatory.

Hypotonicity can occur in any pathologic edema-forming state.[1,37,38,48] Early in the course of these diseases, EABV is usually not sufficiently decreased to limit the amount of fluid delivered to the diluting sites or to increase the secretion of ADH, and, consequently, hypotonicity is unusual. However, as the underlying disease progresses and EABV declines further, fluid delivery to the diluting sites progressively declines, and, in some patients, circulating ADH levels increase. Consequently, ingested water is retained, and progressive dilution of body fluids occurs. The mechanisms underlying the hypotonicity that is associated with increased total body sodium in the pathologic edema-forming states and with decreased total body sodium are very similar. In both cases, decreased EABV limits renal water excretion.

However, the therapy of the two states differs markedly. Therapy for the hypotonic edematous patient generally includes both water and sodium restriction. Resolution of hypotonicity is ultimately dependent on the resolution of the underlying disease process. For example, in the hypotonic patient with congestive heart failure, therapy should be directed at improving myocardial function in order to increase EABV and thereby improve renal water excretion. The use of isotonic or hypertonic saline to treat hypotonicity in edematous patients is irrational, since it provides only a transient improvement in EABV. Sodium-containing fluid rapidly equilibrates throughout the entire ECF, thereby worsening the edema. In addition, pulmonary edema is a threat when such solutions are administered to edematous patients. Consequently, when hypertonic saline must be employed in the emergency treatment of the symptomatic, water-intoxicated, edematous patient, potent diuretics generally should be administered simultaneously.

Diuretics represent a double-edged sword for the hypotonic edematous patient. On the one hand, they may be needed to keep edema within tolerable limits and to treat or prevent pulmonary edema. On the other hand, if used to excess, they can produce further decrements in EABV and lead to even more water retention. Diuretics that act in the proximal tubule, such as acetazolamide and metolazone, are helpful to such patients because they increase delivery of fluid to the diluting sites.[9,33,34] However, because these agents are relatively ineffective diuretics when used alone, they are often employed in conjunction with the more potent loop diuretics.

Hypotonicity with Normal Total Body Sodium

Patients who are hypotonic but have normal total body sodium content exhibit no clinically significant symptoms or signs of either ECF volume expansion or depletion. For practical purposes, their hypotonicity and hyponatremia can be considered to result solely from an increase in TBW. The latter can be due to excessive water intake, as in psychogenic polydipsia, to abnormal renal water retention, as in SIADH, or to a combination of these disorders. In reality, at least in patients with SIADH, total body sodium levels are slightly decreased. However, this decrease is not associated with ECF volume depletion, because the sodium deficit is more than compensated for by excessive retention of water.

Since the normal maximal rate of electrolyte-free water excretion by the kidney is around 20 ml/min, patients with psychogenic polydipsia generally have to ingest more than 20 to 30 liters/day of water in order to develop significant degrees of hypotonicity. The diagnosis should be suspected whenever a patient presents with hyponatremia and a minimal urine osmolality of less than 100 mOsm/kg. The treatment of patients with psychogenic polydipsia consists of water restriction.

SIADH is common in the surgical patient. Because ADH release is not suppressed, renal water excretion is impaired, and hypotonicity develops.[49,50] Patients with SIADH present with the following signs:

1. Hypotonicity and hyponatremia (plasma osmolality < 280 mOsm/kg)
2. Inappropriately concentrated urine (urine osmolality > 100 mOsm/kg)
3. High urine sodium concentration (except during sodium restriction)
4. Absence of sodium excess or depletion
5. Normal renal, cardiac, hepatic, adrenal, and thyroid function.

It is particularly difficult to make a definitive diagnosis of SIADH in patients with pathologic edema-forming states, since all of these disorders are characterized by EABV-related defects in renal water handling.

Anterior pituitary insufficiency and hypothyroidism can also be associated with hypotonicity and many of the features of SIADH.[51-53] Normal circulating levels of cortisol appear to be necessary for the hypotonicity-related inhibition of ADH release. When there is no cortisol, ADH release is increased despite prevailing body-fluid hypotonicity.[54] In addition, when cortisol is absent, the permeability of the collecting duct to water may be abnormally high.[55]

Water restriction remains the cornerstone of therapy for the asymptomatic or only mildly symptomatic patient with SIADH. This is particularly true in postoperative patients in whom the abnormality in ADH secretion is generally short-lived. If the syndrome is chronic and if water restriction is poorly tolerated, the drug of choice is demeclocycline, which inhibits ADH-induced water reabsorption in the distal nephron and thereby causes nephrogenic diabetes insipidus.[56-58]

A variant of SIADH is the syndrome of the reset osmostat. Unlike patients with classic SIADH, patients with this disorder generally have mild hyponatremia with a serum sodium concentration of rarely less than 125 mEq/liter and can dilute urine normally when given a water load. These patients defend the concentration of their body fluids at a lower tonicity than normal; their osmostat is reset downwards. They are usually elderly and suffer from chronic debilitating diseases. Since hyponatremia is mild and usually asymptomatic, therapy should be directed at the underlying disorder.[59]

Manifestations and Emergency Therapy of Symptomatic Hypotonicity

Hypotonicity is associated with cellular overhydration and, most importantly, with cerebral edema. Mild or moderate degrees of hypotonicity, if chronic, are generally asymptomatic and can be treated conservatively. More severe degrees of hypotonicity with serum sodium concentrations of less than 120 mEq/liter, especially if acute, can be life-threatening. The signs and symptoms of severe acute hypotonicity include changes in mental status ranging from mild confusion to frank coma, seizures, muscle weakness, cramps, and myoclonus. Deep tendon reflexes may be increased or decreased. Focal neurologic findings, although unusual, are occasionally obtained.[60] The emergency therapy of severe symptomatic hypotonicity, irrespective of etiology, is directed at rapidly raising ECF tonicity in order to shift water from the ICF to the ECF and ameliorate cerebral edema.

If the patient's symptoms are mild, ECF tonicity can be safely and effectively raised over a period of 6 hr to 12 hr by the concomitant administration of a potent loop diuretic, such as furosemide, and isotonic saline. By inhibiting the reabsorption of sodium chloride at the medullary diluting site, furosemide effects the production of a large volume of hypotonic urine, and, over a period of several hours, body-fluid tonicity returns to normal. Isotonic saline is employed to maintain ECF volume and delivery of fluid to the site of diuretic action. This mode of therapy is relatively simple, but care must be taken to maintain ECF volume and to replete urinary potassium losses.

If the clinical situation is more grave, immediate therapy with hypertonic 3% or 5% saline or hypertonic mannitol is indicated. Since water distributes freely across cell membranes, the amount of solute to be administered is calculated on the basis of TBW. For example, if a patient weighing 70 kg has a serum sodium concentration of 105 mEq/liter and a plasma glucose concentration of 108 mg/dl, his calculated body-fluid tonicity would be $(2 \times 105) + \left(\dfrac{108}{18}\right) = 216 \, \text{mOsm/kg}$. This means that every liter of TBW is deficient by $(286 - 216) = 70$ mOsm of solute or $(140 - 105) = 35$ mEq of sodium. If the patient's TBW is estimated to be 42 liters, or 60% of 70 kg, he has a total body osmolal deficit of $(42 \times 70) = 2940$ mOsm and a total body sodium deficit of $(42 \times 35) = 1470$ mEq.

An infusion of 3% saline should be started immediately and symptoms monitored closely. The calculated sodium or osmolal deficit is approximate at best but gives a rough estimate of how much solute is needed to correct life-threatening hypotonicity. To replace the sodium deficit, $\dfrac{1470}{0.5}$ or 2940 ml of 3% saline containing 0.5 mEq of sodium/ml is theoretically needed. However, it generally takes less than half the calculated deficit to reverse life-threatening hypotonicity.

Two major problems can arise with this form of therapy. The first is rapid volume expansion and acute pulmonary edema. This complication should be anticipated and potent loop diuretics used as needed.[61] The second is rapid ICF volume contraction, which may lead to abrupt shrinkage of the brain and intracranial hemorrhage. This complication can be avoided by discontinuation or marked reduction of the administration of the hypertonic saline as soon as symptomatic improvement is evident.

Hypertonic States

Hypertonicity is always associated with cellular dehydration. When hypertonicity develops rapidly, all cells, regardless of type, dehydrate rapidly. When hypertonicity develops more slowly, some cells, such as red blood corpuscles, maintain their volume by taking on ECF; however, most cells dehydrate and decrease in size, albeit at a slower rate than in the acute state.[62]

The brain is particularly vulnerable to volume loss, because rapid cerebral dehydration may lead to rupture of the blood vessels that penetrate the layers of connective tissue surrounding the brain. The neurologic changes that occur in hypertonicity are similar to those seen in hypotonic states; however, focal symptoms and signs are more common.[60,63]

Like hypotonicity, hypertonicity can occur in association with normal, increased, or decreased total body sodium (Table 17-4). Hypertonicity only rarely results from pure water loss or pure solute gain. Much more commonly, the hypertonic state is the result of water losses in excess of sodium losses. Hypertonicity is therefore most often associated with decreased total body sodium.

Hypertonicity with Normal Total Body Sodium

Pure water deficits result from inadequate water intake in the face of ongoing insensible cutaneous and pulmonary water losses or excessive losses of relatively electrolyte-free water in the urine, as in diabetes insipidus. Since primary hypodipsia is extremely uncommon, inadequate water intake generally results from an inability of the patient to obtain water in the face of normal or increased insensible or renal water losses. This is common in surgical patients, in whom meticulous attention to replacement of ongoing water losses is necessary.

Diabetes insipidus. Diabetes insipidus may result either from a deficiency of ADH (central diabetes insipidus) or from

Table 17-4. Evaluation of Hypertonic States

Total Body Sodium	Pathophysiology		Edema	$U_{Na} + V$	Condition
$\downarrow$	H_2O deficit > Na^+ deficit	Renal fluid loss	−	$\uparrow$	See text
		GI fluid loss Cutaneous fluid loss	−	$\downarrow$	See text
$\uparrow$	Na^+ excess > H_2O excess	Hypertonic fluid administration	±	$\uparrow$	Table 17-6
Normal	Pure H_2O deficit	$\uparrow$ Insensible losses	−	$\updownarrow$	Hyperthermia Hyperventilation
		$\uparrow$ Renal H_2O loss	−	$\updownarrow$	Diabetes insipidus

$U_{Na} + V$ = Urinary sodium excretion; GI = gastrointestinal.
(After Geheb M, Singer I, Cox M: In McDonald FD (ed): Progress in Clinical Kidney Disease and Hypertension. New York, Thieme-Stratton, 1980)

renal unresponsiveness to the action of ADH (nephrogenic diabetes insipidus). Diabetes insipidus need not be associated with hypertonicity; the latter is dependent on the existence of a concomitant defect in thirst or lack of access to water.

Absolute and relative lack of circulating ADH results in complete and partial central diabetes insipidus, respectively. Damage to the hypothalamic neurons that synthesize ADH or to the posterior pituitary gland is presumed to be the mechanism in central diabetes insipidus resulting from head trauma, pituitary surgery, tumors (especially pituitary adenomas and craniopharyngiomas), vascular disorders, granulomatous diseases, meningitis, and encephalitis.[41,65] However, approximately 50% of cases of central diabetes insipidus are idiopathic in nature.

Nephrogenic diabetes insipidus is often multifactorial in etiology, with defects in several biochemical processes at the cellular level. Many of the disorders that produce nephrogenic diabetes insipidus are also associated with defects in the corticopapillary osmotic gradient, which is essential for normal urinary concentration. Such defects contribute to polyuria. In addition to electrolyte disorders, several

drugs and certain systemic disorders interfere with the action of ADH.[66,67] Causes of diabetes insipidus include the following:[1]

Central diabetes insipidus
    Essential hypernatremia
    Tumors (pituitary adenoma, craniopharyngioma, metastatic breast cancer)
    Vascular disorders (aneurysms, cavernous sinus thrombosis, postpartum pituitary infarction)
    Granulomatous diseases (sarcoidosis)
    Infections (meningitis, encephalitis)
    Head trauma
    Surgical ablation of the pituitary
    Familial
    Idiopathic
Nephrogenic diabetes insipidus
    Electrolyte disorders (hypercalcemia, potassium depletion)
    Drugs (lithium, demeclocycline, methoxyflurane, amphotericin B)
    Systemic disorders (Sjogren's syndrome, amyloidosis)
    Hereditary

Complete diabetes insipidus, whether central or nephrogenic, is characterized by massive polyuria and polydipsia and an inability to concentrate urine. Urine osmolality is generally less than 200 mOsm/kg. However, even when ADH is completely absent, the volume-depleted patient with central diabetes insipidus may have a urine osmolality as high as 300 to 400 mOsm/kg because of decreased tubular fluid flow rate. Partial diabetes insipidus of either type is associated with more modest degrees of polyuria and polydipsia, and renal concentration ability is less severely impaired. However, when stressed by prolonged water deprivation, patients with partial diabetes insipidus are unable to maximally concentrate urine. The diagnosis of diabetes insipidus should be suspected in any patient with polyuria whose urine is relatively solute-free.[68] The diagnosis of diabetes insipidus can be confirmed by a standard dehydration test.[69]

Ongoing renal water losses in patients with complete central diabetes insipidus can generally be controlled with 5 units to 10 units of aqueous vasopressin given intramuscularly every 2 hr to 6 hr as required. The long-term control of polyuria in these patients can be achieved either with long-acting parenteral preparations of vasopressin, such as subcutaneous vasopressin tannate in oil, or long-acting synthtic analogs of vasopressin, such as 1-desamino-8-d-arginine vasopressin (DDAVP), which is administered in a nasal spray. Similar hormonal therapy can be employed to control milder polyuria in central diabetes insipidus. In addition, agents that either enhance ADH release, such as chlorpropamide and clofibrate, or increase ADH action, such as chlorpropamide, can be used alone or in conjunction with hormonal therapy (Table 17-5).[68]

Therapy for reversible forms of nephrogenic diabetes insipidus consists of treatment of the underlying disorder or discontinuance of the offending drug. Since patients with nephrogenic diabetes insipidus are refractory to the action of ADH, therapy of the irreversible forms of this syndrome is limited to dietary solute restriction and use of a thiazide diuretic. Dietary protein and sodium restriction, by reducing obligate urinary solute and therefore water excretion, can markedly reduce the degree of polyuria. Thiazide diuretics, by decreasing ECF volume and consequently increasing proximal tubular fluid reabsorption, further decrease urine volume.

Repletion of pure water deficits. Therapy for hypertonicity due to pure water depletion has three basic objectives: to replace water deficits, to match ongoing losses, and to treat the underlying disease process.

Because total body solute (TBW × plasma osmolality) has not changed, the resultant hypertonicity is directly proportional to the total body water deficit. Therefore,

$$(\text{normal TBW}) \times (\text{normal P}_{osm}) = (\text{present TBW}) \times (\text{present P}_{osm}).$$

Since the serum sodium concentration is more likely to be rapidly available than the plasma osmolality, the calculation can instead be based on the serum sodium concentration. This avoids the potential for error that exists when azotemia elevates plasma osmolality but not plasma tonicity. The equation then becomes

$$(\text{normal TBW}) \times (\text{normal P}_{Na}) = (\text{present TBW}) \times (\text{present P}_{Na}),$$

or

$$\text{present TBW} = (\text{normal TBW}) \times \left(\frac{\text{normal P}_{Na}}{\text{present P}_{Na}}\right).$$

Table 17-5. Treatment of Diabetes Insipidus

Therapy	Dose	Route	Onset	Duration	Comments
Hormonal Therapy					
Aqueous vasopressin (Pitressin) (arg & lys VP; 20 U/ml)	5–10 U	SC, IM IV*	30–60 min	4–6 hr	For diagnostic use only. *IV route investigational.
Vasopressin tannate (Pitressin-in-oil) (arg & lys VP; 5 U/ml)	2–5 U	SC, IM	2–4 hr	24–72 hr	Emulsion must be shaken and warmed before use. Vasoconstriction and smooth muscle contraction frequent side-effects.
Synthetic vasopressin (Lypressin; Diapid) (lys VP; 50 U/ml)	5–10 U	Nasal spray	30–60 min	4–6 hr	Replaced pituitary "snuff," since it is relatively nonallergenic and nonirritating.
DDAVP (1-desamino-8-d-arg-VP; 100 μg/ml)	5–20 μg	Nasal spray	30–60 min	12–24 hr	Drug of choice for complete central diabetes insipidus.
Adjunctive Therapy					
Hydrochlorothiazide (Hydrodiuril; 50 mg/tab)	50–100 mg/ day (daily)	PO	—	12–24 hr	Has usual thiazide side-effects; can be used in central or nephrogenic diabetes insipidus.
Chlorpropamide (Diabinese; 250 mg/tab)	250–750 mg/ day (daily)	PO	—	24–36 hr	May be given as a single dose. Start at 250 mg; increase 1 tab q 3–4 days; expect hypoglycemia over 500 mg/d. Can be used only in partial central diabetes insipidus.
Clofibrate (Atromid S; 250 mg/tab)	250–500 mg (q 6–8 hr)	PO	—	6–8 hr	Needs to be given frequently; may produce GI distress, myositis, abnormal liver function tests. Can be used only in partial central diabetes insipidus.

VP = vasopressin; U = units; SC = subcutaneous; IM = intramuscular; IV = intravenous; PO = per os (Singer I: Med Clin North Am 65:303, 1981)

The water deficit is then equal to normal TBW minus present TBW. For example, if a patient normally weights 70 kg and currently has a serum sodium concentration of 170 mEq/liter when the normal concentration is 140 mEq/liter,

present TBW = $(0.6 \times 70) \times \left(\dfrac{140}{170}\right)$

= 34.6 liters. The water deficit is therefore (42 − 34.6) or 7.4 liters.

The rapidity with which water deficits are replaced depends on the severity of the hypertonicity and the patient's symptoms. If water deficits are replaced too rapidly, there is danger of cerebral edema. No more than half of the calculated deficit should be replaced as 5% dextrose in water over a period of a few hours while the patient's neurologic status is carefully monitored. The remainder of the deficit can then be replaced during the next 24 to 48 hr. Pure water should never be infused intravenously, since it produces severe hemolysis.

Hypertonicity with Increased Total Body Sodium

An important cause of hypertonicity due to pure solute excess is inadvertent or intentional administration of hypertonic solutions, as shown in Table 17-6. Large amounts of 7.5% sodium bicarbonate solutions are frequently used in patients who have had a cardiac arrest or are suffering from severe metabolic acidosis. Inadvertent administration includes mistaken intravenous instead of intra-amniotic administration of hypertonic saline during therapeutic abortions.

As in any hypertonic state, the resultant

Table 17-6. Therapeutic Hypertonic Solutions

Solute	Molecular Weight (g)	Concentration (%)	Water (mOsm/kg)	Usual Container Size (ml)	Use
Sodium chloride	58.5	3	1026	500	Emergency treatment
		5	1711	500	of hypotonic states
		20	6845	250	Intra-amniotic instillation for therapeutic abortion
Sodium bicarbonate	84	5	1190	500	Metabolic acidosis,
		7.5	1786	50	hyperkalemia, and cardiopulmonary arrest
Dextrose	198	10	505	500, 1000	Caloric agent
		20	1010	500	
		50	2525	50, 500	Treatment of hypoglycemia
Mannitol	182	10	549	500, 1000	Osmotic diuresis,
		20	1099	250, 500	acute renal failure,
		25	1374	50	cerebral edema, and acute glaucoma
Glycerol	92	50	5435	120	Cerebral edema and
		75	8152	120	acute glaucoma

(Feig PU, McCurdy DK: N Engl J Med 297:1444, 1977)

cerebral dehydration can be life-threatening. In addition, ECF volume expansion is a serious complication. Since seizures, intracranial hemorrhage, and pulmonary edema are not uncommon, immediate treatment is crucial. However, although acute cerebral dehydration is life-threatening, the necessarily rapid administration of large amounts of water expands ECF volume and can worsen already compromised cardiac and pulmonary function. Consequently, therapy must include both water administration and removal of excess solute.

In order to estimate the amount of water needed to correct hypertonicity, one must calculate the theoretical water deficit. For example, for a 70-kg woman with a TBW volume of 42 liters, the inadvertent administration of 1 liter of 5% saline instead of 5% dextrose in water represents an extra volume of 1 liter of water and 1709 mOsm of sodium chloride. The total amount of osmotically active solute equals the sum of the pre-existing solute (TBW $\times$ P_{osm} or 42 $\times$ 300 = 12,600 mOsm) and the administered solute (1709 mOsm), or 14,309 mOsm, and the new TBW volume is 42 + 1 eq 43 liters. Consequently, the new plasma osmolality would be $\frac{14,309}{(42 + 1)}$, or 333 mOsm/g, and the volume of water needed to dilute 14,309 mOsm to normal would be $\frac{14,309}{300}$, of 47.7 liters. Thus, the amount of water needed to correct the hypertonicity or the theoretical water deficit would be (47.7 − 43), or 4.7 liters.

Half of the estimated deficit should be infused as 5% dextrose in water over several hours while neurologic status is carefully monitored. Rapid water administration should continue only until neurologic symptoms improve. Simultaneously, a loop diuretic such as furosemide should be administered to facilitate rapid removal of excess solute and prevent pulmonary edema. In patients with overwhelming pulmonary edema or renal failure, phlebotomy can be employed as a temporizing measure until dialysis can be instituted.

Hypertonicity with Decreased Total Body Sodium

The coexistence of hypertonicity and decreased total body sodium (*i.e.*, ECF volume depletion), implies that the water deficit is greater than the sodium deficit, that is, that hypotonic fluid loss has occurred. The coexistence of hypotension and hypertonicity almost always implies the concomitant loss of sodium. Hypotension is unusual in pure water loss unless the loss is of a large enough magnitude to produce extreme hypernatremia.

Hypotonic fluid can be lost through the skin, gastrointestinal tract, or kidney. Sweat is hypotonic, and, when large volumes are lost, hypertonicity, hypernatremia, and ECF volume depletion can result. With the exception of biliary and pancreatic secretions, most drainage from the gastrointestinal tract is also hypotonic (Table 17-2). For example, prolonged vomiting, nasogastric suction, and diarrhea can all be associated with hypertonicity, hypernatremia, and ECF volume depletion. The hypertonicity and ECF volume depletion that are associated with renal hypotonic fluid losses most commonly result from the use of diuretics or from ongoing osmotic diuresis due to glucose, mannitol, or urea.

Since, by definition, hypotonic fluid loss leads to ECF volume depletion and consequently to decrements in EABV, there is volume stimulus for thirst and ADH release. Consequently, ingestion of larger quantities of water but little sodium can ultimately lead to hypotonicity. The presence of marked hypertonicity with ECF volume depletion therefore implies hypotonic fluid loss in conjunction with either an inappropriately depressed thirst mechanism or, more commonly, an inability to respond to thirst because of age, illness, mental status, or postoperative status.

The first priority in the therapy of the hypertonic volume-depleted patient is restoration of an adequate intravascular volume. Either isotonic saline or, if hypotension is severe, colloid should be used. After blood pressure is stabilized, the correction of hypertonicity can be addressed. Provided that sodium and potassium deficits have been corrected, the water deficit can be calculated as shown above. Full correction of hypertonicity should always be gradual in order for cerebral edema to be avoided.

Diabetes Mellitus and Tonicity Homeostasis

Hypertonicity due to hyperglycemia is a common disorder requiring close attention. Hypertonicity associated with intravenous mannitol or glycerol for the treatment of post-traumatic cerebral edema shares many of the features of hypertonicity due to hyperglycemia. Glucose permeates biologic membranes relatively poorly and, at high plasma concentrations, is a potent osmotic diuretic. Consequently, hyperglycemia produces hypertonicity both directly, by virtue of its presence in the ECF, and indirectly, by virtue of the hypotonic fluid losses it causes. The loss of sodium should lead to ECF volume depletion, but this is sometimes masked, because large amounts of glucose in the ECF can maintain ECF volume by drawing water from the ICF into the ECF compartment. In addition, since hypertonicity generally develops over a period of several days or weeks, there is time for marked sodium, potassium, and water depletion to occur.

Since hyperglycemia tends to lower the plasma sodium concentration by drawing water from the ICF to the ECF compartment, hyponatremia may coexist with hypertonicity. The serum sodium concentration falls by 1.6 mEq/liter for each rise of 100 mg/dl above normal in blood glucose concentration. For example, if blood glucose is 900 mg/dl, or approximately 800 mg/dl above normal, the expected decrement in serum sodium concentration would be 8 × 1.6, or 13 mEq/liter. Under these circumstances, a "normal" serum sodium concentration of 140 mEq/liter would indicate the presence of a substantial water deficit. The two clinically most important hyperglycemic syndromes are hyperosmolar hyperglycemic nonketosis (HHNK) and diabetic ketoacidosis (DKA).[62,70,71] Treatment is the same for surgical as for medical patients.

DISORDERS OF POTASSIUM HOMEOSTASIS

Fundamental Principles

An understanding of the following fundamental principles is helpful in the analysis of clinical disorders of potassium homeostasis.

1. Potassium is the most abundant cation within cells, and approximately 98% of total body potassium is located intracellularly. The majority of potassium in the body resides in muscle, and total body potassium content varies with muscle mass.

2. Total body potassium content is determined by external potassium balance, the difference between potassium intake and potassium excretion in the urine and feces.

3. The ECF potassium concentration is a function of two variables, total body potassium content and "internal" potassium balance.

4. Internal potassium balance is determined by net flux of potassium across cell membranes. Since the quantity of potassium located outside cells is so small, relatively minor alterations in internal potassium balance can produce large changes in the plasma potassium concentration.[72]

5. When potassium is lost from the body, the proportional decrease in plasma potassium concentration exceeds the proportional decrease in total body potassium (Figure 17-2). Similarly, as potassium is gained by the body, the proportional increase in plasma potassium concentration exceeds the proportional increase in total body potassium.

6. The ECF potassium concentration may not provide a reliable indication of body potassium stores. Hyperkalemia may exist with increased, normal, or decreased body potassium stores: hypokalemia is most commonly associated with decreased potassium stores (Table 17-7).

Internal Potassium Balance

The distribution of potassium between cells and the ECF compartment is affected by acid–base balance, several hormones (insulin, aldosterone, epinephrine), body-fluid tonicity, a variety of pharmacologic agents, and acute changes in cell mass, as listed below.[72,73]

Hyperkalemia
Acid–base disturbances
 Metabolic acidosis
  Mineral acids (e.g., renal insufficiency)
  (?) Respiratory acidosis
Hormonal deficiency states
 Insulin (diabetes mellitus)
 (?) Aldosterone (Addison's disease, selective hypoaldosteronism)
 (?) Epinephrine
Disorders of body-fluid tonicity
 Hypertonicity
  Hyperglycemia (diabetes mellitus with or without associated selective hypoaldosteronism)
Pharmacologic agents
 Beta-adrenergic antagonists
 Digitalis glycosides
 Succinylcholine
 Arginine and lysine hydrochloride
Acute cell necrosis
 Rhabdomyolysis
 Hemolysis
 Burns
 Chemotherapy of myelo- and lymphoproliferative disorders
Hyperkalemic periodic paralysis

Hypokalemia
Acid–base disturbances
 Metabolic alkalosis
 (?) Respiratory alkalosis
 (?) Hyperbicarbonatemia
Pharmacologic agents
 Insulin (treatment of hyperkalemia or uncontrolled diabetes mellitus)
 $NaHCO_3$ (treatment of hyperkalemia or metabolic acidosis)
 Beta-adrenergic agonists
Acute increase in cell synthesis
 Treatment of severe megaloblastic anemias (with vitamin B_{12}, folate)
 Intravenous hyperalimentation
Hypokalemic periodic paralysis

Table 17-7. Relationship of ECF Potassium Concentration to Total Body Potassium Content in Selected Disorders of Potassium Homeostasis

Serum Potassium Concentration	Total Body Potassium Content	Mechanism(s)	Examples
↑	↑	Decreased renal K^+ excretion	High K^+ intake associated with renal insufficiency Hypoaldosteronism K^+-sparing diuretics
↑	↔	Redistribution	Acidosis associated with renal insufficiency Succinylcholine Hyperkalemic periodic paralysis
↑	↓	Effects of redistribution predominate despite increased renal K^+ excretion and TBK depletion.	Diabetic ketoacidosis
↓	↓	Increased renal or gastrointestinal K^+ excretion	Kaliuretic diuretics Hyperaldosteronism Renal tubular acidosis Protracted vomiting
↓	↔	Redistribution	Administration of excessive amounts of insulin or bicarbonate to treat hyperkalemia in patients with normal TBK (see above) Hypokalemic periodic paralysis
↓	↑	Effects of redistribution predominate despite decreased renal K^+ excretion.	Administration of excessive amounts of insulin or bicarbonate to treat hyperkalemia in patients with increased TBK (see above)

K^+ = serum potassium concentration; TBK = total body potassium content.

Acid–Base Balance

The generalizations that acidemia invariably produces hyperkalemia as potassium exits from cells in exchange for hydrogen ions and that alkalemia always produces hypokalemia as potassium enters cells in exchange for hydrogen ions are not entirely correct. In particular, the effects of metabolic acid–base disturbances on internal potassium balance differ considerably from those of respiratory acid–base disturbances.[74]

One of the most important factors that influences the effect of metabolic acidosis on the internal potassium balance is the nature of the acid inducing the disturbance.[75] The effects of mineral acids such as hydrochloric, phosphoric, and sulfuric acids differ from those of organic acids such as lactic, acetoacetic, and beta-hydroxybutyric acids. Although experimentally induced mineral acidemia is associated with hyperkalemia, experimentally induced organic acidemia generally is at best associated with a much smaller increment in plasma concentration, if any at all. The metabolic acidosis associated with acute or chronic renal failure, due largely to retention of sulfuric and phosphoric acids, probably contributes to the hyperkalemia that is characteristic of these disorders. In contrast, patients with lactic acidosis, which is seen with seizures and acute pulmonary edema, on administration of phenformin, or with alcoholic ketoacidosis, are not usually hyperkalemic.[76–78] In addition, although patients with diabetic ketoacidosis are generally hyperkalemic, their hyperkalemia may be primarily due to insulin deficiency or hypertonicity and not to acidemia per se.

The effect of metabolic alkalosis on internal potassium balance has not been extensively studied and is complicated by the additional influence of this acid–base disturbance on external potassium balance, since chronic metabolic alkalosis is generally associated with an ongoing kaliuresis and severe total body potassium depletion. Although metabolic alkalosis may be associated with a shift of small amounts of potassium into cells, hypokalemia, commonly seen in patients with chronic metabolic alkalosis, predominantly reflects negative external balance.[72]

Respiratory acid–base disturbances appear to have less effect on internal potassium balance than their metabolic counterparts. Acute respiratory acidosis may cause a redistribution of potassium out of cells under certain circumstances, but chronic respiratory acidosis is generally not associated with hyperkalemia.[72,73] Consequently, hyperkalemia in patients with chronic respiratory acidosis should not be ascribed to acidemia unless other causes of hyperkalemia have been excluded. Finally, although clinically significant hypokalemia has been reported as a consequence of extreme degrees of respiratory alkalosis, most studies of both acute and chronic respiratory alkalosis have shown this acid–base disturbance to have no effect on plasma potassium concentration.[72]

Internal potassium balance also appears to be directly influenced by changes in ECF bicarbonate concentration independent of concurrent changes in ECF pH.[79] For example, in hyperkalemic patients with renal failure, infusions of sodium bicarbonate decrease the plasma potassium concentration regardless of whether there is a concomitant change in arterial blood pH.[80]

In summary, attempts to calculate the magnitude of the change in plasma potassium concentration caused by a change in ECF pH are relatively nonproductive. The rule of thumb that, for every 0.1-unit change in pH, the plasma potassium concentration changes by approximately 0.6 mEq/liter, should be discarded. In evaluating an abnormal plasma potassium concentration in a patient with an acid–base disturbance, careful consideration must be given to a variety of factors, including the exact nature and duration of the disturbance, the effect of the disturbance on renal potassium excretion, pre-existing body potassium stores, and the presence of any other factors that could potentially influence potassium homeostasis. For example, when renal function is normal, chronic metabolic acidosis is generally associated with renal potassium wasting and total body potassium depletion. However, because redistribution of potassium out of cells may occur, the plasma potassium concentration may be increased, as in diabetic ketoacidosis, normal, as in lactic acidosis and alcoholic ketoacidosis, or decreased, as in renal tubular acidosis. Thus, the presence of a normal or increased plasma potassium concentration need not imply that potassium replacement is unnecessary. Similarly, the presence of hypo-or normokalemia in a patient with diabetic ketoacidosis generally indicates profound potassium depletion due to ongoing osmotic diuresis and the need for early and vigorous potassium replacement.

Hormones

Several hormones affect internal potassium balance. The effects of insulin are relatively well defined, whereas those of aldosterone and catecholamines are more speculative.[72,73,81]

Since insulin directly stimulates net potassium uptake by muscle and liver, it may have an important role in the normal control of internal potassium balance.[82,83] An experimentally induced insulin deficiency is associated with an increase in plasma potassium concentration and impairs cellular uptake of acutely administered potassium loads.[84] In addition, impaired potassium tolerance in patients with diabetes mellitus can be improved or corrected by insulin replacement.[73,81,85] These observations suggest that a low but critical level of circulating insulin plays a permissive role in maintaining normal internal potassium balance. Since potassium can induce pancreatic insulin release, under certain circumstances, acute elevations in peripheral or portal insulin levels may participate in a feedback control loop in which elevations in plasma potassium concentration stimulate the release of insulin, which, in turn, facilitates net cellular potassium uptake.[73,81]

A variety of other factors may contribute to hyperkalemia in diabetic patients. First, acidemia may be contributory in those with ketoacidosis. However, it is probably not of major importance, because organic acids generally do not produce marked hyperkalemia in other circumstances. Second, hypertonicity may play a role if the blood glucose concentration is markedly elevated. Third, since some patients with diabetes have selective hypoaldosteronism and/or renal insufficiency, abnormalities in external potassium balance may also contribute to hyperkalemia.

Insulin has long been used in the treatment of hyperkalemia. The administration of insulin to humans in amounts that produce graded elevations in circulating insulin levels within both the physiologic and the supraphysiologic ranges is associated with a dose-related reduction in plasma potassium concentration. However, since the maximal hypokalemic effect occurs only when insulin levels exceed basal levels 20 to 40 times, it is best in the treatment of severe hyperkalemia to administer insulin intravenously to achieve high circulating hormone levels.[82]

The role of aldosterone in the control of internal potassium balance is controversial. There is little evidence that a defect in internal potassium balance contributes significantly to the genesis of hyperkalemia in patients with Addison's disease or the syndrome of selective hypoaldosteronism. A variety of other factors probably account for hyperkalemia in these patients. First, hypoaldosteronism is clearly associated with a decrease in renal potassium excretion. Second, in patients with selective hypoaldosteronism and diabetes mellitus, insulin deficiency or hypertonicity may contribute. Third, since hyperchloremic metabolic acidosis is often associated with selective hypoaldosteronism, the resultant acidemia may also play a role.

There is increasing evidence that epinephrine may be instrumental in the physiologic control of internal potassium balance.[72,73] For example, in both animals and humans, physiologic amounts of epinephrine blunt the hyperkalemia that occurs during potassium loading.[86,87] In addition, net cellular potassium uptake is abnormally low in adrenalectomized animals and is restored to normal by physiologic amounts of epinephrine but not by replacement with the other two major adrenal hormones, aldosterone and cortisol.[88]

The effects of catecholamines on internal potassium balance may have important clinical implications. For example, intravenous administration of salbutamol, a specific beta$_2$-adrenergic agonist, produces marked hypokalemia.[89] Therapeutic doses of propranolol and pindolol, both beta-adrenergic antagonists, increase plasma potassium concentration in patients with hypertension; however, in otherwise healthy individuals, this increase averages only about 0.3 mEq/liter and is clinically insignificant.[90]

Body-Fluid Tonicity

Hypertonicity is associated with a net shift of potassium out of cells into the ECF compartment.[91–93] This redistribution of potassium occurs at equal degrees during the infusion of hypertonic sodium chloride and bicarbonate, mannitol, or glucose. In the latter case, the expected rise in plasma potassium concentration is generally masked by the effects of endogenously released insulin on internal potassium balance. Whereas glucose infusion results in hypokalemia in normal persons, administration of hypertonic glucose solutions to correct hypoglycemia in diabetic patients requiring insulin may lead to hyperkalemia.[93–95] However, glucose-induced hyperkalemia is more commonly seen in patients who have multiple defects in potassium homeostasis.[96–99] For example, hyperglycemia may be associated with severe and even lethal hyperkalemia in diabetic patients with selective hypoaldosteronism or in diabetic patients treated with potassium-sparing diuretics.[94,100–102]

The precise contribution of hypertonicity to an elevation in plasma potassium concentration is usually difficult to determine in a given clinical situation. The interplay of multiple factors influencing internal and external potassium balance must be analyzed. These include urinary potassium losses in osmotic diuresis, gastrointestinal potassium losses, acid–base disturbances, and hormonal abnormalities. However, two generalizations are useful: (1) despite normal or low total body potassium content, patients with glucose-related hypertonicity, such as those with diabetic ketoacidosis or hyperosmolar nonketotic coma, may present with severe hyperkalemia; and (2) a normal or low plasma potassium concentration in a severely hypertonic patient implies the possibility of severe underlying total body potassium depletion.

Pharmacologic Agents

Although digitalis glycosides inhibit net cellular potassium uptake, therapeutic levels have only very small and clinically insignificant effects on plasma potassium concentration. However, hyperkalemia is a common finding in severe and lethal digitalis poisoning.[103]

Use of the depolarizing muscle relaxant succinylcholine is associated with an efflux of potassium from muscle cells. Although the resultant increase in plasma potassium concentration is usually only about 0.5 mEq/liter in normal subjects, life-threatening hyperkalemia may occur in patients with severe burns or in those with pre-existing neurologic or muscular disorders.[104] Consequently, nondepolarizing muscle relaxants such as pancuronium or gallamine, which do not produce hyperkalemia, should be used in such persons.

The use of arginine and lysine hydrochloride in the therapy of metabolic alkalosis can result in life-threatening hyperkalemia, particularly if renal function is impaired.[105] The net cellular efflux of potassium produced by these agents is related to specific intracellular effects of these cationic amino acids rather than to changes in body-fluid pH or bicarbonate concentration.

Acute Changes in Cell Mass

Acute cell necrosis due to rhabdomyolysis, massive hemolysis, severe burns, or chemotherapy in myelo- or lymphoproliferative disorders may result in large endogenous potassium loads. In these circumstances, especially if concomitant renal insufficiency due to myoglobinuria, hemoglobinura, or hyperuricemia or shock is present, severe and often lethal hyperkalemia is common.[106,107]

Although much less common, hypokalemia may be caused by an acute increase in cell synthesis. For example, when patients with severe megaloblastic anemias are treated with vitamin B_{12} or folate or both, potassium is used in the production of new cells. Dangerous and even fatal hypokalemia may result unless sufficiently high potassium intake is provided.[108] A similar problem has been described in patients receiving intravenous hyperalimentation.[109]

External Potassium Balance

Since dietary intake is relatively constant and gastrointestinal losses are small, renal excretion in generally the major determinant of external potassium balance.[110–112]

Potassium Intake

Normal dietary potassium intake approximates 80 mEq/day. Although increased potassium intake may cause hyperkalemia, this is distinctly unusual unless renal potassium excretion is concomitantly compromised.[113] For example, in patients with renal insufficiency who are taking diuretics, potassium supplementation may overwhelm the diminished ability of the kidney to dispose of potassium loads.[114–116] Similarly, because the kidneys are able to conserve potassium in an efficient manner, only prolonged potassium deprivation will eventually lead to a decrease in total body potassium and hypokalemia.[117,118] Factors that influence potassium intake include the following:

Increased potassium intake
    Potassium supplementation (oral or intravenous)
    Dietary sodium substitutes
    (Hemolyzed) blood transfusions containing hemolyzed red cells
    Potassium salts of antibiotics (e.g., penicillin)
Decreased potassium intake
    Starvation
    Poor diet ("tea and toast" syndrome)
    Chronic alcoholism
    Anorexia nervosa
    Geophagia.

Renal Potassium Excretion

The normal kidney responds within hours to increases in potassium intake but may require several weeks to respond to decreases.[84,117–120] When fully adapted to high potassium intake, the urinary potassium concentration may exceed 100 mEq/liter. With chronic potassium depletion, the urinary potassium concentration may fall to less than 5 mEq/liter. Most filtered potassium is reabsorbed in the proximal tubule and loop of Henle, and only about 10% to 15% of the filtered load reaches the early distal convoluted tubule. For the most part, control of the amount of potassium excreted in the urine resides in the distal convoluted tubule, cortical collecting tubule, and collecting duct.[110,121,122]

Impairment of renal function is commonly associated with abnormalities in potassium homeostasis. Decreases in renal potassium excretion leading to hyperkalemia may be caused by the following:

Renal insufficiency
    Acute renal failure
    Oliguric chronic renal failure
    Chronic interstitial nephritis
Aldosterone deficiency
    Addison's disease
    Selective hypoaldosteronism
        Diabetes mellitus
        Chronic interstitial nephritis
        Prostaglandin inhibitors
Tubular unresponsiveness to aldosterone
    Spironolactone
    Chronic interstitial nephritis
    Systemic lupus erythematosus
    Sjogren's syndrome
    Amyloidosis
    Renal allografts
Miscellaneous
    Triamterene
    Amiloride.

Severe hyperkalemia is common in acute renal failure, even when oliguria is absent.[13,14] Changes in internal potassium balance, due to the associated metabolic acidosis, and in cellular potassium release, due to enhanced catabolic rate and cell necrosis, may also contribute to the development of hyperkalemia. In contrast, hyperkalemia is uncommon until late in the course of chronic renal failure; at this point, unless potassium intake is excessive or extensive renal medullary disease is the cause of the renal failure, oliguria generally supervenes.[111,112,120,123]

Patients with chronic renal failure can maintain adequate renal potassium excretion because of enhanced potassium secretion by the residual nephron population.[123] The collecting duct secretes more potassium in renal insufficiency. This may explain the frequent occurrence of hyperkalemia in patients with only mild degrees of renal insufficiency resulting from diseases that primarily affect the renal medulla, such as chronic interstitial nephritis of any etiology. Hyperkalemia in patients with mild or moderate obstructive uropathy is due not only to chronic interstitial renal disease but also to the coexistence of selective hypoaldosteronism or tubular unresponsiveness to aldosterone.[124]

A number of factors other than overall renal function are known to affect renal potassium excretion; these include potassium and sodium intake, distal tubular flow rate, circulating aldosterone levels, tubular responsiveness to aldosterone, and acid–base balance.[110–112,121] An understanding of the interactions of these factors with one another is central to the rational analysis of many of the clinically important disorders of external potassium balance.

The kaliuretic response to an acute potassium load is enhanced by prior high dietary potassium intake and is reduced by prior low potassium intake.[121,125] Whether the former adaptation is the result of increased sensitivity of the adrenal glands to the aldosterone-releasing effects of potassium or of increased renal tubular sensitivity to aldosterone is unknown. In the latter case, chronic dietary potassium restriction produces a dramatic decrease in potassium secretion in the late distal convoluted tubule, and this may be due to a reduction in circulating levels of aldosterone and net reabsorption of potassium in the collecting duct.

Administration of oral or intravenous sodium salts produces ECF volume expansion and an increase in the distal tubular flow rate that is associated with a marked kaliuresis due to enhanced potassium secretion in the late distal convoluted tubule. Sodium depletion with a decreased distal tubular flow rate is generally associated with a fall in renal potassium excretion due to a marked accentuation of net potassium reabsorption in the collecting duct. This relationship between flow rate and potassium secretion in the distal convoluted tubule also explains the kaliuresis that is associated with proximally acting diuretics and osmotic diuresis. Patients with glycosuria who are treated with mannitol, large volumes of isotonic or hypertonic sodium chloride, or sodium bicarbonate solutions and patients with obligate urinary losses of poorly reabsorbed anions commonly become potassium-depleted and hypokalemic.[121] In addition, the osmotic diuresis due to urea and/or sodium in the diuretic phase of acute tubular necrosis or after relief of urinary tract obstruction is generally associated with urinary losses of potassium.[11,12] Increased renal potassium excretion leading to hypokalemia may be caused by the following:

Diuretics
Osmotic diuresis
    Uncontrolled diabetes mellitus (glucose)
    Treatment of cerebral edema with mannitol
    Treatment of severe metabolic acidosis with $NaHCO_3$
    Diuretic phase of acute tubular necrosis (sodium, urea)
    Postobstructive diuresis (sodium, urea)
    Nonreabsorbable anions (penicillin, carbenicillin)
Mineralocorticoid excess
    Primary hyperaldosteronism (Conn's syndrome)

Secondary hyperaldosteronism
    Diuretics
    Osmotic diuresis
    Edematous disorders
    Malignant hypertension
    Renal artery stenosis
    Renin-secreting tumors
Other mineralocorticoids
    Ectopic ACTH syndrome
    Cushing's syndrome
    Licorice abuse*
    Congenital adrenal hyperplasia
Acid–base disorders
    Metabolic alkalosis
        Vomiting
        Nasogastric suctioning
        Diuretics
        Mineralocorticoid excess
    Chronic metabolic acidosis
        Renal tubular acidosis

The effects of mineralocorticoids on renal potassium excretion in the late distal convoluted tubule and probably in the collecting duct have long been recognized.[121] Potassium retention and hyperkalemia may result from inadequate circulating levels of aldosterone or renal tubular unresponsiveness to aldosterone. In the former case, the inadequacy of circulating levels of aldosterone may result from generalized adrenal insufficiency (Addison's disease) or from isolated zona glomerulosa insufficiency (selective hypoaldosteronism).[81,126–129] However, a majority of patients with inadequate levels of circulating aldosterone exhibit concomitant hyporeninemia, which is often associated with diabetes, obstructive uropathy, increasing age, and the use of prostaglandin inhibitors such as indomethacin.[124,127,130] Therefore, it is clear that maintenance of renal potassium ex-

---

*Licorice contains glycyrrhizic acid, a compound with mineralocorticoid properties.

cretion is not entirely dependent on mineralocorticoids. For example, hyperkalemia is unusual in patients with Addison's disease or selective hypoaldosteronism unless the renal potassium excretory system is stressed by sodium depletion or excessive potassium intake.

Potassium-sparing diuretics and potassium supplements should be avoided in patients with diabetes mellitus because of the possibility of associated hypoaldosteronism.[81,126,131,132] Patients with interstitial nephritis associated with systemic lupus erythematous, Sjogren's syndrome, renal amyloidosis, obstructive uropathy, and renal transplantation may present with hyperkalemia because of tubular insensitivity to aldosterone.[132–135]

Disorders associated with excessive mineralocorticoid activity are generally also associated with enhanced renal potassium secretion and hypokalemia.[110–112] However, increased potassium secretion under these circumstances is also dependent on adequate fluid delivery to the distal nephron. For example, patients with Conn's syndrome may not present with hypokalemia if their dietary sodium intake is low. Similarly, patients who are sodium-depleted may not manifest enhanced renal potassium excretion despite the presence of secondary hyperaldosteronism. In addition, patients with secondary hyperaldosteronism associated with cirrhosis, congestive heart failure, or nephrotic syndrome may develop severe hypokalemia only after treatment with diuretics, which increase the delivery of fluid to the potassium secretory sites in the distal nephron.

The aldosterone antagonist spironolactone causes significant hyperkalemia only when potassium intake is high or the potassium excretory system is stressed. Triamterene and amiloride have similar

Table 17-8. Changes in Renal Potassium Excretion Due to Changes in Acid–Base Balance

	Potassium Excretion		Potassium Deficits in Steady-State Phase
	Immediate phase	Transient phase	
Respiratory alkalosis	↑	—	Undetectable
Respiratory acidosis	↓	↑	Mild
Metabolic acidosis	↓	↑ ↑	Moderate
Metabolic alkalosis	↑	↑ ↑	Large

(Gennari FJ, Cohen JJ: Kidney Int 8:1, 1975)

effects but do not depend on the presence of aldosterone to inhibit distal tubular potassium excretion.[131]

Alterations in acid–base balance have important effects on renal potassium excretion (Table 17-8).[136] These changes occur in the late distal convoluted tubule.

Chronic alterations in acid–base balance produce changes in renal potassium excretion that differ considerably from those observed during the initial phase of the acid–base disturbance. Chronic respiratory or metabolic acidosis and chronic metabolic alkalosis are all associated with potassium depletion. The immediate antikaliuresis associated with acute acidemic states is therefore short-lived and is followed by a more sustained increase in renal potassium excretion. In contrast, the immediate kaliuresis that occurs during the induction of metabolic alkalosis is maintained. Consequently, chronic metabolic alkalosis is most likely to be associated with marked total body potassium deficits. Whereas acute respiratory alkalosis results in a mild and short-lived immediate kaliuresis, chronic respiratory alkalosis is the one acid–base disturbance that does not lead to potassium depletion. Most states characterized by metabolic acidosis are relatively short-lived, so that there is little time for significant renal losses of potassium to occur as a direct result of the acidemia *per se*. The most notable exception is renal tubular acidosis, in which stable moderate degrees of acidemia and hypokalemia may persist for years.[137]

Another clinically important interrelationship between acid–base balance and potassium homeostasis is illustrated by patients with hypokalemia following excessive losses of gastric fluid.[18] The hypokalemia reflects (1) total body potassium wasting from direct losses of potassium in gastric fluid and renal potassium wasting and (2) a possible redistribution of potassium into cells as a result of the associated metabolic alkalosis. Renal potassium wasting due to enhanced potassium secretion plays a dominant role. Increased potassium secretion is the result of chronic metabolic alkalosis due to losses of gastric hydrocholric acid as well as of sodium depletion and secondary hyperaldosteronism due to losses of sodium in vomitus and urine.

Gastrointestinal Potassium Excretion

Gastrointestinal excretion of potassium may be due to the following:

Diarrhea
Non-insulin-secreting islet-cell tumors
Villous adenoma
Laxative abuse
Ureterosigmoidostomy
Obstructed ileal loops
Vomiting
Nasogastric suction

Under normal circumstances, fecal potassium excretion is small. Net colonic potassium excretion increases dramatically with diarrhea and malabsorption. It may also increase in renal insufficiency when potassium excretion by the kidney is reduced, or as a result of persistently elevated circulating levels of mineralocorticoids. Particularly severe potassium deficiencies occur in patients with non-insulin-secreting islet-cell tumors of the pancreas or villous adenomas of the colon and in persons who abuse laxatives.[138–140]

Ureterosigmoidostomies may also be associated with increased fecal potassium losses; however, they are now only infrequently performed.[141] More commonly, the ureters are diverted to an ileal loop, which is then brought out to the skin. An obstructed or overly long ileal loop may lead to potassium depletion and hyperchloremic metabolic acidosis through gastrointestinal reabsorption of sodium chloride and concomitant secretion of potassium bicarbonate into the lumen.

Potassium depletion is a common result of surreptitious or overt vomiting or nasogastric suction and is largely due to renal potassium wasting with contributory direct losses of potassium in gastric fluid.[18] Unlike patients with diarrhea, who are potassium-depleted but usually not hypoaklemic because of associated metabolic acidosis, patients with protracted upper gastrointestinal fluid losses are generally both potassium-depleted and hypokalemic. Hypokalemia in these patients is largely a reflection of a total body potassium deficit, but redistribution of potassium into cells as a result of the associated metabolic alkalosis may also contribute.

Hyperkalemia

The ECF potassium concentration can be considered identical to the concentration of potassium in plasma. Under most circumstances, serum and plasma potassium concentrations differ by less than 10% and, for clinical purposes, are equal. Exceptions to this generalization in which plasma or serum potassium concentration or both do not provide a valid estimate of the ECF potassium concentration include (1) prolonged tourniquet application combined with fist clenching, in which potassium is released from ischemic exercising muscle, elevating both plasma and serum concentration; (2) *in vitro* hemolysis, which also raises both plasma and serum concentrations; and (3) release of potassium from platelets or leukocytes during *in vitro* clotting of blood in patients with thrombocythemia or leukemia, which elevates the serum but not the plasma concentration.[134–136,142,143] The latter phenomenon has been called pseudohyperkalemia and can be readily distinguished from true hyperkalemia by simultaneous measurement of serum and plasma potassium concentrations.

Once increased potassium intake, alterations in internal potassium balance, and renal insufficiency per se have been excluded as primary causes of hyperkalemia, the remaining possibilities can largely be divided into those disorders that are characterized by aldosterone deficiency and those disorders that are characterized by end-organ unresponsiveness to aldosterone. Associated clinical findings often provide important clues as to which of the two situations applies in a particular patient. Addison's disease is easily excluded by the performance of a standard ACTH stimulation test. The definitive diagnosis of selective hypoaldosteronism of any etiology is usually based on the finding of an abnormally low level of aldosterone in urine or blood under circumstances in which it should be high, as

in intravascular volume depletion induced by chronic sodium restriction or by administration of furosemide. The urinary potassium concentration in patients with hyperkalemia is usually greater than 40 mEq/liter. However, if the hyperkalemia is due to hypoaldosteronism or tubular unresponsiveness to aldosterone, it is generally less than 20 mEq/liter. In the latter situation, hormone deficiency can generally be distinguished from lack of hormone effect by administration of exogenous mineralocorticoid.

The clinical manifestations of hyperkalemia primarily affect neuromuscular and cardiovascular function.[111] The neuromuscular effects of hyperkalemia are complex. Both increased and decreased muscle excitability can occur, but the latter effect usually predominates. However, generalized muscle weakness is not commonly observed, because cardiac arrest frequently supervenes. The cardiac effects of hyperkalemia are best evaluated by electrocardiography. Initially, the amplitude of the T wave in the precordial leads increases. As the plasma potassium concentration rises further, the amplitude of the R and P waves decreases, and the duration of the QRS complex and the PR interval increases. Finally, the P wave disappears, atrioventricular dissociation occurs, and the QRS complex and the T wave merge into the classic sine wave pattern of severe hyperkalemia. Ventricular arrhythmias or cardiac arrest may occur at any time during this progression. Severe cardiac abnormalities are more commonly associated with acute than with chronic hyperkalemia. Although the plasma potassium concentration at which electrocardiographic manifestations are first evident varies considerably from patient to patient, in any given person, the electrocardiogram is a reliable indicator of the severity of hyperkalemia, the necessity for immediate therapy, and the response to therapy.

Therapy

If the plasma potassium concentration is less than 6.5 mEq/liter and there are no indications or only early signs of cardiac toxicity, the hyperkalemia can be treated conservatively by simple correction of the underlying problem. If more advanced electrocardiographic changes are present or the plasma potassium concentration is greater than 8.0 mEq/liter, more aggressive therapy is in order (Table 17-9).

The most rapidly acting therapeutic agent for reversing the cardiac manifestations of hyperkalemia is calcium. It exerts a direct action on the heart and does not affect the plasma potassium concentration or total body potassium content. One-gram ampules of calcium gluconate and calcium chloride contain 4.5 mEq and 13.6 mEq of elemental calcium, respec-

tively. When rapidly infused in undiluted form, these agents should be given through a central venous line, since peripheral administration is associated with local venous calcification and phlebitis. Calcium acts rapidly, but its effect lasts only about 30 min.

Redistribution of potassium from the ECF to the ICF compartment, also an effective treatment of hyperkalemia, is generally instituted immediately after infusion of calcium or, if myocardial dysfunction is not very threatening, as first-line therapy. Redistribution can be achieved with intravenous sodium bicarbonate administered as 1 to 2 ampules containing 50 mEq to 100 mEq of bicarbonate or with regular insulin administered as 10 units in 500 ml of 10% glucose. Both regimens act within 15 to 30 min and exert their effects for several hours. The effect of bicarbonate is not dependent on a change in ECF pH. Insulin should be given only by the intravenous route in or-

Table 17-9. Treatment of Hyperkalemia

Treatment	Mechanism	Effects on $[K^+]ECF$	TBK	Onset	Duration	Limitations
Calcium	Direct antagonism	None	None	Immediate	~ 30 min	↑ Ca^{2+}
NaHCO₃	Direct antagonism Redistribution	↓	None	15–30 min	Few hours	↑ ECF volume Hypernatremia Alkalosis
Glucose and insulin	Redistribution	↓	None	15–30 min	Few Hours	↑ ↓ Blood sugar ↑ ECF volume
NaCl	Renal excretion Dilution	↓	↓	< 1 hr	Few hours	↑ ECF volume
Kayexelate	GI excretion	↓	↓	Few hours	Few hours	GI tolerance Diarrhea
Hemodialysis	Direct removal	↓	↓	Few minutes	Few hours to few days after end	Dialysis
Peritoneal dialysis	Direct removal	↓	↓	Few hours	Few hours to few days after end	Dialysis

$[K^+]ECF$ = extracellular fluid potassium concentration; TBK = total body potassium content.

der for a reliable, prompt, and maximal therapeutic effect to be obtained. Expansion of the ECF with isotonic sodium chloride is usually reserved for those special instances in which hyperkalemia is the result of inadequate renal perfusion and oliguria. This measure is generally effective within 1 hr and lowers the plasma potassium concentration by increasing renal potassium excretion and diluting extracellular potassium.

Potassium can be removed from the body with ion-exchange resins such as sodium polystyrene sulfonate (Kayexelate) or by dialysis. Kayexelate can be administered orally or rectally in combination with sorbitol, which facilitates excretion of the resin and increases potassium excretion by producing diarrhea. Although the amount varies considerably depending on the situation, 1 g of Kayexelate removes approximately 1 mEq of potassium from the body. Kayexelate in a dose of 25 g to 50 g is administered with 50 ml to 100 ml of sorbitol orally or as a retention enema. It takes several hours to exert its effect, but administration can be repeated as needed. Hemodialysis is effective in removing potassium from the body but is rarely employed for treating hyperkalemia alone. Peritoneal dialysis is less effective than either hemodialysis or ion-exchange resins.

Hypokalemia

Most patients with hypokalemia are total body-potassium-depleted. The existence of abnormalities in internal potassium balance can generally be easily determined from the clinical situation and an arterial blood gas assay. Attention can then be turned to an analysis as to whether the hypokalemia is the result of decreased intake or increased excretion or a combination of these factors.

The potential for excessive renal losses of potassium may not be immediately evident. Although routine clinical evaluation usually uncovers potassium wasting due to osmotic diuresis, other etiologies, such as diuretic abuse, excess mineralocorticoid states, surreptitious vomiting, and renal tubular acidosis, may present diagnostic difficulties. Diuretic abuse, vomiting, and excess mineralocorticoid states are all generally associated with metabolic alkalosis. Many but not all mineralocorticoid excess states are accompanied by hypertension. Urinary screening tests for diuretics may help to pinpoint the cause of hypokalemia.

The urinary potassium concentration is not as helpful in the evaluation of hypokalemia as in that of hyperkalemia. It is increased in patients with excessive losses of gastric fluid as well as in patients with renal potassium-wasting. In patients with diarrhea, it may not be low, either because of volume-related hyperaldosteronism or because maximal renal adaptation to potassium depletion has not had sufficient time to develop.

Hypokalemia causes a wide variety of arrhythmias and potentiates those induced by digitalis. The electrocardiographic effects of potassium deficiency are less predictable than those associated with hyperkalemia and, apart from arrhythmias, include flattened T waves, development or accentuation of U waves, and prolongation of the PR interval. Apparent lengthening of the QT interval may occur; however, in reality, this is due to the T wave being flattened and the U wave being mistaken for the T wave. The apparent QT interval is in fact the QU interval.

Modest degrees of hypokalemia are associated with mild skeletal muscle weakness and ileus, but more marked degrees of hypokalemia lead to flaccid paralysis. In general, chronic potassium depletion results in fewer and less severe neuromuscular changes than acute hypokalemia. In severe cases, respiratory muscle paralysis may cause apnea and death. Severe hypokalemia with a plasma potassium concentration of less than 2.0 mEq/liter can lead to rhabdomyolysis and acute renal failure.

Potassium deficiency has important effects on the kidney. Renal concentrating ability and responsiveness to antidiuretic hormone are both reduced. Potassium deficiency also results in increased hydrogen ion secretion and development of maintenance of metabolic alkalosis. In addition, potassium deficiency is an important stimulus to renal ammoniagenesis and increases in urinary ammonium excretion, ammonia concentrations in the renal vein, and systemic circulation. The increase in ammonia production is important in patients with severe hepatic cirrhosis in whom potassium deficiency can precipitate hepatic coma. In this case, the patient's mental status may improve markedly simply through correction of the potassium deficit. Potassium deficiency also leads to renal structural alterations. Some are reversible, but chronic potassium depletion is probably never the sole cause of serious renal insufficiency.

Therapy

The initial step in the therapy of hypokalemia is determination of whether the hypokalemia is due to redistribution alone or whether, as is usually the case, potassium depletion exists with it. In either case, the underlying cause should be identified and, if possible, corrected while potassium deficits and ongoing losses are replaced. Estimating the magnitude of total body potassium deficits is neither easy nor precise. If there are no confounding abnormalities in internal potassium balance, an estimate of the deficit can be derived from the plasma potassium concentration (Fig. 17-3). However, such an estimate should be used only as a rough guideline to therapy. Total body potassium deficits may become very large before they are recognized and not infrequently amount to many hundreds of milliequivalents of potassium.

For hyperkalemia to be avoided, oral potassium replacement over a period of several days is desirable whenever possible. If intravenous therapy is unavoidable, as in the postoperative patient, potassium in concentrations of no more than 40 to 60 mEq/liter should be administered at a rate of no more than 10 to 20 mEq/hr. If a higher rate is necessary because of life-threatening symptoms in a severely hypokalemic patient, the electrocardiogram should be monitored continuously and frequent determinations of plasma potassium concentration should be made. Particular caution must be exercised in the administration of potassium to patients with renal insufficiency or other defects in renal potassium excretion.

The choice of the potassium salt used to replace the deficit is extremely important. In the usual situation of concomitant metabolic alkalosis, potassium must be replaced as potassium chloride. A bicarbonate salt equivalent such as citrate or gluconate will not correct the deficit because the bicarbonate load leads to further urinary potassium loss. However, when potassium deficiency is associated with metabolic acidosis, as in renal tubular acidosis or diarrhea, potassium bicarbonate or a potassium bicarbonate equivalent can be used effectively.

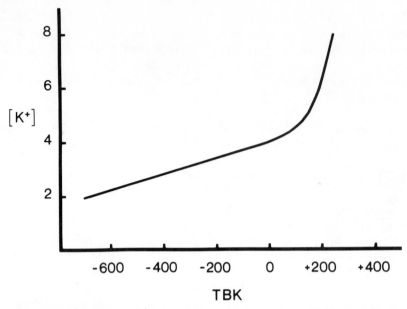

Fig. 17-3. Changes in plasma potassium concentration ($[K^+]$) (meq/liter) due to alterations in total body potassium content *(TBK)* (meq).

SUMMARY

Volume

1. The renal response to surgery and trauma is retention of sodium and water.
2. Intravascular volume depletion can accompany either decreased ECF volume, as in blood loss, third-space sequestration or sodium depletion, or increased ECF volume, as in hypoalbuminemia.
3. Renal sodium depletion can be seen in uncontrolled diabetes, postobstructive diuresis, and recovery from acute tubular necrosis or after the use of mannitol and other diuretics.
4. Surgical patients may suffer extensive sodium losses from the gastrointestinal tract or in serous drainage from wounds or burns.
5. Chronic hypoalbuminemia is generally characterized by a normal intravascular volume and edema. Acute hypoalbuminemia is characterized by hypotension.
6. Therapy of the sodium-depleted patient depends on the magnitude of the deficit, the rapidity of its development, ongoing losses, and associated disturbances in acid–base and potassium homeostasis.
7. Losses should be estimated by calculation of the electrolyte composition and volume of all fluids lost.
8. Dietary and intravenous fluid management should be closely monitored in patients with cardiac, renal, and liver disease in order for intravascular volume expansion to be avoided.
9. Diuretics should be employed with particular caution in patients with hepatic cirrhosis.

Tonicity

1. Hypotonicity usually accompanies hyponatremia. However, if the ECF contains a large amount of glucose, mannitol, lipids, or protein, hyponatremia can exist without hypotonicity.
2. Because surgical patients may not have free access to water and may have changes in ADH release, they may not be able to respond appropriately to changes in tonicity.
3. Hypotonicity can occur in association with decreased, increased, or normal total body sodium content (ECF volume).
4. Therapy for the hypotonic edematous patient includes water and sodium restriction. Diuretics should be used cautiously.
5. The syndrome of inappropriate ADH should be suspected in patients with hyponatremia and a urinary osmolality of more than 100 mOsm/g. All patients exhibiting hypotonicity and normal total body sodium, regardless of cause, should be water-restricted.
6. Serum sodium concentrations of less than 120 mEq/liter can be life-threatening. If symptoms are mild, isotonic saline followed by furosemide should be administered. If symptoms are severe, 3% saline or hypertonic mannitol is indicated. Acute pulmonary edema and intracranial hemorrhage are complications of this therapy.
7. Hypertonicity with normal total body sodium may result from inadequate water intake or diabetes insipidus.
8. Hypertonicity with increased total body sodium is usually produced by hypertonic solutions. Its major risk is cerebral dehydration.
9. Hypertonicity with decreased total body sodium is usually due to gastrointestinal losses, diuretics, or osmotic diuresis.
10. The rapidity with which water deficits are replaced depends on the severity of the hypertonicity. Aggressive treatment can produce cerebral edema. Half the calculated deficit may be replaced as 5% dextrose in water over a few hours; the remainder can be replaced within the next 48 hr. If total body sodium is increased, furosemide should be administered. If total body sodium is decreased, stabilization of blood pressure is paramount.

Potassium

1. Two pre-eminent factors affect potassium homeostasis in the surgical patient: (1) the potential for increased entry of potassium into the ECF compartment resulting from enhanced catabolism or cell necrosis, and (2) the potential for decreased potassium excretion due to either reversible defects (e.g., volume depletion) or more long-term defects (e.g., acute tubular necrosis) in renal function.
2. Internal potassium balance is affected by acid–base status, insulin, aldosterone, epinephrine, body-fluid tonicity, pharmacologic agents, and acute changes in cell mass.
3. A normal or low potassium concentration in a severely hypertonic patient raises the probability of total body potassium depletion.
4. Hypokalemia due to kaliuresis may be caused by ECF volume expansion, diuretics, osmotic diuresis, acute tubular necrosis, hyperaldosteronism, or urinary tract obstruction.
5. Hypokalemia may also result from gastrointestinal losses.

6. Hypokalemia should be treated with oral potassium whenever possible. If intravenous therapy is unavoidable, potassium in concentrations of no more than 60 mEq/liter should be administered no faster than 20 mEq/hr.

7. Situations that aggravate hyperkalemia should be promptly recognized. Exogenous potassium intake should be carefully monitored, particularly in patients with abnormal renal potassium excretion.

8. Patients with impaired renal potassium excretory capacity who become volume-depleted and oliguric almost always develop hyperkalemia. Appropriate attention to volume status is therefore of paramount importance.

9. The cardiac manifestations of hyperkalemia can be most rapidly reversed with calcium. Further treatment is summarized in Table 17-9.

REFERENCES

1. Geheb M, Singer I, Cox M: Clinical disorders of sodium and water homeostasis. In McDonald FD (ed); Progress in Clinical Kidney Disease and Hypertension. New York, Thieme-Stratton, 1980

2. Shizgal HM, Solomon S, Gutelius JR: Body water distribution after operation. Surg Gynecol Obstet 144:35, 1977

3. Irvin TT, Modgill VK, Hayter CJ et al: Plasma volume deficits and salt and water excretion after surgery. Lancet 2:7788, 1972

4. Shires GT, Canizaro PS: Fluid resuscitation in the severely injured. Surg Clin North Am 53:1341, 1973

5. Cochrane JPS: The aldosterone response to surgery and the relationship of this response to postoperative sodium retention. Br J Surg 65:744, 1978

6. Harrington JT, Cohen JJ: Acute oliguria. N Engl J Med 292:89, 1975

7. Seldin DW: Sodium balance and fluid volume. In Bricker NS (ed): The Sea Within Us. Puerto Rico, Searle, 1975

8. Cuono CB: Early management of severe thermal injury. Surg Clin North Am 60:1021, 1980

9. Beck LH: Edema states and use of diuretics. Med Clin North Am 65:291, 1981

10. Gennari FJ, Kassirer JP: Osmotic diuresis. N Engl J Med 291:714, 1974

11. Howards S: Post-obstructive diuresis: A misunderstood phenomena. J Urol 110:537, 1973

12. Beck LH, Stein JH, Earley LE: Obstructive uropathy. In Earley LE, Gottschalk CW (eds): Straus and Welt's Diseases of the Kidney, 3rd ed, Boston, Little, Brown & Co, 1979

13. Anderson RJ, Schrier RW: Clinical spectrum of oliguric and non-oliguric acute renal failure. In Brenner BM, Stein JH (eds): Contemporary Issues in Nephrology, Vol 6. New York, Churchill Livingstone, 1980

14. Grossman RA: Oliguria and acute renal failure. Med Clin North Am 65:413, 1981

15. Danovitch GM, Bourgoigni J, Bricker NS: Reversibility of the "salt-losing" tendency of chronic renal failure. N Engl J Med 296:14, 1977

16. Phillips SF: Water and electrolytes in gastrointestinal diseases. In Maxwell MH, Kleeman CH (eds): Clinical disorders of fluid and electrolyte metabolism. New York, McGraw-Hill, 1980

17. Randall NT: Fluid, electrolyte and acid base balance. Surg Clin North Am 56:1019, 1976

18. Seldin DW, Rector FC: The generation and maintenance of metabolic alkalosis. Kidney Int. 1:306, 1972

19. Tullis JL: Albumin. JAMA 237:355, 1977

20. Worthley LIG: Principles of pre-operative fluid therapy and resuscitation. Anaesth Intensive Care 5:316–332, 1977

21. Davidson, GM: Intra-operative fluid and

electrolyte requirements. Anaesth Intensive Care 5:333, 1977

22. Fisher M: Postoperative intravenous therapy. Anaesth Intensive Care 5:339, 1977

23. Weaver DW, Ledgewood AM, Lucas CE et al: Pulmonary effects of albumin. Arch Surg 113:387, 1978

24. Bouwan DL, Weaver DW, Vega J et al: Effects of albumin on serum protein homeostasis after hypovolemic shock. J Surg Res 24:229, 1978

25. Garella S, Chang BS, Kahn S: Dilution acidosis and contraction alkalosis. Review of a concept. Kidney Int 8:279, 1975

26. Morrison G, Murray T: Electrolyte, acid base, and fluid homeostasis in chronic renal failure. Med Clin North Am 65:429, 1981

27. Agus Z, Goldberg M: Renal function in congestive heart failure. In Levine HJ (ed): Clinical Cardiovascular Physiology. New York, Grune & Stratton, 1976

28. Cannon PJ: The kidney in heart failure. N Engl J Med 296:26, 1977

29. Conn HO: A rational approach to the hepatorenal syndrome. Gastroenterology 65:321, 1973

30. Levy M: The kidney in liver disease. In Brenner BM, Stein JH (eds): Sodium and Water Homeostasis, p 73. New York, Churchill Livingstone, 1978

31. Forrester JS, Waters DD: Hospital treatment of congestive heart failure. Am J Med 65:173, 1978

32. Chatterjee K, Massie B, Rubin S et al: Long-term outpatient vasodilator therapy of congestive heart failure. Am J Med 65:134, 1978

33. Schrier RW, Anderson RJ: Renal sodium excretion, edematous disorders, and diuretic use. In Schrier RW (ed): Renal and electrolyte disorders, 2nd ed. Boston, Little, Brown & Co, 1980

34. Suki WN, Ny RCK: Rational use of diuretics. In McDonald FD (ed): Progress in Clinical Kidney Disease and Hypertension. New York, Thieme-Stratton, 1980

35. Gabow PA, Moore S, Schrier RW: Spironolactone-induced hyperchloremic acidosis in cirrhosis. Ann Intern Med 90:338, 1979

36. Baumber CD, Clark RG: Insensible water loss in surgical patients. Br J Surg 61:53, 1974

37. Goldberg M: Hyponatremia. Med Clin North Am 65:251, 1981

38. Schrier RW, Berl T: Disorders of water homeostasis. In Schrier RW (ed): Renal and electrolyte disorders, 2nd ed. Boston, Little, Brown & Co, 1980

39. Fitzsimons JT: The physiological basis of thirst. Kidney Int 10:3, 1976

40. Andersson B: Regulation of water intake. Phys Rev 58:582, 1978

41. Hays RM: Antidiuretic hormone. N Engl J Med 295:659, 1976

42. Robertson GL, Shelton RL, Athar S: The osmoregulation of vasopressin. Kidney Int 10:25, 1976

43. Zerbe RL, Vinicor F, Robertson GL: Plasma vasopressin in uncontrolled diabetes mellitus. Diabetes 28:503, 1979

44. Sinnatamby C, Edwards CRW, Kitau M et al: Antidiuretic hormone response to high and conservative fluid regimes in patients undergoing operation. Surg Gynecol Obstet 139:715, 1974

45. Robertson GL: The regulation of vasopressin function in health and disease. Recent Prog Horm Res 33:333, 1977

46. Kendler KS, Weitzman RE, Fisher DA: The effect of pain on plasma arginine vasopressin concentrations in man. Clin Endocrinol 8:89, 1978

47. White WA, Berglan RM: Experimental inappropriate ADH secretion caused by positive pressure respirators. J Neurosurg 36:608, 1972

48. Goldberg M: Water control and the dysnatremias. In Bricker NS (ed): The Sea Within Us. Puerto Rico, Searle, 1975

49. Bartter FC: The syndrome of inappropriate secretion of antidiuretic hormone (SIADH). DM November, 1978

50. Zerbe R, Strapes L, Robertson G: Vaso-

pressin function in the syndrome of inappropriate antidiuresis. Annu Rev Med 31:315, 1980

51. Derubertis FR, Michelis M, Bloom ME et al: Impaired water excretion in myxedema. Am J Med 51:41, 1971

52. DiScala VA, Kinney MJ: Effects of myxdema on the renal diluting and concentrating mechanism. Am J Med 50:325, 1971

53. Skowsky WR, Kikuchi TA: The role of vasopressin in the impaired water excretion of myxedema. Am J Med 64:613, 1978

54. Agus ZS, Goldberg M: Role of antidiuretic hormone in the abnormal water diuresis of anterior hypopituitarism in man. J Clin Invest 50:1478, 1971

55. Schwartz MJ, Kokko JP: Urinary concentrating defect of adrenal insufficiency. J Clin Invest 66:234, 1980

56. Forrest JN Jr, Cox M, Hong C et al: Superiority of demeclocycline over lithium in the treatment of chronic syndrome of inappropriate secretion of antidiuretic hormone. N Engl J Med 298:173, 1978

57. Geheb M, Cox M: Renal effects of demeclocyline. JAMA 243:2519, 1980

58. Miller PD, Linas SL, Schrier RW: Plasma demeclocycline levels and nephrotoxicity. JAMA 243:2513, 1980

59. DeFronzo RA, Goldberg M, Agus ZS: Normal diluting capacity in hyponatremic patients. Ann Intern Med 84:538, 1976

60. Epstein FH: Signs and symptoms of electrolyte disorders. In Maxwell MH, Kleeman CR (eds): Clinical disorders of fluid and electrolyte metabolism, 3rd ed. New York, McGraw-Hill, 1980

61. Hantman D, Rossier B, Zohlman R et al: Rapid correction of hyponatremia in the syndrome of inappropriate secretion of antidiuretic hormone. Ann Intern Med 78:870, 1973

62. Feig PU, McCurdy DK: The hypertonic state. N Engl J Med 297:1444, 1977

63. Covey CM, Ariff AI: Disorders of sodium and water metabolism and their effect on the central nervous system. In Brenner BM, Stein JH (eds): Sodium and Water Homeostasis. New York, Churchill-Livingstone, 1978

64. Cox M: Diabetes insipidus In Conn HO (ed): Current Therapy. WB Saunders, Philadelphia, 1978

65. Shucart WA, Jackson I: Management of diabetes insipidus in neurosurgical patients. J Neurosurg 44:65, 1976

66. Forrest JN Jr, Singer I: Drug-induced interference with action of antidiuretic hormone. In Andredi TE, Grantham JJ, Rector FC Jr (eds): Disturbances in Body Fluid Osmolality, p 309. Baltimore, Williams & Wilkins, 1977

67. Barbour GL, Straub KD, O'Neal BL et al: Vasopressin-resistant nephrogenic diabetes insipidus. A result of amphotericin-B therapy. Arch Intern Med 139:86, 1979

68. Singer I: Differential diagnosis of polyuria and diabetes insipidus. Med Clin North Am 65:303, 1981

69. Miller M, Dalakas T, Moses AM et al: Recognition of partial defects of antidiuretic hormone secretion. Ann Intern Med 73:721, 1970

70. McCurdy DK: Hyperosmolar hyperglycemic nonketotic diabetic coma. Med Clin North Am 54:683, 1970

71. Feig PU: Hypernatremia and hypertonic syndrome. Med Clin North Am 65:271, 1981

72. Sterns RH, Cox M, Feig PU et al: Internal potassium balance and the control of the plasma potassium concentration. Medicine (in press)

73. Bia MJ, DeFronzo RA: Extrarenal potassium homeostasis. Am J Physiol 240:F257, 1981

74. Leibman J, Edelman IS: Interrelations of plasma potassium concentration, plasma sodium concentration, arterial pH and total exchangeable potassium. J Clin Invest 38:2176, 1959

75. Oster JR, Perez GO, Castro A et al: Plasma potassium response to acute metabolic acidosis induced by mineral and nonmineral acids. Mineral Electrolyte Metabolism 4:28, 1980

76. Fulop M: Serum potassium in lactic aci-

dosis and ketoacidosis. N Engl J Med 200:1087, 1979

77. Orringer CE, Eustace JC, Wunsch CD et al: Natural history of lactic acidosis after grand-mal seizures. A model for the study of an anion-gap acidosis not associated with hyperkalemia. N Engl J Med 297:796, 1977

78. Rograve HJ, Alabaster S: Lactic acidosis in seizures. N Engl J Med 297:1352, 1977

79. Fraley DS, Adler S: Isohydric regulation of plasma potassium by bicarbonate in the rat. Kidney Int 9:333, 1976

80. Fraley DS, Adler S: Correction of hyperkalemia by bicarbonate despite constant blood pH. Kidney Int 12:354, 1977

81. Cox M, Sterns RH, Singer I: The defense against hyperkalemia: The roles of insulin and aldosterone. N Engl J Med 299:525, 1978

82. DeFronzo R, Felig P, Ferrannini E, Wahren J: Effects of graded doses of insulin on splanchnic and peripheral potassium metabolism in man. Am J Physiol 238:E421, 1980

83. Zierler KL, Rabinowitz D: Effect of very small concentrations of insulin on forearm metabolism: Persistence of its action on potassium and free fatty acids without its effect on glucose. J Clin Invest 43:950, 1964

84. DeFronzo RA, Sherwin RS, Dillingham M et al: Influence of basal insulin and glucagon secretion on potassium and sodium metabolism: Studies with somatostatin in normal dogs and in normal and diabetic human beings. J Clin Invest 61:472, 1978

85. DeFronzo RA, Sherwin RS, Felig P et al: Nonuremic diabetic hyperkalemia. Possible role of insulin deficiency. Arch Intern Med 137:842, 1977

86. Rosa RM, Silva P, Young JB et al: Adrenergic modulation of extrarenal potassium disposal. N Engl J Med 302:431, 1980

87. DeFronzo RA, Birkhead G, Bia M: The effect of epinephrine on potassium homeostasis in man. Kidney Int 16:917, 1979

88. Hiatt N, Chapman LW, Davidson MB et al: Adrenal hormones and the regulation of serum potassium in potassium-loaded adrenalectomized dogs. Endocrinology 105:215, 1979

89. Leitch AG, Clancy LJ, Costello JF et al: Effect of intravenous infusion of salbutamol on ventilatory response to carbon dioxide and hypoxia and on heart rate and plasma potassium in normal man. Br Med J 1:365, 1976

90. Traub YM, Rabinov M, Rosenfeld JB et al: Elevation of serum potassium during beta blockage: Absence of relationship to the renin–aldosterone system. Clin Pharmacol Ther 28:765, 1980

91. Makoff DL, DaSilva JA, Rosenbaum BJ et al: Hypertonic expansion: Acid–base and electrolyte changes. Am J Physiol 218:1201, 1970

92. Makoff DL, Dasilva JA, Rosenbaum BJ: On the mechanism of hyperkalemia due to hyperosmotic expansion with saline and mannitol. Clin Sci 41:383, 1971

93. Tarail R, Seldin DW, Goodyer AVN: Effects of hypertonic glucose on metabolism of water and electrolytes in patients with edema. J Clin Invest 30:1111, 1951

94. Goldfarb S, Cox M, Singer I et al: Acute hyperkalemia induced by hyperglycemia: Hormonal mechanisms. Ann Intern Med 84:426, 1976

95. Santeusio F, Faloona GR, Knochel JP et al: Evidence for a role of endogenous insulin and glucagon in the regulation of potassium homeostasis. J Lab Clin Med 81:809, 1973

96. Viberti GC: Glucose-induced hyperkalemia: A hazard for diabetics. Lancet 1:690, 1978

97. Ammon RA, May WS, Nightingale SD: Glucose-induced hyperkalemia with normal aldosterone levels. Studies in a patient with diabetes mellitus. Ann Intern Med 89:349, 1978

98. Nicolis GL, Kahn T, Sanchez A et al: Glucose-induced hyperkalemia in diabetic subjects. Arch Intern Med 141:49, 1981

99. Popp D, Achtenberg JF, Cryer PE: Hyperkalemia and hyperglycemic increments

in plasma potassium in diabetes mellitus. Arch Intern Med 146:1617, 1980

100. Perez GO, Lespier L, Knowles R et al: Potassium homeostasis in chronic diabetes mellitus. Arch Intern Med 137:1018, 1977

101. Walker BR, Capuzzi DM, Alexander F et al: Hyperkalemia after triamterene in diabetic patients. Clin Pharmacol Ther 13:643, 1972

102. McNay JL, Oran E: Possible perdisposition of diabetic patients to hyperkalemia following administration of potassium-retaining diuretic, amiloride. Metabolism 19:58, 1970

103. Smith TW, Haber E, Yeatman L et al: Reversal of advanced digoxin intoxication with FAB fragments of digoxin-specific antibodies. N Engl J Med 294:797, 1976

104. Gronert GA, Theye RA: Pathophysiology of hyperkalemia induced by succinylcholine. Anesthesiology 43:89, 1975

105. Bushinsky DA, Gennari FJ: Life-threatening hyperkalemia induced by arginine. Ann Intern Med 89:632, 1978

106. Arseneau JC, Bagley CL, Anderson T et al: Hyperkalemia, a sequel to chemotherapy of Burkitt's lymphoma. Lancet 1:10, 1973

107. Grossman RA, Hamilton RW, Morse BM et al: Nontraumatic rhabdomyolysis and acute renal failure. N Engl J Med 291:897, 1974

108. Hesp R, Chanarin I, Tait CE: Potassium changes in megaloblastic anemia. Clin Sci Molec Med 49:77, 1975

109. Vogel CM, Kingsbury RJ, Barre AE: Intravenous hyperalimentation. A review of two and one-half year's experience. Arch Surg 105:414, 1972

110. Cox M: Potassium homeostasis. Med Clin North Am 65:363, 1981

111. Cohen JJ, Gennari FJ, Harrington JT: Disorders of potassium balance. In Brenner BM, Rector FC Jr (eds): The Kidney, 2nd ed, Vol 1, p 908. Philadelphia, WB Saunders, 1981

112. Schultze RG, Nissenson AR: Potassium: Physiology and pathophysiology. In Maxwell MH, Kleeman CR (eds): Clinical Disorders of Fluid and Electrolyte Metabolism, 3rd ed, p 113. New York, McGraw-Hill, 1980

113. Sopko JA, Freeman RM: Salt substitutes as a source of potassium. JAMA 238:608, 1977

114. Lawson DH: Adverse reactions to potassium chloride. Q J Med 43:443, 1974

115. Bostic O, Duvernoy WFC: Hyperkalemic cardiac arrest during transfusion of stored blood. J Electrocardiol 5:407, 1972

116. Moss MH, Rasen AR: Potassium toxicity due to intravenous penicillin therapy. Pediatrics 29:1032, 1962

117. Black DAK, Milne MD: Experimental potassium depletion in man. Clin Sci 11:397, 1952

118. Squires RD, Huth EJ: Experimental potassium depletion in normal human subjects. I. Relation of ionic intakes to the renal conservation of potassium. J Clin Invest 38:1134, 1959

119. Himathongham T, Dluhy R, Williams G: Potassium–aldosterone–renin interrelationships. J Clin Endocrinol Metab 41:153, 1975

120. Gonick ND, Kleeman CR, Rubini ME et al: Functional impairment in chronic renal disease. III. Studies of potassium excretion. Am J Med Sci 261:281, 1971

121. Giebisch G, Malnic G, Berliner RW: Renal transport and control of potassium excretion. In Brenner BM, Rector FC Jr (eds): The Kidney, 2nd ed, Vol 1, p 408. Philadelphia, WB Saunders, 1981

122. Wright FS, Giebesch G: Renal potassium transport: Contributions of individual nephron segments and populations. Am J Physiol 235:F515, 1978

123. Van Ypersele de Strihou C: Potassium homeostasis in renal failure. Kidney Int 11:491, 1977

124. Battle DC, Arruda JAL, Kurtzman NA: Hyperkalemic distal renal tubular aci-

dosis associated with obstructive urop-athy. N Engl J Med 304:373, 1981

125. Silva P, Brown RS, Epstein RH: Adaptation to potassium. Kidney Int 11:466, 1977

126. DeFronzo RA: Hyperkalemia and hyporeninemic hypoaldosteronism. Kidney Int 17:118, 1980

127. Tan SY, Burton M: Hyporeninemic hypoaldosteronism. An overlooked cause of hyperkalemia. Arch Intern Med 141:30, 1981

128. Schambelan M, Sebastian A, Biglieri EG: Prevalence, pathogenesis, and functional significance of aldosterone deficiency in hyperkalemic patients with chronic renal insufficiency. Kidney Int 17:89, 1980

129. Phelps KR, Lieberman RL, Oh MS et al: Pathophysiology of the syndrome of hyporeninemic hypoaldosteronism. Metabolism 29:186, 1980

130. Tan SY, Shapiro R, Franco R et al: Indomethacin-induced prostaglandin inhibition with hyperkalemia. A reversible cause of hyperreninemic hypoaldosteronism. Ann Intern Med 90:783, 1979

131. Gussin RZ: Potassium-sparing diuretics. J Clin Pharmacol 17:651, 1977

132. DeFronzo RA, Cooke CR, Goldberg M et al: Impaired renal tubular potassium secretion in systemic lupus erythematosus 86:268, 1977

133. Luke RG, Allison MEM, Davidson JF et al: Hyperkalemia and renal tubular acidosis due to renal amyloidosis. Ann Intern Med 70:1211, 1969

134. Popovtzer MM, Katz FH, Pinggera WF et al: Hyperkalemia in salt-wasting nephropathy. Study of the mechanism. Arch Intern Med 132:203, 1973

135. DeFronzo RA, Goldberg M, Cooke CR et al: Investigation into the mechanisms of hyperkalemia following renal transplantation. Kidney Int 11:357, 1977

136. Gennari FS, Cohen JJ: Role of the kidney in potassium homeostasis: Lessons from acid–base disturbances. Kidney Int 8:1, 1975

137. Narins RG, Goldberg M: Renal tubular acidosis: Pathophysiology, diagnosis and treatment. DM 23(6):1, 1977

138. Kidd GS, Donowitz M, O'Doriso T et al: Mild chronic watery diarrhea–hypokalemia syndrome associated with pancreatic islet cell hyperplasia. Am J Med 66:883, 1979

139. Hodin E, Remington JH: Villous adenoma with severe electrolyte depletion. Dis Colon Rectum 12:36, 1969

140. Cummings JH, Sladen GE, James OFW et al: Laxative-induced diarrhea: A continued clinical problem. Br Med J 1:537, 1974

141. Stamey TS: The pathogenesis and implications of the electrolyte imbalance in ureterosigmoidostomy. Surg Gynecol Obstet 103:736, 1956

142. Brown JJ: Falsely high plasma potassium values in patients with hyperaldosteronism. Br Med J 2:18, 1970

143. Frank JJ, Bermes EW, Bickel MJ et al: Effect of in vitro hemolysis on chemical values for serum. Clin Chem 24:1966, 1978

144. Chumley LC: Pseudohyperkalemia in acute myelocytotic leukemia. JAMA 211:1007, 1970

145. Hartman RC, Auditore JV, Jackson DP: Studies on thrombocytosis. I. Hyperkalemia due to release of potassium from platelets during coagulation. J Clin Invest 37:699, 1958

146. Myerson RM, Truman AM: Hyperkalemia associated with the myeloproliferative disorders. Arch Intern Med 106:479, 1960

18

Acid–Base Disturbances in the Surgical Patient

ARTHUR GREENBERG
STANLEY GOLDFARB

Acid–base disturbances commonly arise in the perioperative period. Proper therapy requires a thorough understanding of the multiple etiologies and pathophysiology involved. This chapter first reviews basic acid–base terminology and physiology. The various causes and treatment of specific acid–base disturbances are then fully discussed with particular attention to those pertinent to the surgical setting.

ACID–BASE TERMINOLOGY

Blood pH is closely regulated in the range between 7.38 and 7.42. Although there are a number of intracellular and extracellular buffer systems, including hemoglobin, cellular proteins, and bone, the principal extracellular fluid (ECF) buffer system is the carbonic acid–bicarbonate system, which may be depicted as follows.

$$H^+ + HCO_3^- \leftrightharpoons H_2CO_3 \leftrightharpoons CO_2 + H_2O$$

The Henderson–Hasselbalch equation describes the role of this system in regulating blood pH and maintaining it around 7.4.

$$pH = 6.1 + \log \frac{[HCO_3]}{0.03 \times P_{CO_2}}$$

Normally, pH

$$= 6.1 + \log \frac{[24 \text{ mEq/liter}]}{[1.2 \text{ moles/liter}]}$$

$$pH = 6.1 + \log \frac{20}{1} \text{ (or 1.3)} = 7.4$$

The ratio of bicarbonate to dissolved CO_2 must remain 20:1 to ensure normal blood pH. States that tend to alter pH by primarily affecting bicarbonate concentration are *metabolic disturbances*, and those that primarily affect P_{CO_2} are *respiratory disturbances*. Factors that lower pH lead to *acidosis*; those that raise pH bring about *alkalosis*. The terms *acidemia* and *alkalemia* refer to the measured arterial pH and reflect the sum of the effects of acidosis or alkalosis that may be present alone or in combination.

Because it is an open system, carbonic acid–bicarbonate buffering is particularly effective. New CO_2 formed by titration of bicarbonate during metabolic acidosis is rapidly excreted by the lungs, thereby decreasing the perturbation in the HCO_3:CO_2 ratio. The open buffer system allows for respiratory compensation for metabolic disturbances and metabolic compensation for respiratory disturbances. For example, acidemia serves as a potent respiratory stimulant, and reduced blood pH and bicarbonate concentration in metabolic acidosis lead to hyperventilation. The P_{CO_2} decreases and the pH rises toward normal as the HCO_3:CO_2 ratio of 20:1 is re-established. Similarly, hypercapnia increases renal bicarbonate generation. When respiratory failure causes a rise in P_{CO_2} with respiratory acidosis, the kidney compensates by generating more bicarbonate.

In a simple acid–base disturbance, only the primary process, whether metabolic or respiratory, and its expected compensation are operating. The pH reflects the nature of the primary process. In a mixed acid–base disturbance, two or more primary processes are working simultaneously. The pH may be increased, decreased, or normal, depending on the magnitude of each individual disturbance. Since compensation is incomplete, the pH is never normal in a simple disturbance, the sole exception being chronic respiratory alkalosis.

It is important for the physician to identify each acid–base disturbance separately in order to choose the appropriate therapy. McCurdy and Narins and Emmett have elegantly described a method for accurately diagnosing mixed acid–base disturbances.[1,2] A useful short-cut is provided by one of the published acid–base nomograms (Fig. 18-1).[3] If values fall within one of the shaded areas, a simple disturbance is likely. If the point falls outside any of the shaded areas, there is a 95% chance that the disturbance is mixed.

CARDIOVASCULAR EFFECTS OF ACIDEMIA AND ALKALEMIA

Mild acidemia and alkalemia are well tolerated, but marked deviation of the blood pH from normal may profoundly alter cardiovascular function and cellular metabolism.[4,5] Although acidemia reduces myocardial contractility, little clinical effect is seen until the pH falls below 7.2. Since acidemia also induces release of catecholamines, much of the direct depressant effect is mitigated in mild acidemia. However, when the pH is below 7.1, cardiac responsiveness to catecholamines decreases and compensatory inotropy is diminished.

Patients treated with beta adrenergic blocking agents may be more sensitive than normal to mild degrees of acidemia. At low pH, vagal tone increases owing to inhibition of acetylcholinesterase, and, when pH falls below 7.1, the risk of bradycardia and cardiac arrest rises. Hyperkalemia induced by acidosis may further increase the likelihood of these disorders. Acidemia also leads to venoconstriction and may further compromise cardiac function in patients with increased ventricular preload. This effect is partly offset by a decrease in ventricular afterload, since acidemia leads to systemic arterial vasodilation.

The direct effects of alkalemia on cardiac contractility are less striking than those of acidemia. Alkalemia-induced decreases in serum potassium and ionized calcium increase myocardial irritability. This is especially important in digitalized patients, since the effects of digitalis and hypokalemia in producing arrhythmias are additive.

CENTRAL NERVOUS SYSTEM EFFECTS OF ACID–BASE DISTURBANCES

Intracerebral blood flow and intracerebral or cerebrospinal fluid (CSF) pH affect central nervous system (CNS) function and are sensitive to metabolic changes induced by acidosis or alkalosis. Low intracerebral pH decreases cerebrovascular resistance and increases cerebral blood

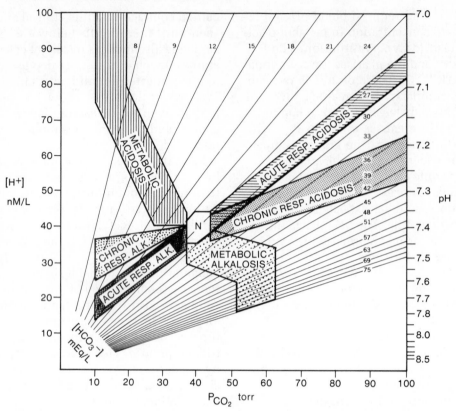

Fig. 18-1. This acid-base nomogram is used to ascertain whether a given set of values, determined by arterial blood gas analysis, represents a simple or a mixed acid-base disturbance. Values for pH, P_{CO_2}, and HCO_3 are provided by the laboratory. The point at which any two values intersect is then evaluated in relation to the shaded areas. These areas represent the confidence limits, as determined by review of the literature, for the predicted response of a group of persons to a given perturbation in P_{CO_2} (respiratory disturbances) or HCO_3 (metabolic disturbances). If a value falls outside a shaded area, a mixed disturbance is likely. The nomogram may also be used to verify that the laboratory has properly calculated the HCO_3 value from the directly measured pH and P_{CO_2} values. See Goldberg et al[3] for details regarding the use of the nomogram.

flow, whereas elevated intracerebral pH has the opposite effect.[4] The blood-brain barrier permits free diffusion of dissolved CO_2 but retards passage of bicarbonate. During periods of rapid systemic acid–base changes, P_{CO_2} rather than systemic pH or bicarbonate concentration is the principal determinant of the pH of the CSF and ce-

rebral interstitium. When P_{CO_2} falls, pH and vascular resistance rise, and cerebral blood flow decreases. Impaired oxygen delivery and CNS dysfunction may therefore follow rapidly developing respiratory alkalosis or rapid respiratory compensation for acute metabolic acidosis with a fall in P_{CO_2}. Independent of changes in cerebral blood flow, a decrease in CSF pH leads to cerebral dysfunction. Therefore, acute respiratory acidosis can affect CNS function despite its effect in increasing cerebral blood flow. Findings in this disorder include decreased mentation, personality changes, asterixis, lethargy, and coma.

With time, there is equilibration of bicarbonate across the blood-brain barrier. Cerebrovascular tone and CSF pH then reflect what is shown systemically by both serum bicarbonate concentration and P_{CO_2}. Although blood flow is increased by chronic respiratory or metabolic acidosis, the low pH alone may depress brain function. In chronic respiratory or metabolic alkalosis, diminished blood flow and elevated pH lead to CNS dysfunction.

METABOLIC ALKALOSIS

The generation and maintenance of metabolic alkalosis occur as separate processes.[6] Although metabolic alkalosis may develop as a transient response to rapid administration of base or loss of acid, it persists only if renal excretion of excess base is deficient. The factors responsible for generation and maintenance of metabolic alkalosis are listed below.

GENERATION
Gain of alkali
    $NaHCO_3$: oral or parenteral
    Infusion of organic acid anions
        Lactate (lactated Ringer's solution)
        Citrate (acid citrate dextrose anticoagulated blood)
        Acetate (intravenous hyperalimentation, purified protein fraction)
    Rapid correction of hypercapnia

Loss of acid
    Renal (mineralocorticoid excess with potassium depletion)
        Primary hyperaldosteronism
        Secondary hyperaldosteronism
        Bartter's syndrome
    Gastrointestinal
        Nasogastric suctioning
        Vomiting
MAINTENANCE
    Decreased filtration of bicarbonate (renal failure)
    Increased reabsorption of bicarbonate
        Volume depletion
        Potassium depletion with mineralocorticoid excess
        Severe potassium deficiency
        Chloride depletion
        Elevated P_{CO_2}

Oral or parenteral administration of alkali in the form of bicarbonate or as organic anions such as acetate, citrate or, lactate, which are readily metabolized to bicarbonate, raises serum bicarbonate levels. Given that 1 mEq of bicarbonate is produced for each milliequivalent of gastric acid secreted, loss of gastric acid by vomiting or gastric aspiration has a similar effect.

The kidney is another source of bicarbonate production. In the distal nephron, sodium is reabsorbed in exchange for secreted potassium or hydrogen ions. Since secreted hydrogen ion is buffered by phosphate as titratable acid or by ammonia as ammonium ion, 1 mEq of bicarbonate is retained for each milliequivalent of hydrogen ion secreted. Volume depletion stimulates sodium reabsorption directly, as does hypermineralocorticism, whether due to primary aldosteronism, secondary aldosteronism from volume depletion or hyperreninism, or exogenously administered mineralocorticoid or glucocorticoid.

Potassium depletion frequently complicates hypermineralocorticism or diuretic-induced volume depletion. In this circumstance, potassium is less readily available for secretion than normal, and acid excretion is further enhanced.

In patients who develop severe hypercapnia, bicarbonate concentration in the blood rises through compensatory renal generation. If the hypercapnia is corrected rapidly with mechanical ventilation, bicarbonate levels remain elevated despite normalization of P_{CO_2}. This phenomenon, termed posthypercapnic metabolic alkalosis, resolves over 2 to 3 days, provided that bicarbonaturia is unimpaired. It is a common problem in patients in medical or surgical intensive care units.

It has been suggested that contraction of the extracellular volume around a fixed quantity of bicarbonate may generate a "contraction" alkalosis. Garella and co-workers have shown that this should increase bicarbonate concentration by no more than 3 or 4 mEq/liter, various buffer systems preventing a greater rise.[7] "Contraction alkalosis" more likely develops through one of the mechanisms described above for generating "new" bicarbonate.

Implicit in the maintenance of metabolic alkalosis is the failure of normal renal homeostatic mechanisms to excrete excess bicarbonate. An important cause of impaired bicarbonate excretion is severe renal failure. Schwartz and his co-workers have emphasized the importance of tubular factors and particularly the relative roles of chloride and potassium deficiency in the maintenance of hypochloremic hypokalemic metabolic alkalosis.[8–10]

Ordinarily, an increase in serum bicarbonate concentration is corrected by a reduction in renal bicarbonate reabsorption. In the proximal nephron, bicarbonate reabsorption occurs as a consequence of secretion of hydrogen ion in exchange for luminal sodium. Conversely, sodium reabsorption occurs in exchange for hydrogen ion or in parallel with chloride reabsorption. ECF volume depletion stimulates proximal tubular sodium reabsorption. As chloride depletion accompanies sodium depletion, availability of chloride anions to be transported with sodium is decreased. Consequently, exchange of sodium for hydrogen ion increases, and the rate of bicarbonate reabsorption rises. Hypokalemia and hypercapnia also stimulate bicarbonate reabsorption.

Therefore, if volume depletion, chloride depletion, hypokalemia, or hypercapnia is present, the kidney may be unable to excrete excess bicarbonate, and metabolic alkalosis will be maintained. A decrease in "effective arterial volume" as seen with congestive heart failure or hepatic failure has an effect on proximal tubular reabsorption identical to that seen with true extracellular volume depletion. A conceptually trivial but clinically important cause of impaired bicarbonate excretion is severe renal failure. A fall in the glomerular filtration rate (GFR) with a reduction in filtered solute load to a level below the rate of new bicarbonate formation will lead to an elevation in the serum bicarbonate level.

Clinical Characteristics

Metabolic alkalosis is encountered frequently postoperatively.[11,12] In one report, it developed as an isolated disturbance in 15% and in combination with respiratory alkalosis in 51% of patients with organ trauma admitted to a surgical service.[13]

The diagnosis of metabolic alkalosis is made on the basis of an elevation in the serum bicarbonate concentration when primary respiratory acidosis is absent. Bicarbonate is measured as total CO_2 by automated analysis of venous blood or is calculated from the Henderson–Hasselbalch equation after arterial pH and P_{CO_2} have been measured. The values obtained by the two methods are similar; however, the venous blood bicarbonate level is 1 to 2 mEq higher than that calculated from arterial blood gas determinations, and venous pH is slightly lower and P_{CO_2} slightly higher than arterial values. Respiratory compensation for metabolic alkalosis is incomplete, and the P_{CO_2} rises by 3 to 4 torr for each rise of 10 mEq in serum bicarbonate level. A P_{CO_2} value above 55 torr suggests the presence of concomitant respiratory acidosis due to pulmonary disease, although there are reports of P_{CO_2} values in excess of 60 torr in patients with pure metabolic alkalosis receiving supplemental oxygen.[14]

Causes

The frequent use of nasogastric tubes postoperatively makes metabolic alkalosis a common problem. The electrolyte content of normal gastric fluid is shown in Table 18-1.[15] Gastric aspiration can produce acid losses of about 400 to 500 mEq/day of hydrogen ion. Concurrent chloride and sodium losses in the gastric fluid and renal potassium wasting due to secondary hyperaldosteronism serve to maintain a high level of renal bicarbonate reabsorp-

tion and sustain the alkalosis. In patients with renal failure, prolonged gastric acid aspiration invariably results in alkalosis unless the accumulated bicarbonate is removed by dialysis or neutralized by acid production or exogenous acid infusion. Cimetidine may be a useful adjunct for reducing gastric acid secretion, but its efficacy has not been proven in controlled studies.[16]

Mild metabolic alkalosis of little clinical significance frequently occurs after cardiopulmonary bypass and has been attributed to the administration of acid citrate dextrose, an anticoagulant for blood used to prime the membrane oxygenator or infused during transfusion.[17] In one prospective study, the degree of alkalosis was decreased by administration of the carbonic anhydrase inhibitor acetazolamide.[18] However, if renal function is normal and neither volume nor potassium depletion is present, the accumulated bicarbonate is excreted promptly.

Excessive bicarbonate administration during cardiopulmonary resuscitation or treatment of lactic acidosis may lead to rebound alkalosis once tissue perfusion is restored and accumulated organic anions are metabolized to bicarbonate. During cardiopulmonary resuscitation, bicarbonate should be given at a dosage no greater than 1 ampule containing 44 mEq every 5 min after an initial dose of 2 ampules. For rebound alkalosis and severe hyper-

Table 18-1. Composition of Gastrointestinal Fluids

	Na (mEq/liter)	K (mEq/liter)	Cl (mEq/liter)	HCO$_3$ (mEq/liter)	pH
Gastric Fluid	20–100	5–10	120–160	—	1–7
Bile	150–250	5–10	40–80	20–40	7–8
Pancreatic Fluid	120	5–10	10–60	80–120	7–8
Colonic Fluid	135	15	80	70	7–8

(After Phillips SF: In Maxwell MH, Kleeman CR (eds): Clinical Disorders of Fluid and Electrolyte Metabolism, 3rd ed. New York, McGraw Hill, 1980) osmolality to be avoided, the subsequent rate of administration should be determined on an individual basis by measurement of arterial pH and bicarbonate concentration during the course of the resuscitation.[19]

Since stored blood contains both citric and lactic acids, measured lactate and citrate levels rise after rapid transfusion.[20] Routine bicarbonate administration to patients who have received many transfusions has been advocated.[21] However, more recent studies have shown that the clinical acidosis in this situation is insignificant and that frank alkalosis may occur if bicarbonate is given.[22-24]

Several commercially available plasma protein fractions are relatively hypochloremic and contain more than 40 mEq/liter of acetate. Infusion of large volumes of these fluids in patients with renal failure has caused significant alkalosis.[25]

Volume depletion is a frequent cause of metabolic alkalosis in patients undergoing surgery. Evidence of extracellular volume depletion should be carefully sought in any surgical patient with metabolic alkalosis. Common causes of volume depletion include diarrhea, accumulation of ECF in the third space created by adynamic ileus, hemorrhage, loss of gastrointestinal fluid through aspiration, and administration of diuretics. A urinary chloride concentration of less than 20 mEq/liter suggests that volume depletion is a factor in maintaining metabolic alkalosis. The urinary sodium concentration is less reliable, because acute rises in serum bicarbonate concentration may transiently overwhelm the renal bicarbonate resorptive capacity and cause the excretion of sodium despite volume depletion.[26]

Diuretics are used frequently postoperatively and are often implicated in the generation or maintenance of hypochloremic hypokalemic metabolic alkalosis. Whether these agents primarily inhibit sodium reabsorption (thiazides, mercurials, metolazone) or chloride reabsorption (furosemide, ethacrynic acid) or produce osmotic diuresis (mannitol), they all cause loss of sodium, chloride, and potassium. If these losses are not carefully replaced, resultant deficits may lead to metabolic alkalosis by mechanisms described above.

Since losses of potassium often parallel those of sodium, potassium depletion is a frequent concomitant of volume depletion. Potassium losses should be anticipated in patients with vomiting or diarrhea and in those requiring nasogastric aspiration, diuretics, or mineralocorticoids. Although chloride depletion accompanying volume depletion is a crucial factor in the maintenance of metabolic alkalosis, alkalosis may not be corrected by sodium chloride repletion alone in patients with profound potassium deficits of 400 mEq to 500 mEq. Urinary chloride concentrations in excess of 40 mEq/liter may be found in these "chloride-resistant" alkalotic patients. Presumably, increased proximal tubular bicarbonate reabsorption is maintained by potassium depletion itself and not by volume depletion. Therefore, inducing bicarbonate excretion and correcting the alkalosis may not be possible until potassium has been replaced.[27]

Primary hyperaldosteronism (Conn's syndrome) and secondary aldosteronism due to hyperreninemia associated with renovascular disease or Bartter's syndrome also lead to increased distal tubular acid excretion and metabolic alkalosis. Exogenous mineralocorticoid or high-dose glucocorticoid administration may have the same effect. Since the ECF volume in patients with these conditions tends to be increased, urinary chloride and sodium excretion are often high, and this may provide an important diagnostic clue.

Approach to the Surgical Patient with Metabolic Alkalosis

Successful treatment of metabolic alkalosis begins with accurate identification of those factors that first led to the generation of a high serum bicarbonate concentration and of those that are maintaining the disturbance. After a careful search for etiologic factors outlined above, determination of urinary chloride concentration is useful in corroborating the presence of ECF volume contraction with levels of less than 20 mEq/liter or the presence of diuretic use, severe potassium depletion, or mineralocorticoid excess in which levels are greater than 30 mEq/liter.

In a given surgical patient with metabolic alkalosis, the etiology of the disturbance is often multifactorial. For example, in the patient undergoing cardiac surgery, the disorder may be generated by transfusion of acid citrate dextrose (ACD)-anticoagulated blood and by gastric aspiration. A diminished GFR due to low cardiac output and diuretic-induced volume and potassium depletion maintain the alkalosis.

Treatment must always be based on identification and correction of all factors responsible for both maintenance and generation of alkalosis. In patients with normal renal function, metabolic alkalosis is usually mild, with a blood pH below 7.5 and a bicarbonate concentration below 40 mEq/liter. Correction of ECF volume and potassium deficits leads to increased bicarbonate excretion with correction of pH within 36 to 48 hr. When more rapid correction is necessary because of severe

alkalemia with compensatory hypoventilation or CNS depression, hydrogen ion may be administered as dilute hydrochloric acid. Acid administration requires insertion of a central venous catheter; peripheral administration can cause sclerosis of veins and hemolysis. Acid may be given as 0.1 N HCl in 5% dextrose in water at a rate of no greater than 0.2 mEq/kg/hr.[29] Since the chloride space equals 20% of total body weight, the required dose of acid in milliequivalents equals total body weight $\times$ 0.2 $\times$ (103 mEq/liter − present [Cl] mEq/liter). If the GFR is near normal, excess renal bicarbonate reabsorption may be decreased by the infusion of acetazolamide in a dose of 250 mg to 500 mg every 4 hr to 6 hr. This therapy is particularly useful in post-hypercapnic alkalosis.

In patients with acute or chronic renal failure, renal excretion of bicarbonate may be impaired, and correction of severe alkalosis requires treatment with hydrochloric acid or dialysis against low-acetate dialysate.[32,33]

METABOLIC ACIDOSIS

Daily nonvolatile acid production from dietary acid precursors such as methionine-containing proteins and phosphoproteins and from incomplete metabolism of neutral food stuffs approximates 1 mEq of hydrogen ion per kilogram of body weight. This load is excreted each day through the kidney by secretion of hydrogen ions, which are buffered by compounds such as phosphate and creatinine to produce titratable acid or are combined with ammonia as ammonium ion. In contrast to the kidney's great capacity to excrete bicarbonate, its ability to enhance total acid excretion is limited to only a two- to threefold increase. This capacity to excrete acid may be impaired or overwhelmed in a number of disorders, making metabolic acidosis a frequent clinical condition.

Clinical Characteristics

Metabolic acidosis is characterized by a fall in the serum bicarbonate concentration and pH. Several of the conditions that lead to metabolic acidosis may independently stimulate ventilation, and a primary respiratory alkalosis may therefore accompany the disturbance. It is essential to distinguish between this mixed acid–base disturbance and simple metabolic acidosis with respiratory compensation. From a series of patients with pure metabolic acidosis due to diarrhea, Winters developed a regression formula that predicts within 95% confidence limits the expected degree of respiratory compensation as expressed by the P_{CO_2}:[34]

expected P_{CO_2}

$$= (1.5 \times [HCO_3]) + 8 \pm 2$$

If the P_{CO_2} is less than this calculated value, primary respiratory alkalosis is present. If the P_{CO_2} exceeds this predicted value, respiratory acidosis may be inferred, even if the P_{CO_2} is not elevated above 40 torr.

Calculation of the serum-undetermined anion concentration or "anion gap" is invaluable in the diagnosis of metabolic acidosis:[35]

anion gap (mEq/liter) = [Na] mEq/liter
− ([Cl] mEq/liter + [HCO₃] mEq/liter)

The normal anion gap is 12 ± 4 and is made up of phosphate, sulfate, and other unmeasured organic or inorganic acid anions that are buffered by bicarbonate and cause a decrease in serum bicarbonate concentration. An increased anion gap thus indicates an excess of these anions and is suggestive of metabolic acidosis. In contrast, hyperchloremic metabolic acidosis due to retention of hydrochloric acid or loss of bicarbonate depresses the serum bicarbonate concentration without increasing the anion gap. The common etiologies of metabolic acidosis with a normal anion gap are the following:

Bicarbonate loss
   Renal disease: interstitial nephritis, renal tubular acidosis
   Drugs: acetazolamide, mafenide, cholestyramine, spironolactone (cirrhosis)
   Urinary diversion: ureterosigmoidostomy, ileal loop with stasis
   Gastrointestinal: diarrhea, pancreatic drainage, jejunoileal bypass
Acid gain
   Acid administration: NH_4Cl, HCl, cationic amino acids

Causes of metabolic acidosis with an increased anion gap include the following:

Diabetic or alcoholic ketoacidosis
Uremia
Lactic acidosis
Toxin ingestion: salicylate, methanol, paraldehyde, ethylene glycol

Once the physician has distinguished between high and normal anion-gap acidosis, the specific diagnosis is usually evident from clinical signs.

Causes

Metabolic Acidosis with a Normal Anion Gap

Specific impairment of renal acid excretion is an early finding in mild chronic renal failure.[38] Impaired renal genesis of ammonium or type 4 renal tubular acidosis is responsible for this defect and often accompanies tubulointerstitial diseases, including those due to analgesic abuse, lupus erythematosus, diabetes, lead nephropathy, and obstructive uropathy. The abnormal bicarbonaturia in proximal, or type 2, renal tubular acidosis and the impaired urinary acidification in classic, or distal type 1, renal tubular acidosis both lead to a decrease in serum bicarbonate concentration. Since the GFR is relatively normal in these disorders, anions of fixed acids can be excreted normally. Because these anions do not accumulate in the plasma, the anion gap is not increased. A hyperchloremic acidosis is thus produced.

Tubulointerstitial renal disease, a common disorder, is a frequent cause of metabolic acidosis in surgical patients. The acidosis is usually mild with serum bicarbonate concentrations in the range of 18 to 22 mEq/liter. No specific treatment is required. However, since these patients with mild postoperative metabolic acidosis are unable to increase acid excretion through tubular mechanisms, severe acidosis may result if a minimal increase in acid generation occurs. Although rare, severe baseline acidosis may be seen in type 1 renal tubular acidosis.[39]

High-capacity bicarbonate reabsorption in the proximal tubule is dependent on the enzyme carbonic anhydrase. Inhibition of this enzyme results in bicarbonaturia and hyperchloremic acidosis. This effect is exploited when the carbonic anhydrase inhibitor acetazolamide (Diamox) is given to correct post-hypercapneic metabolic alkalosis. The topical antibiotic mafenide (Sulfamylon) is systemically absorbed when used in the treatment of burns and may produce a hyperchloremic acidosis. Cholestyramine, a cationic resin that binds bile salts in the gut, also binds

bicarbonate and may cause metabolic acidosis by inducing gastrointestinal bicarbonate loss.

The intestinal lumen, particularly that of the colon, can secrete bicarbonate in exchange for chloride. As a result, hyperchloremic acidosis is a frequent complication of ureterosigmoidostomy. This procedure has therefore been abandoned in favor of the ileal conduit. Metabolic acidosis less frequently complicates the latter procedure but may result if stasis occurs in an ileal segment that is too large or strictured.

The electrolyte content of pancreatic fluid, bile, and diarrhea are listed in Table 18-1. Pancreatic or biliary tract drainage, diarrhea, or even excessive preoperative bowel cleansing may result in the loss of bicarbonate and severe metabolic acidosis.[40] This may also occur after jejunoileal bypass, in which case up to 300 mEq/day of bicarbonate or even reanastomosis may be required.[41]

Two types of amino acid mixtures are currently used in intravenous hyperalimentation; casein or fibrin hydrolysates, and synthetic mixtures of amino acids (Freamine, Neoaminosol, Travasol). Early synthetic mixtures contained a high percentage of cationic amino acids such as lysine, arginine, and histidine as their hydrochloride salts. When metabolized, these amino acids yielded 1 mEq of hydrogen ion for each millimole administered and often produced a metabolic acidosis. Protein hydrolysates contain fewer cationic amino acids, and modification of synthetic mixtures has essentially obviated the problem of acidosis.[42] However, modern synthetic mixtures and hydrolysates may produce acidosis in patients unable to augment acid excretion.[43] Acidosis can be readily detected if serum electrolyte concentrations in patients receiving intravenous hyperalimentation are followed closely. Substitution of sodium acetate for sodium chloride in the electrolyte mixture provides a rapid and simple means of correction.

Metabolic Acidosis with a High Anion Gap

Diagnosis of high anion-gap acidosis depends upon identification of the retained anion. Underlying disorders producing this disturbance are usually more severe than those causing hyperchloremic acidosis, and early recognition and treatment are mandatory.

The high anion-gap acidosis of renal failure results from accumulation of anions of strong acids such as sulfate and phosphate. It occurs when the GFR falls to less than 20 ml/min as evidenced by a rise in the serum creatinine concentration to greater than 4 mg/dl. Characteristically, the serum bicarbonate concentration remains above 15 mEq/liter, and the anion gap is less than 25 mEq/liter. Acidosis developing in postsurgical acute renal failure is poorly tolerated, in part because of the hemodynamic problems induced by the acidosis itself and in part because of the hypercatabolism and hyperkalemia that accompany it. Although the acidosis of acute renal failure may be managed conservatively, early dialysis is often the preferred treatment (see Chapter 15). Patients with chronic renal failure tolerate acidosis well and carry little increased risk during surgery if their blood pH is above 7.3. Attempts to correct acidosis rapidly with sodium bicarbonate can result in ECF volume overload. Management of the surgical patient with chronic renal failure is discussed in Chapter 16.

Free fatty acids and their ketoacid metabolites accumulate during states of insulin lack. Ketoacidosis is a frequent complication of diabetes, and combined ketoacidosis and lactic acidosis may be seen in starvation and alcoholism. The diagnosis is usually clinically apparent, but a bedside determination of serum or urine detoacids by the nitroprusside test (Ketostix, Acetest) is easy and rapidly confirmatory. However, in severe ketoacidosis, the intracellular redox state is low, and the mitochondrial NADH:NAD$^+$ ratio is high. Because these conditions favor reduction of acetoacetate to beta-hydroxybutyrate, a nonketoacid that does not react with nitroprusside, the test in this case may be negative or only weakly positive.

Alcoholic ketoacidosis may be seen on admission but rarely develops de novo in hospitalized patients. In contrast, diabetic ketoacidosis is an occasional but completely preventable complication of perioperative stress. Treatment of alcoholic ketoacidosis includes correction of the accompanying extracellular volume depletion and administration of bicarbonate and glucose as necessary. Administration of insulin has been proposed as part of the therapy, but this may produce hypoglycemia and is usually unnecessary.[44,45] Treatment of diabetic ketoacidosis in the surgical setting is discussed in Chapter 11.

A history of drug or toxin ingestion should be sought in any patient with a high anion-gap acidosis. Acidosis is a prominent finding in patients who have ingested methanol or ethylene glycol, and these patients are usually admitted to the medical service when the diagnosis is clear. However, abdominal pain with or without pancreatitis is frequently seen in patients with severe acidosis, and, occasionally, such patients are admitted to the surgical service if the underlying cause goes unrecognized. The diagnosis is also suggested by a discrepancy, called the "osmolar gap," of more than 15 mOsm/liter between measured and calculated serum osmolality. For example, methanol in a concentration of 100 mg/dl raises the measured serum osmolality by 31 mOsm/liter above the osmolality calculated from serum sodium, urea, and glucose concentrations. Like urea, relatively low molecular-weight alcohols readily diffuse across cell membranes and contribute to the measured but not to the "effective" osmolality. Since "effective" hypertonicity is not present, the serum sodium concentration is not depressed. Although less specific, determination of osmolar gap can be accomplished more rapidly than individual plasma toxin assays.

Clinical findings may suggest a specific toxin. Blindness with retinal edema and optic nerve hyperemia points to methanol ingestion. Ethylene glycol ingestion is associated with acute renal failure induced by oxalate, its principal metabolite, and bipyramidal oxalate crystals may be found on urinalysis. Dialysis is required to remove these two toxins. Ethyl alcohol infusion is also a useful treatment, because ethyl alcohol competes for metabolism with ethylene glycol and methanol and reduces production of their toxic metabolites.[46,47]

Salicylate intoxication may occur in hospitalized patients receiving aspirin for rheumatologic disorders or topical methyl salicylate as a keratolytic. The diagnosis is frequently missed with dire consequences. In one series of 73 consecutive patients with salicylate intoxication, delay in diagnosis was documented for as long as 72 hr in 27%. Mortality in this group was 25%, and severe morbidity was 30%.[48] Salicylates stimulate respiration, and coexistent respiratory alkalosis and high anion-gap metabolic acidosis should alert the clinician to the possibility of salicylate intoxication. This complication can often be confirmed by review of medication records and by determination of blood salicylate levels. Dialysis may be required in patients with renal failure or salicylate levels above 80 mg/dl, but forced alkaline diuresis is usually adequate in patients with less severe intoxication.[49] Acetazolamide should be avoided, since acidemia augments salicylate toxicity.[50]

Lactic acidosis is the most severe form of high anion-gap acidosis. Morbidity and mortality depend upon the severity and reversibility of the underlying precipitating cause. In spontaneous lactic acidosis, reported mortality ranges up to 100%. Shock, whether hemorrhagic, cardiogenic, or septic, is the most frequent cause of lactic acidosis. Lactate generation increases when hypoperfusion and inadequate oxygen delivery to tissues lead to increased anaerobic metabolism and impaired hepatic uptake and utilization of lactate. The pathophysiologic mechanisms by which other underlying disorders lead to lactic acidosis have been extensively reviewed.[55,56,57]

The presentation of lactic acidosis is variable. The disorder may develop as a prominent feature in established shock or may be an early finding in developing sepsis. Lactic acidosis is frequently associated with primary respiratory alkalosis, particularly when sepsis is the underlying cause. It may also occur in states of localized hypoperfusion, burns, tumors, and limb or mesenteric arterial occlusion.[51-54] The classic presentation with the dramatic onset of Kussmaul respiration is rare.

Diagnosis of lactic acidosis should be clear if a high anion-gap acidosis is present and uremia, diabetes, and alcohol or toxin ingestion have been excluded. Confirmation can be established by measurement of lactate levels. Freely flowing venous levels above 1.3 mEq/liter or arterial levels above 0.8 mEq/liter are diagnostic. It must be remembered that certain physiologic events such as exercise or catecholamine release may transiently increase lactate levels, and moderate elevation of lactate occurs with the stimulation of glycolysis induced by alkalosis. Lactate levels that remain below 6 mEq/liter are usually not associated with excessive morbidity. Causes of lactic acidosis with a mild elevation in anion gap include the following:

Alkalosis
Carbohydrate infusion
Exercise or seizures
Catecholamines
Diabetic ketosis
Ethanol

Causes of lactic acidosis with a severe elevation in anion gap include the following.

Impaired tissue oxygenation
    Hypotension
    Severe anemia
    Arterial occlusion
    Hypoxia
Glycogen storage diseases
Malignancies
Spontaneous

Treatment consists of vigorous correction of hypoperfusion and acidemia. Rapid administration of blood, colloid, or crystalloid is essential in patients with ECF volume contraction. Despite early reports to the contrary, if transfusion corrects underlying hypotension, the lactate in the stored blood used in transfusion does not lower pH or increase blood lactate levels in patients with hemorrhagic shock.[20,23] In patients with high venous pressures due to cardiac failure, nitroprusside may be of value in improving hemodynamics rather than in altering the lactate metabolism itself.[58,59] Dichloroacetate increases utilization of pyruvate, the precursor of lactate, in the tricarboxylic acid cycle and thereby reduces the concentration of lactate. However, this agent is not available for clinical use.[60] Alkali therapy and the role of dialysis are discussed below.

Approach to the Surgical Patient with Severe Metabolic Acidosis

Treatment of metabolic acidosis requires attention to the pathophysiologic process that led to acidemia and correction of the acidemia itself. Renal disease underlying hyperchloremic acidosis is usually not remediable. In chronic renal disorders, correction of the serum bicarbonate level to approximately 20 mEq/liter is desirable. Once the bicarbonate deficit is corrected, daily bicarbonate requirements are relatively modest, on the order of 1 mEq/kg day. Parenteral or oral sodium bicarbonate (each 325-mg tablet is equivalent to 3.9 mEq) may be given. In patients who experience bicarbonate-induced gastrointestinal discomfort, Shohl's solution, a mixture of sodium citrate and citric acid of which 1 ml is equivalent to 1 mEq of bicarbonate, may be substituted. Care must be taken in prescribing Shohl's solution. Some pharmacies supply a modified solution containing potassium citrate, a formulation that is valuable for patients with renal tubular acidosis but contraindicated in patients with renal failure. Hyperchloremic acidosis due to gastrointestinal bicarbonate loss may be severe. With substantial continuing losses, daily bicarbonate doses must be individualized.

Severe high anion-gap acidosis constitutes a medical emergency. Specific treatment, when available, must be initiated immediately. Insulin rapidly blocks acid production in diabetic ketoacidosis. Dialysis is specific therapy for uremia and toxin ingestion.

Only supportive treatment is available for lactic acidosis. Correction of inadequate perfusion and severe acidemia are the goals of therapy. Careful clinical assessment of intravascular volume as well as measurement of central venous or pulmonary artery wedge pressure are essential. In patients who are volume-contracted, expansion with blood, colloid, and crystalloid should be rapid. Blood pressure maintenance may require catecholamine infusion. When volume overload and renal failure exist, dialysis is indicated to optimize the hemodynamic status and to allow further administration of sodium bicarbonate.

The goal of alkali therapy is to maintain the serum bicarbonate concentration above 10 mEq/liter and the blood pH between 7.15 and 7.20. When the pH is below 7.1, myocardial irritability is markedly increased, and contractility is diminished. With bicarbonate concentrations below 5 mEq/liter small increases in P_{CO_2} lead to profound acidemia and make resuscitation impossible. In high anion-gap acidosis, correction of the serum bicarbonate concentration to normal should not be attempted, because treatment of the underlying process itself facilitates rapid metabolism of accumulated ketoacids or lactate to bicarbonate, and overly vigorous treatment with bicarbonate can result in severe alkalemia. The initial bicarbonate deficit can be estimated with the assumption that the bicarbonate space is 50% of total body weight:

$$\text{Bicarbonate deficit (mEq)} = 0.5$$
$$\times \text{ total body weight (kg)}$$
$$\times \text{ [desired (HCO}_3\text{) mEq/liter}$$
$$- \text{ actual (HCO}_3\text{) mEq/liter]}$$

Sodium bicarbonate is the alkali salt of choice in the therapy of metabolic acidosis. In practice, therapy must be individualized, with frequent determinations of blood pH and serum bicarbonate concentrations. The bicarbonate space is greater than 50% of the total body weight in severe acidosis, and continuing acid production may make it seem infinite.[61] In lactic acidosis, several hundred milliequivalents of bicarbonate may be required in the first 4 hr. Bicarbonate may be given in hyperosmolar intravenous bolus infusions (44 mEq/ampule) or in a continuous drip (3 ampules of bicarbonate in 1 liter of 5% dextrose in water is equivalent to 132 mEq/liter).

Since lactic acidosis is frequently complicated by oliguria due to renal failure or by congestive heart failure, the high sodium and osmolar load imposed by bicarbonate administration is often poorly tolerated. The role of early dialysis in this setting cannot be overemphasized. Lactate or acetate-buffered dialysate is usually satisfactory, allowing for removal of sodium and permitting further intravenous administration of bicarbonate. Occasionally, bicarbonate dialysis is required.[62] Preparation of bicarbonate containing dialysate is time-consuming, and dialysis should begin with standard dialysate while the pharmacy is preparing special fluids.

RESPIRATORY ALKALOSIS

Respiratory alkalosis is the result of abnormal stimulation of ventilation with a consequent reduction in P_{CO_2} and increase in pH. Simultaneous metabolic acidosis and respiratory alkalosis should be suspected whenever the P_{CO_2} is lower than anticipated for a given decrease in bicarbonate concentration. As already discussed, Winters' formula is useful for this purpose. A partial list of the causes of respiratory alkalosis appears below.

Anxiety, hysteria, pain
Fever
Salicylism
CNS Disease (cerebrovascular accident, infection, trauma, tumor)
Congestive heart failure
Pneumonia
Pulmonary embolus
Hypoxemia
Hepatic insufficiency
Sepsis
Mechanical ventilation at excessive rates

Respiratory alkalosis occurs frequently postoperatively. In one series, it occurred as an isolated disturbance in 34% of patients with severe trauma and together with metabolic alkalosis in 51%.[13] This disorder frequently accompanies obvious pulmonary disease, such as pneumonia or pulmonary emboli; its underlying causes are often more subtle. An unexplained respiratory alkalosis may be the only early clue to developing sepsis or hepatic encephalopathy. It is therefore imperative that every effort be made to identify the cause.

Respiratory alkalosis can produce a rapid rise in blood pH and profound clinical deterioration. A sudden fall in P_{CO_2} from 40 torr to 20 torr in a patient with a serum bicarbonate concentration of 24 mEq/liter results in a pH in excess of 7.7. Paresthesias, tetany, and seizures may result. Although CO_2 rebreathing or mild sedation may be useful in anxiety-induced hyperventilation, treatment of the alkalosis itself is usually unrewarding. When pulmonary disease, CNS abnormalities, hepatic dysfunction, or sepsis is the cause, treatment with opiates or other respiratory depressants is clearly contraindicated. Instead, treatment should be directed at the underlying condition. Hypokalemia and hypophosphatemia due to intracellular shifts of potassium and phosphate are frequent complications of respiratory alkalosis and may necessitate phosphate administration.[63]

RESPIRATORY ACIDOSIS

Respiratory acidosis is caused only by alveolar hypoventilation with consequent CO_2 accumulation. Clinically relevant causes are listed below.

Acute
General anesthesia
Sedation, overdose
Cardiac arrest
Pneumothorax
Pulmonary edema
Severe pneumonia
Bronchospasm
Laryngospasm
Aspiration
Mechanical ventilation
Respiratory nerve damage
Guillain–Barré syndrome
Hypophosphatemia
Hypokalemia
Chronic
Chronic obstructive pulmonary disease
Primary alveolar hypoventilation
Brain tumor
Neurologic diseases of respiratory muscles (polio, myasthenia gravis)
Primary myopathy of respiratory muscles
Restrictive disease of the thorax
Burns
Scleroderma
Severe pneumonia

Respiratory acidosis is recognized by a rise in P_{CO_2} and a fall in blood pH. Bicarbonate retention occurs as a compensatory response, and the rise in serum bicarbonate level averages 4 to 5 mEq/liter for every increase of 10 torr in P_{CO_2}. The serum bicarbonate concentration seldom exceeds 38 mEq/liter in pure respiratory acidosis; higher levels suggest concomitant metabolic alkalosis. Since the serum potassium concentration rises in acidemia, a low serum potassium level provides a clue to the presence of vomiting or diuretic-induced hypokalemic metabolic alkalosis. The combination of respiratory acidosis and metabolic alkalosis is also a frequent finding in patients with chronic obstructive lung disease who receive diuretics as treatment for cor pulmonale or other conditions that cause sodium retention.

As in respiratory alkalosis, the major effort of therapy is treatment of the underlying cause of respiratory failure. Although narcotic antagonists such as naloxone are useful in reversing respiratory depression due to opiate administration, respiratory stimulants and analeptics have no role. Progressive hypercapnia is an indication for emergent endotracheal intubation and control of ventilation. A more extensive discussion of respiratory failure and its management is presented in Chapter 25.

SUMMARY

1. It is important to identify each acid–base disturbance separately in order to determine appropriate therapy. An acid–base nomogram may be helpful.
2. Mild acidemia and alkalemia are well tolerated; marked deviations alter cardiovascular and CNS function and cellular metabolism.
3. Metabolic alkalosis is a common finding in surgical patients. Its etiology is usually multifactorial.
4. In patients with volume depletion and alkalosis, bicarbonaturia and correction of alkalemia do not occur until volume deficits are replaced.
5. Urinary chloride concentrations are useful for differentiating ECF volume contraction (a concentration of less than 20 mEq/liter) from diuretic use, potassium depletion, or mineralocorticoid excess (a concentration of greater than 30 mEq/liter).
6. Acid administration is rarely required for metabolic alkalosis. The indications are severe alkalemia with compensatory hypoventilation or CNS depression.
7. The causes of normal and high anion-gap acidoses are listed in the section on "Metabolic Acidosis."
8. Severe high anion-gap metabolic acidosis is a medical emergency. Treatment varies with the underlying pathology. Because myocardial irritability is greatly increased when the *p*H falls below 7.1, sodium bicarbonate should be administered.
9. Respiratory alkalosis is common postoperatively and may be accompanied by hypokalemia and hypophosphatemia.
10. Respiratory acidosis is caused by alveolar hypoventilation. Progressive hypercapnia is an indication for emergent intubation.

REFERENCES

1. McCurdy DK: Mixed metabolic and respiratory acid–base disturbances: Diagnosis and treatment. Chest (Suppl) 62S:35, 1972
2. Narins RG, Emmett M: Simple and mixed acid–base disorders: A practical approach. Medicine 59:161, 1980

3. Goldberg, M, Green SB, Moss ML et al: Computer-based instruction and diagnosis of acid–base disorders. JAMA 223:269, 1973

4. Mitchell JH, Wildenthal K, Johnson RL Jr: The effects of acid–base disturbances on cardiovascular and pulmonary function. Kidney Int 1:375, 1972

5. Relman AS: Metabolic consequences of acid–base disorders. Kidney Int 1:347, 1972

6. Seldin DW, Rector FC Jr: The generation and maintenance of metabolic alkalosis. Kidney Int 1:306, 1972

7. Garella S, Chang BS, Kohn SI: Dilution acidosis and contraction alkalosis: Review of a concept. Kidney Int 8:279, 1975

8. Kassirer JP, Berkman PM, Lawrenz DR et al: The critical role of chloride in the correction of hypokalemic alkalosis in man. Am J Med 38:172, 1965

9. Kassirer JP, Schwartz WB: The response of normal man to selective depletion of hydrochloric acid. Am J Med 40:10, 1966

10. Kassirer JP, Schwartz WB: Correction of metabolic alkalosis in man without repair of potassium deficiency. Am J Med 40:19, 1966

11. Berman IR, Moseley RV, Doty DB et al: Post-traumatic alkalosis in young men with combat injuries. Surg Gynecol Obstet 133:11, 1971

12. Lyons JH Jr, Moore FD: Posttraumatic alkalosis: Incidence and pathophysiology of alkalosis in surgery. Surgery 60:93, 1966

13. Wilson RF, Gibson D, Percinel AK et al: Severe alkalosis in critically ill surgical patients. Arch Surg 105:197, 1972

14. Webb J: Severe hypercapnia associated with non-respiratory alkalosis. Br J Dis Chest 72:62, 1978

15. Phillips SF: Water and electrolytes in gastrointestinal diseases. In Maxwell MH, Kleeman CR (eds): *Clinical Disorders of Fluid and Electrolyte Metabolism*, 3rd ed. New York, McGraw Hill, 1980

16. Barton CH, Vaziri ND, Ness RL et al: Cimetidine in the management of metabolic alkalosis induced by nasogastric drainage. Arch Surg 114:70, 1979

17. Weygandt GR, Roos A: The effects of citrated blood and hypothermia on acid–base balance during cardiopulmonary bypass. Anesthesiology 36:268, 1972

18. Grigor KC, Blair JI, Hutchison JRS: The effect of acetazolamide on post-perfusion metabolic alkalosis. Br J Anaesth 43:352, 1971

19. Mattar JA, Weil MH, Shubin H et al: Cardiac arrest in the critically ill. II. Hyperosmolal states following cardiac arrest. Am J Med 56:162, 1974

20. Schweizer O, Howland WS: Significance of lactate and pyruvate according to volume of blood transfusion in man. Ann Surg 162:1017, 1965

21. Howland WS, Schweizer O, Boyan CP: The effect of buffering on the mortality of massive blood replacement. Surg Gynecol Obstet 121:777, 1965

22. Kahn RL, Jascott D, Carlon GC et al: Massive blood replacement: Correlation of mixed calcium, citrate and hydrogen ion concentration. Anesth Analg (Cleve) 58:274, 1979

23. Collins JA, Simmons RL, James PM et al: Acid–base status of seriously wounded combat casualties. II. Resuscitation with stored blood. Ann Surg 173:6, 1971

24. Miller RD, Tong MJ, Robbins TO: Effects of massive transfusion of blood on acid–base balance. JAMA 216:1762, 1971

25. Rahilly GT, Berl T: Severe metabolic alkalosis caused by administration of plasma protein fraction in end-stage renal failure. New Engl J Med 301:824, 1979

26. Harrington JT, Cohen JJ: Measurement of urinary electrolytes—Indications and limitations. New Engl J Med 293:1241, 1975

27. Garella S, Chazan JA, Cohen JJ: Saline resistant metabolic alkalosis or "chloride-wasting nephropathy." Ann Int Med 73:31, 1970

28. Worthley LIG: The rational use of IV hydrochloric acid in the treatment of meta-

bolic alkalosis. Br J Anaesth 49:811, 1977

29. Wagner CW, Nesbit RR, Mansberger AR: The use of intravenous hydrochloric acid in the treatment of 34 patients with metabolic alkalosis. Am Surg 46:140, 1980

30. Shavelle HS, Parke R: Postoperative metabolic alkalosis and acute renal failure: Rationale for the use of hydrochloric acid. Surgery 78:439, 1979

31. Swartz RD, Rubin SE, Brown RS et al: Correction of postoperative metabolic alkalosis and renal failure by hemodialysis. Ann Intern Med 86:52, 1977

32. Barcenas CG, Fuller TJ, Knochel JP: Metabolic alkalosis after massive blood transfusion. JAMA 236:953, 1976

33. Ayus JC, Olivero JJ, Androqué HJ: Alkalemia associated with renal failure: Correction by hemodialysis with low-bicarbonate dialysate. Arch Intern Med 140:513, 1980

34. Albert MD, Dell RB, Winters RW: Quantitative displacement of acid–base equilibrium in metabolic acidosis. Ann Intern Med 66:312, 1967

35. Emmett ME, Narins RG: Clinical use of the anion gap. Medicine 56:38, 1977

36. Madias NE, Ayus JC, Androqué HJ: Increased anion gap in metabolic alkalosis. The role of plasma–protein equivalency. New Engl J Med 300:1421, 1979

37. Gabow PA, Kaehny WD, Fennessey PV et al: Diagnostic importance of an increased serum anion gap. New Engl J Med 303:854, 1980

38. Widmer B, Gerhardt RE, Harrington JT et al: Serum electrolyte and acid–base composition. The influence of graded degrees of chronic renal failure. Arch Intern Med 139:1099, 1979

39. Narins RG, Goldberg M: Renal tubular acidosis: Pathophysiology, diagnosis and treatment. DM 23:1, 1977

40. Hurdley J: Unexpected metabolic acidosis during rectal surgery. Anaesthesia 33:478, 1978

41. Fuller, TJ, Garg LC, Harty RF et al: Severe hyperchloremic acidosis complicating jejunoileal bypass. Surg Gynecol Obstet 46:567, 1978

42. Heird WC, Dell RB, Driscoll JM Jr et al: Metabolic acidosis resulting from intravenous alimentation mixtures containing synthetic amino acids. New Engl J Med 287:943, 1972

43. Fraley DS, Adler S, Bruns F et al: Metabolic acidosis after hyperalimentation with casein hydrolysate. Ann Intern Med 88:352, 1978

44. Levy LJ, Duga J, Girgis M et al: Ketoacidosis associated with alcoholism in nondiabetic subjects. Ann Intern Med 78:213, 1973

45. Fulop M, Hoberman HD: Alcoholic ketosis. Diabetes 24:785, 1975

46. Gonda A, Gault H, Churchill P et al: Hemodialysis for methanol intoxication. Am J Med 54:749, 1978

47. Underwood F, Bennett WM: Ethylene glycol intoxication. Prevention of renal failure by aggressive management. JAMA 226:1453, 1973

48. Anderson RJ, Potts DE, Gabow PA et al: Unrecognized adult salicylate intoxication. Ann Intern Med 85:745, 1976

49. Winchester JF, Gelfand MC, Knepshield JH et al: Dialysis and hemoperfusion of poisons and drugs-update. Trans Am Soc Artif Intern Organs 23:761, 1977

50. Hill JB: Salicylate intoxication. New Engl J Med 288:1110, 1973

51. Eggleston FC, Feierabend TC: The early acidosis of burns: Its relationship to extent of burn and management. Surgery 77:641, 1975

52. Spechler SJ, Esposito A, Koff RS et al: Lactic acidosis in oat cell carcinoma with extensive hepatic metastases. Arch Intern Med 138:1633, 1978

53. Fisher RD, Fogarty TJ, Morrow AG: Clinical and biochemical observations of the effect of transient femoral artery occlusion in man. Surgery 68:323, 1970

54. Brooks DH, Carey LC: Base deficit in superior mesenteric artery occlusion. An aid to early diagnosis. Ann Surg 177:352, 1973

55. Oliva PB: Lactic acidosis. Am J Med 48:209, 1970

56. Ritz E, Heidland A: Lactic acidosis. Clin Nephrol 7:231, 1977

57. Kreisberg RA: Lactate homeostasis and lactic acidosis. Ann Intern Med 92:227, 1980

58. Taradash MR, Jacobson LB: Vasodilator therapy of idiopathic lactic acidosis. New Engl J Med 293:468, 1975

59. Brezis M, Rowe M, Shalev O: Reversal of lactic acidosis associated with heart failure by nitroprusside administration. Br Med J 2:1399, 1979

60. Relman AS: Lactic acidosis and a possible new treatment. New Engl J Med 298:564, 1978

61. Garella S, Dana CL, Chazan JA: Severity of metabolic acidosis as a determinant of bicarbonate requirements. New Engl J Med 289:121, 1973

62. Vaziri ND, Ness R, Wellikson L et al: Bicarbonate-buffered peritoneal dialysis. An effective adjunct in the treatment of lactic acidosis. Am J Med 67:392, 1979

63. Knochel JP: The pathophysiology and clinical characteristics of severe hypophosphatemia. Arch Intern Med 137:203, 1977

19

Postoperative Gastrointestinal Bleeding

GARY M. LEVINE

Gastrointestinal (GI) bleeding is an important complication in the surgical patient and can occur without symptoms or prior history of bleeding. Whether it is directly related to the operative procedure is often difficult to assess. Wound pain, postoperative ileus, and narcotic administration all may compound the difficulty of evaluation and treatment. Nevertheless, determination of the cause of bleeding is crucial and will result in decreased morbidity and mortality.[1,2]

The occurrence of postoperative GI bleeding depends largely on the overall status of the patient. Bleeding is encountered most often in patients with multisystem failure, sepsis, severe burns, and central nervous system (CNS) injury or surgery. In these groups, the incidence of upper GI bleeding is at least 25%.[3] Mortality in high-risk patients, directly attributed to or associated with bleeding, may range up to 50% for patients with stress ulcers and may exceed 90% for patients with mesenteric vascular disease.[4–6]

The early literature concerning GI bleeding in postoperative patients is flawed. Until the advent of accurate diagnostic techniques, the causes of bleeding and their relative incidence could not be accurately assessed. The diagnosis of "stress ulcer" was therefore erroneously made for many patients with bleeding in the postoperative period. Furthermore, with advances in anesthesia and more aggressive surgical techniques, patients who used to be considered poor risks are undergoing surgery more frequently. Thus, a marked alteration in patient population may have resulted in a change in the natural history and patterns of etiology of GI bleeding in the postoperative period.

This chapter reviews the incidence, pathogenesis, diagnosis, and treatment of postoperative GI bleeding.

UPPER GASTROINTESTINAL BLEEDING

The etiology of GI bleeding in the postoperative patient differs from that in the general population. Stress is probably the most important cause of upper GI bleeding in patients with sepsis, burns, and head injury. Extensive studies in these groups form the basis for our understanding of the pathogenesis of stress bleeding.

The term "stress ulcer" has been applied to a diverse group of lesions in surgical patients with GI bleeding. However, it should be restricted to those patients who initially demonstrate acute superficial ulceration, which may progress to deep ulceration and even perforation.[7] Such lesions are usually found in the upper two-thirds of the stomach, although they can occur in the antrum, duodenum, and, rarely, in the esophagus. The word "stress" implies that the patient has experienced a preceding causative episode of sepsis, trauma, hypotension, burns, or multisystem failure. The definition of stress ulcer should not be extended to include patients who bleed from known peptic ulcer disease reactivated by stress.[7]

The development and outcome of stress-induced upper GI lesions was initially discussed by Lucas and his co-workers.[4] They performed serial endoscopic examinations beginning within 12 hr of trauma, sepsis, or shock. Acute mucosal lesions were regularly found within the first 24 hr. GI bleeding from these lesions developed in 25% of patients.

The pathogenesis of stress lesions has been the subject of many excellent investigations. Although several factors have been implicated, two major hypotheses predominate. First, when there is shock, anoxia, or sepsis, mucosal blood flow decreases.[8] Menguey and his colleagues demonstrated that hypoperfusion decreased gastric mucosal energy metabolism and substrate availability, leading to anoxic necrosis of the mucosa and impairment of regenerative ability.[9] However, although mucosal metabolism decreases, acid secretion may be preserved. Endotoxin, released into the blood during an episode of sepsis, may lead to a decrease in mucosal perfusion with resultant stress ulceration.

The second theory involves back diffusion of acid from the gastric lumen into the GI mucosa and submucosa.[10] The resulting low tissue pH leads to mucosal damage, inflammation, and necrosis. Back diffusion may be increased by reflux of bile salts and pancreatic enzymes and by gastric mucosal secretion of the potent proteolytic enzyme pepsin.[11] Aspirin, indomethicin, and nonsteroidal anti-inflammatory agents also disrupt the gastric mucosal barrier and increase back diffusion.[12] One study has suggested that bicarbonate, produced as an obligatory by-product of carbonic acid hydrolysis and secreted into gastric mucus from the gastric glands, may protect the stomach from ulceration by forming an adherent mucosal barrier. A decrease in bicarbonate secretion may be the critical factor mediating stress ulceration.[13]

GI bleeding is second only to sepsis as a major complication and cause of death in burn patients. The association of GI bleeding and burns was first reported by Curling in 1842.[15] The incidence of bleeding increases from 10 to 20% for burns involving 35% of the body surface to 40 to 50% for those covering more than 70% of the surface area.[16] Studies in burn patients have documented that disruption of the gastric mucosal barrier precedes development of mucosal erosions and ulcerations.[17]

A prospective endoscopic study of the natural history of upper GI mucosal lesions reveals that, within hours of the burn injury, the gastric and duodenal mucosa begin to develop microscopic hemorrhagic lesions that progress to erosions and frank ulceration. Bleeding can develop at any stage but is often present by the time erosions are visible.[18] Multiple erosions were found in 86% of patients with burns covering more than 50% of the body surface area, and approximately 25% of this group developed a gastric ulcer at the site of the most intense superficial erosive disease. Mucosal disruption and bleeding were greatest in those patients whose course was one of continuing deterioration. Duodenal ulcer often accompanied gastric mucosal disease and further complicated management.

Harvey Cushing first described GI bleeding following intracranial injury or neurosurgery in 1932.[19] The incidence of GI bleeding after CNS injury may exceed 25%.[20] Patients with trauma in addition to head injury have the highest risk of bleeding. The progression of mucosal disease in patients with CNS injury follows a similar endoscopic progression as that in burn patients. In addition to the causes of stress ulceration discussed above, neurally mediated factors may be important in patients with CNS injury. Increased gastric acid and pepsin secretion results directly from increased vagal tone and indirectly from vagus-mediated release of gastrin, a potent stimulant of gastric acid secretion.[21-23] These factors stimulate the parietal cell mass to secrete acid even when gastric mucosal blood flow is very low.[9] Hyperacidity and disruption of the gastroduodenal mucosal barrier due to hypotension, hypoxia, and sepsis frequently precipitate bleeding.

Prophylactic measures against GI bleeding have been well studied in stressed patients.[3,17] Although most studies use well-defined criteria for the presence of GI bleeding, the diagnosis of stress ulcer as the cause often has been inferential. Nevertheless, several groups have demonstrated the protective value of antacids in preventing GI bleeding in stressed patients. Skillman and Silen advocate hourly installation of antacids in sufficient doses to keep the gastric pH above 3.5, a value at which hydrogen ion concentration is reduced by more than 90%.[7] Two randomized controlled studies show that antacid prophylaxis is effective in re-

ducing the incidence of GI bleeding in stressed patients from 25% to less than 5%.[3,24]

Antacids are also effective in preventing bleeding in burn patients.[25,26] McAlhaney and colleagues found that only 1 of 27 patients bled after antacid therapy, compared to 7 of 21 controls.[17] Although antacids did not prevent mucosal erosions, overt bleeding did not occur in the antacid group. Nutritional supplementation has also been shown to prevent stress ulcers in burn patients.[26] Intragastric installation of a chemically defined diet provides calories and protein required for wound healing, and such a diet has a pH of 6 or greater that may buffer gastric acid almost as well as antacids.

The use of cimetidine as prophylaxis against stress bleeding is controversial. Two studies found it to be ineffective; however, it does prevent stress-induced bleeding in certain well-defined situations.[24,27] In one study of patients with hepatic failure, cimetidine dramatically decreased the incidence of GI bleeding but did not change mortality.[28] Another prospective study in patients with CNS injury also showed cimetidine to have protective value.[29] Lastly, in a third study, cimetidine prevented GI bleeding in patients undergoing renal transplantation.[30] The controversy surrounding cimetidine in preventing stress bleeding may be due to several factors. The dose of the agent administered in some studies was not always titrated to reduce the gastric pH to a given level, whereas antacid administration was regulated to assure hypochlorhydria.[3,24] In addition, cimetidine may have been ineffective because its antisecretory effect blocked gastric bicarbonate production as well as acid secretion.

The treatment of bleeding from stress ulceration is generally unsatisfactory, with mortality rates as high as 50% reported in the literature.[4,7] Vigorous antacid therapy is recommended initially, and Silen and co-workers have demonstrated the efficacy of antacid treatment for stress bleeding.[3,24] In a randomized double-blind study of treatment with cimetidine and antacid, cimetidine alone was as effective as cimetidine with antacid in the treatment of acute bleeding. However, only 33% of patients responded to either regimen. The same study also demonstrated that cimetidine and antacid were superior to antacid alone in preventing rebleeding and in decreasing mortality.[31]

Intra-arterial vasopressin is recommended for acute gastric mucosal hemorrhage unresponsive to gastric lavage and antacids. In a retrospective analysis of 50 patients with gastric bleeding of varying etiologies, it was found that this method produced control of hemorrhage in 84%. Of patients who could not be infused, 80% required surgery to control bleeding.[32]

Other causes of upper GI bleeding must also be considered. Postoperative patients are at risk for development of the Mallory–Weiss syndrome from repeated wretching, emesis, and coughing.[33] Of all upper GI bleeds, 10% to 20% are attributable to superficial mucosal tears.[34] Maneuvers like straining, coughing or vomiting generate intra-abdominal pressures of greater than 200 torr and can cause a tear at the gastroesophageal junction.[35] Such a pressure gradient across the narrow diameter of the diaphragmatic hiatus creates shearing force on the mucosa that can lead to laceration and bleeding.[36] The diagnosis of the Mallory–Weiss syndrome is easily made endoscopically. Although bleeding from most tears is self-limited, 10% of patients may require angiographic control or surgical intervention.[37]

Peptic ulcer, predominantly duodenal, is a common disease with a prevalence exceeding 4% in the United States.[38] Of particular interest to the physician caring for the postoperative patient is the high incidence of peptic ulcer disease in renal transplant patients.[39] Studies have shown that the natural history of peptic ulcer disease is one of repeated exacerbations.[40,41] Many patients are asymptomatic; the presence of an ulcer correlates poorly with symptoms. Ulcer symptoms may disappear with therapy, but the lesion may still present on radiographic or endoscopic examination.[42] Prophylaxis of surgical patients with known peptic ulcer disease or a history of a recent exacerbation is recommended, but its effectiveness is largely unproved except in studies in which small doses of cimetidine appear to prevent recurrence in ambulatory patients.[42,43]

Bleeding from esophagitis in postoperative patients is a consequence of either reflux of gastric contents through the lower esophageal sphincter or candidiasis.[34] Endoscopy shows that reflux esophagitis produces erythematous friable mucosa occasionally associated with focal areas of peptic ulceration. Candidiasis produces plaques of whitish exudate varying in size from several millimeters to larger confluent areas with surrounding erythema. Microscopic examination of the exudate with 10% potassium hydroxide reveals yeast and mycelia.[47] Nasogastric tubes, prolonged bed rest, and recent abdominal surgery may all produce reflux.[44,45] The use of multiple antibiotics or immunosuppressives, debility, and postoperative malnutrition facilitate the invasion of candida.[46] Symptoms of esophagitis may be minimal, and, in some reports, fewer than half of the patients found to have esophagitis complained of significant substernal burning, dysphagia, or odynophagia.[47]

Initial therapy for esophagitis is aimed at eliminating predisposing causes of reflux. Nasogastric tubes should be removed and the patient encouraged to assume an upright posture. Cimetidine has been shown in several controlled trials to be effective in the treatment of reflux esophagitis.[48,49] Antacids are useful for symptomatic relief. Most patients with candidiasis respond to oral nystatin in the form of viscous gargle or suppositories. For severely affected patients, especially those with underlying hematologic problems, low doses of intravenously administered amphotericin have been advocated and found to be successful.[50]

The postoperative patient on anticoagulants may be at high risk for bleeding into the intestinal lumen or bowel wall. In the case of patients with GI bleeding who are on anticoagulants maintained within the therapeutic range, diagnostic evaluation reveals a structural lesion in 85%.[51] Patients who bleed as a result of excessive anticoagulation usually do not have a demonstrable lesion and may have diffuse mucosal bleeding. Reversal or better regulation of anticoagulation usually suffices for control of bleeding.

LOWER GASTROINTESTINAL BLEEDING

Determining the etiology of postoperative lower GI bleeding can be facilitated by the presence or absence of abdominal pain. This may be difficult to assess in the postoperative period when the patient often complains of generalized discomfort. Abdominal pain and lower GI bleeding suggest an inflammatory or ischemic process.

Pseudomembranous colitis has become a frequent cause of lower GI bleeding since the advent of potent broad-spectrum antibiotics. An incidence of 3% to 10% has been reported after administration of clindamycin and lincomycin.[52,53] Pseudomembranous colitis has also been described with administration of almost all other antibiotics, including cephalosporin, chloramphenicol, tetracycline, amoxicillin, ampicillin, and penicillin. Antibiotic treatment for at least 1 week but occasionally only 2 or 3 days can produce disease. Pseudomembranous colitis can occur as much as 3 to 4 weeks after cessation of therapy, and the length of illness and severity of the disease can be worse than usual in patients with onset after cessation of antibiotics. The disorder has not been reported with the usual antibiotics used for prophylaxis before bowel surgery.

Pseudomembranous colitis has a variable clinical spectrum ranging from mild, watery diarrhea to a severe illness characterized by fever, abdominal pain, rebound tenderness, bloody diarrhea, and leukocytosis. The diagnosis is easily made by proctoscopic examination, which reveals innumerable 2 to 5-mm whitish plaques covering the colonic mucosa with surrounding erythema and friability on swabbing.[52]

Pseudomembranous colitis can be seen in postoperative sepsis and staphylococcal infection and in the debilitated patient.[55] The underlying mechanism of pseudomembranous colitis is change in the *milieu* of normal bowel flora with overgrowth of *clostridia*. *Clostridium difficile* produces a toxin that causes the disease.[56,57]

Responsible antibiotics should be discontinued. Seriously ill patients should receive either oral vancomycin or a binding resin such as colestipol or cholestyramine. Vancomycin is effective in killing the responsible organisms, whereas the binding resins appear to bind the toxin and allow healing.[58]

One of the most dramatic and serious complications that can occur in the postoperative patient is mesenteric vascular insufficiency. This can range from complete bowel infarction to localized ischemic colitis. GI bleeding may not be a prominent part of the presentation, but it is invariably present.[59] The two major causes of mesenteric vascular disease in the postoperative patient are emboli and nonocclusive infarction. Patients with recent cardiac surgery, a history of rheumatic heart disease, or atrial fibrillation are particularly at risk for emboli. When emboli go to the abdominal vessels, the superior mesenteric artery is most commonly involved.[60] Nonocclusive ischemic disease occurs primarily in patients with congestive heart failure, sepsis, hypoxia, and shock. It is also associated with arteriosclerotic vascular disease, diabetes, hypertension, and digitalis administration.[61]

Since there is no characteristic presentation of mesenteric ischemia, the physician must suspect the disease in the postoperative patient with unexplained abdominal pain, hypotension, hemoconcentration, acidosis, or the development of an acute abdomen. Symptoms characteristically exceed physical findings. The findings of an airless abdomen and thickened mucosal folds or bowel wall on radiographic examination and of intramural air on flat-plate examination suggest the diagnosis.[62]

Acute mucosal necrosis of the colon occurs in 1% to 2% of patients after aortic surgery. Resection of an aneurysm or re-construction of the aortoiliac vessels usually includes interruption of the interior mesenteric artery for technical reasons.[63] One-half to two-thirds of patients with mucosal necrosis require partial colectomy, which has a mortality rate of approximately 40%.[64] Patients undergoing renal transplantation are also at high risk for ischemic disease of the colon.[65]

The presence of rectal bleeding without pain suggests a noninflammatory process such as a bleeding from a colonic diverticulum or angiodysplasia. Although the postoperative patient is not at particular risk for bleeding from either of these lesions, their common occurrence in the aged and their frequency as a cause of lower GI bleeding make their recognition imperative.[66] The vascular lesions of angiodysplasia are usually located in the cecum. Patients with aortic stenosis may have a higher risk for developing these lesions in the colon and small bowel.[67] Although these lesions were thought to be arteriovenous malformations, recent evidence suggests chronic ischemia or venous outflow obstruction as the cause.[66]

Bleeding from colonic diverticula is a major cause of painless bleeding. Although the distribution of colonic diverticula favors the left side of the colon, bleeding diverticula are more commonly found proximal to the splenic flexure.[68] The extrusion of a diverticulum through the colonic wall with resultant stretching of its arteriole over the dome of the diverticulum leads to bleeding when the vessel is eroded.[69]

MANAGEMENT OF UPPER GASTROINTESTINAL BLEEDING

There are several differences in evaluation between surgical patients with GI bleeding and other patients. Special circumstances relating to surgery may change the relative frequency of lesions causing GI bleeding. The condition of the patient may preclude certain studies, thereby altering the diagnostic approach. For example, a patient who has recently undergone abdominal surgery and has an ileus cannot undergo barium contrast examination.

The first order of priority is to stabilize the patient. Access to the circulation must be provided so that colloid and blood may be provided to maintain tissue perfusion. Although administration of electrolyte solution may maintain blood pressure transiently, it will quickly leak out of the vascular space. Colloid such as 5% albumin or plasma should be used initially until blood is available. Concurrent with resuscitative efforts, a nasogastric tube should be inserted to confirm or rule out upper GI bleeding. The absence of blood or coffee grounds on nasogastric lavage indicates that bleeding is distal to the ligament of Treitz. Only 1% of upper GI bleeders, usually patients with duodenal ulcers, do not reflux bloody duodenal contents into the stomach.[70] If nasogastric lavage is stained with bile and free of blood, gastroduodenal bleeding is essentially ruled out.

The severity of upper GI bleeding should be rapidly assessed. The presence of hematemesis, orthostatic hypotension, or bright red blood on nasogastric lavage that does not clear strongly suggests massive bleeding with a loss of at least 25% of blood volume.[71] The preferred method for nasogastric lavage is passage of a large-bore nasogastric tube such as an Ewald tube. Controversy exists as to whether to use cold or warm saline or water.[5] The use of saline may lead to salt and water overload, and absorbed free water is more easily excreted by the kidneys. Iced or cold solutions should be avoided, since they lead to considerable discomfort with shivering and possible hypothermia. Although cold solutions may cause temporary vasoconstriction, reactive hyperemia occurs on rewarming. Vigorous nasogastric suction should be avoided during lavage, since injury of the gastric mucosa may enhance bleeding or produce artifacts that may confuse the endoscopist. Nasogastric lavage is successful in stopping one-half to two-thirds of bleeding episodes.[72]

In patients with bright red bleeding that fails to clear with tap-water lavage, the addition of levarentrol to the lavage solution may be helpful.[73] Levarentrol, 16 mg diluted in 250 ml of water, is introduced into the stomach, and the tube is clamped. After 15 min to 20 min, lavage is repeated for assessment of adequacy of control. Levarentrol irrigation may be repeated 2 or 3 times, but, if there is no response, should be abandoned. Once bleeding has slowed, endoscopy should be performed for determination of the site of bleeding. Continued massive bleeding may necessitate arteriography without endoscopy.

Endoscopy is excellent in the evaluation of GI bleeding, providing a diagnosis in over 75% of patients.[34,72,74] In all studies comparing the accuracy of endoscopy and barium in upper GI series, endoscopy has been shown to be superior to radiologic examination.[75–77] Endoscopy visualizes small superficial bleeding sites that may not be seen in barium studies. There is still no evidence that double-contrast upper GI studies are as good as endoscopy.[77] The presence of barium may be an impediment to endoscopy and arteriography in the seriously ill postoperative patient.

The major risk of endoscopy is the extremely low likelihood of perforation of the upper pharynx and esophagus on insertion of the instrument.[78] Overinflation of the abdomen during endoscopic examination may lead to respiratory distress and arrhythmias.[79,80] Aspiration during endoscopy and respiratory distress from sedative drugs may also occur.[78] Endoscopy is contraindicated in the uncooperative patient and in the patient with an unstable cardiorespiratory status. In the future, therapeutic endoscopy may become a reality. Research is underway to determine the safest and most effective method for endoscopic techniques to establish hemostasis.

Angiography should be performed if the patient continues to bleed.[81] This may precede endoscopy as noted above or follow endoscopy if bleeding persists. Angiography demonstrates arterial bleeding by showing extravasation of contrast material from the vascular pool into the lumen of the GI tract. Venous lesions that bleed intermittently, such as varices, are difficult to demonstrate by this method.[82] Demonstration of a bleeding arterial lesion usually justifies the use of selective vasopressin infusion. Placement of the angiographic catheter into the appropriate vessle with infusion of vasopressin at a dose of 0.2 to 0.4 units/min will control bleeding in at least 60% and perhaps as many as 90% of patients.[32,83] There is no role for selective vasopressin infusion in the patient with variceal bleeding. In this case, vasopressin is administered peripherally at an initial rate of 0.2 to 0.4 units/min and may cautiously be increased to a maximum of 0.9 units/min. The complications of angiography include hematomas at the site of catheterization and bowel ischemia or infarction. When vasopressin infusion is not feasible or bleeding does not respond, autogenous clot or Gelfoam can be embolized into the bleeding vessel.[84,85] These techniques, however, carry the risk of intestinal infarction.

MANAGEMENT OF LOWER GASTROINTESTINAL BLEEDING

The evaluation of lower GI bleeding should begin with sigmoidoscopy when the condition of the patient has become stable. Painful bleeding secondary to inflammatory or ischemic lesions has a characteristics mucosal appearance. For example, the picture of pseudomembranous colitis is one of innumerable, small, raised, whitish plaques adherent to the mucosa.[52] Sigmoidoscopic findings in the patient with ischemic colitis range from friability and erythema of the mucosa to a more characteristic dusky cyanosis in the rectosigmoid area.[54]

If a diagnosis is not established by sigmoidoscopy and hemorrhaging continues, a bleeding scan should be performed. This technique, which uses intravenous injection of [99m]technetium–sulfur colloid, is rapid and noninvasive. Extravasation of blood containing the isotope into the intestinal lumen is established by a gamma-camera imaging.[86] Although the bleeding scan has its limitations, it appears to be as sensitive if not more so than angiography and may aid the physician in choosing further diagnostic and therapeutic measures. At the Hospital of the University of Pennsylvania, an angiogram is not performed without a prior positive bleeding scan. In a study of over 120 patients with lower GI bleeding, approximately 75% had negative scans. A group of 15 patients with negative scans underwent angiography, and no bleeding site or other abnormality was identified. Of those patients with positive scans who underwent arteriography, more than 50% were found to have bleeding.[87]

Angiography is especially useful in the evaluation of lower GI bleeding when angiodysplasia or diverticuli are suspected. These lesions are notoriously difficult to find because of their size and distribution. In the case of diverticular bleeding, angiography can distinguish which one of hundreds of diverticuli is responsible. The initial preferred management of such vascular bleeding is vasopressin infusion, which is effective in as many as 80% of patients.[68]

SUMMARY

1. Immediate and ongoing management of GI bleeding begins with hemodynamic stabilization of the patient.
2. Assessment focuses first on the rate of bleeding and its approximate location (upper or lower).
3. The work-up of upper GI bleeding usually begins with endoscopy. One of the most commonly encountered lesions in postoperative patients is stress ulceration.
4. Angiography with intra-arterial infusion of vasopressin should be undertaken for severe upper GI bleeding that is unresponsive to conservative measures. Failure of the patient to respond to therapy necessitates surgical intervention, which has an expected high mortality rate.
5. Prophylaxis for stress-related bleeding with hourly administration of antacids to keep the gastric pH above 3.5 is indicated in all patients undergoing major surgery.
6. Lower GI bleeding occurring without pain and with a normal sigmoidoscopic examination suggests a localized vascular lesion best treated by angiography with arterial vasopressin infusion.
7. Painful bleeding suggests an ischemic or inflammatory lesion with the diagnosis usually apparent on sigmoidoscopy.
8. Pseudomembranous colitis, the most common inflammatory lesion responsible for lower GI bleeding in the postoperative patient, is best treated by discontinuation of the responsible antibiotics and administration of oral vancomycin or binding resins such as colestipol or cholestyramine.
9. Ischemic colitis most commonly occurs after abdominal aortic surgery. If it progresses to mesenteric infarction, surgery, which carries a high mortality, is necessary.

REFERENCES

1. Himal HS, Watson WW, Jones CW et al: The management of upper gastrointestinal hemorrhage: A multiparametric computer analysis. Ann Surg 179:489, 1974
2. Hunt PS, Hansky J, Korman MG: Mortality in patients with haematemesis and melena. Br Med J 1:1238, 1979
3. Hastings PR, Skillman JJ, Bushnell LS et al: Antacid titration in the prevention of acute gastrointestinal bleeding: A controlled, randomized trial in 100 critically ill patients. N Engl J Med 298:1041, 1978
4. Lucas CE, Sugawa C, Friend W et al: Therapeutic implications of disturbed gastric physiology in patients with stress ulcerations. Am J Surg 123:25, 1972
5. Moody FG, Cheung LY: Stress ulcers: Their pathogenesis, diagnosis and treatment. Surg Clin North Am 56:1469, 1976
6. Ottinger LW, Austen WG: A study of 136 patients with mesenteric infarction. Surg Gynecol Obstet 124:251, 1967

7. Skillman JJ, Silen W: Stress ulcers. Lancet 2:1303, 1972

8. Harjola PT, Sivula A: Gastric ulceration following experimentally induced hypoxia and hemorrhagic shock. Ann Surg 163:21, 1966

9. Menguey R, Besbaillets L, Masters YF: Mechanisms of stress ulcer: Influence of hypovolemic shock on energy metabolism in the gastric mucosa. Gastroenterology 66:46, 1974

10. Davenport HW, Warner HA, Code CF: Functional significance of gastric mucosal barrier to sodium. Gastroenterology 47:142, 1964

11. Ivey KJ, DenBesten L, Clifton JA: Effects of bile salts on ionic movement across the human gastric mucosa. Gastroenterology 59:683, 1970

12. Smith MB, Skillman JJ, Edwards BG et al: Permeability of the human gastric mucosa: Alteration by acetyl–salicylic acid and ethanol. N Engl J Med 285:716, 1971

13. Garner A, Flemstrom G: Gastric HCO_3 secretion in the guinea pig. Am J Physiol 234:E535, 1978

14. Cheung LY, Reese RS, Moody FG: Direct effect of endotoxin on the gastric mucosal microcirculation and electrical gradient. Surgery 79:564, 1976

15. Curling TB: On acute ulceration of the duodenum in cases of burn. Medical–Chirurgical Transactions 25:260, 1842

16. Skillman JJ, Gould SA, Chung RSK et al: The gastric mucosal barrier: Clinical and experimental studies in critically ill and normal man and in the rabbit. Ann Surg 172:564, 1970

17. McAlhaney JC, Czaja AJ, Pruitt BA: Antacid control of complications from acute gastroduodenal disease after burns. J Trauma 16:645, 1976

18. Czaja AJ, McAlhaney JC, Pruitt BA: Acute gastroduodenal disease after thermal injury. N Engl J Med 291:925, 1974

19. Cushing H: Peptic ulcer and the interbrain. Surg Gynecol Obstet 55:1, 1932

20. Gordon MD, Skillman JJ, Zervas NJ et al: Divergent nature of gastric mucosal permeability and gastric acid secretion in sick patients with general surgical and neurosurgical disease. Ann Surg 178:285, 1973

21. Norton L, Greer J, Eisman B: Gastric secretory responses to head injury. Arch Surg 101:200, 1970

22. Idjadi F, Robbins R, Stahl WM et al: Prospective study of gastric secretion in stress patients with intracranial injury. J Trauma 11:681, 1971

23. Bowen JC, Fleming WH, Thompson JC: Increased gastrin release following penetrating central nervous system injury. Surgery 75:720, 1974

24. Priebe HJ, Skillman JJ, Bushnell LS et al: Antacid vs. cimetidine in preventing acute gastrointestinal bleeding. N Engl J Med 302:426, 1980

25. Watson LC, Abston S: Prevention of upper gastrointestinal hemorrhage in 582 burned children. Am J Surg 132:790, 1976

26. Solem LD, Strate RG, Fischer RP: Antacid therapy and nutritional supplementation in the prevention of Curling's ulcer. Surg Gynecol Obstet 148:367, 1979

27. Herrmann V, Kaminski DL: Evaluation of intragastric pH in acutely ill patients. Arch Surg 114:511, 1979

28. MacDougall BRD, Basley WJ, Williams R: H_2 receptor antagonists and antacids in the prevention of acute gastrointestinal hemorrhage in fulminant hepatic failure: Two controlled trials. Lancet 1:617, 1977

29. Halloran LG, Zfass AM, Gayle WE et al: Prevention of acute gastrointestinal complications after severe head injury: A controlled trial of cimetidine prophylaxis. Am J Surg 139:44, 1980

30. Jones RH, Rudge CJ, Bewick M et al: Cimetidine: Prophylaxis against upper gastrointestinal hemorrhage after renal transplantation. Br Med J 1:398, 1978

31. Teres J, Bordas JM, Rimola A et al: Cimetidine in acute gastric mucosal bleeding: Results of a double blind randomized trial. Dig Dis Sci 25:92, 1980

32. Athanasoulis CA, Baum S, Waltman AC et al: Control of acute gastric mucosal hemorrhage. N Engl J Med 290:597, 1974

33. Mallory GK, Weiss S: Hemorrhages from lacerations of the cardiac orifice of the stomach due to vomiting. Am J Med Sci 178:506, 1929

34. Katon RM, Smith FW: Panendoscopy in the early diagnosis of acute upper gastrointestinal bleeding. Gastroenterology 65:728, 1973

35. Atkinson MM, Bottrill MB, Edwards AT et al: Mucosa tears at the esophagogastric junction (the Mallory–Weiss syndrome). Gut 2:1, 1961

36. Watts HD: Lesions brought on by vomiting: The effect of hiatus hernia on the site of injury. Gastroenterology 71:683, 1976

37. Knauer CM: Mallory–Weiss syndrome. Characterization of 75 Mallory-Weiss lacerations in 528 patients with upper gastrointestinal bleeding. Gastroenterology 71:5, 1976

38. Kirsner JB: Peptic ulcer: A review of the recent literature on various clinical aspects. Gastroenterology 54:611, 1968

39. Owens ML, Passaro E Jr, Wilson SE et al: Treatment of peptic ulcer disease in the renal transplant patient. Ann Surg 186:17, 1977

40. Bodemar G, Walan A: Maintenance treatment of recurrent peptic ulcer disease by cimetidine. Lancet 1:403, 1978

41. Cargill JM: Very long-term treatment of peptic ulcer with cimetidine. Lancet 2: 1113, 1978

42. Blackwood WS, Maudgal DP, Northfield TC: Prevention by bedtime cimetidine of duodenal ulcer relapse. Lancet 1:626, 1978

43. Gudmand-Høyer E, Birger Jensen K, Krag E et al: Prophylactic effect of cimetidine in duodenal ulcer disease. Br Med J 1:1095, 1978

44. Nagler R, Spiro HM: Persistent gastroesophageal reflux induced during prolonged gastric intubation. N Engl J Med 269: 495, 1963

45. Cohen S, Snape WJ Jr: The pathophysiology and treatment of gastroesophageal reflux disease. New concepts. Arch Intern Med 138:1398, 1978

46. Eras P, Goldstein MJ, Sherlock P: Candida infection of the gastrointestinal tract. Medicine 51:367, 1972

47. Kodsi BE, Wickremesinghe PC, Kozinn PJ et al: Candida esophagitis: A prospective study of 27 cases. Gastroenterology 71:715, 1976

48. Behar J, Brand DL, Brown FC et al: Cimetidine in the treatment of symptomatic gastroesophageal reflux. A double-blind controlled trial. Gastroenterology 74: 441, 1978

49. Wesdorp E, Bartelsman J, Pape K et al: Oral cimetidine in reflux esophagitis: A double-blind controlled trial. Gastroenterology 74: 821, 1978

50. Medoff G, Dismukes WE, Meade RH III et al: A new therapeutic approach to candida infections. Arch Intern Med 130:241, 1972

51. Babb RR, Spittell JA Jr, Bartholomew LG: Gastroenterologic complications of anticoagulant therapy. Mayo Clin Proc 43:738, 1968

52. Tedesco FJ, Barton RW, Alpers DH: Clindamycin-associated colitis—A prospective study. Ann Intern Med 81:429, 1974

53. Pittman FE, Pittman JC, Humphrey CD: Colitis following oral lincomycin therapy. Arch Intern Med 134:368, 1974

54. Pettet JD, Baggenstoss AU, Dearing WH: Postoperative pseudomembranous enterocolitis. Surg Gynecol Obstet 98:456, 1954

55. Goulston SJM, McGovern VJ: Pseudomembranous colitis. Gut 6:207, 1965

56. Bartlett JG, Chang TW, Gurwith M et al: Antibiotic-associated pseudomembranous colitis due to toxin-producing clostridia. N Engl J Med 298:531, 1978

57. Dowell VR Jr: Antibiotic associated colitis. Hosp Pract 14:75, 1979

58. Kreutzer, EW: Treatment of antibiotic associated pseudomembranous colitis with cholestyramine resin. Johns Hopkins Med J 143:67, 1978

59. Williams LF Jr: Vascular insufficiency of the intestines. Gastroenterology 61:757, 1971

60. Kaufman SL, Harrington DP, Siegelman SS: Superior mesenteric artery embolization: an angiographic emergency. Radiology 124:625, 1977

61. Fogarty TJ, Fletcher WS: Genesis of nonocclusive mesenteric ischemia. Am J Surg 111:130, 1966

62. Scott JR, Miller WT, Urso M et al: Acute mesenteric infarction. Am J Roentgenol 113:269, 1971

63. Ottinger LW, Darling RC, Nathan MJ et al: Left colon ischemia complicating aorto-iliac reconstruction. Arch Surg 105:841, 1972

64. Johnson WC, Nasbeth DC: Visceral infarction following aortic surgery. Ann Surg 180:312, 1972

65. Misra MK, Pinkus GS, Birtch AG et al: Major colonic diseases complicating renal transplantation. Surgery 73:942, 1973

66. Boley SJ, Sammartano R, Adams A et al: On the nature and etiology of vascular ectasias of the colon. Degenerative lesions of aging. Gastroenterology 72:650, 1977

67. Galloway SJ, Casarella WJ, Shimkin PM: Vascular malformation of the right colon as a cause of bleeding in patients with aortic stenosis. Radiology 113:11, 1974

68. Casarella WJ, Kanter IE, Seaman WB: Right sided colonic diverticula as a cause of acute rectal hemorrhage. New Engl J Med 286:450, 1972

69. Meyers MA, Volberg F, Katzen B et al: The angioarchitecture of colonic diverticula. Radiology 108:249, 1973

70. Luk, GD, Bynum TE, Hendrix TR: Gastric aspiration in localization of gastrointestinal hemorrhage. JAMA 241:576, 1979

71. Northfield TC, Smith T: Hematemesis as an index of blood loss. Lancet 1:990, 1971

72. Palmer ED: The vigorous diagnostic approach to upper gastrointestinal tract hemorrhage. JAMA 207:1477, 1969

73. Kiselow MC, Wagner M: Intragastric in- stallation of levarterenol. Arch Surg 107:307, 1973

74. Sugawa C, Werner MH, Hayes DF et al: Early endoscopy. A guide to therapy for acute hemorrhage in the upper gastrointestinal tract. Arch Surg 107:133, 1973

75. Morris DW, Levine GM, Soloway RD et al: Prospective randomized study of diagnosis and outcome in acute upper gastrointestinal bleeding: Endoscopy versus conventional radiography. Dig Dis 20:1103, 1975

76. Keller RT, Logan GM Jr: Comparison of emergent endoscopy and upper gastrointestinal series radiography in acute upper gastrointestinal hemorrhage. Gut 17:180, 1976

77. Dronfield MW, Ferguson R, McIllmurray MB et al: A prospective, randomized study of endoscopy and radiology in acute upper gastrointestinal tract bleeding. Lancet 1:1167, 1977

78. Mandelstam P, Sugawa C, Silvis SE et al: Complications associated with esophagogastroduodenoscopy and esophageal dilation. Gastrointest Endosc 23:16, 1976

79. Whorwell PJ, Smith CL, Foster KJ: Arterial blood gas tensions during upper gastrointestinal endoscopy. Gut 17:797, 1976

80. Sturges HF, Krone CL: Cardiovascular stress of peroral gastrointestinal endoscopy. Gastrointest Endosc 19:119, 1973

81. Baum S, Nusbaum M: The control of gastrointestinal hemorrhage by selective mesenteric arterial infusion of vasopressin. Radiology 98:497, 1971

82. Sos TA, Lee JG, Wixon D et al: Intermittent bleeding from minute to minute in acute massive gastrointestinal hemorrhage: Arteriographic demonstration. Am J Roentgenol 131:1015, 1978

83. Conn HO, Ramsby GR, Storer EH et al: Intra-arterial vasopressin in the treatment of upper gastrointestinal hemorrhage: A prospective, controlled trial. Gastroenterology 68:211, 1975

84. Rosch J, Dotter CT, Brown MJ: Selective

arterial embolization. A new method for control of acute gastrointestinal bleeding. Radiology 102:303, 1972

85. Bookstein JJ, Chlosta EM, Foley D et al: Transcatheter hemostasis of gastrointestinal bleeding using modified autogenous clot. Radiology 113:277, 1974

86. Miskowiak J, Nielson SL, Manck O et al: Abdominal scinti-photography with 99mtechnetium-labeled albumin in acute gastrointestinal bleeding. An experimental study and a case report. Lancet 2:852, 1977

87. Alavi A, Ring E, Baum S: Radioisotopic demonstration of acute intestinal bleeding. Gastrointest Radiol (in press)

Medical Complications of Bowel Surgery

WILLIAM M. BATTLE

This chapter considers the common long-term medical complications of gastrointestinal (GI) surgery. These are often chronic or recurrent and require continuous cooperation between the surgeon and internist. The chapter is divided into five sections, covering complications of peptic ulcer surgery, small-bowel resection, colectomy, intestinal bypass, and the postcholecystecomy syndromes (PCS).

PEPTIC ULCER SURGERY

There are several accepted operative procedures for the treatment of peptic ulcer disease, including truncal vagotomy with drainage (pyloroplasty or gastrojejunostomy), truncal vagotomy with antrectomy, and subtotal gastrectomy.[1] More recently, selective or highly selective vagotomy has been introduced.[2,3] Selective vagotomy, unlike truncal vagotomy, preserves all but the gastric branches of the vagus nerves. The highly selective, or proximal, gastric vagotomy leaves hepatic and antral fibers intact with division of only the vagal fibers innervating the parietal cell mass. Surgical treatment of gastric ulcer involves either a hemigastrectomy or a vagotomy with a drainage procedure.[4,5]

It is estimated that half of the patients who undergo surgery for ulcer disease experience some form of chronic disability related to the procedure, and the minority incur serious complications. Long-term complications of peptic ulcer surgery include the following:

Dumping
Gastric stasis
Weight loss
Malabsorption
Blind loop syndrome
Diarrhea
Anemia
Bile gastritis and esophagitis
Recurrent ulcer
Gastric carcinoma
Afferent loop syndrome
Bezoars
Metabolic bone disease
Tuberculosis

The dumping syndrome, common in postgastrectomy patients, consists of a variety of postprandial vasomotor phenomena (flushing, palpitations, diaphoresis, light-headedness, tachycardia, and postural hypotension) and alimentary symptoms (nausea, vomiting, crampy pain, and diarrhea).[6] Dumping symptoms are more frequent and severe after a Billroth II pro-

310

cedure but may complicate any peptic ulcer surgery. Dumping syndrome is seen in 40% of patients immediately after operation, but it persists in fewer than 10%.[7]

The dumping syndrome may consist of early and late postprandial phases. The early phase begins within 30 min after eating and is attributed to contraction of blood volume, autonomic reflexes triggered by intestinal distention, and excessive small-intestinal release of vasoactive hormones such as bradykinin, serotonin, and gastric-inhibitory peptide.[8–12] The late postprandial dumping syndrome may be secondary to hypoglycemia. It is postulated that hyperglycemia and subsequent excessive insulin secretion result from the rapid influx of carbohydrate into the small intestine. The hypersecretion of a GI insulin, secretagogue, may trigger the excessive insulin secretion, and hypoglycemia may result 2 to 3 hr after eating.[13] Increased release of the gut hormone enteroglucagon has been demonstrated in postoperative patients with dumping syndrome, but the role of this hormone in the production of symptoms is still unclear.[14]

The early phase of dumping can be controlled by a high-protein, low-carbohydrate diet taken in multiple small feedings.[15] High-carbohydrate liquids and concentrated sweets are common offenders and should be avoided. Fluids are withheld at mealtime and provided between meals. Anticholinergic drugs may help to slow gastric emptying. Patients who do not respond to dietary management may require revisional surgery, such as insertion of an antiperistaltic jejunal segment or a Roux-en-Y gastrojejunostomy.[16] The late phase of dumping can usually be controlled with restriction of carbohydrate alone. Recent evidence suggests that the ingestion of nonabsorbable polysaccharides such as pectin at mealtimes may help to alleviate symptoms by delaying gastric emptying and carbohydrate absorption.[17]

Delayed gastric emptying is a potential complication of all types of vagotomy. It is most common following complete truncal transection and may occur transiently in the immediate postoperative period as a result of an underlying primary motility disturbance. Solid food may alleviate it by stimulating normal antral motor function more effectively than continued liquid feedings.[18] Gastroscopy should be performed to document gastric outlet obstruction if the need for gastric aspiration persists for more than 3 weeks postoperatively. Medical therapy with metoclopramide or bethanechol should be considered for patients with an underlying primary gastric motility abnormality.[19] Radionuclide methods for measuring gastric emptying are useful in diagnosing gastric atony and following response to treatment.[20] Surgery is usually needed only when significant stenosis is present.

Weight loss from both decreased intake and malabsorption is particularly common following gastrojejunal anastomosis.[21] Factors theorized to explain postgastrectomy malabsorption include loss of gastric protein digestion, diminished cholecystokinin release from the vagally denervated small intestine, ineffective release of cholecystokinin and secretin from the bypassed duodenum, rapid intestinal transit of chyme resulting in poor mixing with pancreatic and biliary secretions, sequestration of these secretions in the afferent loop, and unmasking of gluten enteropathy.[6,22]

Bacterial overgrowth, especially by anaerobes, in the afferent limb of a Billroth II anastomosis or in the blind loop syndrome results from abnormal motility and diminished gastric acid output.[23,24] Rarely, direct seeding of colonic bacterial flora may result from a gastrojejunocolic fistula. Significant bacterial overgrowth occurs in 50% of patients with a Billroth II procedure.[25] Subsequent vitamin B_{12} and fat malabsorption is common; carbohydrate and protein malabsorption is less so.[24] Malabsorption of vitamin B_{12} is the result of bacterial uptake of free or intrinsic factor-bound B_{12}, and fat malabsorption follows bacterial deconjugation of bile salts and defective micellar formation. Mucosal injury may also be an important factor.[24] Deficiency of fat-soluble vitamins (A, D, E, and K) may occur and cause blindness, retinal abnormalities, osteomalacia, or hypoprothrombinemia.[22]

The diagnosis of malabsorption due to bacterial overgrowth is made in the same way in the surgical as in the medical patient. Measurement of serum folate levels may reveal elevation due to bacterial production of folate.[26] The bile acid breath test is another sensitive and noninvasive method of documenting bacterial overgrowth.[27] Another test consists of the oral administration of labeled glycocholic acid, which is deconjugated by intestinal bacteria and expired as labeled CO_2. But this test is not specific, since elevated $^{14}CO_2$ excretion occurs both in small-intestinal bacterial overgrowth and in ileal disease or resection. However, glycocholic acid, a bile salt that is normally absorbed in the terminal ileum, is deconjugated by normal colonic flora, partially absorbed, and expired when the ileum is diseased or absent. Therefore, measurement of labeled glycocholic acid in the stool will generally distinguish bacterial overgrowth from ileal disease. Finally, the ^{14}C-xylose breath test has been proposed as a more specific means of diagnosing bacterial overgrowth, since xylose is normally absorbed in the proximal small intestine.[28]

Broad-spectrum antibiotics usually eliminate the overgrowth of anaerobic bacteria. Intermittent long-term therapy is usually required to prevent recurrence. Revisional surgery may be curative if a fistula is present.

Diarrhea following gastric surgery is usually transient and can be controlled with antispasmodics or other antidiarrheal medications. Severe, persistent diarrhea may be caused by dumping or malabsorption as discussed above, but many other causes have been proposed. Lactose malabsorption has been documented after gastrectomy in patients who were lactose-tolerant preoperatively.[29] Rapid gastric emptying of a large lactose load into the jejunum may override the limited enzymatic capacity of most adults to hydrolyze lactose. In addition, several authors have suggested that loss of gastric acidity may cause increased susceptibility to intestinal infection with *Salmonella* or *Giardia lamblia*.[30,31] Finally, postvagotomy diarrhea may be implicated in the absence of other etiologies. Patients with postvagotomy diarrhea have increased fecal excretion of bile acids and may benefit from cholestyramine.[32–35]

Anemia occurs postoperatively in over 40% of patients who have undergone peptic ulcer surgery but is serious in less than 10%.[36,37] It is more common following gastric ulcer surgery, and its severity is probably proportional to the amount of stomach resected. Iron-deficiency anemia is common and may be related to chronic blood loss, impaired absorption of iron due to duodenal bypass, or decreased reduction of food-bound iron due to hypochlorhydria.[36,37] Vitamin B_{12} and folate deficiencies occur infrequently.[38] Vitamin B_{12} deficiency can result from inadequate dietary intake, defective absorption due to decreased intrinsic factor, or impaired assimilation of B_{12} in food because of pancreatic insufficiency.[37,39–41] Measurements of intrinsic factor in patients who have undergone partial gastrectomy have shown that approximately 30% of the patients do not produce enough intrinsic factor postoperatively to facilitate normal vitamin B_{12} absorption.[42] Folate deficiency may be caused by reduced food intake or rapid transit through the proximal small intestine. Since postoperative anemia may be multifactorial, serum levels of iron, folate, and B_{12} may be misleading. Specific treatment often depends upon examination of the peripheral blood smear and bone marrow aspirate.

Reflux esophagogastritis as a complication of gastric surgery is characterized by epigastric pain, anorexia, pyrosis, and bilious vomiting. It can occasionally result in anemia. It is thought to be due to reflux of bile acids into the stomach and esophagus.[43–45] Symptomatic patients are likely to exhibit severe hyperemia, granularity, and bile staining of the gastric mucosa, with severe inflammation on biopsy.[46] Medical treatment of reflux gastritis and esophagitis is generally unsatifactory, but aluminum hydroxide and cholestyramine, which bind bile acids, may be helpful. A controlled study, however, failed to verify the effectiveness of cholestyramine in the symptomatic treatment of bile reflux gastritis.[47] Roux-en-Y gastrojejunostomy or isoperistaltic jejunal interposition may help patients with refractory symptoms.[48]

Recurrent duodenal ulcer occurs in 7% to 14% of patients after vagotomy with drainage, 1% to 4% after vagotomy with antrectomy, 2% to 5% after subtotal gastrectomy, and 5% after proximal gastric vagotomy.[1,49–53] Recurrent gastric ulcer occurs in 10% to 13% of patients after vagotomy with drainage but is minimal after hemigastrectomy.[4,5] Incomplete vagotomy

or inadequate gastric resection are considered the most common causes of recurrent ulcer following peptic ulcer surgery.[54] Other less common causes include the Zollinger–Ellison syndrome, retained gastric antrum, endocrine disorders associated with hypercalcemia, long afferent loop, and the use of ulcerogenic drugs.

Measurement of a fasting serum gastrin level is useful in determining the cause of recurrent ulcer disease. A markedly elevated level suggests the presence of a gastrinoma or retained antrum. These two conditions can be differentiated by the secretin infusion test, which causes an expected decrease in gastrin with retained antrum and a paradoxical increase with the Zollinger–Ellison syndrome.[55] A technetium radioisotope scan has also been used to confirm the diagnosis of retained antrum.[56,57] Gastric secretory studies may identify patients with hypersecretory states but are technically difficult because of reflux of small-bowel contents. The Hollander insulin test is an imperfect indicator of vagal integrity and a poor discriminator of recurrent ulcer.[54] Although recurrent peptic ulcer is generally considered a surgical disease, recent studies have documented cimetidine as a useful alternative in its treatment.[58,59]

Carcinoma of the gastric remnant may develop as a late complication of peptic ulcer surgery.[60–63] The increased risk begins 10 years postoperatively, although, in most series, an average of 25 years has lapsed from the time of surgery to clinical detection of tumor. Predominance of the disease in males has been reported.[61] The pathogenesis of stump carcinoma is unknown; chronic bile reflux may be a predisposing factor. There is no evidence that histologic findings such as atrophic gastritis, cystic dilation of the gastric glands, or intestinal metaplasia are early indicators of malignant transformation.[61] Some investigators suggest that periodic endoscopy with multiple biopsies be performed 10 to 15 years after surgery.[60–63]

Following a Billroth II gastrojejunostomy, two rare clinical syndromes may develop that involve obstruction of the afferent loop.[64] The acute afferent loop syndrome usually occurs in the immediate postoperative period and is characterized by sudden onset of upper abdominal pain and vomiting with rapid clinical deterioration. Occasionally, hyperamylasemia occurs, and the patient is thought to have acute pancreatitis.[65] Delay in making the correct diagnosis can result in blowout or necrosis of the duodenal stump with fatal peritonitis. The cause of the obstruction is seldom demonstrated but may be related to the sharp angulation at the afferent limb and gastric remnant. The chronic afferent loop syndrome is due to intermittent obstruction of the jejunal limb.[64,66] The patient typically has postprandial projectile bilious vomiting, but the vomitus contains none of the recently ingested food, as is seen in reflux bile gastritis. The condition may be difficult to characterize radiographically because of difficulty in filling the afferent loop with barium. Stenosis of the afferent loop may be demonstrated at endoscopy. Revisional surgery is usually necessary for correction of both syndromes.[67]

Phytobezoars (plant bezoars) may be present following Billroth I and II procedures, especially when these operations are accompanied by vagotomy.[68,69] Treatment includes a liquid diet, nasogastric suction and lavage, and an attempt at endoscopic internal fragmentation.[70] Bezoars carry a high mortality rate and should be treated with gastrotomy if conservative methods fail.

Metabolic bone disease has been documented postoperatively in 15% to 30% of patients who have undergone a partial gastrectomy.[71,72] Osteomalacia appears to be the major bone disorder and is more prevalent than previously suspected. Significant histologic changes have been found without clinical, radiologic, or biochemical abnormalities.[72] Elevated serum alkaline phosphatase levels suggest asymptomatic bone disease. Treatment with calcium and vitamin D supplements should be considered.

Several studies have suggested an increased incidence of pulmonary tuberculosis after gastrectomy.[73–75] This has been attributed to the poor nutritional status of gastrectomy patients.

SMALL-BOWEL RESECTION

The major diseases of the small bowel that require extensive resection include mesenteric thrombosis, mechanical obstruction with bowel infarction, Crohn's disease, tumor, radiation enteritis, and abdominal trauma.[76,77] Mortality is proportional to the length of bowel resected and is especially high if, in addition to the duodenum, less than 2 ft (60 centimeters) of jejunum or ileum remain.[76] Patients undergoing small-bowel resection of greater than 75% have severe nutritional and metabolic problems. The complications of small-bowel resection include the following:

Volume depletion
Electrolyte abnormalities
Steatorrhea
Malabsorption (especially of fat-soluble
  vitamins)
Gastric acid hypersecretion
Cholelithiasis
Nephrolithiasis
Diarrhea

Preservation of the ileocecal valve and

compensation of remaining bowel are among the factors that affect the nature and severity of these derangements.[76,78] Combined ileal and colonic resection predispose to greater volume and electrolyte depletion.[79–81] A massive proximal and small-intestinal resection is better tolerated than an equivalent distal resection because of the remarkable ability of the ileum to assume the absorptive function of the upper small intestine.[82] Although the rate of absorption of iron, calcium, and magnesium is highest in the duodenum, these elements can be absorbed throughout the small intestine. In contrast, ascorbic acid, folic acid, and other water-soluble vitamins, except vitamin B_{12}, are normally absorbed in the jejunum.[78] Secretin and cholecystokinin are synthesized and released from duodenal and jejunal mucosa, and extensive resection of these areas may result in decreased hormonal stimulation of exocrine pancreatic and biliary secretion. The ileum is the selective site for absorption of intrinsic factor-bound vitamin B_{12} and conjugated bile salts. The latter substances not only impair colonic water absorption but may also cause secretion of water and electrolytes.[83,84]

Other metabolic changes may develop after extensive small-bowel resection. Gastric acid hypersecretion is seen in 50% of patients.[77,85] Elevated fasting and meal-stimulated serum gastrin levels may be due to decreased clearance of gastrin or loss of a hormonal inhibitor.[86–88] Many hormones, such as secretin, cholecystokinin, glucagon, vasoactive intestinal polypeptide, and gastric inhibitory peptide, are known to decrease gastric acid secretion, and extensive resection may reduce their levels. Severe ulcer diathesis or hemorrhagic gastritis may develop, necessitating emergency surgery. Gastric hypersecretion may also augment the usual postoperative diarrhea by deactivation of pancreatic enzymes and precipitation of bile salts. Increased acid loads damage the remaining intestinal mucosa, thereby further inhibiting absorption. Fortunately, gastric hypersecretion is usually transient after extensive small-bowel resection, and studies have demonstrated the efficacy of cimetidine in its management.[89,90]

The incidence of cholelithiasis and nephrolithiasis is higher than normal after ileal resection. Cholelithiasis is related to a contracted bile-salt pool that causes secretion of lithogenic bile containing an increased cholesterol concentration.[91,92] A predisposition to calcium oxalate nephrolithiasis is caused by the following process: Hyperoxaluria results from increased binding of calcium to malabsorbed fatty acids, leaving little calcium available to form insoluble calcium oxalate, which is normally excreted in the stool.[93,94] Oxalate therefore remains available for absorption by the colonic mucosa, which exhibits increased permeability induced by exposure to bile salts and fatty acids.[95]

Voluminous diarrhea can be a significant problem in the immediate postoperative period, requiring meticulous replacement of fluid and electrolytes. Possible causes include loss of absorptive surface, shortened transit time, steatorrhea, acquired lactose intolerance, impaired bile-salt absorption, acid hypersecretion, and an overgrowth of bacterial flora.[76–78] The diarrhea can usually be controlled with diphenoxylate and atropine, loperamide, or codeine. Restriction of fat (to less than 30 g/day) and lactose is also required. Broad-spectrum antibiotics are helpful in the treatment of bacterial overgrowth, especially if the ileocecal valve has been removed. Cholestyramine in a dose of 8 to 12 g/day may improve bile salt-induced diarrhea in patients with less than 100 cm of ileum resected.[96,97] After more extensive resections, cholestyramine may aggravate the situation by further depleting the bile-salt pool and thereby worsening the steatorrhea. This will result in increased delivery of unabsorbed fatty acids into the colon to stimulate water and electrolyte secretion.

During the first several months after surgery, the remaining small intestine undergoes adaptation. Jejunal biopsies in the postoperative period have documented epithelial cell hyperplasia.[98] Animal studies have shown not only mucosal cell hyperplasia but also increased villus height and crypt depth as well as an increase in segmental absorption of nutrients, electrolytes, and water.[82] Luminal nutrients are important in initiating and maintaining these adaptive responses.[99,100] During the period of intestinal adaptation, patients should be supported with total parenteral nutrition. In patients with extensive resections, plans for life-long home parenteral nutrition may be necessary.[101,102] The transition to oral feedings may take several months and may initially aggravate postoperative diarrhea. Enteral hyperalimentation with elemental diets is helpful in initiating feedings approximately 1 to 3 weeks after surgery.[103] Long-term management will require supplementation of fat-soluble vitamins, calcium, magnesium, and trace elements such as zinc. Deficiencies of water-soluble vitamins are uncommon unless a significant length of jejunum in addition to ileum has been resected.[104] Periodic parenteral injection of vitamin B_{12} may be necessary in patients with extensive ileal resection.[104,105]

INTESTINAL BYPASS SURGERY

Intestinal bypass is frequently employed in the treatment of obese patients weighing more than twice ideal weight.[106,107] Jejunocolic bypass, the earliest of these operative procedures, has been abandoned. Instead, jejunoileal and gastric bypass operations are now performed.[106–108] The jejunoileal bypass consists of a jejunoileostomy in which only a 50-cm functional segment of small bowel (40 cm of jejunum and 10 cm of ileum) remains in continuity.[106] In the gastric bypass, a fundic pouch is created by transection or stapling of the stomach, and a gastrojejunostomy is formed that bypasses the body and antrum.[108] The small pouch produces early satiety.

Follow-up studies document a high incidence of complications following jejunoileal bypass, and many authorities feel this is not an acceptable treatment for morbid obesity.[109,110] Although few adequate follow-up studies have been done for gastric bypass, the incidence of serious complications appears lower with this operation. Mortality for the jejunoileal bypass ranges from 2% to 10%, and major complications occur in over 50% of patients.[106,107,109,110] Many of the complications associated with the jejunoileal bypass are similar to those that follow extensive small-bowel resection. The mechanisms and management of postoperative diarrhea, nutritional and electrolyte deficiencies, cholelithiasis and nephrolithiasis are similar to those discussed above.

Progressive liver disease is the most significant complication associated with intestinal bypass surgery.[109,110] Clinically recognizable hepatic disease has been noted in up to 17% of patients and carries a significant rate of mortality.[111] The hepatic lesion is characterized by extensive triglyceride accumulation (steatosis), which increases during the period of maximal weight loss from 2 to 8 months after surgery.[111,112] Those patients who lose weight most rapidly are at greater risk for this complication. Patients may develop acute hepatic failure or experience insidious progression to cirrhosis.[111] It is generally agreed that progressive hepatic damage is an indication for restoration of small-bowel continuity. Nonoperative treatment with parenteral hyperalimentation has been successful in a few cases.[115,116]

An inflammatory process known as bypass enteropathy may occur in the excluded small-bowel segment.[117] Patients develop abdominal distention and an exacerbation of diarrhea associated with gas fluid levels in the large and small bowels. The clinical picture resembles intestinal pseudo-obstruction and is frequently associated with arthritis, fever, and skin lesions. Clinical improvement may follow treatment with broad-spectrum antibiotics such as metronidazole or with restitution of small-bowel continuity, suggesting bacterial overgrowth in the excluded segment as the cause of bypass enteropathy.

Musculoskeletal symptoms are frequent following intestinal bypass surgery.[118–120] The arthritis is usually transitory, nondeforming, and responsive to treatment with anti-inflammatory agents.[120] Circulating immune complexes related to absorbed intestinal bacterial antigens may activate complement pathways to cause these joint symptoms.[119,120]

Malnutrition after bypass surgery may be associated with abnormal immunoreactivity, which predisposes patients to infection. Patients with accelerated weight loss, lymphadenopathy, and unexplained fever and chills should be evaluated for tuberculosis.[121,122]

Metabolic bone disease following jejunoileal bypass is caused by malabsorption and steatorrhea.[123,124] Steatorrhea impairs the absorption not only of dietary vitamin D but also of 25-hydroxy-vitamin D_3. Bone biopsy demonstrates osteomalacia and impaired osteoblast function.[124] Vitamin D and calcium supplementation may help to prevent severe bone demineralization in patients with metabolic bone disease.

COLECTOMY

Total proctocolectomy and resultant ileostomy cause a chronic, salt-losing state.[125] The colon is normally a major site of sodium and water absorption and possesses a large reserve capacity.[81] During periods of salt depletion, the colon avidly conserves salt. After the loss of the colon, functioning ileostomies put out 500 to 600 g/day of effluent, 90% of which is water.[126] A necessary loss of 30 to 40 mEq/day of sodium and the inability of the small intestine to augment salt and water absorption predispose the patient to dehydration and electrolyte imbalance.[127] Chronic oliguria and nephrolithiasis develop in some patients.[128,129]

In recent years, a continent ileostomy called a Koch pouch has been developed.[130] Although this pouch is more appealing esthetically than conventional ileostomies, its stomal output is not significantly different.[131] Chronic stasis within the pouch predisposes to anaerobic bacterial overgrowth and a stagnant loop syndrome with malabsorption of B_{12}.[132] A colitic type of arthropathy may also occur.[133]

POSTCHOLECYSTECTOMY SYNDROME

PCS is a general term used to describe symptoms ranging from mild dyspepsia to severe attacks of colicky abdominal pain after cholecystectomy. Of all cholecystectomy patients, 30% to 40% report some symptoms postoperatively, and 15% are significantly disabled.[134,135] Patients who undergo surgery for classic biliary colic are more likely to obtain symptomatic relief than those whose major preoperative complaint is dyspepsia.[136,137] The most common cause of this syndrome may be an erroneous preoperative diagnosis of biliary tract disease. Proposed causes of PCS are listed below.

Reflux esophagitis
Diffuse esophageal spasm
Peptic ulcer disease
Irritable bowel syndrome
Pancreatitis
Choledocholithiasis
Biliary stricture
Cystic duct remnant
Stenosis of the sphincter of Oddi
Biliary dyskinesia
Psychosomatic disorders

Choledocholithiasis due to residual or recurrent stones may cause postoperative discomfort. Concomitant choledocholithiasis is found in 15% of patients operated upon for cholelithiasis.[138] Half of all common-duct stones encountered during cholecystectomy were asymptomatic preoperatively.[139] The postoperative cholangiogram shows stones in 2% to 5% of cases, despite a negative operative cholangiogram and thorough common-duct exploration.[139,140] About one-fourth of patients who present with common-duct stones following cholecystectomy do so more than 10 years after surgery, suggesting formation of the stones after removal of the gallbladder.[141–142]

Reoperation for removal of common-duct stones is necessary in about 2% of patients who have undergone cholecystectomy.[139] Extraction of stones with a Dormia basket may be feasible if the patient has a T tube in place.[143,144] Infusion of solvents through the T tube or administration of oral bile acids may dissolve the stones; however, these methods are limited by side-effects and the need for prolonged therapy.[145] A large collective European experience suggests that the morbidity and mortality rates of endoscopic retrograde sphincterotomy compare favorably with those of surgical choledochotomy and that the former procedure may be especially useful in poor surgical candidates.[146]

Bile-duct strictures after cholecystectomy occur in 0.2% of patients.[137] Hepaticojejunal anastomosis with a Y loop may be necessary to treat extended or high strictures.

A long cystic-duct remnant greater than 1 cm or a residual portion of gallbladder may occasionally cause recurrent symptoms because of bile stasis and recurrent stone formation. However, if the presence of stones is not demonstrable, this is an unlikely cause of PCS.[137,147]

Papillary stenosis and functional disorders of the bile-duct musculature or sphincter of Oddi (biliary dyskinesia) have long been topics of controversy. Provocative diagnostic maneuvers such as the administration of morphine and neostigmine have proved nonspecific.[148–151] A high rate of false-positive results among controls was found as well as a poor correlation with pressure measurements and operative findings. These provocative maneuvers are not reliable for evaluating patients with suspected biliary dyskinesia or papillary stenosis.

Although several studies have revealed psychosomatic disorders in 40% to 50% of patients with PCS, this remains an etiology of exclusion.[152,153] A thorough diagnostic evaluation must be pursued.

In addition to routine radiographic studies, certain diagnostic modalities are especially helpful in the evaluation of a patient with PCS. Upper endoscopy may reveal previously unsuspected esophagitis, gastritis, or ulcer disease. Esophageal manometry and the acid perfusion (Bernstein) test can detect major disorders, such as diffuse esophageal spasm or an incompetent lower esophageal sphincter predisposing to repeated gastroesophageal reflux. Endoscopic retrograde cholangiopancreatography (ERCP) allows demonstration of common-duct stricture or stone, large cystic-duct remnant, or pancreatic disease. ERCP manometry provides direct pressure measurement in the sphincter of Oddi, common bile duct, and pancreatic duct and may help identify patients with papillary stenosis who would benefit from sphincterotomy.[154] However, the expertise and capability necessary for performance of ERCP manometry is presently limited to only a few centers.

SUMMARY

1. **One-half of patients undergoing surgery for peptic ulcer disease have some form of chronic disability, including dumping, delayed gastric emptying, weight loss, malabsorption, diarrhea, anemia, reflux, recurrent ulcer, tuberculosis, and metabolic bone disease.**
2. **Early postprandial dumping can usually be controlled by high-protein, low-carbohydrate, small meals. Late postprandial dumping can usually be controlled by restriction of carbohydrate alone.**
3. **A fasting serum gastrin level should be checked in patients with recurrent ulcer disease.**
4. **Rare complications of ulcer surgery include carcinoma of the gastric rem-**

nant, the afferent loop syndrome, and phytobezoars. All have a high mortality rate without specific treatment.
5. **Medical complications of small-bowel resection include malabsorption, fluid, electrolyte, and vitamin loss, gastric acid hypersecretion, diarrhea, cholelithiasis, and nephrolithiasis.**
6. **During the postoperative period of intestinal adaptation, patients should be supported with total parenteral nutrition. Feedings should begin 1 to 3 weeks postoperatively with elemental diets.**
7. **The major problem following colectomy is salt and water loss.**
8. **PCS occurs in 40% of patients and should be evaluated.**

REFERENCES

1. Jordan PH: Elective operations for duodental ulcer. N Engl J Med 287:1329, 1972
2. Kennedy T, Connell AM, Love AHG et al: Selective or truncal vagotomy. Five-year results of a double-blind, randomized, controlled trial. Br J Surg 60:944, 1978
3. Kronborg O, Madsen P: A controlled randomized trial of highly selective vagotomy versus selective vagotomy and pyloroplasty in treatment of duodenal ulcer. Gut 16:268, 1975
4. Madsen P, Kronborg O, Hart H et al: Billroth I gastric resection versus truncal vagotomy and pyloroplasty in treatment of gastric ulcer. Acta Chir Scand 142:151, 1976
5. Duthie HL, Kwong NK: Vagotomy or gastrectomy for gastric ulcer. Br Med J 4:79, 1973
6. Meyer JH: Chronic morbidity after ulcer surgery. In Sleisenger MH, Fordtran JC (eds). Gastrointestinal Disease, p 947. Philadelphia, WB Saunders, 1978
7. Smith FW, Jeffries GH: Late and persis-

tent postgastrectomy problems. In Sleisenger MH, Fordtran JS (eds). Gastrointestinal Disease, p 822. Philadelphia, WB Saunders, 1973

8. Machella TE: Symposium on some aspects of peptic ulcer: Mechanisms of postgastrectomy dumping syndrome. Gastroenterology 14:237, 1950

9. Stahlgren LH, Fronek K: The rule of jejunal distention in the initiation of the dumping syndrome. Ann Surg 176:139, 1972

10. Jesseph JE: Serotonin and the dumping syndrome. Surgery 63:536, 1968

11. Cuschieri A, Onabanjo OA: Kinin release after gastric surgery. Br Med J 3:565, 1971

12. Woodward ER: The early postprandial dumping syndrome: Clinical manifestations and pathogenesis. In Bushkin FL, Woodward ER (eds): Postgastrectomy Syndromes, p 1. Philadelphia, WB Saunders, 1976

13. Shultz KT, Neelon FA, Nilseh LB et al: Mechanism of postgastectomy hypoglycemia. Arch Intern Med 128:240, 1971

14. Bloom SR, Royston CMS, Thomson JPS: Enteroglucagon release in the dumping syndrome. Lancet 2:789, 1972

15. Unser HL: Principles of diet therapy for postgastrectomy dumping syndrome. Major Probl Clin Surg 20:159, 1976

16. Miranda R, Steffes B, O'Leary JD et al: Surgical treatment of the postgastrectomy dumping syndrome. Am J Surg 139:40, 1980

17. Jenkins DJ, Gassull MA, Leeds AK et al: Effect of dietary fiber on complications of gastric surgery: Prevention of postprandial hypoglycemia by pectin. Gastroenterology 72:215, 1977

18. Koelz HR, Gerwertz BL: The Stomach. I. Vagotomy. Clin Gastroenterol 8(2):305, 1979

19. Metzger WH, Cano R, Sturdevant RA: Effect of metoclopramide in chronic gastric retention after gastric surgery. Gastroenterology 71:30, 1976

20. Kroop HS, Long WB, Alavi A et al: Effect of water and fat on gastric emptying of solid meals. Gastroenterology 77:997, 1979

21. Alexander–Williams J, Hoare AM: The Stomach. II: Partial gastric resection. Clin Gastroenterol 8:321, 1979

22. King CE, Toskes PP: Malabsorption following gastric resection. In Bushkin FL, Woodward ER (eds): Postgastrectomy Syndromes, p 129. Philadelphia, WB Saunders, 1976

23. Donaldson RM: Small bowel bacterial overgrowth. Adv Intern Med 16:191, 1970

24. King CE, Toskes PP: Small intestine bacterial overgrowth. Gastroenterology 76:1035, 1979

25. Browning GG, Buchan KA, Mackay C: The effect of vagotomy and drainage of the small bowel flora. Gut 15:139, 1974

26. Hoffbrand AV, Tabaqchali S, Booth CC et al: Small intestinal bacterial flora and folate status in gastrointestinal disease. Gut 12:27, 1971

27. Sherr HP, Sasaki Y, Newman A et al: Detection of bacterial deconjugation of bile salts by a convenient breath analysis technique. N Engl J Med 285:656, 1971

28. King CE, Tuskes PP, Spivey JC et al: Detection of small intestine bacterial overgrowth by means of a ^{14}C-D-xylose breath test. Gastroenterology 77:75, 1979

29. Condon JR, Westerholm P, Tanner NC: Lactose malabsorption and postgastrectomy milk intolerance, dumping and diarrhea. Gut 10:311, 1969

30. Waddell WR, Kunz LJ: Association of salmonella enteritis with operations on the stomach. N Engl J Med 255:555, 1956

31. Yardley JH, Takano J, Hendrix TR: Epithelial and other mucosal lesions of the jejunum in giardiasis. Jejunal biopsy studies. Bull Johns Hopkins Hosp 115:389, 1964

32. Allan JG, Gerskowitch VP, Russell RI: The role of bile acids in the pathogenesis of postvagotomy diarrhea. Br J Surg 61:516, 1974

33. Condon JR, Robinson V, Suleman MI et al: The cause and treatment of postvagotomy diarrhea. Br J Surg 62:309, 1975

34. Allan JG, Russell RI: Cholestyramine in treatment of post-vagotomy diarrhea. Double-blind controlled trial. Br Med J 1:674, 1977

35. Duncombe VM, Bolin TD, Davis AE: Double-blind trial of cholestyramine in postvagotomy diarrhea. Gut 18:531, 1977

36. Pryor JP, O'Shea MJ, Brooks PL et al: The long-term metabolic consequences of partial gastrectomy. Am J Med 51:5, 1971

37. Shafer RB, Ripley D, Swaim WR et al: Hematologic alterations following partial gastrectomy. Am J Med Sci 266:240, 1973

38. Baird IM, Blackburn EK, Wilson GM: The pathogenesis of anemia after partial gastrectomy. Q J Med 28:21, 1959

39. Hines JD, Hoffbrand AV, Mollin DL: The hematological complications following partial gastrectomy. Am J Med 43:555, 1967

40. Toskes PP, Deren JJ: Vitamin B_{12} absorption and malabsorption. Gastroenterology 65:662, 1973

41. Mahmud K, Ripley D, Swaim WR et al: Hematologic complications of partial gastrectomy. Ann Surg 177:432, 1973

42. Doscherholmen A, Swaim WR: Impaired assimilation of egg ^{57}CO vitamin B_{12} in patients with hypochlorhydria and after gastric resection. Gastroenterology 64:913, 1973

43. Hoare AM, Keighley RB, Starkey B et al: Measurement of bile acids in fasting gastric aspirates: An objective test for bile reflux after gastric surgery. Gut 19:166, 1978

44. Gadacz TR, Zuidema GD: Bile acid composition in patients with and without symptoms of postoperative reflux gastritis. Am J Surg 135:48, 1978

45. Tolin RD, Malmud LS, Stelzer F et al: Enterogastric reflux in normal subjects and patients with Billroth II gastroenterostomy. Gastroenterology 17:1027, 1979

46. Hoare AM, Jones EL, Alexander–Williams J et al. Symptomatic significance of gastric mucosal changes after surgery for peptic ulcer. Gut 18:295, 1977

47. Meshkinpour H, Elashoff J, Stewart H et al: Effect of cholestyramine on the symptoms of reflux gastritis. A randomized double-blind crossover study. Gastroenterology 73:441, 1977

48. Reber HA, Way LH: Surgical treatment of late postgastrectomy syndromes. Am J Surg 129:71, 1975

49. Price WE, Grizzle JE, Postlethwait RW et al: Results of operation for duodenal ulcer. Surg Gynecol Obstet 131:233, 1970

50. Howard RJ, Murphy WR, Humphrey EW: A prospective randomized study of the elective surgical treatment for duodenal ulcer. Two- to ten-year follow-up study. Surgery 73:256, 1973

51. Postlethwait RW: Five-year follow-up results of operations for duodenal ulcer. Surg Gynecol Obstet 137:387, 1973

52. Jordan PH: A follow-up report of a prospective evaluation of vagotomy–pyloroplasty and vagotomy–antrectomy for treatment of duodenal ulcer. Ann Surg 180:259, 1974

53. Van Heerden JA, Kelly KA, Dozois RR et al: Proximal gastric vagotomy. Mayo Clin Proc 55:10, 1980

54. Stabile BE, Passaro E: Recurrent peptic ulcer. Gastroenterology 70:124, 1976

55. Korman MG, Scott DF, Hansky J et al: Hypergastrinemia due to an excluded gastric antrum: A proposed method for differentiation from Zollinger–Ellison syndrome. Aust NZ J Med 2:266, 1972

56. Sciarreta G, Malaguri P, Turba E et al: Retained gastric antrum syndrome diagnosed by ^{99m}Tc-pertechnetate scintiphotography in man: Hormonal and radioisotope study of two cases. J Nucl Med 19:377, 1978

57. Chaudhuri TK, Shiragi SS et al: Radioisotopic scan, a possible aid in differentiating retained gastric antrum from Zollinger–Ellison syndrome in patients with recurrent peptic ulcer. Gastroenterology 65:697, 1973

58. Gugler R, Lindstaedt H, Miederer S et al: Cimetidine for anastomotic ulcers after partial gastrectomy. N Engl J Med 301:1077, 1979

59. Festen HPM, Lamers CBE, Driessen WM et al: Cimetidine in anastomotic ulceration after partial gastrectomy. Gastroenterology 76:83, 1979

60. Osnes M, Lotveit T, Myren J et al: Early gastric carcinoma in patients with a Billroth II partial gastrectomy. Endoscopy 9:45, 1977

61. Domellöf L, Eriksson S, Janunger KG: Carcinoma and possible precancerous changes of the gastric stump after Billroth II resection. Gastroenterology 73:462, 1977

62. Domellöf L, Janunger KG: The risk for gastric carcinoma after partial gastrectomy. Am J Surg 134:581, 1977

63. Schrumpf E, Serck–Hanssen A, Stadaas J et al: Mucosal changes in the gastric stump 20–25 years after partial gastrectomy. Lancet 2:467, 1977.

64. Bushkin FL, Woodward ER: Postgastrectomy Syndromes, pp 34–48. Philadelphia, WB Saunders, 1976

65. Hinshaw DB, Carter R, Baker H et al: Postgastrectomy afferent loop obstruction simulating acute pancreatitis. Ann Surg 151:600, 1960

66. Mitty WF, Grossi C, Nealon TF: Chronic afferent loop syndrome. Ann Surg 172:996, 1970

67. Brooke-Cowden GL, Braasch JW, Gibb SP et al: Postgastrectomy syndromes. Am J Surg 131:464, 1976

68. Amjad H, Kumar GK, McCaughey R: Postgastrectomy bezoars. Am J Gastroenterol 64:327, 1975

69. Wortzel E, Ferrer JP, DeLuca RF: Medical treatment of the postgastrectomy bezoar. Am J Gastroenterol 67:565, 1977

70. McKechnie J: Gastroscopic removal of a phytobezoar. Gastroenterology 62:1047, 1972

71. Eddy R: Metabolic bone disease after gastrectomy. Am J Med 50:442, 1971

72. McKechnie J: Gastroscopic removal of a phytobezoar. Gastroenterology 62:1047, 1972

71. Eddy RL: Metabolic bone disease after gastrectomy. Am J Med 50:442, 1971

72. Garrick R, Ireland AW, Posen S: Bone abnormalities after gastric surgery. A prospective histological study. Ann Intern Med 75:221, 1971

73. Frucht H, Kunke P: Pulmonary tuberculosis following gastric resection. Ann Intern Med 46:696, 1957

74. DiBenedetto A, Diamond P, Essig HC: Tuberculosis following subtotal gastrectomy. Surg Gynecol Obstet 134:586, 1972

75. Steiger Z, Nickel WO, Shannon GJ et al: Pulmonary tuberculosis after gastric resection. Am J Surg 131:668, 1976

76. Weser E: The management of patients after small bowel resection. Gastroenterology 71:146, 1976

77. Krejs GJ: The small bowel. I. Intestinal resection. Clin Gastroenterol 8:373, 1979

78. Weser E, Fletcher JT, Urban E: Short bowel syndrome. Gastroenterology 77:572, 1979

79. Cummings JH, James WPT, Wigging HS: Role of the colon in ileal-resection diarrhea. Lancet 1:344, 1973

80. Mitchell JE, Breuer RI, Zuckerman L et al: The colon influences ileal resection diarrhea. Dig Dis Sci 25:33, 1980.

81. DeBongnie JC, Phillips SF: Capacity of the human colon to absorb fluid. Gastroenterology 74:698, 1978

82. Williamson RLN: Intestinal adaptation. 1. Structural, functional, and cytokinetic changes. 2. Mechanisms of control. N Engl J Med 298:1393; 1444, 1978

83. Ammon HV, Phillips SF: Inhibition of colonic water and electrolyte absorption by fatty acids in man. Gastroenterology 65:744, 1973

84. Mekhjian HS, Phillips SF, Hoffman AF: Colonic secretion of water and electrolytes induced by bile acids: Perfusion studies in man. J Clin Invest 50:1569, 1971

85. Buxton B: Small bowel resection and gastric hypersecretion. Gut 15:229, 1974

86. Straus E, Gerson CD, Yalow RS: Hypersecretion of gastrin associated with the short bowel syndrome. Gastroenterology 66:175, 1974

87. Becker HD, Reeder DD, Thompson SC: Extraction of circulating endogenous gas-

trin by the small bowel. Gastroenterology 65:903, 1973

88. Wright HK, Tilson MD: The short gut syndrome. Pathophysiology and treatment. Curr Probl Surg, June:3, 1971

89. Cortot A, Fleming CR, Malagelada JR: Improved nutrient absorption after cimetidine in short bowel syndrome with gastric hypersecretion. N Engl J Med 300:79, 1979

90. Murphy JP, King DR, Dubois A: Treatment of gastric hypersecretion with cimetidine in the short bowel syndrome. N Engl J Med 300:80, 1979

91. Dowling RH, Bell GD, White J: Lithogenic bile in patients with ileal dysfunction. Gut 13:415, 1972

92. Vlahcevic ZR, Prazich J, Swell L: Evidence that a diminished bile acid pool precedes the formation of cholesterol gallstones in man. Surg Gynecol Obstet 136:961, 1973

93. Hoffman AF, Thomas PJ, Smith LH et al: Pathogenesis of secondary hyperoxaluria in patients with ileal resection and diarrhea. Gastroenterology 58:960, 1970

94. Earnest DL, Johnson G, Williams HE et al: Hyperoxaluria in patients with ileal resection: An abnormality in dietary oxalate absorption. Gastroenterology 66:1114, 1974

95. Dobbins JW, Binder HJ: Effect of bile salts an fatty acids on the colonic absorption of oxalate. Gastroenterology 70:1096, 1976

96. Hoffman AF, Poley JR: Cholestyramine treatment of diarrhea associated with ileal resection. N Engl J Med 281:397, 1969

97. Hoffman AF, Poley JR: Role of bile acid malabsorption in pathogenesis of diarrhea and steatorrhea in patients with ileal resection. I. Response to cholesytramine or replacement of dietary long chain triglyceride by medium chain triglyceride. Gastroenterology 62:1077, 1973.

98. Porus, RL: Epithelial hyperplasia following massive small bowel resection. Gastroenterology 48:753, 1965

99. Levine GM, Deren JJ, Steiger E et al: Role of oral intake in maintenance of gut mass and disaccharide activity. Gastroenterology 67:975, 1974

100. Levine GM, Deren JJ, Yezdimir E: Small bowel resection: Oral intake is the stimulus for hyperplasia. Am J Dig Dis 21:542, 1976

101. Jeejeebhoy KN, Zohrab WJ, Langer B et al: Total parenteral nutrition at home for 23 months without complication and with good rehabilitation. A study of technical and metabolic features. Gastroenterology 65:811, 1973

102. Heizer WD, Orringer EP: Parenteral nutrition at home for five years via arteriovenous fistulae: Supplemental intravenous feeding for a patient with severe short bowel syndrome. Gastroenterology 72:527, 1977

103. Heymsfield SB, Bethel RA, Ansley JD et al: Enteral hyperalimentation: An alternative to central venous hyperalimentation. Ann Intern Med 90:63, 1979

104. Scheiner E, Shils ME, Vanamee P: Malabsorption following massive intestinal resection. Am J Clin Nutr 17:64, 1965

105. Allcock E: Absorption of vitamin B_{12} in man following extensive resection of the jejunum, ileum, and colon. Gastroenterology 40:81, 1961

106. Bray GA, Barry RE, Benfield JR et al: Intestinal bypass operation as a treatment for obesity. Ann Intern Med 85:97, 1976

107. Scott HW, Dean RH, Shull HJ et al: Results of jejunoileal bypass in two hundred patients with morbid obesity. Surg Gynecol Obstet 145:661, 1977

108. Buckwalter JA, Herbst CA: Complications of gastric bypass for morbid obesity. Am J Surg 139:55, 1980

109. Iber FL, Cooper M: Jejunoileal bypass for the treatment of massive obesity. Prevalence, morbidity, and short and long term consequences. Am J Clin Nutr 30:4, 1977

110. Halverson JD, Wise L, Wazna MF et al: Jejunoileal bypass for morbid obesity. Am J Med 64:461, 1978

111. Peters RL: Patterns of hepatic morphology in jejunoileal bypass patients. Am J Clin Nutr 30:53, 1977

112. Holzbach RT, Wieland RG, Lieber CS et al: Hepatic lipid in morbid obesity. N Engl J Med 290:296, 1974

113. Peters RL, Gay T, Reynolds TB: Postjejunal bypass hepatic disease, its similarity to alcoholic liver disease. Am J Clin Pathology 63:318, 1975

114. Moxley RT, Pozefsky T, Lockwood DH: Protein nutrition and liver disease after jejunoileal bypass for morbid obesity. N Engl J Med 290:921, 1974

115. Heimberger SL, Steiger E, Logerfo P et al: Reversal of severe fatty hepatic infiltration after intestinal bypass for morbid obesity by calorie free amino acid infusion. Am J Surg 129:229, 1975

116. Ames FC, Copeland EM, Leeb DC et al: Liver dysfunction following small bowel bypass for obesity. JAMA 235:1249, 1976

117. Drenick EJ, Ament ME, Finegold SM et al: Bypass enteropathy: An inflammatory process in the excluded segment with systemic complications. Am J Clin Nutr 30:76, 1977

118. Buchanan RF, Wilkens RF: Arthritis after jejunoileostomy. Arthritis Rheum 15:644, 1972

119. Wands JR, LaMont JT, Mann E et al: Arthritis associated with intestinal bypass procedure for morbid obesity. N Engl J Med 294:121, 1976

120. Ginsberg J, Quismorio FP, Dewind LT et al: Musculoskeletal symptoms after jejunoileal shunt surgery for intractable obesity. Am J Med 67:443, 1979

121. Bruce RM, Wise L: Tuberculosis after jejunoileal bypass for obesity. Ann Intern Med 87:574, 1977

122. Harris JO, Wasson KR: Tuberculosis after intestinal bypass operation for obesity. Ann Intern Med 86:115, 1977

123. Teitelbaum SL, Halverson JD, Bates M et al: Abnormalities of circulating 25-OH vitamin D after jejunoileal bypass for obesity. Ann Intern Med 86:289, 1977

124. Parfitt AM, Miller MJ, Frame B et al: Metabolic bone disease after intestinal bypass for treatment of obesity. Ann Intern Med 89:193, 1978

125. Philips SF: Life with an ileostomy. In Sleisenger MH, Fordtran JS (eds): Gastrointestinal Disease, p 1653. Philadelphia, WB Saunders, 1978

126. Kanaghinis T, Lubran M, Coghill NF: The composition of ileostomy fluid. Gut 4:322, 1963

127. Phillips SF: Absorption and secretion by the colon. Gastroenterology 56:966, 1969

128. Clarke AM, Chirnside A, Hill GL et al: Chronic dehydration and sodium depletion in patients with established ileostomies. Lancet 2:740, 1967

129. Clarke AM, McKenzie RG: Ileostomy and the risk of urinary uric stones. Lancet 2:395, 1969

130. Kock NG, Dare N, Kewenter J et al: The quality of life after proctocolectomy and ileostomy: A study of patients with conventional ileostomies converted to continent ileostomies. Dis Colon Rectum 17:287, 1974

131. Jagenburg R, Dotenvall G, Kewenter J et al: Absorption studies in patients with intraabdominal ileostomy reservoirs and in patients with conventional ileostomies. Gut 12:437, 1971

132. Schjonsby H, Halvorsen JF, Hofstadt T et al: Stagnant loop syndrome in patients with continent ileostomy (Intra-abdominal ileal reservoir). Gut 18:795, 1977

133. Hawley PR, Ritchie JK: The colon. I. Complications of ileostomy and colostomy following excisional surgery. Clin Gastroenterol 8:403, 1979

134. Bodvall B: The postcholecystectomy syndromes. Clin Gastroenterol 2:103, 1977

135. Stephani P, Carboni M, Petrassi N et al: Factors influencing the long term results of cholecystectomies. Surg Gynecol Obstet 139:734, 1974

136. Gunn A, Keddie N: Some clinical observations on patients with gallstones. Lancet 2:239, 1972

137. Tondelli P, Gyr K, Stalder G et al: The biliary tract. Cholecystectomy. Clin Gastroenterol 2:487, 1979

138. Wilson ID, Delaney JP, Duane WC et al: Choledocholithiasis. Gastroenterology 75:120, 1978

139. Way LW, Admirand WH, Dunphy JE:

Management of choledocholithiasis. Ann Surg 176:347, 1972

140. Glenn F: Retained calculi within the biliary ductal system. Ann Surg 179:528, 1974

141. Thurston OG, McDougall RM: The effect of hepatic bile on retained common duct stones. Surg Gynecol Obstet 143:625, 1976

142. Soloway RD, Trotman BW, Ostrow JD: Pigment gallstones. Gastroenterology 72:167, 1977

143. Burhenne HJ: Nonoperative extraction of retained common duct stones. Adv Surg 10:121, 1976

144. Mazzariello RM: Residual biliary tract stones: Nonoperative treatment of 570 patients. Surg Annu 8:113, 1976

145. Key PH, Schoenfield LJ: Medical dissolution of gallstones: Current status. In Berk JE (ed): Developments in Digestive Diseases, p 111. Philadelphia, Lea & Febiger, 1977

146. Safrany L: Duodenoscopic sphincterotomy and gallstone removal. Gastroenterology 72:338, 1977

147. Bodvall B, Overgaard B: Cystic duct remnant after cholecystectomy. Ann Surg 163:382, 1966

148. Holtzer JD, Hulst SG: Confirmation of postcholecystectomy biliary dyskinesia by elevation of serum transaminases (GOT and GPT) after injection of morphine. Acta Med Scand 194:221, 1973

149. Nardi GL: Papillitis and stenosis of the sphincter of Oddi. Surg Clin North Am 53:1147, 1973

150. Logiudice JA, Geenen JE, Hogan WJ et al: Efficacy of the morphine–prostigmin test for evaluating patients with suspected papillary stenosis. Dig Dis Sci 24:455, 1979

151. Steinberg WM, Salvato RF, Toskes PP: The morphine–prostigmin provocative test—Is it useful for making clinical decisions? Gastroenterology 78:728, 1980

152. Christiansen J, Schmidt A: The postcholecystectomy syndrome. Acta Chir Scand 137:789, 1971

153. Kakizaki G, Kato E, Fujiwana Y et al: Postbiliary surgery complaints. Psychosomatic aspects. Am J Gastroenterol 66:62, 1976

154. Bar–Meir S, Geenen JE, Hogan WJ et al: Biliary and pancreatic duct pressures measured by ERCP manometry in patients with suspected papillary stenosis. Dig Dis Sci 24:209, 1979

Anesthesia and Surgery in the Patient with Liver Disease

FRANK H. BROWN
YIH-FU SHIAU
GARY C. RICHTER

Acute and chronic liver disease are among the most prevalent underlying disorders found in surgical patients. Patients with liver disease frequently require surgery for complications of their disease and have an increased incidence of associated conditions that require surgical intervention, including hernias, cholelithiasis, and peptic ulcer disease.[1,3] Many abuse ethanol or drugs with the attendant risks of trauma and infection. Some investigators estimate that 5% to 10% of all patients with liver disease undergo surgery in the last 2 years of their lives, and two large reviews state that between 4% and 16% of all cirrhotics die from postoperative complications.[3–5]

Evaluation of the surgical patient with hepatic disease is complex because of the multiple synthetic and metabolic functions of the liver that are essential in maintaining homeostatic balance during the stress of surgery. This chapter deals with the pathophysiologic effects of anesthesia and surgery on hepatic function and reviews the evidence that patients with acute and chronic liver disease have higher than normal risk of operative morbidity and mortality. The use of preoperative evaluation and preparation to assess and modify this risk and the diagnosis and management of postoperative complications are also discussed. Detailed discussions of specialized procedures, including portasystemic shunting, hepatic resection, and liver transplantation, are omitted, but some relevant data from studies of patients who have undergone these procedures are presented.

EFFECTS OF ANESTHESIA AND SURGERY

Multiple studies have shown that postoperative abnormalities in one or more liver function tests are found in a large though highly variable percentage of patients.[6–21] Interpretation of these studies is often difficult. Frequently, the effect of the underlying disease, the anesthetic technique or agent used, and the operative procedure done cannot be clearly defined. Furthermore, many early studies used tests of liver function that have now been abandoned as unreliable. Many suffer from small sample size, inadequate controls, or lack of statistical analysis. Most often, changes in hepatic function are small and of questionable clinical significance.

Surgery is often precipitated by uncontrolled infection, hemorrhage, or extensive trauma. Several studies have shown that fever, sepsis, burns, multiple trauma, hemorrhage, and shock can in themselves cause liver dysfunction.[22–29] Thus, hepatic function in the surgical patient may be compromised even before surgery begins.

Anesthesia

Anesthesia has long been suspected as a cause of hepatic dysfunction, but its contribution to frequently noted disturbances in postoperative liver function tests remains unclear and is difficult to separate from the effects of the operative procedure itself.[30–33] Brouhoult and Gillquist evaluated the effect of anesthesia alone by measuring postanesthetic serum transaminase levels in patients who had received halothane for angiography and found no abnormalities.[34] Stevens and co-workers addressed the problem by administering various anesthetics to healthy volunteers not undergoing surgery and found subsequent small abnormalities in liver function after using several agents.[35]

The effects of various anesthetic techniques, whether local, regional, spinal, or general, have been studied in patients undergoing similar operations. Some investigators have suggested that local and spinal anesthesia interfere less with liver function than general anesthesia, but others have been unable to demonstrate statistically significant differences among techniques, concluding that factors other than anesthesia are probably more important. [6,11,17,36,37]

There is in fact little evidence that any anesthetic agent, with the possible exception of chloroform, is a direct hepatotoxin as defined by Klatskin.[38] The idea that anesthetics are not hepatotoxic is supported by some studies that have failed to show a correlation between duration of anesthesia and postoperative liver function test abnormalities and by others that have not detected significant differences among various inhalational anesthetics in their effect on hepatic function. [9,11,13,14,17, 19,21,37,39,40]

Although none of the anesthetic agents in current use is a true hepatotoxin, all cause a reduction in hepatic splanchnic blood flow by various mechanisms. Cyclopropane reduces hepatic blood flow by approximately one-third by increasing splanchnic vascular resistance through its effect on the sympathetic nervous system. Halothane leads to a similar reduction in hepatic blood flow, not by its effect on splanchnic blood flow, but by causing systemic vasodilation and a decrease in cardiac output. Methoxyflurane lowers systemic and splanchnic perfusion pressure and may cause portal venoconstriction, thereby reducing hepatic blood flow by approximately 50%. Similarly, spinal and lumbar epidural agents reduce hepatic blood flow by reducing arterial pressure while causing little or no change in splanchnic vascular resistance.[41–43]

The significance of these reductions in hepatic blood flow is unclear. Although all anesthetics decrease splanchnic oxygen consumption, they cause a relatively greater reduction in hepatic blood flow, resulting in lower hepatic vein oxygen content and possible liver hypoxia.[41–43]

Price and associates evaluated this hypothesis by measuring hepatic venous lactate:pyruvate ratios in anesthetized healthy volunters but were unable to demonstrate evidence of hypoxia.[44] However, other factors influence blood flow in patients undergoing surgery.[41-43] Positive-pressure ventilation, hypocapnia, and hypercapnia all increase splanchnic vascular resistance and decrease hepatic blood flow. Hypotension, hemorrhage, systemic hypoxemia, and vasoactive drugs also reduce blood flow. In addition, traction on abdominal viscera during surgery produces reflex-mediated dilatation of splanchnic capacitance vessels, systemic hypotension, and reduced flow.[45]

In summary, although anesthetics themselves may have only minor hepatotoxic and hemodynamic effects, marginal changes in hepatic blood flow and oxygenation may become clinically significant when other intraoperative factors further compromise hepatic perfusion. This may be particularly true for patients with liver disease. Patients with cirrhosis and hepatitis already have decreased hepatic blood flow, and animals demonstrate markedly increased hepatic oxygen consumption after liver injury.[46] Therefore, changes in hepatic blood flow and hepatic hypoxia may account for the mild transient liver function abnormalities that are often seen following anesthesia and surgery and may explain why the frequency and magnitude of these changes are greater in patients with underlying liver disease.[9]

Surgery

In a number of studies, the frequency and magnitude of abnormalities in postoperative liver function tests correlate more closely with the nature and extent of surgery than with the type of anesthesia used.[8,9,47] For example, Killen found postoperative elevations in serum transaminase levels in 35% of patients after herniorrhaphy, in 65% after laparotomy, in 75% after biliary surgery, and in 90% after thoracotomy. Similarly, Hobson and his colleagues found greater than twofold elevations in postoperative levels of serum glutamic oxaloacetic transaminase (SGOT) in 75% of patients who had undergone biliary and upper abdomimal surgery, in 17% of those who had undergone lower abdominal procedures, and in 4% of those who had undergone lesser procedures such as breast biopsy.[15] Similar data pointing to the conclusion that the type and extent of surgery are the most important determinants of postoperative liver function abnormalities have been noted by other investigators.[7-9,48] The high incidence of abnormalities after biliary tract or upper abdominal surgery has been repeatedly emphasized.[10,19,20,39,49,50]

The histologic and functional studies of Zamcheck and associates provide additional evidence that anesthesia and surgery may result in liver damage.[51] Liver biopsies taken at the end of major abdomimal procedures showed evidence of acute inflammation in all 15 patients studied, whereas control biopsies performed at the beginning of the operation were normal. Similar results were reported by Edlund and Zettergren, who concluded that anesthesia of long duration and severe operative trauma may give rise to lesions suggestive of hepatitis.[52]

It is therefore clear that underlying illness, injury, anesthesia, and surgery may all contribute in varying degrees to functional impairment and morphologic changes in the liver. The type and extent of surgery done appear to be more important than the technique and duration of anesthesia or the choice of agent in the pathogenesis of these changes. The hepatic dysfunction seen is generally mild, transient, and usually inconsequential. However, in patients with underlying acute or chronic liver disease, these changes may contribute to clinically apparent hepatic decompensation and, potentially, to greater operative risk.

POSTOPERATIVE MORTALITY

Compromise of the many synthetic and metabolic functions of the liver appears to result in an increased incidence of infection, abnormal hemostasis, abnormal drug metabolism, and impaired protein and glucose synthesis even without the added metabolic burdens of anesthesia and surgery. Frequently, associated anemia, fluid and electrolyte disturbances, malnutrition, or portal hypertension further complicate the situation. Yet there are relatively few data documenting a higher operative risk in patients with liver disease than in healthy control subjects or correlating type and severity of liver disease with postoperative morbidity and mortality rates. Most data are derived from studies of patients undergoing portasystemic shunting procedures, and these patients represent a highly select group undergoing a specific operation that directly affects the liver and hepatic blood flow. Many studies suffer from small sample size, lack of controls, and little or no statistical analysis.

Acute Hepatitis

Medical teaching has stressed the importance of distinguishing between surgical and medical jaundice to avoid both unnecessary laparotomy and prohibitive op-

erative mortality in patients with acute hepatitis. Stone clearly states that "active hepatitis (whether alcoholic or viral) is uniformly associated with a poor prognosis and has therefore become an almost absolute contraindication to surgery."[53] The evidence for this, however, is equivocal. In a study of 3 patients with viral hepatitis undergoing laparotomy, Shaldon and Sherlock documented slow postoperative recovery in all and serious deterioration of hepatic function in 1 and cautioned that "surgery may kill the patient with infective hepatitis."[54] Discussing a paper of Leevy, Byrne cites an operative mortality rate of 33% in patients with hepatitis at Boston City Hospital, and Schmid warns that surgical intervention "may have grave consequences and postoperatively these patients often do poorly."[55] Turner and Sherlock followed 12 patients with viral hepatitis undergoing surgery.[56] Of the 12, 5 died postoperatively, and 4 others suffered hepatic decompensation, developed ascites, and recovered only after protracted illnesses.

Harville and Summerskill reviewed 42 patients with viral hepatitis and 16 patients with drug-induced hepatitis who were taken to laparotomy.[57] Among the patients with viral hepatitis, 4 (9.5%) died, and another 5 (11.9%) suffered major complications. The authors concluded that, although the mortality rate was less than expected, the combined morbidity and mortality rate of 21.4% was high enough to emphasize the importance of avoiding operation in patients with hepatis. Hargrove presented two cases of patients with chronic active hepatitis who died after laparotomy and suggested that surgery and anesthesia may have an adverse effect on the course of the disease.[58] Greenwood and co-workers studied 12 patients with alcoholic hepatitis who underwent open liver biopsy, in some cases during abdominal surgery, and documented a postoperative mortality rate of 58%.[59] Orloff and associates found that patients with an SGOT level of greater than 100 had a higher mortality rate following portasystemic shunt surgery than patients with no evidence of hepatitis.[60] Further evidence that acute inflammation of the liver adversely affects surgical outcome has been presented by Mikkelsen and Kein, who found that the degree of acute hyaline necrosis found on liver biopsy closely correlates with operative death in patients undergoing shunt procedures and should mitigate against surgery.[61,62]

Other investigators, however, have questioned the signifiance of hepatitis as a risk factor. Strauss and colleagues performed elective surgery for common-duct drainage on 73 patients with hepatitis and reported no deaths in the immediate postoperative period.[63] Bourke and co-workers reported that three patients with hepatitis subjected to laparotomy suffered no adverse consequences.[64] Among 14 patients with acute viral hepatitis and 16 patients with chronic active hepatitis operated on by Hardy and Hughes, there were 0 and 2 deaths, respectively.[65] The authors concluded that their "observations do not confirm the view that laparotomy is necessarily dangerous in viral hepatitis, but neither do they suggest that caution is unjustified." Based on the available data, this assessment seems reasonable.

Cirrhosis

Cirrhosis has long been associated with a high operative mortality rate. In 1927, Hughson noted a death rate of 60% in patients with cirrhosis undergoing omentopexy, and, in 1936, Henrikson reported a postoperative mortality rate of 55% in similar patients undergoing various operations.[66,67] More recently, Jackson and co-workers cited a general operative mortality rate of between 6.4% and 5% for major operations.[3] Lindenmuth and Eisenberg studied the results of various operations in 104 patients with cirrhosis and documented a mortality rate of 6.7% and an overall complication rate of 25%, with most complications occurring in patients with more severe disease.[68]

The impact of cirrhosis on operative mortality can only be inferred from evidence presented in studies. Cayer and Sohmer compared a group of cirrhotics dying after nonshunt surgery with groups of survivors and found greater evidence of hepatic dysfunction in those who died, suggesting that severity of cirrhosis correlates with operative death.[69] Similarly, Wirthlin and colleagues reported an overall surgical mortality rate of 57% in cirrhotics with nonvariceal gastroduodenal bleeding and demonstrated a higher death rate in those with more severe disease.[70] Numerous studies of patients with cirrhosis who have undergone portasystemic shunt procedures have also demonstrated that severity of the underlying liver disease is the major determinant of operative death.

RISK OF POSTOPERATIVE COMPLICATIONS

A higher than normal postoperative morbidity rate in patients with liver disease can be expected in four areas: wound healing, bleeding, infection, and deterioration of hepatic function, including encephalopathy.

Wound Healing

Abnormal wound healing can be anticipated because of associated abnormalities in protein synthesis, anemia, and poor nutritional status. Excessive bleeding or infection of surgical wounds may impair healing. Ascites also imposes a mechanical stress on abdominal wounds.

In experimental studies in rats, the presence of jaundice produced histologic evidence of delayed wound healing and decreased wound-burst strength.[71] Ellis and Heddle found 3 cases of abdomimal wound dehiscence and 4 incisional hernias among 21 jaundiced patients, giving a wound failure rate of 33%, compared to one of 5.2% among 305 nonjaundiced controls.[72] Similarly, Irvin and associates noted wound dehiscence or an incisional hernia in 27.1% of their patients undergoing laparotomy for jaundice, whereas only 4.3% of anicteric controls experienced difficulty in wound healing.[73] However, although anemia and hypoproteinemia were found to be significant factors in the review of abdomimal wound dehiscence by Keill and co-workers, jaundice was not.[74] Reitamo and Möller also found that anemia, hypoproteinemia, and factors that increase abdomimal pressure, including ascites, correlated with dehiscence.[75] However, there were too few patients with jaundice or abnormal liver function for significant conclusions to be reached. Marx reported 5 cases of patients with acute viral hepatitis undergoing laparotomy among which there were 2 episodes of dehiscence.[76]

Yonemoto and Davidson examined wound healing in 16 herniorrhaphies in cirrhotic patients and found only 1 wound complication.[1] In Lindenmuth's and Eisenberg's series of 104 operative procedures in cirrhotics, there were 13 wound complications with 5 cases of impaired healing of intestinal anastomoses and 1 case of wound dehiscence.[68] Serum protein levels did not correlate with wound complications, and ascites did not appear to interfere with wound healing.

Excessive Bleeding

Abnormal hemostasis is frequently found in patients with liver disease. The liver produces all clotting factors except factor VIII. Low plasma levels of one or more of factors II, V, VII, IX, and X are found in 70% to 85% of patients with liver disease on presentation at the hospital.[77] Thrombocytopenia frequently occurs because of suppression of platelet production by alchol or hypersplenism. Circulating platelets may be functionally impaired, and abnormal aggregation has been demonstrated.[78] Abnormal fibrin polymerization and increased catabolism of fibrinogen, prothrombin, and plasminogen have also been reported and may contribute to defective coagulation[79,80] Furthermore, portal hypertension may cause increased vascularity and bleeding during abdomimal surgery.

However, there is litle evidence of a significant increase in operative or postoperative bleeding in patients with liver disease. This may reflect careful selection of patients and careful preoperative preparation. In Lindenmuth's series of 28 operations on patients with prothrombin levels of 70% or less, not a single incidence of abnormal bleeding was attributed to lowered prothrombin alone and in none did increases in complications or death result from hemorrhage.[68]

Infection

Although patients with liver disease are thought to have lowered resistance to infection, there is little evidence documenting an increased incidence of wound or other postoperative infections in these patients.[81]

Deterioration of Hepatic Function

The risk of deterioration of hepatic function after surgery in patients with liver disease is not clear. Kiéri-Szántó and Lafleur reviewed their experience with 45,-000 anesthetized patients and found that 60% of the postoperative hepatic complications occurred in 94 patients with pre-existing liver disease.[82] They concluded that preoperative liver disease increased the risk of a postoperative hepatic complication 500-fold. Similar data have been presented by others.[83,84] There are no data on the incidence of hepatic encephalopathy following nonshunt surgery.

PREOPERATIVE EVALUATION AND ESTIMATION OF OPERATIVE RISK

Preoperative evaluation of the patient with liver disease has several objectives. The type and severity of liver disease must be determined and the risk of operation estimated. Potentially reversible disturbances such as encephalopathy or coagulopathy must be sought and treated to minimize operative risk and the risk of postoperative complications. Finally, other significant conditions must be identified. As always, preoperative evaluation must begin with a careful medical history

and physical examination. Particular attention should be paid to the presence of jaundice, hepatosplenomegaly, ascites, and encephalopathy and to assessment of nutritional state. Laboratory evaluation must include an electrocardiogram, chest x-ray, urinalysis, complete blood count, platelet count, prothrombin time, electrolytes, blood urea nitrogen, creatinine, glucose, and a complete set of standard liver function tests. Testing for hepatitis B-associated surface and e antigens is useful in determining the risk of the patient infecting others. Bleeding times and blood ammonia levels are not generally indicated. Some authors have also suggested that arterial blood gas tests, pulmonary function tests, and cardiac output determinations precede portasystemic shunting.[85]

Which elements of the history, physical findings, and laboratory data best predict the magnitude of operative risk? There are two studies of patients with cirrhosis who underwent nonshunt surgery that yield some information. Cayer and Sohmer found that the presence of ascites, hypoalbuminemia, a prolonged prothrombin time, or anemia was correlated with higher than normal operative mortality.[69] The presence of jaundice and other abnormalities of liver function tests was not significant. The presence of hepatomegaly seemed to predict a better prognosis for cirrhotic patients than for patients with small livers; this finding has been suggested by other studies as well.[60,86] In the study by Wirthlin and colleagues of cirrhotic patients who underwent emergency surgery for gastroduodenal bleeding, a significant predictor of death was a history of cirrhosis, varices, or ascites but not the presence of ascites on physical examination.[70] The death rate was directly correlated with serum bilirubin concen-

Table 21-1. Clinical and Laboratory Classification of Hepatic Function—Child's Criteria

Measurements	Class A	Class B	Class C
Functional impairment	Minimal	Moderate	Severe
Serum bilirubin (mg/dl)	< 2	2–3	> 3
Serum albumin (g/dl)	> 3.5	3.0–3.5	< 3
Ascites	None	Easily controlled	Poorly controlled
Neurologic disorders	None	Minimal	Moderate to severe
Nutrition	Excellent	Good	Poor, wasted

(After Child CG III: The Liver and Portal Hypertension. Philadelphia, WB Saunders, 1967)

tration, ammonia concentration, and prothrombin time and was inversely related to the serum albumin level. The serum bilirubin concentration was felt to be the most reliable indicator.

A larger number of studies attempting to predict operative mortality from the findings of preoperative evaluation have been performed in patients undergoing portasystemic shunting, and several authors have proposed multifactorial indices to estimate surgical risk.[60,87–89] The most widely used of these is that proposed by Child.[90] This classification of patients was empirically derived and uses clinical assessment of the state of nutrition, the presence or absence of ascites, and levels of serum bilirubin and albumin to place patients in one of three groups (Table 21-1). Several studies have shown that this classification correlates well with operative mortality in shunt surgery.[90,91]

Although Child's criteria were originally designed to predict the operative risk of patients undergoing portasystemic shunting, Nolan and Stone have asserted that they are equally useful in predicting the outome of any major surgical procedure, including hepatic resection (Table 21-2). Pugh and co-workers have proposed a modification of the Child classification (Table 21-3), adding prolongation of the prothrombin time to the criteria and omitting the assessment of body nutri-

tion.[93] Patients who score 5 to 6 points are considered to be good operative risks (grade A), those with 7 to 9 points moderate risks (grade B), and those with 10 to 15 points poor operative risks (grade C). These clinical classes predicted operative mortality in the authors' series of patients subjected to transection of the esophagus for bleeding varices.

Other investigators have failed to demonstrate a relationship between clinical or laboratory assessment and operative mortality. Welch and colleagues stated that, in a review of liver function values in

Table 21-2. Basic Liver Functions and Operability

Class	Operability
A	No limitations Normal response to all operations Normal ability of liver to regenerate
B	Some limitations to liver function Altered response to all operations, but good tolerance with preoperative preparation Limited ability of the liver to regenerate new hepatic parenchyma; therefore, all sizable liver resections are contraindicated
C	Severe limitations to liver function Poor response to all operations regardless of preparatory efforts Liver resection, regardless of the size, is contraindicated

(Stone HH: Surg Clin North Am 57:411, 1977)

Table 21-3. Grading of Severity of Liver Disease—Pugh's Criteria

Clinical and Biochemical Measurements	Points Scored For Increasing Abnormality		
	1	2	3
Encephalopathy (grade)*	None	1 and 2	3 and 4
Ascites	Absent	Slight	Moderate
Bilirubin (mg/dl)	1–2	2–3	> 3
Albumin (g/dl)	3.5	2.8–3.5	< 2.8
Prothrombin time (sec prolonged)	1–4	4–6	> 6
For primary biliary cirrhosis:			> 10
Bilirubin (mg/dl)	1–4	4–10	

*According to grading of Trey C, Burns DG, Saunders SJ: N Engl J Med 274:473, 1966. (Pugh RNH, Murray–Lyon IM, Dawson JL et al: Br J Surg 60:647, 1973)

their series of 40 patients, no single test or combination of tests proved be a consistent guide to survival.[86] Jackson and associates concluded "that the prognosis for survival in cirrhotics cannot at present be predicted in clinical, laboratory or physiologic studies alone and that the ultimate outcome in an individual patient is not easily determined prior to an operation."[3]

TIMING OF SURGERY

Hepatitis

No elective surgery should be performed on a patient with viral hepatitis.[94] Surgery should be postponed for at least 1 month after liver function tests have returned to normal.[95] In patients with chronic active hepatitis, it has been recommended that the disease be quiescent for at least 3 months prior to operative intervention.[95] Patients with alcoholic hepatitis should have elective surgery postponed until maximum recovery of liver function is determined by serial liver function tests.[95]

Cirrhosis

All patients with cirrhosis should be classified according to Child's or Pugh's criteria. Only those in group A should be considered fit for anesthesia and surgery.[53, 96] Those in group B or C should have elective surgery deferred to allow for preoperative preparation.

PREOPERATIVE PREPARATION

Clotting

The prothrombin time is frequently prolonged in patients with liver disease. Vitamin K-dependent coagulation factors synthesized by the liver include factors II, VII, IX, and X. Deficiencies of these factors are often seen in jaundiced patients and in patients who have received long courses of oral antibiotics for bowel sterilization or treatment of infection or encephalopathy.[95] All patients with a prolonged prothrombin time should receive parenteral vitamin K prior to surgery. Those with severe liver dysfunction do not often respond to vitamin K, and adequate amounts of fresh frozen plasma should be administered with careful attention to the possible effects of a sizable sodium and volume load. Patients with alcoholic bone marrow depression or hypersplenism generally do not require platelet transfusions, but such transfusion can be given for emergency surgery in patients with platelet counts low enough to predispose them to excessive bleeding.

Electrolyte Abnormalities

Patients with chronic liver disease frequently have electrolyte disturbances incluing hyponatremia, hypokalemia, and metabolic alkalosis resulting from secondary hyperaldosteronism or diuretic therapy for ascites. Other factors, such as prolonged vomiting or nasogastric suction, may be important. Since there is some evidence that these disturbances are associated with greater than normal operative risk and may precipitate encephalopathy, they should be treated preoperatively.[60] Treatment includes appropriate water restriction, potassium repletion, and judicious use of diuretics. The diagnosis, management, and significance of these fluid and electrolyte disturbances are discussed more fully in Chapter 17.

Encephalopathy

Evidence of hepatic encephalopathy must be carefully sought. Examination for the presence of asterixis alone is not adequate. If encephalopathy is detected, all but emergency surgery should be deferred until precipitating causes are identified and corrected and treatment is instituted. Frequently, several precipitating causes can be found in the surgical patients, including hypokalemia, metabolic alkalosis, infection, gastrointestinal (GI) bleeding, and the use of potent analgesics. Treatment of encephalopathy includes lactulose or neomycin administered orally or in retention enemas.

Although aggressive preoperative treatment of impending or overt encephalopathy is clearly indicated, preoperative management of nonencephalopathic patients with severe liver disease is less straightforward. Some authors have recommended prophylactic treatment to prevent postoperative encephalopathy.[97,98] Routine bowel preparation for abdominal surgery and the severe protein restriction imposed by the perioperative setting may in themselves reduce the incidence of encephalopathy.

Ascites

Ascites is common in patients with chronic liver disease and complicates anesthesia and surgery. Massive accumulation of ascites impairs diaphragmatic movement, decreases functional residual capacity, and promotes atelectasis. Since ascitic fluid is in equilibrium with fluid in the interstitial and intravascular spaces, sudden decompression of ascites can lead to marked hypotension resulting from fluid shifts and pooling in the splanchnic venous system.[99] Proper control of asites is one of the most important elements of preoperative preparation and is achieved in the usual manner with bed rest, sodium restriction, and the appropriate, careful use of diuretics.

Nutritional Problems

Many patients with chronic liver disease are malnourished. The significance of preoperative nutritional assessment and support is discussed in greater detail in Chapter 14. However, there are problems in nutritional support that are unique to the patient with severe liver disease. Although GI protein absorption is normal in patients with cirrhosis, oral protein supplementation must be limited, because it may precipitate or worsen encephalopathy. Intravenous amino acid supplementation has the theoretical advantage of bypassing intestinal bacterial degradation, the major source of ammonia production, but, when conventional intravenous amino acid solutions were first given to cirrhotic patients, encephalopathy worsened.[100] However, experimental solutions containing a high concentration of branched-chain amino acids and a low concentration of aromatic amino acids have reportedly been well tolerated in animals and humans with encephalopathy, although some investigators have failed to confirm this.[101,102] Similarly, experiments in animals have suggested that the ketoanalogues of animo acids are incorporated into protein and cause positive nitrogen balance without the hazard of encephalopathy.[103]

The use of high-fat diets as a method of caloric supplementation is also limited in patients with cirrhosis because impaired bile-salt synthesis results in impaired fat digestion and absorption. Substitution of medium-chain triglycerides is not recommended because of recent studies documenting elevated serum octanoate concentrations in encephalopathic patients.[104] This elevation may result from the inability of the body to utilize medium-chain fatty acids or incomplete oxidation of long-chain fatty acids.

Although there are encouraging experimental studies that may find clinical application in the future, current nutritional support of patients with severe liver disease is limited to the provision of adequate carbohydrate as a calorie source and maximal tolerable protein. This is especially important in these patients, since tissue protein catabolism can precipitate encephalopathy. It is also important to recognize that these patients have little or no hepatic glycogen stores. Glucose infusions should be begun prior to surgery to prevent intraoperative hypoglycemia.

POSTOPERATIVE COMPLICATIONS

A number of postoperative complications are common in the patient with liver disease. Problems with wound healing, wound infection, and bleeding at the operative site generally require surgical intervention and will not be discussed here. The diagnosis and management of hepatic encephalopathy in the postoperative setting is the same in the nonsurgical patient.[105] It should be emphasized that potent analgesics for postoperative pain should be given with caution because hypoalbuminemia and impaired drug metabolism can result in more prolonged or pronounced effects than normal and precipitate overt encephalopathy.

Pulmonary complications occur frequently, particularly in patients with ascites. The approach to this problem is presented in Chapter 23. The usual management of ascites and electrolyte disturbance does not differ significantly for the postoperative patient with liver disease. Upper GI bleeding is sufficiently common in these patients for prophylactic treatment with cimetidine or antacids to be recommended. Recent evidence suggests that, of the two, antacids may be more effective.[106]

Acute renal failure (ARF) is a not uncommon postoperative complication in patients with liver disease. Although the differential diagnosis is much the same in these patients as in other surgical patients as discussed in Chapter 15, several specific clinical conditions deserve mention. Aminoglycoside nephrotoxicity should be considered in patients receiving neomycin for hepatic precoma. Although this is generally considered a nonabsorbable antibiotic, as much as 3% of the neomycin dose can be absorbed.

Hepatorenal syndrome refers to progressive oliguria and azotemia in patients with severe decompensated liver disease in whom other causes of renal failure have been excluded. It is characterized by a concentrated urine, a low urinary sodium concentration of less than 10 mEq/liter and a benign urine sediment. The pathogenesis is uncertain but appears to be related to an abnormal distribution of renal blood flow with a marked decrease in perfusion of the cortex despite normal total renal blood flow. This may be due to vasoconstriction of cortical vessels with intrarenal shunting of blood. Renal histology is normal, and affected kidneys function normally when transplanted into patients without liver disease, suggesting a functional basis for the disorder.[107] This theory is further supported by case reports of improved renal function after liver transplantation.[108] Various treatment regimens for hepatorenal syndrome have been used, including volume expansion with colloid, prostaglandin inhibitors, dopamine, portasystemic shunting, and hemodialysis, but with little success.[109–112] Peritoneojugular shunting has been reported to be effective, but its value remains unproved.[113] Currently, the hepatorenal syndrome is regarded as irreversible.

Many investigators report a high incidence of postoperative renal failure in patients with obstructive jaundice.[114] This is regarded by some as a distinct entity and by others as part of the hepatorenal syndrome. A direct nephrotoxic effect of bilirubin or bile salts has been postulated as the cause, as has a nephrotoxic effect of endotoxin absorbed from the bowel because of decreased bile-salt excretion. Dawson has studied this particular variant of renal failure and has found a significant correlation between preoperative bilirubin levels and postoperative falls in creatinine clearance.[115] Deterioration in renal function may be prevented by forced diuresis with mannitol, the prophylactic use of which Dawson strongly recommends in these patients. Another type of ARF following hepatic artery ligation for hepatic tumors has also been described.[116]

SUMMARY

1. **Abnormalities in one or more liver function tests are frequently found following anesthesia and surgery in patients with normal livers. These abnormalities occur with greater frequency and are of greater magnitude in patients with pre-existing liver disease. There appears to be little or no relation of anesthetic technique, anesthetic agent, or duration of anesthesia to postoperative liver function abnormalities. The type and extent of surgery appear to be more important determinants. These abnormalities are generally mild, transient, and of little clinical significance.**

2. **None of the anesthetic agents in current use is a direct hepatotoxin. All reduce hepatic blood flow, which may be further compromised by other factors that are present frequently during surgery. Reduction in hepatic blood flow may be related to postoperative liver function abnormalities and histologic changes.**

3. **Although the data are not conclusive, patients with both acute and chronic liver disease appear to have a higher than normal risk of postoperative complications and death. The magnitude of the operative risk for patients with acute hepatitis may not be as great as previously feared. The magnitude of operative risk for patients with cirrhosis is directly related to the severity of their disease.**

4. **Preoperative evaluation of the patient with liver disease should include a careful history and physical examination. Laboratory evaluation must include a platelet count, prothrombin time, and full set of liver function tests. In patients with acute hepatitis**

or unexplained chronic liver disease, appropriate hepatitis serologies should be done.

5. No elective surgery should be performed in patients with acute, viral, or alcoholic hepatitis.

6. Patients with chronic liver disease should be classified by Child's or Pugh's criteria. Only those in group A should be considered fit for elective surgery. Those in group B or C should be prepared preoperatively to minimize risk.

7. Preoperative preparation should focus on treatment of clotting abnormalities, electrolyte disturbances, and hepatic encephalopathy. Attempts should also be made to reduce ascites and improve nutritional status.

8. Postoperative complications that occur with a greater frequency in patients with liver disease than in other patients include atelectasis and pneumonia, upper GI bleeding, and deterioration of hepatic function. Wound complications and ARF also occur frequently. Most patients should receive prophylactic antacids postoperatively. The prophylactic use of mannitol has also been recommended for patients with obstructive jaundice.

9. Although patients with liver disease have higher than normal risk of postoperative death or complications, careful preoperative assessment and preparation and aggressive treatment of postoperative complications will minimize their risk and allow more of them to tolerate major surgery.

REFERENCES

1. Yonemoto RH, Davidson CS: Herniorrhaphy in cirrhosis of the liver with ascites. N Engl J Med 255:733, 1956

2. Nicholas P, Rinaudo PA, Conn HO: Increased incidence of cholelithiasis in Laennec's cirrhosis. Gastroenterology 63:112, 1972

3. Jackson FJ, Christopher EB, Peternel WW et al: Preoperative management of patients with liver disease. Surg Clin North Am 48:907, 1968

4. Wallach JB, Hyman W, Angrist AA: The cause of death in patients with Laennec's cirrhosis. Am J Med Sci 234:56, 1957

5. Ratnoff OD, Patek AJ: Natural history of Laennec's cirrhosis. Medicine 21:259, 1942

6. Geller W, Tagnon H: Liver dysfunction following abdominal operation. Arch Intern Med 86:908, 1950

7. Tagnon HJ, Robbins GJ, Nichole MP: The effect of surgical operations on the bromosulfalein retention test. N Engl J Med 238:356, 1948

8. Engstrand L, Friberg O: On function of liver as affected by various operations and anesthetics. Acta Chir Scand Suppl 97:104, 1945

9. French AB, Bares TP, Fairlie CS et al: Metabolic effects of anesthesia in man. Ann Surg 135:145, 1952

10. Ayres PR, Williard RB: Serum glutamic oxaloacetic transaminase level in 266 surgical patients. Ann Intern Med 52:1279, 1960

11. Fairlie CW, Bares TP, French AB et al: Metabolic effects of anesthesia in man. IV A comparison of the effects of certain anesthetic agents on the normal liver. N Engl J Med 244:615, 1957

12. Evans C, Evans M, Pollack AJ: The incidence and causes of postoperative jaundice. Br J Anaesth 46:520, 1974

13. Dawson B, Adson MA, Dockerty MB et al: Hepatic function tests: Postoperative changes with halothane or diethyl ether anesthesia. Mayo Clin Proc 41:599, 1966

14. Little DM, Barbour CM, Given JB: The effects of fluothane, cyclopropane, and ether anesthesia on liver function. Surg Gynecol Obstet 107:712, 1958

15. Hobson RW, Conant C, Fleming A et al: Postoperative serum enzyme patterns. Milit Med 136:624, 1971

16. Killen DA: Serum enzyme elevations: A diagnostic test for acute myocardial infarction during the early postoperative period. Arch Surg 96:200, 1968

17. Pohle FJ: Anesthesia and liver function. Wis Med J 47:476, 1948

18. Thompson DS, Geifenstein FF: Enzyme patterns reflecting hepatic response to anesthesia and operations. South Med J 67:69, 1974

19. Kalow B, Rogoman E, Sims FH: A comparison of the effects of halothane and other anesthetic agents on hepatocellular function in patients submitted to elective operation. Can Anaesth Soc J 23:71, 1976

20. Person DA, Judge RD: Effect of operation on serum transaminase levels. Arch Surg 77:892, 1958

21. Akdikman SA, Flanagan TV, Landmesser CM: A comparative study of SGPT changes following anesthesia with halothane, methoryflurane and other inhalational agents. Anesth Analg (Cleve) 45:819, 1966

22. Hicks MH, Holt HP, Guerrant JL et al: The effect of spontaneous and artificially induced fever on liver function. J Clin Invest 27:580, 1948

23. Eley A, Hargrove T, Lambert HD: Jaundice in severe infections. Br Med J 2:75, 1965

24. Hartman FW, Romence HL: Liver necrosis in burns. Ann Surg 118:402, 1943

25. Walker J, Saltonstall H, Rhoads JE et al: toxemia syndrome after burns. Arch Surg 52:177, 1946

26. Gilmore JP, Roggard HA: Liver function following thermal injury. Am J Physiol 198:491, 1960

27. Shoemaker WC, Szanto PB, Fitch LB et al: Hepatic physiologic and morphologic alteration in hemorrhagic shock. Surg Gynecol Obstet 118:828, 1964

28. Ellenberg M, Osserman KE: The role of shock in the production of central liver necrosis. Am J Med 11:170, 1951

29. Nunes G, Blaisdell W, Margurettin W: Mechanism of hepatic dysfunction following shock and trauma. Arch Surg 100:546, 1970

30. Defalque RJ: The first delayed chloroform poisoning. Anesth Analg (Cleve) 47:374, 1968

31. Little DM, Welstone HJ: Anesthesia and the liver. Anesthesiology 25:815, 1964

32. Carney FMT, Van Dyke RA: Halothane hepatitis: A critical review. Anesth Analg (Cleve) 51:135, 1972

33. Dykes MH (ed): Anesthesia and the liver. Int Anesthesiol Clin 8:175, 1970

34. Brouhoult J, Gillquist J: Serum ornithane carbanyl transferase activity in man after halothane and spinal anesthesia with and without systolic blood pressure fall. Acta Chir Scand 135:113, 1969

35. Stevens WC, Egar EI, Joas TA et al: Comparative toxicity of isoflurane, halothane, fluoroxene, and diethyl ether in human volunteers. Can Anaesth Soc J 20:357, 1973

36. Schmidt CR, Unrich RJ, Chesky JE: Clinical studies of liver function. I. The effect of anesthesia and certain surgical procedures. Am J Surg 57:43, 1942

37. Collins WL, Fabian LW: Transaminase studies following anesthesia. South Med J 57:55, 1964

38. Klatskin G: Symposium on toxic hepatitis. Gastroenterology 38:789, 1960

39. Kelley JL, Campbell DA, Brandt RL: The recognition of myocardial infarction in the early postoperative period. Arch Surg 94:673, 1967

40. Dodson ME, Richards TG: A prospective study of changes in liver function after operation under two forms of general anesthesia. Br J Anaesth 44:47, 1942

41. Ngai SH: Current concepts in anesthesiology: Effect of anesthetics on various organs. N Engl J Med 302:564, 1980

42. Cooperman LH: Effects of anaesthetics on the splanchnic circulation. Br J Anaesth 44:967, 1972

43. Batchelder BM, Cooperman LH: Effects of anesthetics on splanchnic circulation and metabolism. Surg Clin North Am 55:787, 1975

44. Price HL, Davidson IA, Clement AJ et al: Can general anesthesia produce splanchnic visceral hypoxia by reducing regional blood flow? Anesthesiology 27:24, 1966

45. Torrance HB: Liver blood flow during op-

eration on the upper abdomen. JR Coll Surg Edinb 2:216, 1957

46. Brauer RW, Lesing GF, Holloway RJ: Oxygen uptake and hypoxia in the isolated rat liver preparation. Fed Proc 20:286, 1961
47. Griffiths HWC, Ozguc L: Effects of chloroform and halothane anesthesia on liver function in man. Lancet 1:246, 1964
48. Nickell WK, Albritten FF: Serum transaminase content related to tissue injury. Surgery 42:240, 1957
49. Fisk AA, Thomas RG, Maurukas J: Serum transaminase values after cholecytectomy, hysterectomy, and operation on the fractured hips. Am J Med Sci 236:33, 1958
50. Craig HK, Butch WL, McGowan JM: Effect of biliary operation on the liver. Arch Surg 37:609, 1938
51. Zanicheck N, Chalmers TC, Davidson CS: Pathologic and functional changes in the liver following upper abdominal operations (abstr). Am J Med 7:409, 1949
52. Edlund YA, Zettergren LSW: Microstructure of the liver in biliary tract disease and notes on the effect on the liver of anesthesia, intubation, and operation trauma. Acta Chir Scand 113:201, 1957
53. Stone HH: Preoperative and postoperative care. Surg Clin North Am 57:409, 1977
54. Shaldon S, Sherlock S: Virus hepatitis with features of prolonged retention. Br Med J 2:734, 1957
55. Leevy CM: Intrahepatic cholestasis. Am J Surg 97:132, 1959
56. Turner MD, Sherlock S: In Smith R, Sherlock S (eds): Surgery of the Gallbladder and Bile Ducts. London, Butterworth & Co, 1964
57. Harville DD, Summerskill WHJ: Surgery in acute hepatitis. JAMA 184:257, 1963
58. Hargrove MD: Chronic active hepatitis: Possible adverse effects of exploratory laparotomy. Surgery 68:771, 1970
59. Greenwood SM, Leffler CT, Minkowitz S: The increased mortality rate of open liver biopsy in alcoholic hepatitis. Surg Gynecol Obstet 134:600, 1972
60. Orloff MJ, Chandler JG, Carters AC et al: Emergency portacaval shunt treatment for bleeding esophageal varices. Arch Surg 108:293, 1974
61. Mikkelsen WP, Kein WH: The influence of acute hyaline necrosis in survival after emergency and elective portacaval shunt. Major Prob Clin Surg 14:233, 1974
62. Mikkelsen WP: Therapeutic portacaval shunt: Preliminary data on controlled trial and morbid effects of acute hyaline necrosis. Arch Surg 108:302, 1974
63. Strauss AA, Strauss SF, Schwartz AH et al: Decompression by drainage of the common bile duct in subacute and chronic jaundice. A report of 73 cases with hepatitis or concomitant biliary duct infection as cause. Am J Surg 97:137, 1959
64. Bourke JB, Cannon P, Retchie HD: Laparotomy for jaundice. Lancet 2:521, 1967
65. Hardy KJ, Hughes ESR: Laparotomy in viral hepatitis. Med J Aust 1:710, 1968
66. Hughson W: Portal cirrhosis with ascites and its surgical treatment. Arch Surg 15:418, 1927
67. Henrikson EC: Cirrhosis of the liver. Arch Surg 32:413, 1936
68. Lindenmuth WW, Eisenberg MM: The surgical risk in cirrhosis of the liver. Arch Surg 86:235, 1963
69. Cayer D, Sohmer MF: Surgery in patients with cirrhosis. Arch Surg 71:828, 1955
70. Wirthlin LS, Urk HV, Malt RB et al: Predictors of surgical mortality in patients with cirrhosis and nonvariceal gastroduodenal bleeding. Surg Gynecol Obstet 139:65, 1974
71. Bayer I, Ellis HJ: Jaundice and wound healing: An experimental study. Br J Surg 63:392, 1976
72. Ellis H, Heddle R: Does the peritoneum need to be closed at laparotomy? Br J Surg 64:733, 1977
73. Irvin TT, Vassilakis JS, Challopadhyiay DK et al: Abdominal wound healing in

jaundiced patients. Br J Surg 65:521, 1978

74. Keill RH, Keitzer WF, Nichols WK et al: Abdominal wound dehiscence. Arch Surg 106:573, 1973

75. Reitamo J, Möller C: Abdominal wound dehiscence. Acta Chir Scand 138:170, 1972

76. Marx GF: Unsuspected preoperative hepatic dysfunction. Int Anesthesiol Clin 8:369, 1970

77. Losowsky M, Simmons AV, Mitoszewski K: Coagulation abnormalities in liver disease. Postgrad Med 53:117, 1973

78. Ballard HS, Marcus AJ: Platelet aggregation in portal cirrhosis. Arch Intern Med 136:316, 1976

79. Green G, Thompson JM, Dymock IW et al: Abnormal fibrin polymerization in liver disease. Br J Haematol 34:427, 1976

80. Verstroete M, Vermglen J, Collen D: Intravascular coagulation in liver disease. Annu Rev Med 25:447, 1974

81. Gaines KC, Sonell MF: Host resistance in liver disease—Its evaluation and therapeutic modification. Med Clin North Am 63:495, 1979

82. Kiéri-Szántó M, Lafleur F: Postanesthetic liver complications in a general hospital: A statistical study. Can Anaesth Soc J 10:531, 1963

83. Dykes MHM, Walzer SG: Preoperative and postoperative hepatic dysfunction. Surg Gynecol Obstet 124:747, 1967

84. Marx GF, Nagayoski M, Shoukos JA et al: Unsuspected infectious hepatitis in surgical patients. JAMA 205:169, 1968

85. Kaplan JA, Betner RL, Bripps RD: Hypoxia hyperdynamic circulation and the hazards of general anesthesia in patients with hepatic cirrhosis. Anesthesiology 35:427, 1971

86. Welch HF, Welch CS, Carter JH: Prognosis after surgical treatment of ascites: Results of side-to-side shunt in 40 patients. Surgery 56:75, 1964

87. Linton RR: The selection of patients for portacaval shunts. Ann Surg 134:433, 1951

88. McDermott W: The double portacaval shunt in the treatment of chronic ascites. Surg Gynecol Obstet 110:457, 1960

89. Malt RA: Portasystemic venous shunts. N Engl J Med 295:24, 1976

90. Child CG: The liver and portal hypertension in major problems in clinical surgery. Philadelphia, WB Saunders, 1964

91. Turcotte JG, Lambert MJ: Variceal hemorrhage, hepatic cirrhosis, and portacaval shunts. Surgery 73:810, 1973

92. Nolan JP: The management of the surgical patient with chronic liver disease. In Siegel JH, (eds): The Aged and High Risk Surgical Patient. New York, Grune and Stratton, 1976

93. Pugh RNH, Murray–Lyon IM, Dawson JL et al: Transection of the oesophagus for bleeding oesophageal varices. Br J Surg 60:646, 1973

94. Leibowitz S: Guidelines to clearing patients with liver disease for surgery. Mt Sinai J Med (NY) 44:539, 1977

95. Iwatsuki S, Geis WP: Hepatic complications. Surg Clin North Am 57:1335, 1977

96. Stunin I: Preoperative assessment of the patient with liver dysfunction. Br J Anaesth 50:25, 1978

97. Seifkin AD, Bolt RJ: Preoperative evaluation of the patient with gastrointestinal or liver disease. Med Clin North Am 631:1309, 1979

98. Editorial: Liver Disease and Anesthesia. Br Med J 1:1374, 1978

99. Cooperman LH, Wollman H, Marsh ML: Anesthesia and the liver. Surg Clin North Am 57:421, 1977

100. Fisher JE, Yoshimina N, Aguirre A et al: Plasma amino acids in patients with hepatic encephalopathy: Effect of amino acid infusion. Am J Surg 127:40, 1974

101. Fisher JE, Rosen HM, Ebeid AM et al: The effect of normalization of plasma amino acids on hepatic encephalopathy in man. Surgery 80:77, 1976

102. Freund H, Yoshimina N, Fisher JE:

Chronic hepatic encephalopathy: Long-term therapy with a branched chain amino acid enriched elemental diet. JAMA 242:347, 1979

103. Maddreg WC, Weber FL, Coulter AW et al: Effect of keto analogues of essential amino acids in portal-systemic encephalopathy. Gastroenterology 71:190, 1976

104. Rabinowitz JL, Staeffen J, Aumonier P et al: A method for serum octanoate in hepatic cirrhosis and hepatic encephalopathy. Clin Chem 23:2202, 1977

105. Najarian JS, Harper HA, McCorkle HJ: The diagnosis and clinical management of hepatic coma in surgical patients. Am J Surg 96:172, 1958

106. Priebe HJ, Skillman JJ, Bushnell LS et al: Antacid versus cimetidine in preventing acute gastrointestinal bleeding. N. Engl J Med 302:426, 1980

107. Kamel MH, Cobuin JW, Mimis MM et al: Transplantation of cadaveric kidney from patients with hepatorenal syndrome: Evidence for the functional nature of renal failure in advanced liver disease. N Engl J Med 280:1367, 1969

108. Iwutsuki S, Popovitzer MM, Corman JL et al: Recovery from hepatorenal syndrome after orthotopic liver transplantation. N Engl J Med 289:1155, 1973

109. Tristani FE, Cohn JN: Systemic and renal hemodynamics in oliguric hepatic failure: Effect of volume expansion. J Clin Invest 46:1894, 1967

110. Bennet WM, Keefe E, Melnyk C et al: Response to dopamine hydrochloride in hepatorenal syndrome. Arch Intern Med 135:964, 1975

111. Fisher JE, Foster GS: Survival from acute hepatorenal syndrome following splenorenal shunt. Ann Surg 184:22, 1976

112. Aregan S, Sweeney T, Keistein MD: Hepatorenal syndrome: Recovery after portacaval shunt. Ann Surg 181:847, 1975

113. LeVeen HH, Wapnick S, Grosberg S et al: Further experience with peritoneo-venous shunt for ascites. Ann Surg 184:574, 1976

114. Dawson JL: The incidence of postoperative renal failure in obstructive jaundice. Br J Surg 52:663, 1965

115. Dawson JL: Postoperative renal function in obstructive jaundice: Effect of a mannitol diuresis. Br Med J 1:82, 1965

116. Kim DK, Penneman R, Kallum B et al: Acute renal failure after ligation of the hepatic artery. Surg Gynecol Obstet 143:391, 1976

22

Postoperative Liver Dysfunction

JULIUS J. DEREN

Clinical jaundice and hyperbilirubinemia in the postoperative patient may be the first signs of severe complications or only transient abnormalities with no prognostic implications.[1–6] The evaluation of jaundice and liver function abnormalities after surgery requires an understanding of the effects of surgery and anesthesia on bilirubin metabolism and hepatic function. Many putative factors may be present in the patient with postoperative jaundice, and it is frequently difficult to ascribe hepatic injury to only one of them. The incidence of postoperative increases in serum concentrations of hepatic enzymes or bilirubin varies with the nature of the surgical procedure, the presence or absence of underlying liver disease, the quantity of blood transfused, and perhaps the anesthetic agents employed.[7]

BILIRUBIN METABOLISM

In the adult, about 250 to 350 mg/day of bilirubin are formed from the breakdown of heme-containing compounds in the reticuloendothelial system.[8–10] The bilirubin enters the circulation and is firmly bound to albumin. Through unclarified

mechanisms, the bilirubin molecule passes across the sinusoidal membrane of the hepatocyte by way of a concentration-dependent, carrier-mediated process and is conjugated with one or two molecules of glucuronic acid to form direct-reacting bilirubin. It is then actively secreted by the hepatocyte across the canalicular membrane into the biliary ducts. The rate-limiting step in the process appears to be the excretion of conjugated bilirubin across the sinusoidal membrane rather than hepatic uptake or hepatic conjugation.[11]

Under normal circumstances, the total serum bilirubin concentration of up to 1.0 or 1.2 mg/dl consists almost exclusively of unconjugated or indirect-reacting bilirubin, although techniques currently used in clinical laboratories might also show a variable quantity of the conjugated or direct-reacting fraction. Routine analytic methods for detecting low concentrations of direct-reacting pigment can also be inaccurate, and, although the concentration of direct-reacting bilirubin is generally less than 15% of the total, in some circumstances it may form a higher fraction of the total.[12] When bilirubin formation is increased by any one of a variety of mechanisms (e.g., hemolysis of autologous or transfused red blood cells), the serum concentration of the unconjugated bilirubin rises, with a resultant increase in hepatic uptake, conjugation, and excretion. If bilirubin formation increases only slightly, up to 2 or 3 times normal, the concentration of unconjugated bilirubin, although increased, may still be within the normal range because of increased hepatic metabolism. With a further increase in pigment load, the unconjugated bilirubin may rise to abnormal levels, but these rarely exceed 5 to 6 mg/dl.

Most conjugated bilirubin is excreted into the bile, but some may reflux back into the circulation.[13,14] When liver disease is not present, this fraction is approximately 15%, as measured by the standard diazo reaction commonly employed in clinical laboratories. When total bilirubin is less than 4 mg/dl, a higher percentage is observed in about 25% of cases. With pre-existing liver disease or in conditions that cause both an increased in pigment load and impairment in hepatic excretory function (e.g., sepsis), there may be an even greater reflux of conjugated bile into the circulation.

There may be a rise in indirect bilirubin even without hemolysis.[15] In a variety of hepatobiliary, cardiac, and hematologic disorders, there may be shunting of blood away from the liver or impairment of the hepatic uptake mechanism with a modest rise in unconjugated bilirubin. In such cases, sophisticated studies have eliminated the possibility that an increased pigment load is the cause of the increase.

Since 500 ml of whole blood yields 2500 mg of bilirubin, modest hemolysis or extravasation of a small amount of blood into extravascular spaces other than the gastrointestinal tract may substantially increase the bilirubin load and lead to jaundice. Transfused blood cells often have a decreased life span, the reduction in which is inversely related to the duration of the blood's storage.[16] Transfusion of blood stored for 2 weeks results in a 10% decrease in the number of red cells within 24 hr after transfusion. A transfusion of 1 unit of 2-week-old blood results in a twofold increase in the bilirubin load.

A fraction of the direct-reacting bilirubin is filtered through the glomerulus and appears in the urine.[17] This route of excretion assumes greater importance when hepatic excretory function is impaired.[18–20]

EFFECT OF SURGERY AND ANESTHESIA ON HEPATIC FUNCTION

Many anesthetic agents decrease hepatic blood flow by 25% to 50%.[21] This may be secondary to a fall in cardiac output (nitrous oxide, halothane, enflurane, methoxyflurane), an increase in splanchnic resistance (cyclopropane), or a combination of the two (methoxyflurane). Intermittent positive-pressure ventilation, hypocarbia, and sympathetic activation are also likely to increase splanchnic vascular resistance and lead to a decrease in splanchnic blood flow.[22]

Anesthesia and surgery are accompanied by a drop in hepatic oxygen consumption, although the magnitude of this drop does not match that of the decrease that occurs in hepatic blood flow.[23] Decreased oxygen delivery with a lesser fall in oxygen consumption may lead to regions of hypoxia. There is no increase in lactate production during surgery and anesthesia. Nevertheless, these vascular changes are dramatic and may explain the frequent minor increases in serum transaminase levels that follow surgery.[24–27]

A rise in serum levels of hepatic transaminases in the postoperative period is common.[2,25-30] Serum glutamic oxaloacetic transaminose (SGOT) is present not only in the liver but also in heart and skeletal muscle; serum glutamic pyruvate transaminase (SGPT) is a more specific hepatic marker. In one study, a mild elevation in SGPT was noted 2 to 7 days after surgery in 25% of patients who had undergone a variety of surgical procedures with different anesthetic agents.[27] Halothane and methoxyflurane were associated with a higher frequency of postoperative abnormalities than cyclopro-prane. There was a similar incidence of SGPT elevation in patients who had undergone spinal anesthesia, although the magnitude of the increase was smaller. In general, upper abdominal procedures, particularly those involving the gallbladder and common duct, were associated with both a higher incidence and a greater magnitude of rise in SGPT than other procedures.[29]

INCIDENCE OF POSTOPERATIVE LIVER DYSFUNCTION

A rise in the serum concentration of hepatic transaminases, not uncommon in postoperative patients, has been estimated to occur in 20% to 25% of cases.[24, 29,30] It is thought to indicate hepatocyte injury with increased cellular permeability. A rise in bilirubin after surgery is distinctly less common, with an incidence of less than 1%.[31]

The incidence of clinically detectable jaundice following surgery is low. Several prospective series encompassing a large number of patients who had undergone minor surgical procedures such as cystoscopy or breast biopsy under general anesthesia failed to demonstrate a single patient with post-operative jaundice. However, in one series of consecutive patients who had undergone major surgery, the incidence of postoperative increases in bilirubin above 1.5 mg/dl was 20.2%, with 3.7% of the patients demonstrating a rise of greater than 4 mg/dl.[28] An incidence rate of 8.6% was observed in one study of patients who had undergone open-heart surgery for congenital or acquired heart disease. The magnitude of the surgical procedure correlated well with the likelihood of postoperative jaundice; 53% of patients who underwent triple-valve replacement developed postoperative jaundice, and almost 50% of patients with cirrhosis who received portacaval shunts develop jaundice after surgery.[7,32,33]

POSTOPERATIVE CAUSES OF HEPATIC DYSFUNCTION

Drugs

The risk of halothane-induced hepatic injury on first exposure is 1 in 10,000. The risk increases to 7 in 10,000 after multiple exposures. Retrospective controlled trials have failed to document a higher than normal risk of fulminant hepatic failure after halothane anesthesia, but surveys of patients anesthetized with halothane have estimated the incidence of severe liver damage to be between 1 in 22,000 and 1 in 35,000.[34-41] Several cases of recurrent hepatitis after rechallenge with halothane leave no doubt about this agent's hepatotoxic potential.[42-44] Recent evidence suggests an immunologic mechanism of injury.[45] Other halogenated anesthetic agents such as methoxyflurane and fluroxene may also precipitate liver disease.[46-48]

The clinical picture of halothane-induced hepatic injury may range from a mild elevation in transaminases to fulminant hepatic failure.[49] The estimated fatality rate in icteric cases is 20%, with a higher fatality rate among patients who develop fulminant hepatic failure.[39,50] Cases of chronic liver disease have also been described, although recovery is usually complete if the disease does not prove fatal.[51,52] There is little evidence to suggest that the diseased liver is more susceptible to halothane-induced injury than the normal liver.

Although hepatitis may develop after the first exposure, a previous exposure to halothane has been observed in 50% of the cases. The first exposure may have been tolerated without apparent adverse effect, although unexplained fever, eosinophilia, or mild transaminase elevation may have occurred. In general, the onset of fever or jaundice following the initial exposure occurs later than that following subsequent exposure. Fever occurs 8 to 14 days after the first exposure but only 1 to 11 days after repeated exposure. Similarly, jaundice occurs 10 to 28 days after the initial exposure but only 3 to 17 days after subsequent exposure. Obese persons and females appear to be especially predisposed to hepatic injury. There are no histologic features on liver biopsy to allow for unequivocable diagnosis of halothane-associated hepatitis.

A variety of other drugs commonly used in the surgical patient can induce hepatic injury. Many alter hepatic function without inducing change in the usual laboratory tests employed in clinical medicine. However, drug-induced alterations in hepatic function may contribute to the development of postoperative jaundice and liver dysfunction and constitute the major etiologic factor. Besides halothane, alpha-methyldopa and isoniazid (INH) are most frequently associated with hepatic injury. However, a wide variety of agents can induce hepatic injury. The pattern may simulate hepatitis (INH, alpha-methyldopa) or cholestasis (methyltestosterone, norethandrolone, chlorpromazine, or erythromycin estolate). Evaluating the postoperatively jaundiced patient requires a precise and detailed listing of drugs received before, during, and after surgery. Since so many drugs have been implicated in liver injury, referral to standard texts or review of articles on drug-induced hepatic dysfunction may clarify the picture.[53]

Infection

The development of jaundice in patients with severe infection is common. When infection involves the biliary tree or liver, as in cholangitis or liver abscess, the cause of the liver dysfunction is often apparent. In other instances, abnormalities in serum concentration of bilirubin or transaminases in the patient with infection may represent hemolysis due to sepsis, development of congestive heart failure as a result of increased oxygen demands associated with infection, hypoxemia associated with pulmonary infection, vascular injury to the liver consequent to sepsis-induced cardiac collapse, or effects of pharmacologic or surgical therapy used to treat the infection. However, there are patients with severe infections not involving the hepatobiliary tree in whom jaundice or abnormal liver function tests develop without any of the aforementioned factors.[54-57] The predominant pattern of liver dysfunction is one of increased total and conjugated bilirubin without rising serum levels of transaminase or alkaline phosphatase. Recently, a marked elevation of alkaline phosphatase alone has been observed with systemic infection.[58] Liver biopsies in these cases displayed evidence of canalicular injury with bile plugging.

Other

The high rate of oxygen utilization by the liver makes this organ vulnerable to the effects of oxygen deprivation. Hepatocytes around the central veins appear to be particularly liable to injury, since they are perfused with blood with lower oxygen tension than hepatocytes closer to arterial sources.[59] Congestion in the hepatic veins, low oxygen delivery rates due to central hypoxia, or poor perfusion suppresses a variety of hepatic functions. Since circulatory abnormalities occur in complicated clinical settings in which more than one factor is present, it is often difficult to pinpoint the exact abnormality responsible for liver dysfunction. The pathologic characteristic of the liver lesion seen in these circulatory abnormalities is centrilobular necrosis or necrosis around the central vein with congestion of the centrilobular sinusoids.[60] In most cases, a mild elevation in serum bilirubin concentration is noted, but severe hepatocellular injury with marked increases in bilirubin and transaminases may also accur.[61–64] On occasion, liver function abnormalities may even simulate obstructive jaundice. Recent case reports have convincingly demonstrated that low cardiac output without significant right-sided heart failure or central hypoxemia may lead to profound hepatocellular injury and even liver coma due to hepatic encephalopathy.[65,66]

EVALUATION OF HEPATIC DYSFUNCTION

The generally employed division of jaundice into prehepatic jaundice, hepatocellular jaundice, and bile secretory failure or cholestasis provides a useful framework for approaching the patient with postoperative jaundice. The fractionation of bilirubin, extent of transaminase elevation, and magnitude of rise in serum alkaline phosphatase concentration measured place the postoperative patient in one of the above categories (Table 22-1).

Prehepatic Jaundice

Prehepatic jaundice is characterized by a direct-reacting fraction of less than 15% of the total bilirubin concentration, absence of bilirubin in the urine, and normal serum transaminase levels. These findings clearly indicate that the jaundice is due to an excessive pigment load. The direct fraction may sometimes constitute more than 15% of total bilirubin owing to laboratory inaccuracy or regurgitation of conjugated bilirubin into the bloodstream. Under these circumstances, an excretory defect may be falsely diagnosed. In addition, the minor transient elevation in serum transaminase concentration seen so frequently in postoperative patients may lead the physician to the erroneous conclusion that the clinical jaundice is the result of hepatocellular disease.

The suspicion that jaundice is due to prehepatic factors is supported by clinical and laboratory evidence of hemolysis, recent blood transfusions, or extensive bleeding into extravascular sites. The patient with Gilbert's syndrome undergoing surgery is the one exception. Many persons with this inborn error of hepatic bil-

Table 22-1. Differential Diagnosis of Postoperative Jaundice

Category	Laboratory Features				Pathogenesis
	Bilirubin as Direct Fraction (%)	Serum Transaminase Level	Serum Alkaline Phosphatase Concentration	Status of Extrahepatic Duct	
Prehepatic	<15	Normal	Normal	Nondilated	Increase in bilirubin load from endogenous sources (hemolysis, pulmonary emboli, hematoma, or hemolysis of transfused red cells)
Hepatocellular	>15	Elevated (up to greater than 1000 U/liter)	Slightly elevated (less than twice normal)	Nondilated	Hypoxemia, viral hepatitis, drug-induced hepatitis (including by halothane), and total parenteral nutrition
Cholestatic	>15	Normal or slightly elevated	Elevated (more than twice normal)	Nondilated	Canalicular injury due to sepsis, shock, or "benign postoperative jaundice"
				Dilated	Major bile duct tumors, stones, pancreatitis, or stricture

irubin uptake and conjugation are only mildly or intermittently jaundiced and are usually unaware of the diagnosis. The total bilirubin concentration rarely rises above 5 mg/dl during infections, fasting, or stress, and the liver remains normal in size and in histologic appearance. Surgery, too, may increase the bilirubin concentration postoperatively.[67,68] Table 22-2 contains a complete listing of processes that can cause unconjugated hyperbilirubinemia in the postoperative patient.

Factors related to surgery frequently suppress hepatic excretory function, so the maximal transport of conjugated bilirubin from the hepatocyte into the bile canaliculus is decreased, and direct-reacting bilirubin regurgitates into the bloodstream. Under these circumstances, clinical diagnosis of the predominant process, increased pigment load or hepatic excretory suppression, is most easily made by a search for evidence of hemolysis with a reticulocyte count, serum haptoglobin concentration, and Coombs' test, documentation of previous transfusions, and a search for signs of extravasation of blood into extravascular sites.

Hepatocellular Jaundice

Hepatocellular injury is characterized by a direct-reacting fraction bilirubin of greater than 15% of the total serum bilirubin concentration, elevated serum transaminase levels, and an alkaline phosphatase concentration of less than twice normal. These findings are indicative of

Table 22-2. Differential Diagnosis of Unconjugated Hyperbilirubinemia

Process	Supportive Data
Congenital abnormalities in bilirubin uptake (e.g., Gilbert's syndrome)	Family history, previous history of intermittent jaundice, failure of bilirubin to decline to normal levels after acute episode
Increased bilirubin load from hemolysis of autologous red cells (e.g., glucose-6 phosphate dehydrogenase deficiency, sickle-cell anemia)	Increased reticulocyte count, anemia
Increased bilirubin load from breakdown of extravasated red cells	Evidence for pulmonary embolus, retroperitoneal bleeding, hemorrhage into operative site
Increased bilirubin load from shortened survival of transfused red cells	Transfusions
Unconjugated hyperbilirubinemia without hemolysis	No history of transfusions, absence of anemia or reticulocytosis, return of bilirubin to normal after acute episode

direct injury to hepatocytes. A minimally elevated alkaline phosphatase concentration under these circumstances generally implies that the biliary tract from the bile canaliculi to the ampulla of Vater has escaped major injury and that cholestasis is absent.

There are two important limitations to this general rule. First, although virtually all patients with chronic injury to bile ducts have elevated serum alkaline phosphatase levels, acute injury to the biliary tree, such as that caused by a stone entering the common duct postoperatively, may not provoke an immediate rise in the concentration of this enzyme. Bile duct injury induces synthesis of alkaline phosphatase with resultant regurgitation of the enzyme into the vascular compartment, and this process may lag behind the rise in serum bilirubin concentration or the release of hepatic transaminases into the circulation. A second exception to the rule that alkaline phosphatase and transaminase levels can distinguish between hepatocellular injury and cholestasis is the observation that an occasional patient with acute biliary obstruction, especially that associated with biliary infection, may develop a striking elevation in serum transaminase concentration.[69–72]

Although a rise in serum transaminase levels usually indicates hepatocellular damage, it does not define the mechanism of liver injury. A thorough review of the patient's past history and complete perioperative course may lead to a suspected cause. Table 22-3 lists the major causes of hepatocellular injury with a description of pertinent clinical and laboratory findings for each. Vascular injury is suggested by clinical evidence of right-heart failure, hypoxemia, shock, or low cardiac output in the perioperative period.

In general, post-transfusion hepatitis does not enter into the differential diagnosis of jaundice in the period of up to 1 month after surgery. With the advent of blood-donor screening for hepatitis B and an increase in the number of volunteer donors, the incidence of hepatitis B infection has been all but eliminated. Hepatitis A is a rare cause of post-transfusion hepatitis. Most post-transfusion hepatitis is due to another virus, which is currently classified as non-A, non-B.[73]

The incubation period from the time of

Table 22-3. Causes of Postoperative Hepatocellular Injury

Etiologic Factor	Supportive Clinical and Laboratory Findings
Vascular injury	Right-sided heart failure, hypoxemia, shock, low cardiac output
Viral hepatitis (particularly post-transfusion hepatitis)	Suitable incubation period, serologic evidence of acute hepatitis B, A, non-A, non-B, cytomegalovirus, or Epstein–Barr virus infection
Drugs (including halothane)	Ingestion of drug known to cause hepatocellular injury; injury usually occurs within 2 to 4 weeks after initiation of drug administration
	Previous exposure to halothane, particularly in the setting of unexplained postoperative fever
Total parental nutrition	Prolonged parenteral hyperalimentation
Obstruction (?cholangitis)	Suspicion of acute biliary obstruction, particularly in association with cholangitis

transfusion to the beginning of the rise in serum transaminase concentration averages 7 to 8 weeks, although increases in enzyme levels may be detected as early as 2 weeks after transfusion. Jaundice occurs in only 25% of cases and follows the rise in serum transaminase levels by 1 to 4 weeks. If a patient requires transfusion before surgery, viral hepatitis must be considered as a possible cause of liver dysfunction or jaundice in the postoperative period.

The pattern of change seen in serum levels may provide a diagnostic clue, because elevated transaminase concentrations usually return to normal within several days in ischemic injury but decline more gradually in virus-induced injury. In some instances, liver biopsy may further clarify the specific cause of hepatic damage. Liver biopsy in the patient with vascular injury shows necrosis predominantly around the central vein with or without congestion of the perivenular sinusoids. Hepatic damage due to drugs or virus produces an indistinguishable histologic picture that consists of a more diffuse pattern of panlobular cellular necrosis.

Treatment of jaundice due to hepatocellular damage is supportive, directed toward eliminating those factors that are contributing to the hepatic injury. There is little evidence of benefit from steroid therapy in the acute phase of the illness.[74,75]

Cholestasis

Cholestatic injury is characterized by a fraction of direct-reacting bilirubin greater than 15% of the total serum bilirubin concentration, minor elevations in serum transaminase levels, and a rise in serum alkaline phosphatase concentration to more than twice normal. This biochemical pattern indicates injury in the bile canaliculi or larger biliary radicals.

Findings in drug-induced liver injury, sepsis, and sometimes virus-related hepatic injury occasionally mimic a cholestatic pattern. In addition, postoperative cholestasis with intact extrahepatic bile ducts may occur without a clear cause.[76,77] This syndrome has been generally observed in elderly patients who have undergone extensive and difficult surgery with significant postoperative complications. The biliary excretory apparatus is adversely affected in such patients by ill-defined mechanisms; the result is cholestasis and bile-plugging, seen on liver biopsy, and accumulation of bilirubin in the serum.

The predominant consideration in the jaundiced postoperative patient with an elevated serum alkaline phosphatase concentration and normal or near normal serum transaminase levels is exclusion of the possibility of the presence of extrahepatic biliary obstruction. On occasion, the cause may be fortuitous, as in the progression of an overlooked pancreatic neoplasm, but extrahepatic obstruction is usually indicative of postoperative cholecystitis, with stones present in only 50% of cases, common-duct stones, biliary tract injury, or postoperative pancreatitis and bile duct compression.[78–82]

There are numerous techniques available for evaluation of the integrity of the biliary tract. Abdominal gray-scale ultrasonography is one such diagnostic modality that can be performed at the bedside. However, a technically satisfactory study may not be possible, because clips, scar tissue, ileus, or ascites may be present. Furthermore, although abdominal ultrasonography is sensitive and specific for gallstones, less than 25% of common-duct stones are detected by this method. Because the common duct dilates slowly, incomplete obstruction may cause only modest dilatation. Therefore, although a dilated common duct observed on ultrasonography almost certainly indicates biliary obstruction, the presence of a normal common duct does not exclude a surgically correctable cause for jaundice.

The recently developed radioisotopic compounds that are readily excreted by the liver allow good visualization of the extrahepatic biliary tree. Demonstration of a markedly dilated common duct without passage of isotope into the gastrointestinal tract means obstruction of major bile ducts but does not indicate the cause of the process or whether surgical correction is required. Furthermore, the small images obtained do not allow the physician to make an accurate estimate of mild or moderate bile duct dilatation or to reliably detect common-duct stones.

Injection of radiopaque material into the common duct in percutaneous transhepatic cholangiography or endoscopic retrograde cholangiopancreatography (ERCP) allows for definitive detection of the bile duct dilatation. Liver biopsy is not generally useful for distinguishing between intrahepatic cholestasis and extrahepatic obstruction. The presence of bile lakes, particularly in the portal area, provides definitive evidence of bile duct obstruction but offers no etiologic information.

Treatment of the patient with intrahepatic cholestasis due to canilicular injury is supportive, with elimination of pertinent etiologic factors such as sepsis or drugs.[83] Therapy of extrahepatic obstruction depends on the cause. Postoperative pancreatitis generally subsides with time. Bile duct strictures, common-duct stones, and obstruction by tumor require eventual surgical intervention with immediate treatment of associated cholangitis. The timing of surgical correction, whether accomplished by means of standard laparotomy, peroral endoscopy, or percutaneous transhepatic catheter manipulation, must be individualized.

SUMMARY

1. **The major issue in the patient who develops postoperative jaundice, as in any patient, is to decide whether the cause of the jaundice is surgically cor-**

rectible. This is particularly important in the patient who has undergone surgery of the biliary tree, since retained common-duct stones or biliary injury are always possible.

2. The first step in the assessment of postoperative jaundice is a review of the patient's previous medical history, the present illness that led to surgery, the intraoperative course (with special attention to blood transfusions, anesthetic agents, and cardiovascular stability), and the time sequence of the development of liver function abnormalities after surgery.

3. Laboratory features of prehepatic, cholestatic, and hepatobiliary jaundice are listed in Table 22-1.

4. Differentiating hepatocellular disease from obstruction as a cause of jaundice may be difficult. High serum transaminase concentrations, a minimally elevated serum alkaline phosphatase level, and the absence of dilatation of biliary radicals seen in ultrasonography suggest that the jaundice is due to hepatocellular damage. Minimal elevation in the serum transaminase level with a high serum alkaline phosphatase concentration is seen in obstruction. Since treatment of canalicular injury can only be supportive whereas that of major bile duct obstruction must be surgical, a precise diagnosis is needed. Percutaneous transhepatic cholangiography or ERCP may clarify the structure of the bile duct to afford the crucial etiologic distinction.

REFERENCES

1. Lamont JT, Isselbacher KJ: Post-operative jaundice. New Engl J Med 268:305, 1973

2. Koff RS: Post-operative jaundice. Med Clin North Am 59:823, 1975

3. Lamont JT: Post-operative jaundice. Surg Clin North Am 54:637, 1974

4. Iwatsuki S, Geis WP: Hepatic complications. Surg Clin North Am 57:1335, 1977

5. Strasberg SM, Silver MD: Post-operative hepatogenic jaundice. Surg Gynecol Obstet 132:81, 1971

6. Babior BM, Davidson CS: Post-operative massive liver necrosis. New Engl J Med 276:645, 1967

7. French AB, Barss TP, Fairlie CS et al: Metabolic effects of anesthesia in man. V. A comparison of the effects of ether and cyclopropane anesthesia on the abnormal liver. Ann Surg 135:145, 1952

8. Schmid R, McConough AF: Hyper-bilirubinemia. In Stanbury JB, Wyngaarden JB, Fredrickson DS (eds): The Metabolic Basis of Inherited Disease. New York, McGraw-Hill, 1978

9. Barrett PVD, Berk PD, Menken M et al: Bilirubin turnover studies in normal and pathological state utilizing bilirubin-C^{14}. Ann Intern Med 68:355, 1968

10. Berk PD, Howe RB, Bloomer JR et al: Studies of bilirubin kinetics in normal adults. J Clin Invest 48:2176, 1969

11. Arias I, Johnson L, Wolfson S: Biliary excretion of injected conjugated and unconjugated bilirubin by normal and GUNN rats. Am J Physiol 200:1091, 1961

12. Tisdale WA, Klatskin G, Kinsella ED: The significance of the direct-reacting fraction of serum bilirubin in hemolytic jaundice. Am J Med 26:214, 1959

13. Schlam L, Weber A: Jaundice with conjugated bilirubin in hyperhemolysis. Acta Med Scand 176:549, 1964

14. Snyder AL, Satterlee W, Robinson SH et al: Conjugated plasma bilirubin in jaundice caused by pigment overload. Nature 213:93, 1967

15. Levine R, Klatskin G: Unconjugated hyperbilirubinemia in the absence of overt hemolysis. Importance of acquired disease as an etiologic factor in 366 adolescent and adult subjects. Am J Med 36:541, 1964

16. Valeri CR: Viability and function of preserved red cells. N Engl J Med 284:81, 1971

17. Fulop M, Sandson J, Brazeau P: Dialyzability, protein binding, and renal excretion of plasma conjugated bilirubin. J Clin Invest 44:666, 1965

18. Fulop M, Sandson J, Brazeau P: Bilirubinemia. Gastroenterology 49:464, 1965

19. Cameron JL, Filler RM, Iber FL et al: Metabolism and excretion of C^{14} labeled bilirubin in children with biliary atresia. N Engl J Med 274:231, 1966

20. Fulop M, Katz S, Lawrence C: Extreme hyperbilirubinemia. Arch Intern Med 127:254, 1971

21. Ngai SH: Effects of anesthetics on various organs. N Engl J Med 302:564, 1980

22. Batchelder BM, Cooperman LH: Effects of anesthetics on splanchnic circulation and metabolism. Surg Clin North Am 55:787, 1975

23. Cooperman LH, Wollman H, Marsh ML: Anesthesia and the liver. Surg Clin North Am 57:421, 1977

24. Dawson B, Adson MA, Dockerty MB et al: Hepatic function tests: Post-operative changes with halothane or diethyl ether anesthesia. Mayo Clin Proc 41:599, 1966

25. Geller W, Tagnon HJ: Liver dysfunction following abdominal operations. The significance of post-operative hyperbilirubinemia. Arch Intern Med 86:908, 1950

26. Thompson DS, Greifenstein FE: Enzyme patterns reflecting hepatic response to anesthesia and operation. South Med J 67:69, 1974

27. Ayres PR, Williard TB: Serum glutamic oxalacetic transaminase levels in 266 surgical patients. Ann Intern Med 52:1279, 1960

28. Evans C, Evans M, Pollack AV: The incidence and causes of post-operative jaundice. Br J Anaesth 46:520, 1974

29. Kalow B, Rogoman E, Sims FH: A comparison of the effects of halothane and other anesthetic agents on hepatocellular function in patients submitted to elective operations. Can Anaesth Soc J 23:71, 1976

30. McEwan J: Liver function tests following anaesthesia. Br J Anaesth 48:1065, 1976

31. Morgenstern L: Post-operative jaundice: An approach to a diagnostic dilemma. Am J Surg 128:255, 1974

32. Sanderson RG, Ellison JH, Benson JA et al: Jaundice following open-heart surgery. Ann Surg 165:217, 1965

33. Lockey E, McIntyre N, Ross ON et al: Early jaundice after open-heart surgery. Thorax 22:165, 1967

34. Wright R, Chisholm M, Lloyd B et al: Controlled prospective study of the effect of liver function of multiple exposures to halothane. Lancet 1:817, 1975

35. Carney FMT, Van Dyke RA: Halothane hepatitis: A critical review. Anesth Analg (Cleve) 52:135, 1972

36. National Halothane Study: Summary of the National Halothane Study: Possible association between halothane anesthesia and post-operative hepatic necrosis. JAMA 197:775, 1966

37. Inman WHW, Mushin WW: Jaundice after repeated exposure to halothane: A further analysis of reports of the Committee on Safety of Medicines. Br Med J 2:1455, 1978

38. Sherlock S: Halothane hepatitis. Lancet 2:364, 1978

39. Sherlock S: Halothane hepatitis. G 12:324, 1971

40. Mushin WW, Rosen M, Jones EV: Post-halothane jaundice in relation to previous administration of halothane. Br Med J 3:18, 1971

41. Strunin L: The Liver and Anesthesia. Philadelphia, WB Saunders, 1977

42. Tygstrup M: Halothane hepatitis. Lancet 2:466, 1963

43. Belfrage S, Ahlgren I, Axelson S: Halothane hepatitis in an anesthetist. Lancet 1:1466, 1966

44. Klatskin G, Kimberg DV: Recurrent hepatitis attributable to halothane sensitization in an anesthetist. N Engl J Med 280:515, 1969

45. Vergani D, Mieli-Vergani G, Alberti A et al: Antibodies to the surface of halothane-altered rabbit hepatocytes in patients with

severe halothane-associated hepatitis. N Engl J Med 303:66, 1980

46. Joshi PH, Conn HO: The syndrome of methoxyflurane-associated hepatitis. Ann Intern Med 80:395, 1974

47. Brenner AI, Kaplan MM: Recurrent hepatitis due to methoxyflurane anesthesia. N Engl J Med 284:961, 1971

48. Reynolds ES, Brown BR, Vandam LD: Massive hepatic necrosis after fluroxene anesthesia—A case of drug interaction? N Engl J Med 286:530, 1972

49. Conn HO: Halothane-associated hepatitis. Isr J Med Sci 10:404, 1974

50. Moult PJA, Sherlock S: Halothane-related hepatitis. Q J Med 44:99, 1975

51. Thomas FB: Chronic aggressive hepatitis induced by halothane. Ann Intern Med 81:487, 1974

52. Miller DJ, Dwyer J, Klatskin G: Halothane hepatitis: Benign resolution of a severe lesion. Ann Intern Med 89:212, 1978

53. Ludwig J: Drug effects on the liver: A tabular compilation of drugs and drug-related hepatic diseases. Dig Dis Sci 24:785, 1979

54. Miller DJ, Keeton GR, Webber BL et al: Jaundice in severe bacterial infection. Gastroenterology 71:94, 1976

55. Vermillion SE, Gregg JA, Baggenstoss AH: Jaundice associated with bacteremia. Arch Intern Med 124:611, 1969

56. Fahrlander H, Huber F, Gloor F: Intrahepatic retention of bile in severe bacterial infections. Gastroenterology 47:590, 1964

57. Eley A, Hargreaves T, Lambert HP: Jaundice in severe infection. Br Med J 2:75, 1965

58. Fang MH, Ginsberg AL, Dobbins WO: Marked elevation in serum alkaline phosphatase activity as a manifestation of system infection. Gastroenterology 78:592, 1980

59. Bynum TE, Boitnott JK, Maddrey WC: Ischemic hepatitis. Dig Dis Sci 24:129, 1979

60. Cohen JA, Kaplan MM: Left-sided heart failure presenting as hepatitis. Gastroenterology 74:583, 1978

61. Rueff B, Benhamou JP: Acute hepatic necrosis and fulminant hepatic failure. G 14:805, 1970

62. Novel O, Henrion J, Bernuau J et al: Fulminant hepatic failure due to transient circulatory failure in patients with chronic heart disease. Dig Dis Sci 25:49, 1980

63. Kaymakcalan H, Dourdourekas D, Szanto PB et al: Congestive heart failure as a cause of fulminant hepatic failure. Am J Med 65:384, 1978

64. Ellenberg M, Osserman KE: The role of shock in the production of central liver cell necrosis. Am J Med 2:170, 1951

65. Refsum HE: Arterial hypoxaemia, serum activities of GO-T, GP-T, and LDH, and centulobular liver cell necrosis in pulmonary insufficiency. Clin Sci 25:369, 1963

66. Sherlock S: Liver in heart failure: Relation of anatomical, functional and circulatory changes. Br Heart J 13:273, 1957

67. Powell LW, Hemingway E, Billing BH et al: Idiopathic unconjugated hyperbilirubinemia (Gilbert's syndrome). N Engl J Med 277:1108, 1967

68. Felsher BF, Rickard D, Redeker AC: The reciprocal relation between caloric intake and the degree of hyperbilirubinemia in Gilbert's syndrome. N Engl J Med 283:170, 1970

69. Ginsberg AL: Very high levels of SGOT and LDH in patients with extrahepatic obstruction. Am J Dig Dis 15:803, 1970

70. Mossberg SM, Ross G: High serum transaminase activity associated with extrahepatic biliary disease. Gastroenterology 45:345, 1963

71. Gardner B: Marked elevation of serum transaminases in obstructive jaundice. Am J Surg 3:575, 1966

72. Abbruzzese A, Jeffrey RL: Marked elevations of serum glutamic oxalacetic transaminase and lactic dehydrogenase activity in chronic extrahepatic biliary disease. Am J Dig Dis 14:332, 1969

73. Aach RD: Post transfusion hepatitis: Current prospective. Ann Intern Med 92:539, 1980

74. Report from the European Association for the Study of the Liver: Randomised trial of steroid therapy in acute liver failure. G 20:620, 1979

75. Ware AJ, Jones RE, Shorey JW et al: A con-

trolled trial of steroid therapy in massive hepatic necrosis. Am J Gastroenterol 62:130, 1974

76. Kantrowitz PA, Jones WA, Greenberger NJ et al: Severe post-operative hyperbilirubinemia simulating obstructive jaundice. N Engl J Med 276:591, 1967

77. Schmid M, Hefti ML, Gattiker R et al: Benign post-operative intra-hepatic cholestasis. N Engl J Med 272:545, 1965

78. Ottinger LW: Acute cholecystitis as a post-operative complication. Ann Surg 184:162, 1976

79. Howard RJ, Delaney JP: Post-operative cholecystitis. Am J Dig Dis 17:213, 1972

80. Donaldson GA, Allen AW, Bartlett MK: Post-operative bile-duct strictures. Their etiology and treatment. N Engl J Med 254:50, 1956

81. Saidi F, Donaldson GA: Acute pancreatitis following distal gastrectomy for benign ulcers. Am J Surg 105:87, 1963

82. Mahaffey JH, Howard JM: The incidence of post-operative pancreatitis in 131 surgical patients utilizing the serum amylase concentration. Arch Surg 70:348, 1975

83. Lindor KD, Fleming CR, Abrams A et al: Liver function values in adults receiving total parenteral nutrition. JAMA 241:2398, 1979

23

Preoperative Pulmonary Evaluation and Preparation

RANDALL D. CEBUL
WILLIAM G. KUSSMAUL

The primary goals of preoperative pulmonary evaluation are to identify patients who have an increased risk of developing respiratory complications, to establish the extent of the risk, and, when possible, to reduce the risk before surgery. In some instances, it may be appropriate to recommend postponement or cancellation of surgery or the use of alternative methods of anesthesia. This chapter provides guidelines for the estimation of preoperative risk and the preparation of high-risk patients for surgery. Little emphasis is placed on postoperative pulmonary embolism, cardiac arrhythmias related to pulmonary dysfunction, and exacerbations of pre-existing bronchitis. When a tenuous clinical relationship exists between preoperative factors and postoperative pulmonary complications, recommendations are based on known pathophysiologic changes that occur in the postoperative period.

PULMONARY PATHOPHYSIOLOGY IN THE POSTOPERATIVE PATIENT

Whether or not patients have normal pulmonary function before surgery, their pulmonary status changes in the perioperative period. The changes may be seen in four areas: (1) lung volume, (2) ventilatory pattern, (3) gas exchange, and (4) lung defense mechanisms.[1]

Virtually all static lung volumes and most dynamic measures of pulmonary function decrease postoperatively. Depending on the type of surgical procedure carried out, total lung capacity and each of its subdivisions—forced vital capacity (FVC), tidal volume (TV), residual volume (RV), functional residual capacity (FRC), and expiratory reserve volume (ERV)—may decrease by up to 50% and become most evident by the fourth postoperative day.[1,2] Barring complications, most of these changes, as well as changes in forced expiratory volume (FEV_1) and maximal mid-expiratory flow rate ($FEF_{25-75\%}$), will return to preoperative levels within 2 weeks after surgery.[1]

In general, the magnitude of change that occurs in lung volume correlates with the location of the surgical incision. In decreasing order, operations that affect lung volume are thoracic, upper abdominal, lower abdominal, and peripheral surgical procedures.[1,3] Contributing factors to the decrease in lung volume include placement in the recumbent position, abdominal distention, sedation, the use of restrictive bandages, and postoperative pain.

The importance of these changes becomes clearest when considered in relation to the closing volume (CV). The CV is a measure of the lung volume at which, during expiration, the balance of inflation pressures and elastic forces causes small airways to close and collapse. Closure of small airways causes mismatch of perfusion and ventilation and contributes to hypoxemia. In young, normal subjects, the CV occurs above the RV and below the end-tidal point. As long as the CV is smaller than the ERV, airways close normally. Conditions that either raise the CV, such as smoking and age, or lower the ERV, such as obesity, predispose the patient to early closure of airways and atelectasis in the postoperative state. A graphic depiction of these relationships is given in Figure 23-1. Multiple factors may promote atelectasis simultaneously, as exemplified by the obese (decreased ERV), aged smoker (increased CV).

After abdominal surgery, there is a decrease in TV, an increase in respiratory rate, and an absence of periodic hyperinflation. This pattern promotes atelectasis by interfering with surfactant production.[5] Pulmonary compliance, a measure of the ease with which the lungs can be inflated, is generally decreased after abdominal surgery, probably as a result of airway closure and atelectasis.[6] This decrease is most marked in patients with chronic bronchitis. Deep breathing has been shown to return compliance toward normal, presumably by reopening small airways.[1] Flow-volume curves in postoperative patients also show a pattern consistent with restriction.[2] In addition, patients with pre-existing chronic obstructive pulmonary disease show an increase in airway resistance that is possibly due to

the accumulation of interstitial edema around small airways.[6]

Arterial hypoxemia is almost universal in the postoperative period and pathophysiologically results from abnormalities in ventilation:perfusion (V/Q) ratios, which, in turn, are due to the altered lung volumes and their relationships to the CV discussed above.[7] Anatomically, hypoxemia generally indicates atelectasis. The ratio of dead space to TV increases after abdominal surgery because of tachypnea.[8] Pulmonary regional blood flow is altered, but reflex changes in local airways probably prevent this mechanism from contributing significantly to V/Q mismatch.[5] Following abdominal surgery, arterial hypoxemia may persist for at least 3 days, leading some authors to recommend the routine use of postoperative oxygen therapy.[6]

Cough and deep breathing are both impaired after surgery. Normal ciliary function is decreased, and hypoxemia reduces the clearance of bacteria from airways.[1] The degree to which these alterations contribute to postoperative pulmonary complications is unclear, but decreased mucociliary clearance predictably precedes and accompanies atelectasis.[9]

The most commonly recognized respiratory complication after surgery is atelectasis. Most authors accept the concept that "microatelectasis," or that not detected on physical examination or roentgenogram, is nearly universal and accounts for most postoperative hypoxemia.[1] Pathophysiologic mechanisms that contribute to the development of atelectasis include decreased clearance of secretions, absence of periodic hyperinflation, and decreased FRC in relation to CV. "Macroatelectasis" is more common after upper abdominal than lower abdominal or nonabdominal surgery.[7] It occurs in 20% to 40% of patients who have undergone

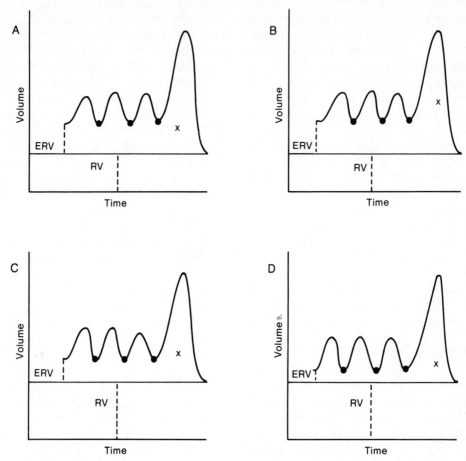

Fig. 23-1. Relationships between closing volume (x) and expiratory reserve volume (ERV) in different conditions. (A) Normal relationship in a young adult. Normal closing volume (CV) is less than ERV and below the end-tidal point. (B) Effects of age or smoking. Increased CV that is larger than the normal ERV and above the end-tidal point. (C) Effects of obesity. Decreased ERV that is lower than the normal CV. (D) Normal relationship in patient in postoperative state. Decreased ERV (magnitude dependent on type of surgery, use of binders, etc.) that is lower than the normal CV. Somewhat decreased RV. Obese, aged smokers have a compounded risk. RV = residual volume; ● = end-tidal point. (After Tisi GM: Am Rev Respir Dis 119:293–310, 1979)

upper abdominal procedures and in 10% to 20% of patients who have had lower abdominal surgery.[10] It rarely occurs after operations outside the chest and abdomen.[11]

RISK OF POSTOPERATIVE PULMONARY COMPLICATIONS

Clinical Factors

Definitions vary as to what postoperative pulmonary events constitute complications. Depending on the definition, the incidence ranges from 0.1% to 70%.[10] Postoperative lung collapse may vary from minimal to massive, and a small temperature elevation may be viewed as either a normal response to surgery or an indication of atelectasis or pulmonary infection.[10] In a recent review, Tisi categorized postoperative pulmonary complications as either infectious or noninfectious, with atelectasis standing out as the primary noninfectious complication.[1]

Latimer and co-workers found macroatelectasis (defined radiographically or by a 3°F postoperative temperature elevation associated with altered physical findings in the lungs) in 37% of postoperative patients, and microatelectasis (defined as a 1°F to 2°F postoperative temperature elevation and changed physical findings without radiographic changes) in 28%.[10] Only 24% of this unselected population of adult patients escaped postoperative pulmonary complications. Comparable studies have reported the incidence of postoperative pneumonia to be in the range of 1% to 15% or more of patients.[12–14]

The type and duration of surgery and anesthesia affect the incidence of postoperative pulmonary complications. Tisi placed surgical procedures into five categories of increasing risk: (1) nonabdominal, nonthoracic; (2) lower abdominal; (3) upper abdominal; (4) thoracic surgery without resection of functional lung; and (5) thoracic surgery with resection of functional lung. The literature supports such a gradation of operative risk by type of procedure. The risk of peripheral or nonabdominal, nonthoracic surgical procedures approximates that of anesthesia alone and is usually less than 1%.[10] Upper abdominal procedures confer approximately the same risk of postoperative complications as thoracic procedures without resection of functional lung, and 30% to 60% of patients who undergo these operations experience some type of postoperative pulmonary problem.[1,3] Lower abdominal operations are followed by pulmonary complications in 10% to 30% of cases.[1,3] In thoracic surgery, including resection of functional lung, risk also depends on the presence or absence of chronic lung disease, the amount of functional lung resected, and the degree to which the bellows function of the lung is affected.[1]

Longer operations impart a greater risk of postoperative pulmonary complications and death than do shorter procedures, although the magnitude of this increased risk is unclear. Dripps and Deming reported that procedures lasting longer than 3 hr conferred over twice the risk of pulmonary complications of procedures lasting less than 3 hr.[15] Other studies using different "critical time periods" and reporting different outcomes support the notion that, in general, postoperative complication rates vary directly with duration of anesthesia.[3,14]

Anesthesia itself may promote postoperative pulmonary complications by virtue of its carry-over effects into the postoperative period.[1] Theoretical arguments favor spinal over general anesthesia in high-risk patients, and clinical studies have been done that support the use of regional anesthesia for such patients.[16] However, data to the contrary may also be found and Tisi warns that "all too often, medical diligence and care are relaxed because a patient is subjected to spinal rather than general anesthesia."[1,10,17]

With this knowledge at hand, the consultant is often confronted by a patient for whom an independent estimate of preoperative pulmonary risk must be made. It is important to realize that ostensibly "normal" individuals are not risk-free and that all gradations of risk exist, from that imposed by anesthesia alone to that imparted by functional lung resection in a patient with chronic obstructive pulmonary disease. It follows that preoperative evaluation must be tailored to the individual patient; no single method of assessment is equally applicable to all persons for all operations. Similarly, preoperatively pulmonary preparation should optimally be directed at minimizing relevant risk factors in individual patients.

Cigarette Smoking, Bronchitis, and Dyspnea

The relationship between smoking and respiratory disease is well established. Cigarette usage has been convincingly implicated in the development of chronic obstructive pulmonary disease, bronchitis, respiratory infection, and bronchogenic carcinoma. Although each of these conditions in turn may increase the risk of postoperative complications, a more difficult question to answer relates to the independent contribution of smoking to poor pulmonary outcome after surgery. In the absence of its associated conditions, does cigarette smoking per se impart an

increased risk of postoperative complications for the patient? If so, what is the magnitude of this risk for which outcomes? Is recent smoking or chronic usage more important in defining this risk? And, finally, if recent smoking is deleterious, what is the role of short-term abstinence in preoperative preparation?

Cigarette smoking has several effects on respiratory tract physiology that might lead to the development of postoperative pulmonary complications. Lung defense mechanisms are impaired by chronic and, to a more variable degree, acute cigarette smoke inhalation.[18] Cigarette smoke impairs the respiratory tract mucociliary transport system, which is necessary for clearance of certain particulate matter, including bacteria.[19] Concomitantly, tracheobronchial secretions may increase in both quantity and viscosity, making clearance more difficult.[18]

The chronic effects of smoking on pulmonary physiology were discussed in the previous section. Small-airways disease may exist in asymptomatic smokers and even in nonsmokers chronically exposed to tobacco smoke.[20,21] The Framingham study demonstrated that smoking has an inverse relationship to FVC and FEV_1. The association between smoking and increased CV and the possible relationship of increased CV to the development of postoperative atelectasis have already been reviewed.

Some of the changes in respiratory physiology that are caused by smoking may be reversible with the cessation of cigarette use. The data from the Framingham study showed that the FVC of ex-smokers became more like that of nonsmokers over a 5-year period.[22] Whether short-term preoperative abstinence may be similarly beneficial is not as clear. Camner and Philipson demonstrated a significant improvement in tracheobronchial clearance of particulates in smokers after abstinence of only 3 months; no effect was noted after 1 week.[23] Similarly, whereas small-airway dysfunction in smokers, as measured by $FEF_{25-75\%}$, may be reversed after abstinence of 1 month, cessation of smoking for 1 week appears to afford no comparable benefit.[24,25]

The results of several surgical series suggest that cigarette smoking is associated with an increased incidence of postoperative atelectasis and pulmonary infections.[10,26,27] The reported relative risk for postoperative complications in smokers has varied from 2 to 6 times that of nonsmokers, depending primarily on the type of surgery done and the definitions used for complications.[21,28] When these data are scrutinized, however, it becomes clear that, in most series, there has been no appropriate control for other important risk factors such as symptoms of chest disease, age, and duration of anesthesia.

A few well-designed studies support the idea that symptoms of respiratory tract disease impart a significantly higher risk of postoperative pulmonary complications than does cigarette smoking per se.[10,12,28] It appears that productive cough or dyspnea, sometimes reflected by severe preoperative impairment in pulmonary function tests (PFTs), confers virtually all of the risk assigned to cigarette smoking.[10,12] In 1974, Presley and Alexander–Williams reported the results of a prospective study of 200 patients undergoing abdominal procedures.[14] Age, sex, smoking history, and symptoms of cough, sputum production, and dyspnea were recorded. Postoperative complications were defined as a productive cough and fever associated with new physical signs on chest examination within 3 days of operation. Preoperative bronchitis or dyspnea was associated with a significant increase in complications regardless of smoking habits. Individuals with a history of smoking and chest symptoms had a twofold greater risk of complications than smokers without chest symptoms. Asymptomatic smokers had no increased risk of developing postoperative pulmonary complications. These findings are supported by data from other studies.[28,29] Presley also noted that the occurrence of clinical complications was associated with an increase of 3 days in length of hospital stay.

Wheatley and co-workers studied the effects of preoperative abstinence from smoking for 5 days on incidence of postoperative clinical pulmonary complications and duration of hospital stay.[30] Patients were carefully matched for history of smoking, cough, and sputum production, surgical procedure done, and type of anesthesia used. No difference in complication rate or length of hospital stay was noted between patients who abstained from smoking and those who did not. This is not surprising, given the known length of abstinence required to effect changes in respiratory tract physiology.[22–25] Critical reviews of the topic suggest that 2 to 4 weeks of abstinence from smoking may be required to cause discernible differences in postoperative outcome.[12,30,31]

Age

The effect of advanced age on postoperative morbidity and mortality is discussed in detail in Chapter 38. There are several theoretical reasons to suspect a positive correlation between operative risk and age. The normal physiologic effects of aging include decreases in static lung volumes, FEV_1, and $FEF_{25-75\%}$, pulmonary elastic recoil, and PaO_2.[32–37] The duration of exposure to environmental toxins and cigarette smoke may increase with age and predispose the patient to further pathologic changes in the lungs. In addition, advanced age may bring with it general debility or specific cardiopulmonary diseases that independently contribute to risk.

Clinically, the risk for postoperative pulmonary complications does not increase linerarly with age but appears to be significantly higher only in the eighth and ninth decades of life. Only one retrospective study of upper abdominal surgery has suggested that there is an increased risk of postoperative chest infection in the fourth decade, but this study also found that the incidence of this complication decreased in frequency in patients in their seventies.[14]

A prospective study of 46 patients reported by Latimer and co-workers revealed no increased risk for a variety of postoperative pulmonary complications with advanced age when several other preoperative variables were also considered.[10] Larger series, including those reported by Wightman and Tarhan and colleagues, suggest that risk may increase significantly only beyond the age of 70.[2,16] In the latter study of 357 patients with chronic lung disease, the postoperative mortality rate among patients 70 years of age or older was substantially higher than that among patients under age 70, although no linear trends in mortality rate were noted in the younger age groups. The same results were obtained by Ziffren and Hartford in their review of ten years of postoperative experience at the University of Iowa.[38]

Obesity

Obesity appears to confer a significant independent risk of postoperative pulmonary complications, although the magnitude of this risk is far from clear. The

physiologic correlates of obesity include decreased FRC and ERV, which decline as a function of weight independent of age, sex, and height.[32] The ERV in obese patients may be smaller than the CV and cause small-airways closure and secondary increases in the $(A-a)PO_2$ gradient. In addition, excessive fat directly increases the mechanical work of breathing.[39] Clinical correlates may include ineffectual cough, atelectasis, progressive hypoxemia, and potential infectious complications. The risks of obesity are discussed fully in Chapter 13.

Despite these theoretical arguments, clinical data to support obesity as a significant risk factor are few and are often hampered by problems of definition. The definition of obesity should include a comparison of the patient's weight to a standard, generally expressed in relation to height.[40] Studies that report weight only or individual weight compared to average weight in a series of patients overlook this basic but important concept.

In a prospective analysis of 400 patients undergoing cholecystectomy, Pemberton and Manax reported no significant difference in postoperative morbidity between obese and nonobese patients.[41] Measured pulmonary and nonpulmonary complications were similar in the two groups. Criticism of this study has focused on the authors' reporting weights without relating them to height or standard norms. Similar results with comparable definitional problems were reported by Presley and Alexander–Williams in a study of 200 patients undergoing surgery for ulcer or biliary tract disease.[14]

When obesity was defined as weight exceeding by 10% those weights that are presented in standard life insurance weight–height tables, significantly more postoperative pulmonary complications were reported by Latimer and co-workers to occur in obese than nonobese patients.[10] Although age, preoperative pulmonary impairment, and history of smoking were not controlled, 95% of obese patients as compared to 63% of nonobese patients had postoperative pulmonary problems. The authors concluded that, when upper abdominal surgery is contemplated, obesity confers an increased risk of postoperative microatelectasis, macroatelectasis, and a variety of "miscellaneous" pulmonary complications. In his recent review of preoperative pulmonary evaluation, Tisi drew similar conclusions from the available literature.[1]

Other

Other information derived from the patient's history and physical examination may provide data for estimation of the preoperative risk of postoperative pulmonary complications. Although the literature is sparse in this area, specific historical data regarding place of residency, occupation, medications used, and intercurrent pulmonary and cardiac illnesses may all prove informative in the preoperative assessment. Similarly, close attention to cardiopulmonary physical findings is mandatory, and special emphasis on findings likely to be associated with postoperative respiratory difficulties may reveal the need for preoperative pulmonary preparation.

Passive exposure to environmental factors may be associated with cough and progressive pulmonary impairment independent of smoking history.[42] In one population study, urban dwellers had an increased likelihood over rural dwellers of productive cough independent of age, sex, and smoking status.[43] Presley and Alexander–Williams noted a significantly higher rate of adverse outcomes in 42 industrial workers than in 152 professionals and clerical workers.[14] A thorough medication history may also prove helpful in revealing underlying medical conditions that are otherwise clinically inapparent. Knowledge of the ongoing use of digoxin, for example, may uncover a significant preoperative risk in the patient in whom physical examination does not suggest the presence of congestive heart failure.[44] Risk factors that may be revealed by a patient's history include the following:

Definite risks
    Chronic bronchitis with productive cough
    Chronic obstructive pulmonary disease with dyspnea
    Age greater than 70 years
Probable risks
    Cigarette use
    Coexisting cardiac or systemic disease
    Occupational and environmental exposure
    Use of cardiac or pulmonary medications

In addition to weight, pertinent physical findings regarding pulmonary risks include skeletal abnormalities, clubbing, wheezing, signs of pulmonary consolidation, hyperinflation, and congestive heart failure. The "loose cough," a unique physical sign that is predictive of postoperative atelectasis, deserves special mention. Performed by listening to the patient during a forcible cough, the loose cough test is considered positive when a moist "rattle" is heard. It is most useful as an index of chronic bronchitis in situations in which a reliable history of respiratory symptoms is unobtainable.[45] Rapidly learned and simple to perform, this test correlates well with dynamic measures of lung function, and the presence of a loose cough preoperatively has been significantly associated with postoperative macroatelectasis.[46,47] Physical examination risk factors are summarized below.

Generalized debility

Abnormal nutritional status with gross deviation in weight

Positive loose cough test

Abnormal cardiac findings with signs of congestive heart failure and/or pulmonary hypertension

Abnormal pulmonary findings, including clubbing, skeletal abnormalities, wheezing or prolonged expiratory phase, hyperinflation, rhonchi or signs of consolidation

Laboratory Evaluation

Chest Radiographs

There are several potential indications for the performance of routine preoperative chest radiographs. Included among these are "screening" for unsuspected diagnoses such as tuberculosis or lung cancer, measurement of preoperative risk, provision of a baseline for postoperative comparison, and defense against malpractice claims. Weighing against these potential indications are the theoretically small, but definable, risk of radiation exposure, and cost.

When surgeons or anesthesiologists do not insist on routine preoperative chest radiographs, wide variations in practice are found. The Royal College of Radiologists in 1979 reported data on over 10,000 consecutive noncardiopulmonary surgical admissions to eight community and teaching hospitals in England.[48] Severalfold differences in usage of preoperative chest x-rays were noted and did not correlate with patient age or severity of operation. Preoperative radiographs did not appear to influence either the decision to operate or the type of anesthesia used. Furthermore, among patients known to have clinically apparent serious cardiac or pulmonary disease, only half had preoperative x-rays, and these patients fared no worse than those who did not have them. Whether these data represent suboptimal utilization and management practices or are true reflections of the marginal benefit to be derived from routine preoperative chest x-rays is the subject of considerable controversy.

General agreement exists that the age of the patient affects the incremental yield of preoperative radiographic screening in cases of noncardiopulmonary surgery. In 1978, Loder reported the results of clinical and radiographic data collected prospectively from 1000 consecutive presurgical admissions classifying chest x-ray results as normal, insignificantly abnormal, or significantly abnormal. Among 437 patients under 30 years of age, there were only 5 (0.23%) significantly abnormal findings, only 1 of which had escaped clinical detection. Similarly, Rees and his co-workers obtained preoperative x-rays for 667 consecutive elective noncardiothoracic surgical patients.[50] Among 108 patients under the age of 30, no significant radiologic abnormalities were noted. Sagel and colleagues classified patients according to clinical suspicion of cardiopulmonary disease.[51] Among patients without suspected cardiopulmonary disease, new diagnoses were made by x-ray in 0 of 521 patients under the age of 20 and in only 9 of 894 patients under the age of 30. The implications of these new diagnoses for the operative management of such patients have been debated.[50]

Radiographic screening for clinically unsuspected disease that would alter or contraindicate surgery, such as tuberculosis or lung cancer, does not appear to warrant independently the cost or risk of the x-ray study. The declining incidence of pulmonary tuberculosis has been reflected in the virtual disappearance of newly discovered active disease found on chest x-rays ordered for screening purposes. Of 39,017 consecutive admissions at Grady Memorial Hospital in 1972, no clinically unsuspected active tuberculosis was diagnosed on screening radiographs.[52] Results reported by Sagel and associates are virtually identical.[51] Screening for lung cancer with routine chest x-rays has been the subject of several studies.[53–55] There is consensus that screening chest x-rays should be obtained for smokers, men over 60, and persons with chronic cough or bronchitis.[53]

Chest x-rays comprise 45% of the radiologic studies performed in the United States, and, in 1970, over 70 million roentgenographic examinations of the chest were performed.[54] At an estimated cost of $20 per examination, it is calculated that nearly $1.5 billion are spent yearly by medical consumers for this examination alone.[51] Although the aggregate cost may not significantly influence the management of an individual patient, it is noteworthy that repeated examinations constitute a significant portion of this cost and that satisfactory, recent x-rays are often available for preoperative patients.[50,55]

Repeated radiographic studies impose on the patient a definable risk of radiation exposure.[56,57] In a study by Rees and coworkers, 38% of consecutive preoperative patients had received a chest radiograph in the previous year. The maximum acceptable bone marrow dose had been exceeded in 12.5% of these patients.

The incremental yield of new information provided by the lateral chest x-ray over that derived from the posteroanterior view alone has received considerable attention.[51,58,59] In Sagel's study, this increased yield was sufficiently low in the 20- to 39-year-old age group to warrant a recommendation that the lateral view not be routinely obtained preoperatively for patients of this age.[51] It is noteworthy that the lateral projection delivers a surface dose approximately 4 times greater than that given by the posteronanterior view. This represents twice the bone marrow integral and gonadal dose.

It is reasonable to conclude that patients undergoing cardiopulmonary procedures, patients over 40 years of age, and patients with symptoms of or with significant risk factors for developing cardiopulmonary disease will benefit from preoperative chest radiographs. The value of preoperative chest films in patients undergoing cardiopulmonary procedures is not debated. Chest x-rays in this population serve to establish or confirm diagnoses, stratify preoperative risk, and provide a baseline for postoperative comparison. In elderly patients with cardiopulmonary risk factors, the concordance between clinical evaluation and radiographic findings is sufficiently low that preoperative x-rays may provide further definition of preoperative risk. The vast majority of clinically inapparent radiographic findings in this population consist of cardiomegaly and chronic obstructive pulmonary disease.[50,51]

In short, preoperative chest radiographs are indicated under the following circumstances:

Definitely indicated
    In all thoracic procedures
    When patient's age ≥ 40 years
    When other significant clinical risk
       factors have been obtained from
       history and physical examination

Probably indicated

    When patient is age 30 to 39 years, especially if an abdominal procedure is planned*

Not routinely indicated

    For screening for clinically unsuspected lung cancer or tuberculosis

    When patient's age ≤ 30 years

Pulmonary Function Tests

The incidence of postoperative complications is higher than normal in patients with abnormal preoperative pulmonary function tests (PFTs).[3] However, it is unclear when preoperative PFTs are indicated and which measures are most predictive of risk. The question of when to obtain spirometric studies has surprisingly not been addressed in surgical candidates other than in those undergoing pulmonary resection. Various recommendations have been made, including encouragement that all smokers, elderly persons, and patients with known chronic obstructive pulmonary disease have complete PFTs.[61]

Once PFTs have been obtained, the literature stands on somewhat firmer ground in assessing their value for predicting postoperative pulmonary complications. The original quadrant diagram of Miller and associates divides pulmonary function into four categories based on a single-breath FVC and $FEV_{0.5}$ determination: normal, obstructive, restrictive, and mixed.[62] Patients in Miller's mixed category have higher than normal risk of postoperative pulmonary complications.[63] A modification of Miller's quadrant diagram has been used to predict postoperative respiratory failure. Observed vital capacity, expressed as a percentage of the predicted

value, is plotted against the ratio $FEV_1:FVC \times 100$ and a "marginal reserve" line drawn (Fig. 23-2). Patients with numbers below this line have an increased operative risk. It should be noted that this classification has not been prospectively evaluated.

Other predictive parameters have also been proposed. An FEV_1 of less than 1 liter is associated with increased surgical risk, but, with appropriate support, patients with such a low FEV_1 can also safely undergo surgery.[65] Age greater than 60 years together with an FEV_1 value of less than 2 liters was similarly associated with increased risk in a study by Boushy and his co-workers.[66] Perhaps more important than the absolute value of the FEV_1 is the FEV_1 expressed as a percentage of predicted value based on height, weight, age, and sex.[34] In a study at the University of Pennsylvania, a value for FEV_1 of less than 75% of the predicted

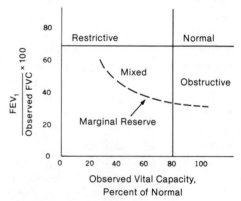

Fig. 23-2. Miller's quadrant system for stratifying preoperative pulmonary risk as modified by Redding.[64] *Dotted line* indicates level below which ventilatory failure may be anticipated. FEV_1 = forced expiratory volume in 1 sec; FVC = forced vital capacity.

---

*Consider posteroanterior view alone if there are no other significant risk factors. Always obtain a history of recent chest x-rays.

value was significantly associated with postoperative macroatelectasis and pulmonary edema.[44] The $FEF_{25-75\%}$, FVC, and maximal voluntary ventilation (MVV) or its equivalent, the maximal breathing capacity (MBC), have also been used as predictors of pulmonary risk.[3,65,67] Of these, the $FEF_{25-75\%}$ is probably the least specific, although Stein and his co-workers found it a useful discriminator of "good" and "poor" preoperative risk.[3,44,68,69]

The literature supports the inclusion of the MVV maneuver with other forced-expiration tests of pulmonary function. Data from the University of Pennsylvania support its routine use in patients undergoing elective thoracic surgery, and Hodgkin has recommended that it be performed if abnormal results are discovered on a routine screen using the FEV_1, FVC, FEV_1:FVC% and $FEF_{25-75\%}$.[44,65] Some authors have suggested that the MVV should in theory correlate best with postoperative pulmonary status.[61] The MVV requires the patient to breathe maximally for 10 sec to 15 sec and therefore reflects both pulmonary function and motivation. In a series of patients undergoing thoracic surgery, Mittman estimated operative risk from electrocardiographic (ECG) findings and measurement of the MVV, using as a cutoff point for the latter 50% of the predicted value.[70] Among 105 patients with normal ECGs and MVVs above the cutoff point, only 5% died. Among 14 patients over 40 years of age with ECG abnormalities and MVVs below 50% of the predicted value, the mortality rate was 71%. Gaensler and co-workers and other investigators have reported similar results in postoperative mortality studies.[71,72] A higher cutoff value of 75% of the expected MVV may be predictive of a wide range of postoperative complications.[44]

Whether PFTs are examined individually or in relation to other spirometric studies, it must be emphasized that their prognostic importance lies in providing information that has not already been obtained from a careful history and physical examination. As sole measures of preoperative risk, their prognostic value is less than that of a focused bedside examination.[44] Furthermore, it is not known whether abnormalities in different PFTs predict different postoperative complications or whether the ideal battery of tests differs for different surgical procedures, as suggested by Block and Olsen.[73] Based on all available data, indications for spirometry and MVV are the following:

All thoracic operations
Upper abdominal operations with other significant clinical risk factors present*
Age of patient greater than 70 with other significant clinical risk factors present
Moderate clinical risk factors present (risk class B), or abnormal chest x-ray

Arterial Blood Gas Determinations

Preoperative determination of arterial blood gas values is generally recommended if clinical evaluation or results of PFTs suggest significant obstructive pulmonary disease.[61] Arterial hypercapnia with an arterial carbon dioxide tension of greater than 45 torr is usually considered substantially more predictive of postoperative respiratory difficulties than arterial hypoxemia.[1,3] An increase in Pa_{CO_2} may be indicative of decreased pulmonary function, minimal respiratory reserve, and advanced lung disease.[1] While hypercapnia alone may be reversible and need not be an absolute contraindication to surgery, its presence implies a high risk of postoperative morbidity. In a study of

*Significant clinical risk factors derived from the bedside examination include productive cough, dyspnea, obesity, positive loose cough test, and abnormal cardiopulmonary physical findings.

63 consecutive preoperative patients reported by Stein and colleagues, 5 patients with elevated Pa_{CO_2} values suffered serious postoperative respiratory problems.[3] None of these patients was thought to have carbon dioxide retention preoperatively, although the method of preoperative clinical assessment was not reported, and all had abnormal spirometric results. Indications for arterial blood gases are the following:

Significant clinical risk factors suggesting obstructive pulmonary disease
Abnormal PFTs
All thoracic procedures with resection of functional lung

Electrocardiograms

As mentioned above, an abnormal ECG association with other clinical and laboratory evidence of pulmonary disease implies increased preoperative risk.[70,72] Although the ECG is not a sensitive indicator of pulmonary compromise, it does reveal multifocal atrial tachycardia, atrial flutter, abnormal P waves, and evidence of right ventricular abnormalities.[74] Ferrer has emphasized that rightward shifts of 30 degrees or more in the QRS axis are substantially more sensitive indicators of obstructive pulmonary disease than right-axis deviation alone.[75] Other findings compatible with right-heart strain due to pulmonary disease include abnormal T waves in the right precordial leads, depressed ST segments in leads II, III, and aVF, and right bundle-branch block.[75] These findings are usually not present without other clinical evidence of pulmonary disease and require no specific therapy; however, their presence in a patient with an otherwise ambiguous history and physical examination, or in a

patient with an abnormal chest x-ray, may mandate further testing or preoperative therapy. It is advisable to perform ECGs routinely for all patients undergoing thoracic procedures, for patients undergoing upper abdominal operations, if other risk factors are present, and for all patients 70 years of age or over.

EVALUATION FOR LUNG RESECTION

Removal of all or part of a lung reduces pulmonary function. Since indications for lung resection usually arise in association with an otherwise diseased lung, useful preoperative indices of lung function should identify patients who have marginal reserve and would therefore risk pulmonary disability or death after resection. The diseased lung may not contribute much to preoperative pulmonary function. The less it contributes, the less change is expected after resection.[1] Such considerations provide the rationale for the measurement of regional or "split" lung function. Preoperative evaluation prior to lung resection using standard spirometry and other readily available tests has been thoroughly reviewed.[67,76,77]

Early work suggested that an MVV of less than 50% to 55% of the predicted value correlates with a perioperative mortality rate of up to 50%.[76,78] Van Nostrand and co-workers compared spirometry, a simple one-flight exercise tolerance test, and measurement of pulmonary artery pressures and found that pressure values, MVV, FVC, FEV_1, and $FEF_{25-75\%}$ did not predict postoperative death better than the exercise test.[79] Reichel performed a more rigorous exercise test and found a greater than 50% incidence of serious cardiorespiratory complications in those patients who were unable to complete the test.[80] Karliner and associates found that FVC and $FEF_{25-75\%}$ did not accurately predict complications.[81] They point out that impaired lung function as determined by spirometry alone should not rule out lung resection, because it does not consistently identify patients at risk.

Why do some patients with diffuse lung disease tolerate resective surgery, whereas others do not? The answer probably resides in regional pulmonary function. The less a diseased lobe contributes to total pulmonary function preoperatively, the less it will be missed after resection. Such reasoning set the stage for measurement of individual lung function and its use as a predictor of resectability. Abnormalities on bronchospirometry, an invasive test that involves intubation of each mainstem bronchus, correlate poorly with loss of VC after resection.[82]

Radionuclide ventilation or perfusion lung scanning has provided a noninvasive and accurate index of individual lung function.[83-85] A split-crystal perfusion lung scan gives the percentage of total perfusion seen in each lung; the percentage attributable to nondiseased lung can be multiplied by preoperative pulmonary function parameters for estimation of postoperative values. Olsen and Block used split-function testing to determine whether operation would be tolerated in patients with impaired pulmonary function as determined by spirometry.[77,85] The test was performed in candidates for lung resection with an FVC of less than 50% of predicted values, an FEV_1 of less than 2 liters, an FEV_1:FVC ratio of less than 50%, an MVV of less than 50% of predicted values, an RV:total lung capacity (TLC) ratio of greater than 50%, a diffusing capacity for carbon monoxide (D_LCO) of less than 50%, or a P_{CO_2} of greater than 45 torr. Split-perfusion and ventilation scans

were carried out, and pulmonary artery pressure was measured during exercise after balloon occlusion of the main pulmonary artery of the diseased lung. Patients were rejected for surgery if the predicted postoperative FEV_1 was less than 0.8 liters and the pulmonary artery pressure after balloon occlusion was equal to or greater than 35 torr during exercise with a fall in PaO_2 to 45 torr or less.

Of 53 patients who were denied operation on the basis of spirometry alone, 28 passed one or more of the split-function criteria and underwent resection, and, of these, 6, or 21%, died. This mortality rate is comparable to that reported in series of patients thought to have acceptable lung function by routine testing. Boysen and colleagues used a similar procedure in a high-risk group of patients with an FEV_1 of less than 2 liters and excluded from surgery patients who had an estimated postpneumonectomy FEV_1 of less than 800 ml.[84] Of 33 patients undergoing surgery, 5, or 15%, died. Another noninvasive test of regional lung function, the lateral position test, does not correlate with bronchospirometric parameters as well as radionuclide lung scanning.[83]

In summary, preoperative spirometric abnormalities correlate with morbidity and mortality rates after lung resection, and the MVV and FEV_1 are the most useful predictive parameters. In patients with marginal pulmonary function, radionuclide scanning can provide an estimate of the contribution to pulmonary function of the involved lung and can be used to define a subgroup of patients with moderate or severe diffuse lung disease who can safely undergo resection. More limited procedures, such as wedge resection, can be used for palliation in selected patients thought unable to tolerate more extensive resection.[86,87]

PREOPERATIVE PULMONARY PREPARATION

On the basis of clinical evaluation and type of surgery planned, patients can be categorized according to pulmonary risk for the purpose of prognostic stratification and diagnostic evaluation. Table 23-1 summarizes one such proposed classification. If preliminary evaluation calls for further diagnostic tests, estimation of risk can be modified (see Fig. 23-3). For example, a patient thought to have a high or severe operative risk because of advanced age and obesity may be reclassified as having only moderate risk if he has a normal chest radiograph, ECG, and spirometry.

If a patient has an increased risk of postoperative pulmonary complications, what can be done preoperatively to minimize this risk? The literature in this area provides some useful information for the establishment of general guidelines, though several important questions remain unanswered. Stein and Cassara evaluated the effects of preoperative pulmonary preparation on one of two groups of patients considered to be poor risks from a pulmonary standpoint.[88] Intensive preoperative chest therapy was uniformly carried out for 23 patients, and 25 other patients matched for severity of preoperative pulmonary dysfunction were treated in the usual manner. Preoperative chest therapy consisted of cessation of smoking, antibiotics, when indicated, bronchodilator drugs, inhalation therapy, segmental postural drainage, and chest physiotherapy 1 to 3 times daily. Surgery was delayed when deemed appropriate by the team of investigators. The treated subjects had a significant reduction in postoperative morbidity and mortality due to pulmonary complications. The incidence of complications in the treated group was

Table 23-1.   Clinical Categories of Preoperative Pulmonary Risk

Risk Class	Level of Risk	Patients Included, after Clinical Evaluation
A	Negligible to very low	Age <30 with no significant clinical risk factors*
B	Mild to moderate	Age <30 with significant clinical risk factors Age >40 with no significant clinical risk factors Upper abdominal surgery with no other significant clinical risk factors
C	Severe	Thoracic surgery Upper abdominal surgery with significant clinical risk factors Age >70 with significant clinical risk factors

*Significant clinical risk factors derived from the bedside examination include productive cough, dyspnea, obesity, positive loose cough test, and abnormal cardiopulmonary physical findings.

close to that in a group of risk-free patients chosen from a prior study, although the severity of complications in the treated poor-risk group was somewhat higher. Comparable results were reported by Tarhan and co-workers in a retrospective study of patients with chronic lung disease.

The benefit of specific interventions, such as cessation of smoking or the administration of antibiotics in particular groups of patients, is unknown. The intensive regimen outlined above may benefit poor-risk patients, but questions regarding deferral of surgery or the benefits of intensive chest physiotherapy in less severely disabled patients have not been addressed. As discussed earlier, abstinence from smoking for 1 week does not appear to reverse the physiologic changes caused by cigarettes. Studies in the surgical literature lend clinical support to this viewpoint, suggesting that abstinence of 2 to 4 weeks may be necessary for differences in postoperative pulmonary outcomes to be discernible.

The data are much less clear regarding routine preoperative antibiotics in bronchitic patients. These patients may be exposed to exogenous reservoirs of gram-negative bacilli from anesthesia equipment and IPPB machines and may harbor these organisms as part of their usual respiratory tract flora.[89] Although prophylactic broad-spectrum antibiotics may eradicate these organisms, their widespread use may also promote colonization and potential infection with more resistant bacteria. Of the few studies addressing this problem, that of Lazlo and his coworkers is most often cited as argument against the routine prophylactic use of antibiotics.[13] In Lazlo's investigation, 52 bronchitic patients were randomly assigned to treated or untreated groups. Those in the former group received 500 mg of parenteral ampicillin 1 to 2 hr before surgery and at 8-hr intervals after surgery for 5 days. Although no increases in postoperative infection with resistant organisms were noted in the treated group, the complication rates in the two groups were virtually identical.

Patients with obstructive pulmonary disease appear to benefit from combined preoperative chest therapy, including inhalation of aerosolized bronchodilators, chest physiotherapy, oral theophylline, and increased fluid intake.[90] The specific benefits of each aspect of this program have been debated, and deletion of certain components may be indicated in any given patient. Useful preoperative therapeutic measures in patients with different

Table 23-2. Preoperative Pulmonary Preparation

Risk Factor	Optimal Therapy
Cigarette smoking	Abstinence for 2 to 4 weeks preoperatively
Bronchitis	Abstinence from smoking, hydration, chest physiotherapy; antibiotics given immediately preoperatively are of no proven benefit
Obesity	Weight reduction to less than 10% above ideal weight
Chronic obstructive pulmonary disease	Intensive chest physiotherapy, inhalation therapy, systemic bronchodilators as indicated, increased fluid intake, abstinence from smoking
Heart failure	Therapy to optimize cardiovascular status

types of pulmonary risk are summarized in Table 23-2.

Patients undergoing surgical procedures other than lung resection have a spectrum of pulmonary risk, and preoperative evaluation and therapy should be individualized. Three categories of risk can be defined clinically, and estimation of risk can be modified by the results of further diagnostic laboratory tests, including radiographs, ECGs, PFTs, and arterial blood gases (see Table 23-1). Figure 23-3 outlines a rational diagnostic and therapeutic approach to these patients.

Young patients without significant historical risk factors or abnormalities on physical examination do not need further preoperative testing unless they are undergoing thoracic or upper abdominal operations. A patient with mild or moderate risk, in class B of Table 23-1, should have a chest x-ray and possibly an ECG,

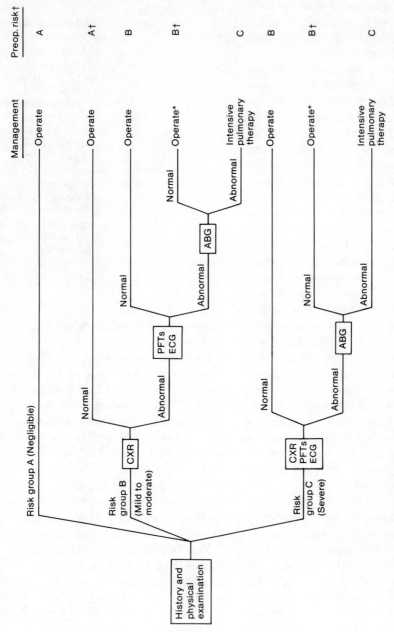

Fig. 23-3. Management algorithm for preoperative pulmonary evaluation and therapy . . . in nonresective procedures. See text for discussion. CXR = chest x-ray; PFTs = pulmonary function tests; ECG = electrocardiogram; ABG = arterial blood gas.

*Some form of pulmonary therapy may be required preoperatively in these patients.
†Preoperative risk after complete evaluation. Patients with (†) after risk group are at a somewhat higher risk.

PFTs, and arterial blood gas analysis to guide preoperative therapy. A more extensive battery of preoperative tests is routinely indicated for patients with severe preoperative clinical risk, in class C of Table 23-1. Depending on the test results, the decision may be made to procede with surgery, to postpone surgery for a period of intensive pulmonary therapy, to choose an alternative route of anesthesia, or to cancel surgery altogether. The decision to procede with surgery in high-risk patients should be accompanied by special vigilance in the postoperative state. Specific postoperative management strategies designed to prevent and treat pulmonary complications are discussed in Chapter 24.

SUMMARY

1. **The bedside history and physical examination are the single most important elements of the preoperative pulmonary evaluation. The history should include questions about exercise tolerance, recent productive cough, the use of cardiac and pulmonary medications, and smoking. Age over 70 probably increases risk. Assessment of nutritional status for gross deviation in relative weight, the presence of a positive loose cough test, and signs of congestive heart failure or pulmonary hypertension should be sought on physical examination. These abnormal findings should guide further diagnostic evaluation and therapeutic interventions designed to reduce risk.**

2. **Chest x-rays should be performed in patients undergoing thoracic surgery, in patients over 40 years of age, and in patients of any age with significant risk factors identified by history and physical examination. If no acute clinical changes have occurred during the immediate preoperative period, chest x-rays performed within 1 month prior to operation should prove adequate for risk stratification. Patients under 40 should have a single posteroanterior x-ray, unless there are significant clinical risk factors.**

3. **Preoperative PFTs should always be obtained for patients considered on the basis of prior clinical evaluation to have a significant risk of postoperative pulmonary complications. Included are patients undergoing thoracic or upper abdominal surgical procedures, patients over age 70 with abnormal cardiopulmonary histories or physical findings suggestive of cardiopulmonary disease, and patients who have chest x-rays showing congestive heart failure, chronic obstructive pulmonary disease, or other significant lung disease. MVV maneuvers should be performed along with forced-expiration tests. Cutoff values for PFTs indicating increased risk have not been definitely established for patients not undergoing lung resection. However, it is likely that an FEV_1 of less than 75% of predicted values, an MVV of less than 50% of predicted values, or values falling below the marginal reserve line in Redding's modification of Miller's quadrant diagram (see Fig. 23-2) all signify an increased likelihood of postoperative pulmonary complications.**

4. **Arterial blood gas determinations should be obtained for all patients undergoing lung resection or when clinical evaluation and the results of PFTs support the diagnosis of significant obstructive pulmonary disease. Arterial hypercapnia ($P_{CO_2} \geq 45$ torr)**

defines a high-risk subgroup in which a high rate of pulmonary complications can be expected and in which extended postoperative respiratory assistance may be anticipated. Intensive preoperative pulmonary therapy should be performed in these patients.

5. All patients who are candidates for lobectomy or pneumonectomy should have preoperative spirometry and arterial blood gas determinations. No further evaluation is necessary for these patients if the MVV is greater than 50% of the predicted value and the FEV_1 is greater than 2 liters. Cessation of smoking for at least 2 weeks and preoperative optimization of pulmonary status should be carried out.

6. Patients with marginal or unacceptable spirometric criteria should have a split-crystal perfusion lung scan with estimation of the fractional contribution to ventilation of the diseased lung. This should be done even if there is only a small lesion apparently confined to one lobe, because unexpected conditions may be found at surgery that mandate more extensive surgical procedures. Lung resection is probably safe if the estimated postpneumonectomy FEV_1 is greater than 800 ml; however, an operative mortality rate of 15% to 20% should be anticipated in this high-risk subgroup.

REFERENCES

1. Tisi GM: Preoperative evaluation of pulmonary function: Validity, indications and benefits. Am Rev Respir Dis 119:293, 1979

2. Drummond GB, Gordon NH: Forced expiratory flow-volume relationships. Anaesthesia 32:464, 1977

3. Stein M, Koota GM, Simon M et al: Pulmonary evaluation of surgical patients. JAMA 181:103, 1962

4. Zikria BA, Spencer JL, Kinney JM et al: Alterations in ventilatory function and breathing patterns following surgical trauma. Ann Surg 179:107, 1974

5. Morton A, Baker AB: Clinical review: Postoperative respiratory dysfunction. Anaesth Intensive Care 6:56, 1978

6. Morton A, Hansen P, Baker AB: Postoperative pulmonary compliance. Anaesth Intensive Care 5:149, 1977

7. Partrey PS, Harte PJ, Quinlan JP et al: Pulmonary function in the early postoperative period. Br J Surg 64:384, 1977

8. Morton A, Mahoney P, Hansen P et al: Postoperative respiratory function: A bentilation-perfusion study. Anaesth Intensive Care 4:203, 1976

9. Harman H, Lillington G: Pulmonary risk factors in surgery. Med Clin North Am 63:1289, 1979

10. Latimer RG, Dickmen M, Day WC et al: Ventilatory patterns and pulmonary complications after upper abdominal surgery determined by preoperative and postoperative computerized spirometry and blood gas analysis. Am J Surg 122:622, 1971

11. Pierce AK, Robertson J: Pulmonary complications of general surgery. Annu Rev Med 28:211, 1977

12. Wightman JAK: A prospective survey of the incidence of postoperative pulmonary complications. Br J Surg 55:85, 1968

13. Lazlo G, Archer GG, Darrell JH et al: The diagnosis and prophylaxis of pulmonary complications of surgical operation. Br J Surg 60:129, 1973

14. Presley AP, Alexander-Williams J: Postoperative chest infection. Br J Surg 61:448, 1974

15. Dripps RD, Deming MV: Postoperative atelectasis and pneumonia. Ann Surg 124:94, 1946

16. Tarhan S, Moffitt EA, Sessler AD et al: Risk of anesthesia and surgery in patients with chronic bronchitis and chronic obstructive pulmonary disease. Surgery 74:720, 1973

17. Babbage ED, McLaughlin CW: Spinal anesthesia: Safety factors and postoperative pulmonary complications in 1,334 consecutive general surgical procedures on naval recruits. Surgery 15:476, 1944

18. Newhouse M, Sanchis J, Bieninstock J: Lung defense mechanisms. N Engl J Med 295:990, 1976

19. Wells WF: Airborne Contagion and Air Hygiene. Cambridge, MA, Harvard University Press, 1955

20. McCarthy DS, Spencer R, Greene R et al: Measurement of "closing volume" as a simple and sensitive test for each detection of small airways disease. Am J Med 52:747, 1972

21. White JR, Froeb HF: Small-airways dysfunction in nonsmokers chronically exposed to tobacco smoke. N Engl J Med 302:720, 1980

22. Ashley F, Kannel WB, Sorlie PD et al: Pulmonary function: Relation to aging, cigarette habit, and mortality. Ann Intern Med 82:739, 1975

23. Camner P, Philipson K: Some studies of tracheobronchial clearance in man. Chest 63:235, 1973

24. McFadden ER, Linden DA: A reduction in maximum midexpiratory flow rate: A spirographic manifestation of small airway disease. Am J Med 52:725, 1972

25. Chodoff P, Margand PMS, Knowles CL: Short term abstinence from smoking: Its place in preoperative preparation Crit Care Med 3:131, 1975

26. Meneely GR, Ferguson JL: Pulmonary evaluation and risk in patient preparation for anesthesia and surgery. JAMA 175:1074, 1961

27. Munro DD: Practical guide to prophylaxis and treatment of lung complications. Recent Adv Surg 68:727, 1970

28. Wiklander O, Norlin U: Effect of physiotherapy on postoperative pulmonary complications. Acta Chir Scand 112:246, 1957

29. Palmer KNV, Gardiner AJS: Effect of partial gastrectomy on pulmonary physiology. Br Med J 1:347, 1964

30. Wheatley IC, Hardy KJ, Barter CE: An evaluation of preoperative methods of preventing postoperative pulmonary complications. Anaesth Intens Care 5:56, 1977

31. Muldoon SM, Rehder K, Didier EP et al: Respiratory care of patients undergoing intrathoracic operations. Surg Clin North Am 53:843, 1973

32. Morris JF, Koski A, Johnson LC: Spirometric standards for healthy nonsmoking adults. Am Rev Respir Dis 103:57, 1971

33. Kuperman AS, Riker JB: The predicted normal maximal midexpiratory flow. Am Rev Respir Dis 107:231, 1973

34. Knudson RJ, Slatin RC, Libowitz MD et al: The maximal expiratory flow-volume curve: Normal standards, variability and effects of age. Am Rev Respir Dis 113:587, 1976

35. Ashley F, Kannel WB, Sorlie PD et al: Pulmonary function: Relation to aging, cigarette habit and mortality. The Framingham Study. Ann Intern Med 82:739, 1975

36. Pierce JA, Ebert RV: The elastic properties of the lungs in the aged. J Lab Clin Med 51:63, 1958

37. Sorbini CA, Grassi V, Solenas E et al: Arterial oxygen tension in relation to age in healthy subjects. Respiration 25:3, 1968

38. Ziffren SE, Hartford CE: Comparative mortality for various surgical operations in older versus younger age groups. J Am Geriatr Soc 20:485, 1972

39. Peters RM: Work of breathing and abnormal mechanics. Surg Clin North Am 54:955, 1974

40. Bray GA: The Obese Patient. Major Problems in Internal Medicine, Vol IX, p 2. Philadelphia, WB Saunders, 1976

41. Pemberton LB, Manax WG: Relationship of obesity to postoperative complications after cholecystectomy. Am J Surg 121:87, 1971

42. Hugh–Jones P, Whimster W: The etiology and management of disabling emphysema. Am Rev Respir Dis 117:343, 1978

43. Gandevia B: A productive cough upon request as an index of chronic bronchitis: The effects of age, sex, smoking habit and environment upon prevalence in Australian general practice. Med J Aust 1:16, 1969

44. Cebul RD, Williams SV, Kussmaul WG et al: Predicting postoperative pulmonary complications after elective thoracic surgery. Presented at the Second Annual Meeting of the Society for Medical Decision-Making, Washington, DC, September, 1980

45. Hall GJL, Gandevia B: Relationship of the loose sign to daily sputum volume: Observer variation in its detection. Br J Prev Soc Med 25:109, 1971

46. Murphy DMF, Fogarty CM, Heyer RA et al: The "loose cough" test—Its relationship to lung function. Am Rev Respir Dis. 119(4):155, 1979

47. Cebul RD, Kussmaul WG: Unpublished observations

48. Royal College of Radiologists: National Study. Preoperative chest radiology. Lancet 2:83, 1979

49. Loder RE: Routine preoperative chest radiography. 1977 compared with 1955 at Peterborough District General Hospital. Anaesthesia 33:972, 1978

50. Rees AM, Roberts CJ, Bligh AS et al: Routine preoperative chest radiography in noncardiopulmonary surgery. Br Med J 1:1333, 1976

51. Sagel SS, Evens RG, Forrest JV et al: Efficacy of routine screening and lateral chest radiographs in a hospital-based population. N Engl J Med 291:1001, 1974

52. Feingold AO: Routine chest roentgenograms on hospital admission do not discover tuberculosis. South Med J 70:579, 1977

53. Kubik A: Screening for lung cancer—High risk groups. Br Med J 2(7):666, 1970

54. Miller AB: Screening for lung cancer. Can J Public Health (Suppl) 64(2):532, 1973

55. Weiss W, Seidman H, Boucot KR: The Philadelphia Pulmonary Neoplasm Research Project. Am Rev Respir Dis 111(3):289, 1975

56. Pochin EE: Radiology now: Malignancies following low radiation exposures in man. Br J Radiol 49:577, 1976

57. Rigler LG: Is this radiograph really necessary? Radiology 129:449, 1976

58. Fraser RG, Paré JAP: Diagnosis of Disease of the Chest. WB Saunders, Philadelphia, 1970

59. Vix VA, Klatte EC: The lateral chest radiograph in the diagnosis of hilar and mediastinal masses. Radiology 96:307, 1970

60. Antoku S, Russell WJ: Dose to the active bone marrow, gonads and skin from roentgenography and fluoroscopy. Radiology 101:669, 1971

61. Auchincloss JH: Preoperative evaluation of pulmonary function. Surg Clin North Am 54:1015, 1974

62. Miller WF, Wu N, Johnson RL: Convenient method of evaluating pulmonary ventilatory function with a single breath test. Anesthesiology 17:480, 1956

63. Williams CD, Brenowitz JB: "Prohibitive" lung function and major surgical procedures. Am J Surg 132:763, 1976

64. Redding JS, Yakaitis RW: Predicting the need for ventilatory assistance. Md State Med J 19:53, 1970

65. Hodgkin JE: Preoperative evaluation of pulmonary function. Am J Surg 138:355, 1979

66. Boushy SF, Belleq DM, North LB et al: Clinical course related to preoperative and postoperative pulmonary function in patients with bronchogenic carcinoma. Chest 59:383, 1971

67. Hodgkin JE, Dines DE, Didier EP: Preoperative evaluation of the patient with pulmonary disease. Mayo Clin Proc 48:114, 1973

68. Appleberg M, Gordon L, Fatti LP: Preoperative pulmonary evaluation of surgical patients using the vitalograph. Br J Surg 61:57, 1974

69. Ferris BG: Epidemiology standardization project. Am Rev Respir Dis 118:72, 1978

70. Mittman C: Assessment of operative risk in thoracic surgery. Am Rev Respir Dis 84:197, 1961

71. Gaensler EA, Cugell DW, Lindgren I et al: The role of pulmonary insufficiency in mortality and invalidism following surgery for pulmonary tuberculosis. J Thorac Cardiovasc Surg 29:163, 1955

72. Didolkar MS, Moore RH, Takita H: Evaluation of the risk in pulmonary resection for bronchogenic carcinoma. Am J Surg 127:700, 1974

73. Block AJ, Olsen GN: Preoperative pulmonary function testing. JAMA 235:257, 1976

74. Kilcoyen MM, Davis AL, Ferrar MI: A dynamic electrocardiographic concept useful in the diagnosis of cor pulmonale. Circulation 42:903, 1970

75. Ferrer MI: Clinical and electrocardiographic correlations in pulmonary heart disease. In Rios JC (ed): Clinical Electrocardiographic Correlations, p 215. Philadelphia, F.A. Davis, 1977

76. Hodgkin JE: Evaluation before thoracotomy. West J Med 122:104, 1975

77. Olsen GN, Block AJ: Pulmonary function testing in evaluation for pneumonectomy. Hospital Practice 8:137, 1973

78. Mittman C: Assessment of operative risk in thoracic surgery. Am Rev Respir Dis 84:197, 1961

79. Van Nostrand D, Kjelsberg MO, Humphrey EW: Preresectional evaluation of risk from pneumonectomy. Surg Gynecol Obstet 127:306, 1968

80. Reichel J: Assessment of operative risk of pneumonectomy. Chest 62:570, 1972

81. Karliner JS, Coomaraswamy R, Williams MH: Relationship between preoperative pulmonary function studies and prognosis of patients undergoing pneumonectomy for carcinoma of the lung. Chest 54:32, 1968

82. Snider GL: A critical evaluation of bronchospirometric measurement in predicting loss of ventilatory function due to thoracic surgery. J Lab Clin Med 64:321, 1964

83. DeMeester TR, Van Heertum RL, Karas JR et al: Preoperative evaluation with differential pulmonary function. Ann Thorac Surg 18:61, 1974

84. Boysen PG, Block AJ, Olsen GN et al: Prospective evaluation for pneumonectomy using the 99mtechnetium quantitative perfusion lung scan. Chest 72:422, 1977

85. Olsen GN, Block AJ, Swenson EW et al: Pulmonary function evaluation of the lung resection candidate: A prospective study. Am Rev Respir Dis 111:379, 1975

86. Peters RM, Clausen JL, Tisi GM: Extending resectability for carcinoma of the lung in patients with impaired pulmonary function. Ann Thorac Surg 26:250, 1978

87. Bennett WF, Smith RA: Segmental resection for bronchogenic carcinoma: A surgical alternative for the compromised patient. Ann Thorac Surg 27:169, 1978

88. Stein M, Cassara EL: Preoperative pulmonary evaluation and therapy for surgery patients. JAMA 211:787, 1970

89. Glover JL, Jolly L: Gram-negative colonization of the respiratory tract in postoperative patients. Am J Med Sci 261:24, 1971

90. Gracey DR, Divertie MB, Didier EP: Preoperative pulmonary preparation of patients with chronic obstructive pulmonary disease. Chest 76:123, 1979

Postoperative Pulmonary Problems in Surgical Patients

GREGORY R. OWENS

Pulmonary complications constitute the leading cause of surgical complication and death. This chapter focuses on the most common postoperative pulmonary problem, atelectasis, and one of the most lethal problems, aspiration of gastric or oropharyngeal contents leading to pneumonia. Aspiration is the major cause of death associated with anesthesia.[1] Three groups of patients have higher than normal risk of developing aspiration and its complications: (1) those with an altered level of consciousness; (2) those with motor disorders of the esophagus or hypopharynx; and (3) those with mechanical disruption of glottic closure (e.g., tracheostomies) or gastroesophageal sphincter function (e.g., nasogastric tubes).[2] It is thus clear that surgical patients are at risk for the development of the clinical sequelae of aspiration in the perioperative period.

It is extremely important to recognize that aspiration pneumonia and aspiration pneumonitis are different syndromes. The etiology, pathophysiology, clinical course, and treatment of each are different and require accurate differentiation by the cli-nician. Aspiration pneumonitis results from aspiration of normally sterile gastric contents, which causes a chemical burn of the tracheobronchial tree and pulmonary parenchyma not usually complicated by bacterial infection. Aspiration pneumonia results from aspiration of mouth contents at physiologic pH, which may lead to bacterial pneumonia.

ASPIRATION PNEUMONITIS

Since the time of Mendelson's description of pulmonary complications following aspiration of gastric contents, the pH of the aspirated material has been viewed as the most important determinant of the extent of damage to the lung.[3] Numerous experimental studies have shown that the extent of lung damage correlates with the volume and pH of the aspirate. Traditionally, it has been felt that a pH of less than 2.5 results in lung damage and that destruction increases with decreasing pH and reaches its maximum at a pH of 1.5.[4,5] Moreover, aspiration of small particles of food creates an inflammatory response comparable to that of acid.[4] Even saline aspiration is associated with transient physiologic changes in the lungs.[6] However, a more recent report casts doubt on the importance of pH as the most important factor in lung destruction and suggests that food particles may constitute the major cause of pulmonary complications in aspiration.[7]

The pathology of gastric aspiration can be divided into two stages based on a typical and repeatable sequence of changes in the lung. The early changes include peribronchial neutrophil accumulation, separation of basement membrane from epithelial cells, the presence of erythrocytes in the alveoli, and pulmonary edema. These changes are seen with aspiration of many fluids, including buffered gastric juice, hypertonic saline, and acid. The aspiration of nonacidic fluids is usually of little or no clinical importance.[3] However, acidic fluids cause progressive damage, with necrosis of type I alveolar cells, alveolar hemorrhage, bronchial mucosal sloughing, and formation of hyaline membranes.[8]

The diagnosis of aspiration pneumonitis is usually clear. Aspiration follows an episode of vomiting or regurgitation, resulting in the abrupt onset of dyspnea and bronchospasm within 1 to 4 hr thereafter. Patients are often hypotensive and may produce thin, frothy sputum that may be mistaken for the fluid seen in pulmonary edema.[9] Except for significant hypoxemia usually associated with hypocapnia, laboratory data are nonspecific.[10] A chest radiograph may be helpful, since aspiration of mouth or gastric contents tends to involve specific lobes of the lung, as determined by gravity and the patient's position. The right lower lobe, particularly the superior segment, the left lower lobe, and the posterior segment of the right upper lobe are commonly affected, but any area of the lung may be involved. The infiltrates are fluffy, mottled, and alveolar in pattern. If the aspiration is massive, the adult respiratory distress syndrome may develop with characteristic, diffuse, bilateral alveolar infiltrates.[11] The morbidity and mortality of aspiration pneumonitis cannot be underestimated. Recent experience appears to differ from that described in Mendelson's classic monograph on the subject. There were no deaths in his series, and all patients recovered within 36 hr. Recent studies, however, have shown mortality rates of 35% to 60%, with rates as high as 100% when the gastric pH was less than 1.75.[5] Although the reason for this difference is not clear, the data suggest that aspiration pneumonitis is a lethal disease with a substantial mortality rate.

Prevention

Measures aimed at preventing aspiration require the diligence and attention of all medical personnel.[12] The agitated, confused, or comatose patient should not be transported or allowed to lie in the prone position; rather, he should be placed in the lateral decubitis position with his head down. The use of nasogatric tubes should be minimized. If such a tube is needed in an unconscious patient, the airway must be protected with an endotracheal tube. Anesthesia personnel must be aware of the danger of vomiting and regurgitation in the early stages of anesthesia and be prepared to safeguard the airway if vomiting occurs. Regional anesthesia may reduce the risk of aspiration.

Another specific preventive measure is the use of antacids. These have been shown to raise the pH of gastric juice in preoperative patients to greater than 2.5

and should decrease the incidence of aspiration pneumonitis.[13,14] Unfortunately, however, no clinical data are available to confirm this supposition. The use of cimetidine to reduce gastric acid production preoperatively has not been evaluated.

Treatment

The damage to pulmonary parenchyma and airways occurs instantly. Thus, there is no rationale for therapeutic interventions designed to evacuate or neutralize the acid.[15] Endotracheal suctioning immediately following an observed aspiration is indicated, since it may remove enough aspirate to clear the upper airway and stimulate cough. Bronchoscopy, either fiberoptic or rigid, is indicated if there is evidence of particulate aspiration suggested by food particles in the suctioned material or if segmental or lobar atelectasis or obstructive emphysema is present on a chest radiograph.[16] There is no clinical or experimental basis for attempted neutralization of acid with bronchial lavage. Experimental evidence suggests that the extent of damage may be increased by this intervention.[17]

Aspiration pneumonitis represents a chemical burn of the tracheobronchial tree and pulmonary parenchyma, and it would therefore seem obvious that immediate use of antibiotics is not indicated. However, there is no consensus on this point in the literature, and numerous authors have strongly advocated the use of antibiotics.[9,10,18] Essentially, all recent well-controlled clinical trials suggest that prophylactic antibiotics are of no value. Their use may in fact select for more virulent organisms and expose the patient to the risk of drug toxicity.[19–21] The most logical approach is to withold antibiotics until clear evidence of bacterial infection is present.

The debate surrounding the use of corticosteroids in gastric aspiration has generated volumes of data but few definitive results. Early studies, usually small and poorly controlled, attempted to claim that pulmonary pathology was decreased and survival improved with corticosteroids.[22–24] However, more recent data from a variety of sources suggest that steroids are of no benefit.[11,25–26] A recent report not only failed to demonstrate improvement with steroids in any of the parameters studied but also showed that patients treated with corticosteroids had a significantly increased incidence of gram-negative pneumonias.[27] This finding is not surprising in view of data showing adverse effects of corticosteroids on leukocyte function and increased susceptibility to infection in steroid-treated animals, including infection with gram-negative bacilli.[28]

Administration of corticosteroids may be justified when an episode of aspiration has been witnessed.[29] If steroids are given immediately after the aspiration, they may reduce the extent of pulmonary damage. Steroids should not be continued for more than 48 hr.

Ventilatory support is the keystone of therapy in aspiration pneumonitis and may determine the ultimate outcome of the disease. Since hypoxemia with hypocapnia usually occurs initially, efforts to improve arterial oxygenation are crucial. Supplementary oxygen given by face mask may suffice in the patient with minimal aspiration. However, positive-pressure ventilation may be required to overcome intrapulmonary shunting and avoid toxic concentrations of inspired oxygen.[30]

Positive-pressure ventilation not only may be a supportive modality that allows the lung time to heal but also may be therapeutic. One group of investigators demonstrated in an experimental model that positive-pressure ventilation prevented the development of pulmonary arterial vasospasm and thrombus formation, which uniformly developed and proved irreversible in control animals.[31] Other studies have confirmed that early positive-pressure ventilation in the treatment of aspiration pneumonitis increases the survival rate.[32,33]

Uncertainties remain about the role of positive end-expiratory pressure (PEEP) in aspiration pneumonitis. There is no doubt that the use of PEEP elevated functional residual capacity and improved ventilation–perfusion matching, allowing better oxygenation in patients with severe hypoxemia. PEEP may also obviate the use of toxic concentrations of inspired oxygen and support the patient while the damaged lung improves. It is not clear, however, that PEEP by itself is therapeutic.

PEEP is associated with complications in as many as 25% of patients.[34] Depression of cardiac output and systemic hypotension are common and reversible problems. They occur at the initiation of PEEP or after an increase in its level and may be the result of decreased venous return to the right side of the heart secondary to constant positive intrathoracic pressure. Patients who develop hypotension on PEEP are usually hypovolemic and respond to increased intravascular volume.[35]

A more serious problem is the development of barotrauma, that is, subcutaneous or mediastinal emphysema or pneumothorax. Although studies have failed to identify patients who are more susceptible than normal to these complications or a level of PEEP above which barotrauma is likely to occur, one study showed that barotrauma is more frequent than normal in patients with aspiration pneumonitis.[36] It was suggested that lung tissue damaged by acid or other necrotizing processes is more susceptible to barotrauma because of decreased supporting structure. Three clinical findings suggest its occurrence: (1) the development of subcutaneous crepitance; (2) the abrupt onset of systemic hypotension; and (3) a precipitous rise in the ventilator pressure required to inflate the lungs. Some groups have advocted the use of prophylactic chest tubes when high levels of PEEP are used, but, in general, this strategy is unnecessary.

Other modalities for delivering positive pressure have been evaluated, two of which deserve special mention. Providing constant positive airway pressure (CPAP) with a tightly fitting face mask, a technique previously used only in infants, causes less depression of cardiac output than PEEP and does not require intubation.[37] In addition, systems have been devised to provide for physiologic negative-pressure inspiration supplemented by positive-pressure ventilation with PEEP.[38] This system of intermittent mandatory ventilation (IMV) with PEEP is effective in the management of patients with a variety of pulmonary disorders, including aspiration pneumonitis.

ASPIRATION PNEUMONIA

Aspiration of contents of the oropharynx is common even in normal persons. It rarely causes clinical sequelae because of its small volume and the intact defense mechanisms of the tracheobronchial tree including the cough reflex, mucociliary transport, and leukocytes and alveolar macrophages. The term "aspiration pneumonia" is usually applied to the development of pneumonia in a patient who has compromised upper airway defenses caused by organisms that inhabit the oropharynx. The clinical syndrome may occur as a primary event or as a complication of the aspiration of gastric contents. Hospitalized patients who develop aspiration pneumonia differ in many respects from patients who develop the disorder outside of the hospital.

The inoculation of oropharyngeal contents into the lung with subsequent development of pneumonia is a common problem. Underlying predisposing factors include alcoholism, seizure disorders, stroke, drug addiction, anesthesia, nasogastric suction, and head trauma. Unlike the sudden onset and fulminant course of aspiration pneumonitis, the clinical course of aspiration pneumonia is usually more slowly paced and occasionally indolent.[39] The episode of aspiration is rarely observed, and the diagnosis may be initially suspected when a predisposed patient develops a pneumonia in a dependent segment of the lung. Signs may include only fever and production of purulent sputum without a predominant organism on Gram staim. Four-smelling sputum is usually absent.[40] As the disease progresses, tissue necrosis may develop in 8 to 14 days. A characteristic lung abscess or necrotizing pneumonia may occur, and, at this time, sputum may become copious and foul-smelling.[41]

Although aspiration pneumonia has been recognized since the 1930s, its pathophysiology has been delineated only in the last ten years. It is now clear that the disorder is caused by aspiration of oropharyngeal contents. The predominant bacteria are anaerobic and belong to several different genera. They number about 10^8 bacteria per milliliter of saliva in nor-

mal persons and can be as many as 10^{11} in persons with poor oral hygiene.[42] Peptostreptococci, Bacteroides melaninogenicus, and Fusobacterium nucleatum account for the majority of isolates, but, in critically ill patients, other organisms may predominate.

The bacteriology of aspiration pneumonia confirms the importance of the mixed oropharyngeal flora. The majority of patients with aspiration pneumonia have mixed infections with three or four organisms. Anaerobes predominate, and the above-mentioned species constitute the major isolates. Aerobic organisms alone are isolated in only 6% of patients but are present as part of a mixed flora in 30%. Those aerobes are usually streptococcal species and Streptococcus pneumonia.

The bacteriology of the oral flora in hospitalized patients is more complex. Several studies have shown that, within 96 hr, the oropharynx becomes colonized by pathogenic aerobic bacteria, including Staphylococcus aureus, Pseudomonas aeruginosa, the Proteus species, and Escherichia coli.[43,44] The change in the normal flora of the oropharynx is associated with the use of antibiotics, a prolonged hospital stay, and the gravity of the underlying illness. About 90% of critically ill patients in intensive care units are colonized with pathogenic aerobic organisms, usually gram-negative rods.[45]

The bacteriology of aspiration pneumonia in hospitalized patients correlates with that of the oropharyngeal contents. Anaerobic organisms are recovered less frequently in nosocomial aspiration pneumonia than in aspiration pneumonias acquired outside of the hospital, and the incidence of pneumonia due to pathogenic aerobic organisms is considerably higher. Anaerobes are isolated in only 30% of patients with hospital-acquired pneumonia and are the sole pathogens in only 10%.[46] Aerobes found most frequently include those mentioned above which colonize the oropharynx. Pneumonias in hospitalized patients are usually not associated with the production of putrid sputum.

Treatment

The implications of these differences in bacteriology on therapy are significant. With the exception of B. fragilis, which is found in 15% to 20% of all aspiration pneumonias, all anaerobic organisms are sensitive to penicillin, the drug of choice for community-acquired infections. The optimal dosage of penicillin is debated, but a reasonable regimen consists of aqueous penicillin, 2 to 5 million units/day in 4 divided doses. For the patient who is allergic to penicillin or who does not respond to penicillin, clindamycin, 300 mg orally or intravenously 4 times a day, is the best alternative. Although B. fragilis is resistant to penicillin by standard in vitro testing, this antibiotic is effective in treating the pneumonia and remains the drug of choice.[47] The reasons for this paradox are not clear, but it has been suggested that continued growth of B. fragilis requires a milieu established by other anaerobes. Elimination of these anaerobes by penicillin alters this milieu.

There are two approaches to the patient with hospital-acquired aspiration pneumonia. Some authors suggest treatment with penicillin, unless the Gram stain shows unequivocal evidence of infection with Staphylococcus aureus or gram-negative rods. Noting the 60% incidence of aerobic organisms and the particular virulence of these infections, other investigators recommend empirical antimicrobial therapy until culture results are available.[41] Regimens consist of an aminoglycoside (gentamicin or tobramycin) combined with a semisynthetic penicillin (oxacillin or nafcillin) or a cephalosporin (cephazolin). These combinations provide broad coverage against most aerobic organisms associated with hospital-acquired aspiration pneumonia. When culture results become available, the appropriate antibiotic with the narrowest spectrum and least toxicity should be chosen.

Both approaches have merit, but there are no data suggesting the superiority of one over the other. Because the toxicity of empirical therapy for 2 or 3 days is minimal, and because these pneumonias cause significant morbidity and mortality, the initial use of broad-spectrum antibiotics until culture results are available may be the more prudent course.

Aspiration Pneumonia as a Complication of Aspiration Pneumonitis

Although the initial pathologic process of aspiration pneumonitis is a chemical burn of the lung, the disorder may be complicated by bacterial superinfection. This sequence of events occurs in approximately 25% to 40% of patients with aspiration pneumonitis.[11] The oropharynx is the origin of the infecting organism, but it is not clear whether these organisms gain entrance to the lung at the time of initial aspiration, through repeated aspiration, or by inhalation at a later time. Regardless of the origin of the bacteria, the damaged respiratory epithelial cells cannot provide normal protection, and the result is bacterial growth and clinical pneumonia.

The diagnosis of this type of pneumonia may be difficult. The signs (fever and rales), symptoms (productive cough and shortness of breath), and findings on chest radiograph (alveolar infiltrates) are the same for aspiration pneumonitis as for aspiration pneumonia complicating aspiration pneumonitis. The Gram stain cannot be relied upon, because colonization of the oropharynx may occur without pneumonia and oropharyngeal contents may contaminate expectorated sputum. Even a transtracheal aspirate may yield confusing results. Fortunately, the clinical course of the patient often indicates the presence of pneumonia due to bacterial infection. There is often a 2-to 4-day time lag between gastric aspiration and development of bacterial pneumonia, and, in this time period, patients who are stable or improving begin to deteriorate.[11] The clinical findings suggesting bacterial infection include recurrent or worsening fever, increased sputum production, more dyspnea, and progression of infiltrates on the chest radiograph. When there is evidence of supervening bacterial pneumonia, antimicrobial therapy should be instituted, dictated by a sputum Gram stain and the condition of the patient. Broad-spectrum antibiotic coverage is appropriate until culture results are available.

There is little data regarding the outcome of aspiration pneumonia, especially in hospitalized patients. However, extrapolating from studies dealing with specific rather than aspiration pneumonias, one can estimate the mortality of anaerobic aspiration pneumonia to be about 10% to 15% and that of aerobic aspiration pneumonia to lie in a range of 18% to 70%.[49–51] There are few studies evaluating long-term sequelae of aspiration pneumonitis and pneumonia. Although pulmonary fibrosis has been noted in a few survivors, pulmonary function tests and chest radiographs generally return to normal.[52]

ATELECTASIS

Postoperative atelectasis, although not usually lethal, is the most common complication of surgery, with an incidence as high as 70% in patients undergoing upper abdominal and thoracic surgery.[53] The extent of atelectasis may vary from "plate-like" with no associated symptoms or physical findings to lobar involvement with significant respiratory compromise.

Efforts to identify patients at greater than normal risk for postoperative pulmonary complications have been made ever since Stein and Cassara showed that diligent preoperative preparation and postoperative care decrease the postoperative complication rate.[54] These investigators found that, when high-risk patients underwent a program consisting of cessation of smoking, bronchodilator therapy, inhalation of humidified air, chest physical therapy, and postural drainage, the incidence of postoperative pulmonary complications dropped from 60% to 22%. Similarly, Dripps and Deming found that the incidence of significant atelectasis decreased by one-half when intensive pre- and postoperative measures relying heavily on chest physical therapy were instituted.[55] It should be recognized that, although factors responsible for atelectasis and pneumonia are similar, no study has shown that atelectasis leads to pneumonia or that postoperative pneumonias develop only in areas of preceding atelectasis.

Numerous additional therapeutic modalities have been proposed for the prevention of postoperative pulmonary complications, specifically of the lung, since it has been demonstrated that repetitive low tidal-volume ventilation is associated with progression alveolar collapse and can be eliminated by periodic hyperinflation.[56,57] Although the list of proposed measures is long, the most commonly discussed are intermittent positive-pressure breathing (IPPB), blow bottles, incentive spirometry, PEEP, and assisted coughing with voluntary deep breathing exercises.

IPPB, the subject of greatest debate, is thought to provide hyperinflation, promote the removal of secretions by shifting their position in the tracheobronchial tree, and decrease the work of breathing in the postoperative patient.[58,59] After its initial use in the therapy of chronic obstructive pulmonary disease, IPPB gained rapid acceptance in pre- and postoperative care in the early 1950s. Since that time, there have been numerous studies initially supporting and later refuting its benefit in this setting.[58,60–65] The majority of recent well-controlled studies fail to show significant benefit when pulmonary function, duration of postoperative fever, atelectasis, and other postoperative pulmonary complications and length of hospital stay are studied. Possible reasons for the failure of IPPB include delivery of pressure to inappropriate areas of the lung, inadequacy of the standard of 4 times a day of use, reliance on delivery of a specific pressure rather than volume, and inability of patients to use the apparatus correctly. Although the controversy is not resolved, the American Thoracic Society (ATS), in its recent conference on the Scientific Basis of In-Hospital Therapy, concluded, "As routinely applied . . . IPPB does not alter the incidence of postoperative pulmonary complications."[66] The use of PEEP as prophylaxis for atelectasis in patients undergoing cardiac surgery has been evaluated and has been found to be no more effective in preventing atelectasis than routine ventilatory care.[67]

The controversy over IPPB has stimulated research on the pathogenesis and mechanism of atelectasis. As noted above, passive hyperinflation of the lungs during surgery has been shown to result in less atelectasis. In addition, several studies have shown that sustained inspiratory maneuvers are effective in preventing or reducing atelectasis in both normal subjects and postoperative patients.[68,69] These data provide the rationale for vigorous postoperative therapy. All preoperative patients should be instructed in deep breathing exercises, and assisted coughing should be performed postoperatively. In the latter, the physician supports the surgical incision with the hand and coaches the patient to cough vigorously in various positions, especially the lateral decubitus.

One of the outgrowths of this research has been the development of incentive spirometry, which induces deep sustained inspiration in the postoperative patient with no emphasis on force or duration of expiration. Spirometric devices provide the patient with a quantitative measure of inspiratory effort. They are less hazardous than IPPB and possibly more effective in the prevention of postoperative atelectasis.[70] Indeed, the ATS recently stated that "the rationale for using incentive spirometry is sound."[66] In a comparison study of several commonly used incentive spirometers, no differences in patient outcome could be found.[71]

In summary, the incidence of postoperative atelectasis can be reduced by perioperative care centered around assisted coughing and induction of deep inspiration. Excellent nursing care coordinated with cessation of smoking and bronchodilator therapy significantly decreases atelectasis.[54] Incentive spirometry, a relatively inexpensive therapeutic modality, may further decrease postoperative pulmonary complications, but further work is needed to confirm this observation.

Treatment

A critical evaluation of various modalities currently used in the treatment of established atelectasis has not been done. This may be due in part to the fact that atelectasis is generally a self-limited pathologic process that usually resolves by the fifth to the seventh postoperative day. Studies supporting the superiority of one therapy over another suffer from lack of control groups and small sample size. Thus, no definitive statements can be made about the relative advantages of IPPB, bronchoscopy, incentive spirometry, or chest physical therapy, and decisions must often be made solely on the basis of clinical presentation. For the asymptomatic or mildly symptomatic patient with atelectasis, a trial of deep breathing maneuvers, assisted cough, and chest physical therapy should be undertaken. If the atelectasis does not clear, either volume (rather than pressure) IPPB, PEEP, or bronchoscopy may be used.[72,73] In significantly symptomatic patients in whom conservative measures prove inefficient, bronchoscopy may quickly alleviate the atelectasis.[74–75]

SUMMARY

1. Aspiration pneumonitis resulting from aspiration of gastric contents is characterized by the abrupt onset of thin sputum production, significant hypoxemia, hypocapnia, and infiltrates on chest x-ray within 4 hr of aspiration.

2. Antibiotics are not recommended in the treatment of aspiration pneumonitis.

3. Corticosteroids are indicated only if given within minutes of observed aspiration.

4. Treatment of hypoxemia with oxygen therapy is mandatory and may obviate intubation. Toxic concentrations of oxygen may be avoided with the use of PEEP; barotrauma and hypotension often accompany PEEP therapy.

5. Aspiration pneumonia resulting from aspiration of oropharyngeal contents is characterized by an indolent course, fever, and purulent sputum.

6. Community-acquired aspiration pneumonia should be treated with 2 to 5 million units/day of intravenous penicillin in 4 divided doses. Clindamycin, 300 mg orally or intravenously 4 times a day, should be given to penicillin-allergic patients.

7. Hospital-acquired aspiration pneumonia requires broad-spectrum antibiotic until culture results are available. Initial empirical therapy should include an aminoglycoside and either a penicillinase-resistant penicillin or cephalosporin.

8. The incidence of postoperative atelectasis is decreased by preoperative preparation consisting of cessation of smoking, bronchodilator therapy, and chest physical therapy and by postoperative measures centered around assisted coughing and sustained inspiratory maneuvers. IPPB provides no benefit in the prophylaxis of postoperative pulmonary complications either in normal subjects or in patients with chronic obstructive lung disease. PEEP is no more effective than routine ventilatory care in preventing atelectasis.

9. If atelectasis develops, conservative measures are generally effective, although bronchoscopy may be needed in serious or persistent clinical situations.

REFERENCES

1. Edwards G, Morton H, Pask E et al: Deaths associated with anesthesia. Anaesthesia 11:194, 1956
2. Arms R, Dines D, Tinstman T: Aspiration pneumonia. Chest 65:136, 1974
3. Mendelson C: Aspiration of stomach contents into the lungs during obstetric anesthesia. Am J Obstetecol Gyn 52:191, 1946
4. Teabeaut J: Aspiration of gastric contents: Experimental study. Am J Pathol 28:51, 1952
5. Hamelberg W, Bosomworth P: Aspiration pneumonitis: Experimental studies and clinical observations. Anesth Analg (Cleve) 43:669, 1964
6. Jones JG, Grossman R, Berry M et al: Alveolar capillary membrane permeability: Correlation with functional, radiographic, and postmortem changes after fluid aspiration. Am Rev Respir Dis 120:399, 1979
7. Schwartz D, Wynne J, Gibbs C et al: The pulmonary consequences of aspiration of gastric contents at pH values greater than 2.5. Am Rev Respir Dis 121:119, 1980
8. Greenfield L, Singleton R, McCaffree D et al: Pulmonary effects of experimental graded aspiration of hydrochloric acid. Ann Surg 170:74, 1969
9. Dines D, Baker W, Scantland W: Aspiration pneumonitis—Mendelson's syndrome. JAMA 176:229, 1961
10. Dines D, Titus J, Sissler A: Aspiration pneumonitis. Mayo Clin Proc 45:347, 1970
11. Bynum L, Pierce A: Pulmonary aspiration of gastric contents. Am Rev Respir Dis 114:1129, 1976
12. Cameron J, Zuidema G: Aspiration pneumonia: Magnitude and frequency of the problem. JAMA 219:1194, 1972
13. Roberts R, Shirley M: Reducing the risk of acid aspiration during cesarean section. Anesth Analg (Cleve) 53:860, 1974
14. Peskett W: Antacids before obstetric anesthesia. Anaesthesia 28:509, 1973
15. Awe W, Fletcher W, Jacob S: The pathophysiology of aspiration pneumonitis. Surgery 50:232, 1966
16. Kim I, Brummitt W, Humphrey A et al: Foreign body in the airway: A review of 202 cases. Laryngoscope 83:347, 1973
17. Taylor G, Pryse–Davies J: Evaluation of endotracheal steroid therapy in acid pulmonary aspiration syndrome. Anesthesiology 29:17, 1968
18. McCormick P: Immediate care after aspiration of vomit. Anaesthesia 30:658, 1975
19. Petersdorf R, Curtin J, Hoeprich P: A study of antibiotic prophylaxis in unconscious patients. N Engl J Med 257:1001, 1957
20. Aldrete J, Liem S, Carrow D: Pulmonary aerobic bacterial flora after aspiration pneumonitis. J Trauma 15:1014, 1975
21. Murray H: Antimicrobial therapy in pulmonary aspiration. Am J Med 66:188, 1979
22. Bannister W, Sattilaro A: Vomiting and aspiration during anesthesia. Anesthesiology 23:251, 1962
23. Lawson D, Defalco A, Phelps J et al: Corticosteriods as treatment for aspiration of gastric contents: An experimental study. Surgery 59:845, 1966
24. Tinstman T, Dines D, Arms R: Postoperative aspiration pneumonia. Surg Clin North Am 53:859, 1973
25. Cameron J, Mitchell W, Zuidema G: Aspiration pneumonia: Clinical outcome following documented aspiration. Arch Surg 106:49, 1973
26. Downs J, Chapman R, Modell J et al: An evaluation of steroid therapy in aspiration pneumonitis. Anesthesiology 40:129, 1974
27. Wolfe J, Bone R, Ruth W: Effects of corticosteroids in the treatment of patients with gastric aspiration. Am J Med 63:719, 1977
28. Kass E, Finland M: Corticosteroids and infection. Adv Intern Med 9:45, 1958
29. Stewardson R, Myhus L: Pulmonary aspi-

ration: An update. Arch Surg 112:1192, 1977

30. Cameron J, Caldini P, Toung J et al: Aspiration pneumonia: Physiologic data following experimental aspiration. Surgery 72:238, 1972

31. Booth D, Zuidema G, Cameron J: Aspiration pneumonia: Pulmonary arteriography after experimental aspiration. J Surg Res 12:48, 1972

32. Cameron J, Sebor J, Anderson R et al: Aspiration pneumonia: Results of positive pressure ventilation in dogs. Surg Res 8:447, 1968

33. Chapman R, Modell J, Ruiz B et al: Effect of continuous positive pressure ventilation and steroids on aspiration of hydrochloric acid (pH 1.8) in dogs. Anesth Analg (Cleve) 53:556, 1974

34. Zwillich C, Pierson D, Creagh CE et al: Complications of assisted ventilation: A prospective study of 354 consecutive episodes. Am J Med 57:161, 1974

35. Sykes M, Adams A, Finlay W et al: The effects of variations in end expiratory inflation pressure on cardiorespiratory function in normo-, hypo-, and hypervolemic dogs. B J Anaesth 42:669, 1970

36. DeLatorre F, Tomasa A, Klamburg J et al: Incidence of pneumothorax and pneumomediastinum in patients with aspiration pneumonia requiring ventilatory support. Chest 72:141, 1977

37. Venus B, Jacobs HK, Lim L: Treatment of the adult respiratory distress syndrome with continuous positive airway pressure. Chest 76:257, 1979

38. Downs J, Klein E, Desautels D et al: Intermittent mandatory ventilation: A new approach to weaning patients from mechanical ventilation. Chest 64:331, 1973

39. Bartlett J, Gorbach S, Finegold S: The bacteriology of aspiration pneumonia. Am J Med 56:202, 1974

40. Bartlett, J: Anaerobic bacterial pneumonitis. Am Rev Respir Dis 119:19, 1979

41. Bartlett J, Gorbach S: The triple threat of aspiration pneumonia. Chest 68:560, 1975

42. Rosebury T: Microorganisms Indigenous to Man. New York, McGraw-Hill, 1966

43. Johanson W, Pierce A, Sanford J: Changing pharyngeal bacterial flora of hospitalized patients. N Engl J Med 281:1137, 1969

44. Tillotson J, Finland M: Bacterial colonization and clinical superinfection of the respiratory tract complicating antibiotic treatment of pneumonia. J Infect Dis 119:597, 1969

45. Johanson W, Pierce A, Sanford J et al: Nosocomial respiratory infections with gram negative bacilli. Ann Intern Med 77:701, 1972

46. Lorber B, Swenson R: Bacteriology of aspiration pneumonia: A prospective study of community and hospital-acquired cases. Ann Intern Med 81:329, 1974

47. Bartlett J, Gorbach S: Treatment of aspiration pneumonia and primary lung abscess: Penicillin G vs. clindomycin. JAMA 234:935, 1975

48. Lewis R, Burgess J, Hampson L: Cardiorespiratory studies in critical illness. Arch Surg 170:74, 1971

49. Bartlett J, Finegold S: Anaerobic infections of the lung and pleural space. Am Rev Respir Dis 110:56, 1974

50. Lerner M, Federman M: Gram negative bacillary pneumonias. J Infect Dis 124:425, 1971

51. Fisher A, Trever R, Curtin A et al: Staphylococcal pneumonia. N Engl J Med 258:919, 1958

52. Sladen A, Zanca P, Hadnott W: Aspiration pneumonia—the sequelae. Chest 59:448, 1971

53. Rudnikoff I, Headland C: Pulmonary changes following cholecystectomy. JAMA 146:989, 1951

54. Stein M, Cassara E: Preoperative pulmonary evaluation and therapy for surgery patients. JAMA 211:787, 1970

55. Dripps R, Deming M: Postoperative atelectasis and pneumonia: Diagnosis, etiology, and management based on 1240 cases of upper abdominal surgery. Ann Surg 124:94, 1946

56. Mead J, Collier C: Relation of volume history of lungs to respiratory mechanics in anesthetized dogs. J Appl Physiol 14:669, 1959

57. Bendixen H, Bullwinkel B, Hedley-Whyte J et al: Atelectasis and shunting during spontaneous ventilation in anesthetized patients. Anesthesiology 25:297, 1964

58. Noehren T, Lasry J, Legters L: Intermittent positive pressure breathing for the prevention and management of postoperative pulmonary complications. Surgery 43:658, 1958

59. Safar P: Respiratory Therapy, p 220. Philadelphia, F.A. Davis, 1965

60. Rudy N, Crepeau J: Role of IPPB preoperatively. JAMA 167:1093, 1958

61. Anderson W, Dossett B, Hamilton G: Prevention of postoperative pulmonary problems. JAMA 186:763, 1963

62. Sands J, Cypert C, Armstrong R et al: A controlled study using routine intermittent positive pressure breathing in the post-surgical patient. Dis Chest 40:128, 1961

63. Baxter W, Levine R: An evaluation of intermittent positive pressure breathing in the prevention of postoperative pulmonary complications. Arch Surg 98:795, 1969

64. Cottrell J, Siker E: Preoperative intermittent positive pressure breathing therapy in patients with COLD: Effect on postoperative complications. Anesth Analg (Cleve) 52:258, 1973

65. Dohi S, Gold M: Comparison of two methods of postoperative respiratory care. Chest 73:592, 1978

66. Pontoppidan H: Mechanical age to lung expansion. Am Rev Respir Dis (Suppl) 122:109, 1980

67. Good J, Wolz J, Anderson J et al: The routine use of positive end expiratory pressure after open heart surgery. Chest 76:397, 1979

68. Ward R, Danziger F, Bonica J et at: An evaluation of postoperative respiratory maneuvers. Surg Gynecol Obstet 123:51, 1966

69. Bartlett R, Hanson E, Moore F: Physiology of yawning and its application to postoperative care. Surg Forum 21:222, 1970

70. Iverson L, Ecker R, Fox H et al: A comparative study of IPPB, the incentive spirometer and blow bottles: The prevention of atelectasis following cardiac surgery. Ann Thorac Surg 25:197, 1978

71. Lederer D, Van De Water J, Indech R: Which deep breathing device should the postoperative patient use? Chest 77:610, 1980

72. O'Donohue W: Maximum volume IPPB for the management of pulmonary atelectasis. Chest 76:683, 1979

73. Fowler A, Scoggins W, O'Donohue W: Positive end expiratory pressure in the management of lobar atelectasis. Chest 74:497, 1978

74. Wanner A, Landa J, Nieman R et al: Bedside bronchofiberoscopy for atelectasis and lung abscess. JAMA 224:1281, 1973

75. Dreisin R, Albert R, Talley P et al: Flexible fiberoptic bronchoscopy in the teaching hospital: Yield and complications. Chest 74:144, 1978

25
The Adult Respiratory Distress Syndrome

PAUL N. LANKEN

The term "adult respiratory distress syndrome" (ARDS) refers to any diffuse lung disorder that is characterized by noncardiac pulmonary edema or that occurs in the absence of left-sided congestive heart failure. ARDS is seen in a number of different clinical situations and has been referred to as shock lung, wet lung, white lung, permeability pulmonary edema, and pulmonary capillary leak syndrome. Pulmonary edema in ARDS forms despite normal pulmonary capillary hydrostatic pressures as a consequence of increased permeability in the alveolar–capillary membrane. Pulmonary edema in left-sided congestive heart failure is the result of excessive filtration of plasma due to high intravascualr hydrostatic pressure.[1–3]

CAUSES

Listed below are a number of clinical conditions which are generally regarded as inciting causes of ARDS and many of which are commonly encountered in the surgical setting.[4]

Injurious agent through bloodstream
    Septic shock
    Multiple trauma with shock
    Acute pancreatitis
    Fat emboli
    Transfusion reaction and shock
Injurious agent through airways
    Gastric acid aspiration
    Viral pneumonia
    Smoke inhalation
    Other diffuse pneumonia
    Oxygen toxicity
Other
    Neurogenic pulmonary edema (head trauma)
    Allergic reactions or heroin pulmonary edema
    Radiation pneumonitis or complications from radiomimetic drugs

Early awareness of developing ARDS in the above conditions may greatly aid in overall patient management. However, strict experimental confirmation that some of these clinical disorders cause permeability pulmonary edema is lacking. For example, increased pulmonary capillary permeability is difficult to demonstrate in simple hemorrhagic shock. Furthermore, the pathogenesis of certain conditions such as neurogenic pulmonary edema probably involves a combination of permeability and hydrostatic mechanisms.[3]

ARDS begins with injury to the alveolar–capillary membrane. The injurious agent may reach the air–blood interface by way of the airway or the bloodstream or through as yet undefined pathways. The injury increases the permeability of the alveolar–capillary membrane to plasma constituents, and protein-rich fluid leaks across the pulmonary capillaries. When the influx of fluid into the lung exceeds the rate of lymphatic drainage, edema fluid accumulates.

Initially, the excessive fluid pools in the pulmonary interstitial space to form interstitial edema causing mild ARDS. With greater leakage into the lung, fluid floods beyond the interstitium into the alveoli, causing alveolar edema. Extensive alveolar edema in turn causes the respiratory failure of severe acute ARDS. This process represents the final common pathway response by pulmonary gas-exchanging units to a variety of injuries.

Loss of alveolar surfactant may also be involved in the pathogenesis of ARDS, but its importance in adults remains unclear. This contrasts with the respiratory distress syndrome in premature infants, in which inadequacy of surfactant in the immature lung appears to underlie the process leading to respiratory failure. In ARDS, two different mechanisms may lead to decreased alveolar surfactant. Fluid flooding into the alveolar spaces may simply wash surfactant out of alveoli. In contrast, injury to alveolar type II pneumocytes (type II cells), which normally produce and secrete surfactant, may lead

to decreased synthesis. The two major cell types comprising the alveolar–capillary membrane, alveolar type I pneumocytes and pulmonary capillary endothelial cells, are less resistant to injury than type II cells. In addition, type II cells commonly proliferate after type I cell loss. Therefore, the second mechanism may come into play after especially severe alveolar injuries such as those seen in influenza pneumonia. Loss of surfactant probably contributes to the physiologic abnormalities and clinical respiratory failure that are seen in ARDS. However, it is probably not the primary pathogenetic factor in ARDS but rather a consequence of alveolar–capillary injury.

CLINICAL PRESENTATION

Patients presenting with ARDS exhibit rapid and shallow respirations. On physical examination, they may have scattered inspiratory rales without other signs of congestive heart failure. Aside from dyspnea, there may be a few other associated pulmonary symptoms, such as cough, sputum production, chest pain, or hemoptysis.[5] In mild cases, chest roentgenograms often reveal no abnormalities or only increased interstitial markings. In severe cases, radiographs characteristically show diffuse lung consolidation without cardiac silhouette enlargement or a "white-out" of the pulmonary parenchyma. In all but the mildest cases, arterial blood gases show hypoxemia, hypocarbia, and a primary respiratory alkalosis. In severe ARDS, hypoxemia becomes marked and does not improve with simple supplemental oxygen administration.

It is important to recognize that the clinical presentation of patients with ARDS may be dominated not by the above findings but by associated injuries or life-threatening conditions such as major trauma with hemorrhagic or septic shock. It is often only during the resuscitation of such patients that ARDS becomes manifest. The clinical presentation in ARDS varies not only with its many causes but also with the degree of lung injury. In mild ARDS, for example, in some cases of fat emboli after long bone fractures, the disease may be clinically inapparent and resolve spontaneously. However, in severe ARDS, like that seen after gastric acid aspiration, fulminant respiratory failure may follow.

CHANGES IN PULMONARY FUNCTION

Mild ARDS produces tachypnea, low tidal volumes, and a mild defect in alveolar oxygen transfer.[6] Nonchemical stimuli are probably responsible for the tachypnea, because the Pa_{CO_2} is low even when the PaO_2 is normal. The tachypnea is thought to be mediated by pulmonary J receptors along vagal afferent pathways in the lung. J receptors, which are located in the alveolar–capillary membrane, are stimulated by deformation of the interstitial space by interstitial edema.

Low tidal volume reflects a decrease in lung compliance or an increase in lung stiffness due to the interstitial edema. Shallow breathing is typical in this and other restrictive disorders with decreased lung volumes and low compliance.

Decreased oxygen transfer in mild ARDS results in a normal or minimally decreased PaO_2 and the decreased Pa_{CO_2} of alveolar hyperventilation. Inadequate oxygenation is confirmed by an increased alveolar–arterial oxygen difference of $P(A-a)O_2$. If the Pa_{CO_2} were normal at 40

torr, the PaO_2 would fall into the hypoxemic range. P_AO_2, or mean alveolar PO_2, is calculated from the ideal alveolar gas equation. PaO_2, or the arterial O_2, is directly measured in the arterial blood. The alveolar gas equation is $P_AO_2 = 713(F_iO_2) - Pa_{CO_2} \times 1.25$. On room air, this simplifies to $P_AO_2 = 150 - Pa_{CO_2} \times 1.25$. The figure 713 equals barometric pressure minus the saturated partial pressure of water vapor at sea level. F_iO_2 is the fraction of inspired oxygen. The normal range for $P(A-a)O_2$ on room air is 10 torr to 20 torr. The increased $P(A-a)O_2$ in mild ARDS is generally attributed to ventilation–perfusion (V/Q) abnormalities in which there are more alveoli with low V/Q ratios than in normals. An increased $P(A-a)O_2$ is not specific for ARDS and occurs commonly in many other pulmonary diseases.

In severe ARDS, the dominant respiratory problems are those of excessively stiff lungs and severe hypoxemia. Stiff lungs are due to widespread alveolar and interstitial edema as well as loss of alveolar surfactant. Lung stiffness is reflected by low compliance in the respiratory system, including the lungs and chest bellows. This system has a normal static compliance in the range of 50 to 100 ml/cm H_2O. Patients with severe ARDS supported with mechanical ventilation have a static compliance of 25 ml/cm H_2O and require high inspiratory pressures and flows.

In a patient with normal lungs and a respiratory system compliance of 100 ml/cm H_2O who is mechanically ventilated with a tidal volume of 1000 ml without positive end-expiratory pressure (PEEP), the end inspiratory pressure will be 10 cm H_2O (compliance = $\dfrac{\Delta \text{ volume}}{\Delta \text{ pressure}}$, or Δ pressure = $\dfrac{\Delta \text{ volume}}{\text{compliance}}$ = 1000 ml/cm H_2O = 10 cm H_2O). In contrast, in a patient with ARDS whose respiratory system static compliance is 25 ml/cm H_2O, the same tidal volume requires an end-expiratory pressure of 40 cm H_2O above the usual required setting of 5 to 15 cm H_2O. The ventilator must develop even greater peak inspiratory pressures because of resistance to flow of gas from machine to alveoli. Pressure-cycled ventilators easily capable of ventilating normal lungs are inadequate for ventilating the stiff lungs of patients with severe ARDS, and volume-cycled ventilators with high pressure capacities are necessary.

Severe hypoxemia in ARDS is associated with a high right-to-left shunt because of numerous fluid-filled alveoli that cannot be ventilated and hence have V/Q ratios of 0. The percentage of shunt can be estimated on the basis of 100% oxygen. Shunt increases 5% for every 100-torr decrease in PaO_2 below 700. This estimate becomes inaccurate when the PaO_2 falls below 100 torr. Normal subjects may have right-to-left shunts of up to 5%. Patients with mild ARDS have shunts of 5% to 15%, and patients with severe ARDS requiring mechanical ventilation usually have shunts in the range of 20% to 50%. Increased shunting underlies the impossibility of improving hypoxemia with simple supplemental oxygen administration or even oxygen concentrations of up to 100%. Under these circumstances, management is aimed at decreasing the shunt fraction. The large proportion of fluid-filled gas-exchanging units in the lungs of patients with ARDS is also reflected in a markedly decreased functional residual capacity and other lung volumes.

The movement of fluid through the walls of pulmonary capillaries is determined by two main factors, the inherent permeability of the capillary wall or conductance and the balance among intravascular and extravascular hydrostatic and oncotic pressures.[7] In the normal state, there is a small flow of lymph that leaves the lung $(+Q)$, creating a positive flow of fluid across pulmonary capillaries. Permeability pulmonary edema is the result of increased net fluid flow from the pulmonary capillaries into the lung due to increased capillary conductance. Pulmonary edema due to left-sided congestive heart failure is explained by increased net fluid flow into the lung as a result of a greatly increased pulmonary capillary hydrostatic pressure.

The association between permeability pulmonary edema and low plasma colloid oncotic pressure has been questioned. A recent experimental study found that lowering colloid osmotic pressure without changing pulmonary capillary wedge pressure does not produce alveolar edema.[8] Decreases in colloid oncotic pressure of the lung interstitial fluid and increases in lung lymph flow were sufficient to balance the reduction in plasma oncotic pressure and prevent alveolar edema. At present, it remains unclear what the effects of acute or chronic reductions in plasma colloid oncotic pressure are on the genesis of clinical pulmonary edema.

PATHOLOGY

Morphological findings in the lungs of patients with ARDS vary strikingly as the disorder progresses.[4,9] Severe ARDS develops through two major phases, an initial exudative phase associated with acute injury and a later fibrotic phase associated with lung repair. At the initiation of the exudative phase, coincident with the onset of lung injury, there may be no morphological changes seen histologically or ultrastructurally other than edema of the alveolar interstitial space. Excessive permeability of the pulmonary capillaries may occur without identifiable cellular destruction of the alveolar–capillary membrane. Further progression of the exudative phase results in alveolar edema, which may be so severe that lungs from patients with ARDS dying of acute hypoxemia may weigh several times more than normal lungs. On histologic examination, these lungs are found to have protein-rich edema filling most of the alveoli as well as variable evidence of acute lung injury and inflammatory cells, depending on the nature of the injurious agent. Of particular pathologic significance in the exudative phase is the presence of hyaline membranes. Hyaline membranes contain fibrin strands and often form a pseudoepithelium over denuded alveolar basement membranes. These are initially located adjacent to the alveolar ducts and subsequently may extend along alveolar walls. Hyaline membranes indicate excessive leakage of fibrinogen, a molecule of high molecular weight, into the alveolar space and support the theory that excessive alveolar–capillary membrane permeability is the cause of ARDS.

The second major pathologic phase in the course of ARDS was described when development of intensive respiratory support became available and helped to prolong the clinical course of ARDS. Previously, patients with ARDS died during the exudative phase from massive pulmonary edema. The onset of the reparative stage probably begins shortly after the initial lung injury, and evidence of repair can be documented histologically about 1 to 2 weeks after the onset of ARDS. The repair process causes marked changes in the injured alveolar–capillary membrane.

First, the thin delicate lining of squamous alveolar epithelium, normally composed of type I pneumocytes, is replaced by a thicker, cuboidal layer of alveolar type II pneumocytes. The type II cells proliferate after injury to the type I pneumocytes and eventually differentiate into type I pneumocytes to reconstitute the alveolar epithelium. Secondly, the earlier edema in the alveolar–capillary interstitium is followed by interstitial fibroblast proliferation and formation of new collagen, resulting in interstitial fibrosis. These fibrotic changes are predominant in ARDS patients who undergo prolonged ventilator support before death.

Death during this phase often results from irreversible respiratory failure due to progressive interstitial fibrosis and obliteration of gas-exchanging units. The immediate cause of death is usually unremitting hypoxemia. A less common cause of death is failure to achieve adequate alveolar ventilation with resultant hypercarbia, which is often associated with development of a bronchopleural fistula through which a large proportion of tidal volume exits from the lung through chest tubes. Other complications of prolonged mechanical ventilation that may be fatal include tension pneumothorax and nosocomial pneumonias, especially those due to gram-negative bacilli, such as *Pseudomonas* or *Serratia*.

Oxygen toxicity may contribute to the pathologic changes of ARDS. Its role is difficult to define, since patients with ARDS are treated with high concentrations of oxygen, and oxygen toxicity itself is a well-established cause of ARDS. Interpretation of pathologic changes is difficult, because safe upper limits of oxygen concentration have not been well defined for either normal or diseased lungs. Evidence supporting a role for oxygen toxicity includes a large series of patients with severe ARDS in whom the severity of pathologic changes at autopsy correlated better with the duration of respiratory therapy than with the duration of the underlying illness causing ARDS.[9]

Multiple thromboemboli may contribute to the development of ARDS in some patients. However, only some patients with ARDS are found to have such emboli at autopsy. Moreover, emboli are often found in critically ill patients without ARDS.

DIFFERENTIAL DIAGNOSIS

Since the initial clinical manifestations of mild ARDS are nonspecific, diagnosis may be difficult. The differential diagnosis includes mild left-sided congestive heart failure, pulmonary emboli, postoperative atelectasis, and bacterial sepsis. Careful clinical and laboratory assessment and frequent monitoring of respiratory dysfunction may help the physician reach an accurate diagnosis in this phase.

The differential diagnosis of severe ARDS includes left-sided congestive heart failure and, rarely, diffuse pulmonary hemorrhage and diffuse aspiration of blood. Aside from severe ARDS, the differential diagnosis in patients with clinical and radiographic evidence of diffuse alveolar consolidation is limited. All the diseases involved in differential diagnosis result in fluid-filled alveoli that alter lung mechanics and gas transfer in a similar manner and may not be easily separable on the basis of physiologic derangements. Clinical clues pointing to a diagnosis of congestive heart failure can often be obtained from the patient's history, the size of the cardiac silhouette on the chest roentgenogram, and the presence or absence of a third heart sound on auscultation. Clinical response and rapid resolution of infiltrates after diuretic therapy is more consistent with congestive heart failure than with ARDS.

In patients with severe pulmonary edema, the distinction between ARDS and congestive heart failure can be made on the basis of whether the left-ventricular filling pressure is elevated.[10] In intensive care units, measurement of the pulmonary capillary wedge pressure has become a standard bedside diagnostic technique. Wedge pressures above 28 torr to 30 torr are associated with widespread alveolar edema due to increased hydrostatic forces. Conversely, with only rare exceptions, wedge pressures below 20 torr support the diagnosis of ARDS. One exception is the case of the patient who has undergone brisk diuresis in the interval between performance of the chest roentgenogram demonstrating pulmonary edema and determination of the wedge pressure.

As already mentioned, less common disorders in the differential diagnosis of severe ARDS include diffuse pulmonary hemorrhage and extensive aspiration of blood following hemoptysis or hematemesis, both of which cause the presence of blood in the alveolar spaces. A falling hematocrit without other obvious sources of blood loss is helpful in documenting pulmonary hemorrhage. There may be coincident renal abnormalities consistent with rapidly progressive glomerulonephritis or Goodpasture's syndrome. The clinical circumstances surrounding extensive aspiration of blood are usually obvious. Unlike the course of ARDS, the resolution of pulmonary infiltrates in hemorrhage occurs relatively rapidly, often within several days.

TREATMENT

Patients who have mild ARDS with shunts of 5% to 15% are often hypoxemic and may suffer progression to severe ARDS. They can usually be managed successfully without endotracheal intubation and mechanical ventilation. Arterial oxygenation can be safely maintained by supplemental oxygen administration by way of nasal prongs or simple masks in which the inspired oxygen percentage is generally less than 50%. If the arterial PaO_2 remains below 55 torr, the FiO_2 can be increased by the use of face masks with rebreathing or nonrebreathing reservoir bags. If tightly fitting, they can provide an oxygen concentration of 100%. Close monitoring of patients requiring such a high FiO_2 is essential and is best performed in an intensive care setting. Unnoticed removal of the mask by a confused patient on a general care unit would rapidly lead to severe arterial oxygen desaturation.

There is no effective treatment to restore capillary permeability after injury. However, decreasing pulmonary capillary hydrostatic pressure will reduce fluid flow into the lung despite the elevated capillary conductance, even if pulmonary capillary pressures are not elevated. For this reason, diuretic therapy is often used in the treatment of mild ARDS. Decreased influx of fluid allows lung lymphatics to drain accumulated interstitial fluid.

In some cases, diuretic therapy may be contraindicated because of its concomitant effects of decreasing left ventricular preload and cardiac output. If the patient is in shock and reduction of cardiac output would clearly be hazardous, careful monitoring of pulmonary capillary wedge pressure during resuscitation efforts helps to ensure adequate cardiac preload and avoid excessive elevation of the wedge pressure beyond 15 torr to 18 torr; such elevation would worsen transcapillary fluid flux into the lung. In these cases, therapy should be directed at reversing the primary cause of shock and maintaining cardiac and urinary output with infusions of pressor and inotropic agents such as dopamine while aiming for wedge pressures of 15 torr to 18 torr.

Because of its high mortality, severe ARDS is a medical emergency. Goals of therapy include cessation of further primary injury to the lung by treatment of the inciting cause and avoidance of oxygen toxicity by limitation of exposure to high inspired oxygen concentrations. Clinicians generally become concerned about oxygen toxicity when inspired oxygen concentrations exceed 70% for prolonged periods. However, the lungs of patients with ARDS may be more sensitive to higher oxygen levels than the lungs of normals and may develop oxygen toxicity at concentrations lower than 70% and after shorter periods of exposure. Problems in the management of these patients arise both from the effects of lung injury and resultant pulmonary edema and from the concomitant failure of other organ systems. The same principles for treating respiratory failure apply to other systems as well. The inciting cause should be treated and supportive care given until the organ recovers as much function as possible.

As in the treatment of mild ARDS, diuretic therapy in severe ARDS has been found to be helpful, probably by reducing pulmonary capillary wedge pressures and diminishing the flux of fluid into the lung. Combined with continued lung lymphatic drainage, diuretics improve oxygenation and lung compliance.

Intravascular volume expansion may be necessary to maintain blood pressure.

Packed red blood cells stay in the intravascular space and are the preferred form of volume replacement in the case of hemorrhage. Both crystalloid and colloid intravenous solutions are redistributed during and after infusion, and only a fraction remains in the intravascular space. The argument has been made that massive crystalloid infusions should be avoided because they lead to a reduction of plasma oncotic pressure by diluting plasma proteins. Infusions of colloid have been recommended to increase plasma oncotic pressure and draw out pulmonary edema fluid. However, the effects of infusions on lung fluid balance depend on the resultant changes in interstitial hydrostatic and oncotic pressures. In severe ARDS, there is probably rapid re-equilibration of plasma albumin between lung edema fluid and plasma. There is little evidence that dilution of plasma proteins by crystalloids causes pulmonary edema except when the pulmonary capillary wedge pressure is elevated. This re-emphasizes the need for accurate monitoring of intravascular volume by pulmonary capillary wedge pressure measurements. Avoidance of excessively elevated wedge pressures may be more important than the choice of fluid administered in severe ARDS.

Mechanical ventilation in severe ARDS is best carried out in an intensive care unit staffed by experienced personnel. Ventilation is accomplished with a volume-cycled ventilator with high flow and pressure capabilities to deliver high tidal volumes and sighs despite low respiratory system compliance. These ventilators provide a continuous range of FiO_2, an integral PEEP mechanism, and alarms to ensure continued safe mechanical ventilation.

Patients with severe ARDS may have been intubated solely because of severe hypoxemia and not because of hypercarbia or ventilatory insufficiency. In these cases, some clinicians use the mechanical ventilator to provide continuous positive airway pressure (CPAP) during spontaneous breathing. This has two theoretical advantages over conventional mechanical ventilation. First, it provides less of an adverse effect on cardiac preload, because inspiratory pleural pressures are generated by the patient, and high positive-peak inspiratory pressures delivered by the ventilator are avoided. Second, it reduces the chances of barotrauma with resultant tension pneumothorax because of lower peak inspiratory pressures. CPAP has the disadvantage of increasing minute oxygen consumption because of the increased work of breathing and lack of ventilator-generated sighs of large tidal volume. However, this problem can be remedied by use of an intermittent mandatory ventilation mode (IMV) in which a number of machine breaths can be given each minute to a spontaneously breathing but intubated patient. Techniques like CPAP and IMV have been used empirically; no controlled clinical trials have been done to confirm the efficacy of one mode of therapy over another.

In the acute exudative phase of ARDS, the main problem is hypoxemia due to massive pulmonary edema. Simple oxygen administration fails to reverse the hypoxemia because of a high right-to-left shunt. Instead, hypoxemia must be treated with oxygen at a high inspired FiO_2 delivered by mechanical ventilation utilizing PEEP. Although a complete understanding of the action of PEEP is lacking, its physiologic effects in improving arterial oxygenation in ARDS are clearly recognized. The aim of treatment with PEEP is to maintain tissue oxygenation using the lowest possible FiO_2, thereby avoiding further injury to the lung parenchyma by toxic concentrations of oxygen.

PEEP has several known effects on respiratory function. It elevates the passive end-expiratory position of the lungs and chest wall and therefore increases the functional residual capacity of the lung. It inflates previously fluid-filled alveoli and expands partially fluid-filled alveoli with more gas. By decreasing the number of alveoli with low or zero V/Q ratios, it decreases shunt fraction and improves oxygenation. In addition, PEEP has been found to improve lung and respiratory system compliance, which makes it possible for the same tidal volumes to be delivered at lower pressures. However, the concept that PEEP acts by "pushing" edema fluid out of the alveolar spaces into lung lymphatics is unproved. Indeed, careful physiological studies in normal lungs indicate that PEEP may actually induce slight fluid retention.

In severe cases, PEEP is begun with the patient on 100% oxygen, while, in milder cases, PEEP allows for an early decrease in FiO_2. Increasing PEEP raises the PaO_2 and thereby the oxygen content of arterial blood (CaO_2). PEEP also causes cardiac output to fall because of decreased venous return to the thorax. The term "best PEEP" refers to that level of PEEP which gives the highest value of the product of cardiac output and CaO_2. For determination of this level, PEEP is applied in increments of 3 to 5 cm H_2O from 0 to 15 cm H_2O. After 15 to 20 min at each incremental PEEP level, PaO_2 and cardiac output are determined. CaO_2 is calculated by multiplication of 1.34 ml O_2/g hemoglobin (Hgb) $\times$ g Hgb/dl $\times$ percent saturation as determined from the PaO_2. Cardiac output is measured with a balloon-tipped catheter by the thermodilution method. The product of cardiac output and CaO_2 is then calculated for each PEEP level, the highest value representing the best PEEP for the patient at that time.[11] Diuretic or inotropic therapy may subsequently alter cardiac output, and the best PEEP may change during the course of therapy.

Measurement of compliance in relation to increments in PEEP was found in one study to be a good noninvasive method for determination of best PEEP. The best PEEP obtained by this method correlated well with that determined by CaO_2 and cardiac output determination.[11] However, the patients studied in this report had relatively mild ARDS with shunt fractions of only 15% to 20%. The question therefore arises as to whether these patients could have been managed successfully without PEEP. In patients with more severe ARDS and higher shunt fractions, the PEEP level that yields the best compliance may not correspond to the PEEP level that provides overall improvement in respiratory function.

While on mechanical ventilation at high inflation pressures and especially at high PEEP levels, the patient with severe ARDS often develops a pneumothorax, which may become a tension pneumothorax. Pneumothorax presents as a sudden elevation in inspiratory pressure, hypotension, and subcutaneous emphysema over the chest. Immediate insertion of a chest tube is the treatment of choice. Prophylactic chest tube placement to prevent tension pneumothorax may be dangerous, because the lung in ARDS does not collapse as readily as the normal lung when the pleural space is opened to atmospheric pressure.

Persistent air leaks commonly occur after chest tube placement, indicating the presence of a bronchopleural fistula. Leakage of a substantial fraction of the tidal volume through such a fistula may cause inadequate ventilation and death. Spontaneous closure of a bronchopleural fistula is uncommon while the patient is receiving tidal volumes at high pressures and high levels of PEEP. The best approach to this problem is achievement of full lung expansion by suction through chest tubes and subsequent weaning of the patient from PEEP as ARDS improves. However, neither may be possible if the ARDS does not improve. Surgical closure of the air leak is usually not attempted if the patient's clinical condition is poor and parenchymal lung disease extensive.

Management of the late phase of severe ARDS, the reparative phase, follows the same course as that detailed above. During this period, the clinical problem remains hypoxemia complicated not by shock or acute renal failure, as in the exudative phase, but by oxygen toxicity and nosocomial pulmonary infections. There is no specific therapy to prevent or reverse the development of interstitial fibrosis in this phase. It is irreversible pulmonary fibrosis that prevents successful weaning of the patient from high concentrations of inspired oxygen. The overall prognosis for patients with severe ARDS is poor, with a mortality of about 90%.[12,13]

SUMMARY

1. **Document hypoxemia by arterial blood gas determinations and pulmonary edema by chest x-ray and physical examination.**
2. **Determine pulmonary capillary wedge pressure to differentiate ARDS (pressure less than 20 torr) from congestive heart failure (pressure greater than 30 torr). Measurements between 20 torr and 30 torr should be treated as congestive heart failure and followed closely.**
3. **Increase FiO_2 to keep the PaO_2 at a minimum of 55 to 60 torr.**
4. **Move the patient to an intensive care unit when an FiO_2 above 50% is required.**
5. **Use diuretics to decrease pulmonary capillary hydrostatic pressures. Begin with furosemide at a dose of 20 mg in an intravenous (IV) bolus, and continue to double the dose up to 480 mg or until satisfactory diuresis occurs.**
6. **Insert a Swan–Ganz catheter to monitor wedge pressure in all but the mildest cases. Aim for a wedge pressure below 15 torr.**
7. **Consider a radial artery cannula for continuous blood pressure monitoring and frequent arterial blood gas sampling.**
8. **Intubate and mechanically ventilate patients with shunts of 20% or greater.**
9. **Set the ventilator as follows:**
   a. **Tidal volume: 10–12 ml/kg ideal body weight**
   b. **Sigh volume: 50% greater than tidal volume**
   c. **Sigh frequency: at least 5 times/hr**
   d. **FiO_2: start at $FiO_2 = 1.0$, which will yield an estimate of the shunt fraction. (On 100% oxygen, there is a 5% shunt for every 100 torr PaO_2 below 700 torr. The method is not accurate if PaO_2 is less than 100 torr.)**
   e. **Respiratory rate: The assist-mode with the patient triggering the respirator will usually keep the Pa_{CO_2} below 40 torr. If the patient needs to be sedated or paralyzed in order to be ventilated, adjust the machine rate to keep the Pa_{CO_2} between 30 torr and 40 torr.**
   f. **PEEP: If the patient requires an FiO_2 greater than 50% to maintain a PaO_2 of 55 torr, determine the best PEEP as described above.**

g. Adjust peak flow to ensure an inspiratory:expiratory ratio of less than 1:1.

10. If there is insufficient urine output after maximum challenge with diuretics in a patient with apparently adequate perfusion, begin peritoneal dialysis or hemodialysis to reduce wedge pressure to the desired level.

11. Treat hypotension with volume expansion first. Replace volume in the following order of preference: packed red blood cells (bring the hematocrit up to at least 30%), albumin, and normal saline.

12. Add pressors if the systolic blood pressure is less than 85 torr. Dopamine can be used as an IV drip at 1 to 3 ug/kg/min; raise the dosage until an adequate perfusion pressure of about 85 torr to 100 torr systolic is reached. While administering pressors, attempt to lower the pulmonary capillary wedge pressure with diuretics or dialysis as far below 15 torr as possible without compromising blood pressure and urine output.

13. Obtain chest roentgenograms to watch for pneumothorax and pneumonias. Insert a chest tube to treat pneumothorax.

14. Defer tracheostomy until after the tenth day of naso- or endotracheal intubation. With low-pressure cuffed tubes, 2 to 3 weeks of prolonged intubation may be safe.

15. Avoid glucocorticoids in the treatment of ARDS.

16. Treat pulmonary infections as indicated by clinical findings and Gram stains of tracheal secretions. Do not treat simple tracheostomy site colonization with antimicrobial agents.

17. The weaning process should be slow, with emphasis on decreasing FiO_2 below 50% before dropping PEEP levels.

REFERENCES

1. Fishman AP: Shock lung. A distinctive non-entity. Circulation 47:921, 1973
2. Robin ED: Pulmonary edema. N Engl J Med 288:239, 1973
3. Fishman AP: Pulmonary edema. The water-exchanging function of the lung. Circulation 46:390, 1972
4. Teplitz C: The core pathology and integrated medical science of adult respiratory insufficiency. Surg Clin North Am 56:1091, 1976
5. Petty TL: The adult respiratory distress syndrome. Clinical features, factors influencing prognosis and principles of management. Chest 60:233, 1971
6. Pontoppidan H: Acute respiratory failure in the adult. N Engl J Med 287:690, 1972
7. Staub NC: Pulmonary edema due to increased microvascular permeability to fluid and protein. Circ Res 43:143, 1978
8. Zarins CK: Lymph and pulmonary response to isobaric reduction in plasma oncotic pressure in baboons. Circ Res 43:925, 1978
9. Pratt PC: Pulmonary morphology in a multi-hospital collaborative extracorporeal membrane oxygenation project. I. Light microscopy. Am J Pathol 95:191, 1979
10. Unger KM: Detection of left ventricular failure in patients with adult respiratory distress syndrome. Chest 67:9, 1975
11. Suter PM: Optimum end expiratory airway pressure in patients with acute pulmonary failure. N Engl J Med 292:284, 1975
12. Zapol WM: Extracorporeal membrane oxygenation in severe acute respiratory failure. A randomized prospective study. JAMA 242:2193, 1979
13. Springer RR: The influence of PEEP on survival of patients in respiratory failure. A retrospective analysis. Am J Med 66:196, 1979

Thromboembolic Disease and Fat Embolism in the Surgical Patient

MARK A. KELLEY

Thromboembolic disease is a major cause of complications and death in the surgical patient.[1] Clot in the deep venous system of the lower extremities can be documented by radioactive fibrinogen scanning in over 40% of surgical patients.[2] Certain subgroups are at higher risk, with an incidence of 50% both in patients over age 60 and in patients with malignancy.[3–5] Of patients who undergo hip surgery and open prostatectomy, 70% and 40% develop deep-vein thrombosis (DVT), respectively.[4,6–8] In some cases, deep venous clot dislodges and migrates to the pulmonary circulation, causing the life-threatening complication of pulmonary embolism. It is estimated that over 500,000 cases of pulmonary embolism occur annually in the United States, with surgical patients forming the majority of this group.[9]

The precise incidence of pulmonary embolism in the surgical population is not known. A large well-controlled prospective study showed the prevalence of fatal pulmonary embolism in general surgery patients to be 1%.[10] Although high-risk patients have a mortality rate as high as 7% the incidence of nonfatal pulmonary embolism in surgical patients is unknown.[10] One limited study suggests that as many as 18% of patients demonstrate new perfusion defects on lung scan.[11] When untreated, pulmonary embolism carries a mortality of 30%, but only 8% of those treated die of the disorder.[9] Little of this data comes from controlled studies, but the weight of circumstantial evidence supports these estimates.

The diagnosis of thromboembolic disease is difficult, particularly in the surgical patient, when other processes may confuse the clinical picture. Treatment with anticoagulants may also be complex in this population because of the danger of wound bleeding. Finally, there are a bewildering number of recommendations about prevention of thromboembolism in the surgical patient. In this chapter, we examine each of these problems.

PATHOPHYSIOLOGY

Clot formation in the deep venous system is associated with a number of conditions. Except in rare coagulation disorders, it is difficult to demonstrate a hypercoagulable state in patients with thromboembolism. Malignancy, trauma, and surgery may activate the clotting cascade, but the exact mechanism is unclear. Immobilization is a major predisposing factor for venous clot formation, probably because of sluggish venous blood flow and platelet aggregation.[12] Pre-existing venous disease may also cause stasis and local inflammation. Other conditions that are associated with thromboembolism include congestive heart failure, pregnancy, the use of oral contraceptives, stroke, and obesity. Oral contraceptives may directly affect coagulation; however, most other conditions predispose to thrombosis probably because of immobilization rather than through other specific machanisms.[12]

Whether surgery predisposes the patient to a hypercoagulable state is unknown. With fibrinogen scanning, clot formation can be detected before surgery, during anesthesia, and well after the surgical procedure.[2,13,14] This may be associated in part with a decrease in fibrinolytic activity during and for 2 days after anesthesia.[15] Except in orthopedic injuries and procedures, direct trauma to veins plays a relatively minor role in the pathogenesis of venous thrombosis.

Clots that embolize to the lung generally migrate from the large capacitance veins of the lower extremities or from larger vessels in the abdomen.[16] DVT below the knee is felt to be clinically important only if it progresses to involve larger, more proximal vessels. However, there is some evidence that even calf vein thrombi may embolize.[16]

Once a clot has embolized to the lung, a series of poorly understood events occurs.[17] The patient often becomes acutely dyspneic through reflex stimulation of lung receptors or release of local mediators such as serotonin from the clot. Arterial PO_2 may fall because of local changes in the ventilation–perfusion (V/Q) relationship, which are again mediated by these mechanisms. Pulmonary artery pressure is not significantly elevated in the normal patient until at least 50% of the pulmanary circulation has been occluded by clot.[9] However, a patient with pre-existing cardiopulmonary disease may already have an elevated pulmonary artery pressure or a limited pulmonary capillary bed, and a relatively small volume of clot may elevate pulmonary artery pressure. In either case, right-heart failure can occur when pulmonary artery pressure is excessively high, but a large volume of clot, usually from several emboli, is needed to produce cor pulmonale in the patient who does not have substantial underlying cardiopulmonary disease.

Death from pulmonary embolism occurs for several reasons. A fragile patient with underlying cardiopulmonary disease may not tolerate the additional stress of hypoxemia or increased work of breathing. In many fatal cases, a large volume of clot blocks the pulmonary circulation and produces pulmonary hypertension and cor pulmonale. Rarely, this may be the result of a single massive clot migrating suddenly to the pulmonary artery. More commonly, multiple pulmonary emboli are unrecognized over a period of days or weeks until the pulmonary vasculature is nearly obliterated and the patient succumbs to the next clot. Once a clot has lodged in the pulmonary artery, it does not remain static. Slow lysis of clot occurs over days or weeks, and some large clots may fragment within hours.

DIAGNOSIS

Venous Thrombosis

The clinical diagnosis of DVT is difficult. Although the classic picture of tenderness and swelling of the calf suggests the diagnosis, only 50% of patients with such findings have DVT on a venogram. In addition, about 50% of patients with DVT on a venogram may display few clinical signs[18]. Therefore, the diagnosis of DVT must be made with laboratory tests. Since DVT occurs in 40% of surgical patients, there are major logistical problems in screening and correctly diagnosing all cases.[1]

There are four methods for diagnosing venous thrombosis: radioactive fibrinogen scanning, impedance plethysmography (IPG), Doppler ultrasonography, and contrast venography (Table 26-1). As previously described, radioactive fibrinogen scanning has been used extensively to study venous thrombosis in surgical patients. The scan requires active clot formation in the leg so that injected fibrinogen is incorporated into the thrombus and can be localized by an external radiation detector. The accuracy of this technique is lost when the method is applied to large vessels above or in the thigh.[12,18] Overlying soft tissue may shield radioactivity or, in cases or surgery near the thigh or hip, radioactive fibrinogen may be deposited in areas of inflammation outside the venous system. These limitations cast doubt on the diagnostic usefulness of the fibrinogen scan for detecting large-vein thrombosis. Most pulmonary emboli arise in large veins at or above the knee in areas where fibrinogen scanning is least useful. Furthermore, the risk or pulmonary embolism with calf vein thrombosis is not known, and the indications for anticoagulation are therefore unclear in a patient with a positive fibrinogen scan of the calf. This is particularly important in the postoperative period when treatment by anticoagulation may be risky.

IPG and Doppler ultrasonography are noninvasive techniques that indirectly measure the patency of the large vessels of the upper leg and abdomen.[18,19] The IPG measures electrical resistance in the leg before and after venous compression. Differences in resistance reflect changes in venous capacitance; in turn, these changes give an indirect measure of venous blood flow. With better equipment and standardization than venography, IPG has an accuracy of 80% to 90%. The Doppler technique, which uses ultrasound to detect flow patterns in large vessels, is less reliable and requires experience in interpretation. In both methods, venous obstruction from ascites or right-heart failure can lead to false-positive results. False-negative results are common in vessels below the knee. However, for detecting clots in large vessels above the knee, IPG and Doppler ultrasonography are quite useful.

Venography is the most invasive but also the most reliable method of documenting DVT.[18] Although easy to perform, it requires experience for interpretation. There is controversy over the risk of dye-induced phlebitis, but, in some centers, careful technique and reduced dye concentrations have eliminated the problem. Nevertheless, the venogram is the stan-

Table 26-1. Diagnostic Tests for Deep-Vein Thrombosis

	Accuracy	Technical Complexity
Venography	Excellent	Moderate
Fibrinogen scan	Excellent for calf veins Poor for larger veins	Moderate
Impedance plethysmogram Doppler ultrasound	Good for large veins	Small

dard against which all other diagnostic tests for venous thrombosis are compared. Venography also provides a measure of clot volume and extent of thrombosis.

Fibrinogen scanning is not widely available and may give misleading information. At least 1 day is required for fibrin deposition to occur. The Doppler and IPG methods are safe, easy tests with encouraging results reported in the literature. However, many hospitals have not had enough experience with these techniques to make them widely applicable diagnostic tools.

Pulmonary Embolism

The majority of pulmonary emboli probably are unrecognized, because clinical signs and symptoms are easily confused with other conditions. In surgical patients, pneumonia, postoperative atelectasis, bronchospasm, and congestive heart failure can mimic pulmonary embolism. The classic syndrome of acute shortness of breath, pleuritic chest pain, and acute right-heart failure is rarely seen.[20] Instead, the patient may be more dyspneic than usual or experience a new type of chest pain or arrhythmia, problems that can occur for a variety of reasons.

Congestive heart failure and pneumonia are particularly common in the perioperative period. However, lack of firm evidence for these processes or failure to respond to treatment should alert the clinician to the possibility of pulmonary embolism. The presence of new chest pain, pleuritic or nonpleuritic, or a sudden unexplained drop in blood pressure strongly suggests pulmonary embolus. Less common presentations of pulmonary embolism include new and persistent tachycardia or arrhythmias. Fever can occur but is almost never greater than 102°F

and is usually accompanied by other signs or symptoms.[12]

Physical examination is not often helpful in the diagnosis of pulmonary embolism.[12] Rarely, there are signs of right-heart strain with a right ventricular heave or gallop and elevated jugular venous pressure, and, sometimes, there is evidence of new pulmonary hypertension with accentuation of the pulmonic component of the second heart sound. Usually, however, there are only nonspecific findings such as increased respiratory rate often accompanied by rales. A pleural rub is present in less than 5% of patients.[20] Signs of phlebitis are found in about one-third of patients, but these signs are not specific for DVT.

Least Helpful Tests

Since history and physical examination provide little information, the diagnosis of pulmonary embolism depends on laboratory tests, particularly on radiologic techniques (Table 26-2). Conventional laboratory data are not very helpful.[12] Unless there is accompanying infection, the white blood cell count in pulmonary embolus is normal or slightly elevated. Serum enzyme determinations are of little value. The combination of elevated serum lactic dehydrogenase and bilirubin levels and a normal serum transaminase concen-

Table 26-2. Diagnostic Tests for Pulmonary Embolism

Useless	Sometimes Helpful	Very Helpful	Diagnostic
Complete blood count	Arterial blood gases	Lung scan	Angiogram
Enzymes	Electrocardiogram		
Fibrin split products	Chest x-ray		

tration was once thought to be useful in the diagnosis of pulmonary embolism, but the sensitivity and specificity of this triad are low.

Measurement of fibrim degradation products enjoyed brief popularity as a useful adjunct for detection of pulmonary emboli. The methods of detecting these circulating by-products of coagulation and fibrinolysis have not been well standardized, and conflicting reports about the sensitivity and specificity of this test have cast doubt on its clinical value.[12] Furthermore, it is useless in postoperative patients or in patients who have suffered trauma in whom active fibrinolysis is occurring in healing tissue.[21]

The electrocardiogram (ECG) provides little diagnostic information.[22] The most common finding in pulmonary embolism is that of nonspecific ST–T changes, which usually reflect underlying cardiac disease. Although often considered a hallmark of pulmonary embolism, atrial fibrillation is actually uncommon. Premature atrial or ventricular beats are seen more often but can be the result of other disease processes. Evidence on ECG of acute right-heart strain with new right-axis deviation, right bundle-branch block, or ST–T changes in the early precordial leads is unusual but strongly suggests the diagnosis of pulmonary embolism.

Moderately Helpful Tests

Arterial blood gas determinations have a limited role in diagnosing pulmonary embolus.[23] Much of the confusion about arterial blood gases in pulmonary embolism stems from an incomplete understanding of the pathophysiology of the disorder. Because most emboli, unless massive, cause transient V/Q abnormalities, arterial blood gases taken some time after embolism has occurred may be unimpressive, particularly in normal patients. Nevertheless, it is unusual for patients with significant pulmonary emboli to have absolutely normal blood gas determinations, though abnormal results may be misleading in patients with underlying cardiopulmonary disease.

The chest radiograph can provide helpful information but is also limited. Pulmonary embolism rarely produces the classic x-ray finding of "Hampton's hump," a peripheral wedge-shaped infiltrate that is indicative of pulmonary infarct. Instead, the roentgenogram may show infiltrate, atelectasis, effusion, or some combination thereof.[24] The differential diagnosis of these findings includes pneumonia, postoperative effusion, and splinting from pain. About 20% of patients have a normal x-ray, and such a finding may simplify interpretation of the lung scan. A very large embolus may obliterate perfusion in one lung and, rarely, cause diminished vascular markings on the affected side.

Most Helpful Tests

The radionuclide lung scan is probably the most useful but misunderstood test for diagnosing pulmonary embolism. This safe and widely available tool employs two techniques. The perfusion scan detects infused labeled albumin after it has lodged in the pulmonary capillary bed. The ventilation scan detects the distribution of inhaled radioactive gas, usually xenon. Together, these two techniques provide a radiographic image of the V/Q pattern of the lung.

Several technical aspects of lung scanning are important. First, the latest scanning devices employ gamma cameras for radionuclide imaging. Gamma cameras give much better resolution and accuracy than the old rectilinear scanners, and all current statistics on lung scanning are based on gamma-camera technology. Second, experience in interpretation of lung scans is essential for diagnostic accuracy and should be supported by comparison of lung scan readings with pulmonary angiogram results.

Much of the controversy about lung scanning stems from unfair expectations of the technique's accuracy. Although lung scanning cannot absolutely confirm or exclude the presence of pulmonary embolism, it is very helpful in estimating its likelihood. Furthermore, the considerable controversy that exists about lung scan interpretation stems from a lack of uniform criteria in reading the scans. Certain lung scan patterns indicate either a very high or a very low likelihood of pulmonary embolism.[25,26] There is agreement that a totally negative perfusion lung scan with no defects rules out clinically important embolic disease. Other scan patterns are read according to their probabilities of indicating pulmonary embolism. For example, a high-probability perfusion scan would demonstrate segmental or lobar defects in areas of normal lung parenchyma on chest x-ray. A low-probability perfusion scan would demonstrate one or several small, nonsegmental defects. The accuracy of these perfusion scan readings ranges from 60% to 80%.[25-27] This relatively poor accuracy is the result of underlying cardiopulmonary disorders, such as obstructive lung disease or congestive heart failure, which are often seen on chest x-ray. Such disorders can alter V/Q relationships in the lung and produce perfusion defects. Obviously, these defects can also be produced by any condition that produces a pulmonary infiltrate.

In most series, addition of data from ventilation scanning improves the accuracy of lung scan interpretation.[25,27,28] Pulmonary emboli usually produce large perfusion defects with little or no change in ventilation. In contrast, most other disorders result in better V/Q matching, suggesting a low probability of pulmonary embolism. When indicative of either a high or a low probability of pulmonary embolism, V/Q scanning has an accuracy of about 85%. Scans with V/Q patterns that do not clearly fall into the high or low-probability categories are read as indeterminate. V/Q defects are often exhibited that exactly correspond to abnormalities on chest x-ray. Up to 25% of patients with indeterminate scans have pulmonary emboli on angiography. For screening purposes, particularly when the chest x-ray is normal, a perfusion scan alone may suffice. A totally normal perfusion scan excludes pulmonary embolus.

The lung scan gives the clinician a reasonably accurate estimate of the likelihood of pulmonary embolus. However, the results of the scan may be inconsistent with the clinical signs, and more invasive studies such as pulmonary angiography may be necessary. A suggested approach to data generated by lung scanning is illustrated in Figure 26-1. A low-probability scan may demand confirmation by angiography in the patient who has serious cardiopulmonary disease and in whom an additional clot could be fatal. Similarly, if anticoagulation is potentially dangerous, a high-probability scan should be supported by angiography.

Pulmonary angiography provides the most accurate though most invasive means of diagnosing pulmonary embolism. With selective injection and magnification, it is safe and reliable. In one large series, there were no documented deaths form pulmonary embolism in patients with negative angiograms.[29] Therefore, although it is argued that angiography can miss very small clots, such an error has no clinical importance. In a seriously ill patient with an equivocal lung scan or complications from anticoagulation, an angiogram may be necessary even if it requires transporting the patient to another institution.

TREATMENT

The treatment of thromboembolic disease is based on several important considera- tion. First, if the patient has tolerated thromboembolism reasonably well, ther- apy with anticoagulants is aimed at pre- venting further clot formation. This should allow clot organization and fibri- nolysis to occur. Most patients with DVT fall into this category. Second, if serious clot formation and migration occur when anticoagulation is adequate, or if antico- agulation is contraindicated, some form of venous interruption should be considered to prevent massive pulmonary embolism. Third, if a massive clot has already filled the pulmonary circulation, thrombolytic therapy may be employed to rapidly dis- solve the clot and reduce right-heart strain. Each of these therapeutic strategies is discussed below.

Anticoagulation

Only one controlled trial has examined the influence of anticoagulation on the mortality of pulmonary embolism.[30] De- spite technical limitations, this study strongly suggests that anticoagulation is beneficial. Much subsequent clinical ex- perience has confirmed this conclusion.[31]

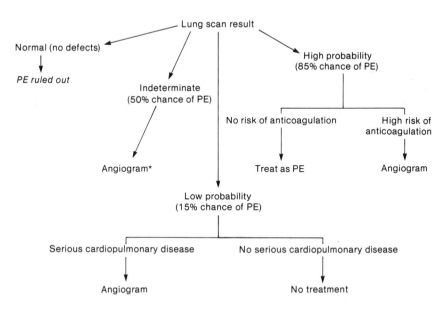

*If a pulmonary angiogram is unavailable, bilateral venograms may be used to document clot in venous system. However, this strategy may miss the 15% of patients with pulmonary emboli who have no demonstrable venous clot. PE = pulmonary embolism.

Fig. 26-1. Application of the lung scan.

The two drugs that are available for anticoagulation are heparin and coumarin. Heparin has the advantage of rapid onset, despite the necessity for parenteral administration. It has direct antithrombin effects, blocks factor IX activation, and inhibits activated factor X. Coumarin reduces the plasma levels of several clotting factors synthesized by the liver. However, this effect requires several days and is less predictable than that of heparin. For this reason, nearly all clinical experience in the acute treatment of thromboembolic disease has been with heparin.[31,32]

For all practical purposes, DVT and pulmonary embolism are treated identically with heparin. The goal in both disorders is to prevent further thrombus formation. There is evidence, most of it indirect, that there is an optimal range of heparin anticoagulation. The activated partial thromboplastin time (PTT) should be 1.5 to 2 times control, or the whole-blood clotting time should be 2 to 3 times control. Patients whose times fall below this anticoagulation range may have a higher recurrence rate of thromboembolic disease than others.[31,32] Anticoagulation beyond this range is associated with a greater number of bleeding complications.

The risk of bleeding on heparin is a major problem in the surgical patient. Significant hemorrhage occurs in 25% of patients who have undergone recent surgery, received intramuscular injections of platelet-suppressive drugs, or suffer from thrombocytopenia, uremia, or an underlying bleeding tendency.[32,33] Even without these conditions, 10% to 15% of surgical patients experience bleeding complications. Therefore, the use of heparin in the surgical population requires considerable clinical skill and judgment. Nonetheless, the risk of bleeding must be weighed against that of life-threatening thromboembolism. Some authors point out that

bleeding, except in special conditions such as intracranial surgery, can be effectively reversed.[31,32]

It is widely accepted that continuous infusion of heparin is associated with a decrease in hemorrhagic complications.[31,34,35] The anticoagulant effect of continuously infused heparin is more predictable than that of bolus therapy, since the latter may produce a temporary anticoagulant effect well beyond the therapeutic range. In addition, the total daily dosage required may be higher with the bolus method.

The recommended starting dosage of heparin for uncomplicated patients is an intravenous bolus of 5,000 units followed by a continuous infusion of 25,000 to 30,000 units in 24 hr. For intermittent infusion, 5,000 to 7,000 units are given every 6 hr. The PTT or whole-blood clotting time is measured 4 hr to 6 hr and 24 hr after the start of therapy and then daily thereafter. Patients with a high risk of bleeding should be started and maintained on somewhat lower doses, with a bolus of 2,000 to 4,000 units and a maintenance dose of 15,000 to 20,000 units over 24 hr. This strategy avoids any anticoagulant effect beyond the therapeutic range, and the dosage can then be adjusted to produce an effect in the lower portion of the range.[31,32] The dosage required to produce a therapeutic effect may fall after several days of treatment, and this should be anticipated. This fall may be due to consumption of heparin by active thrombosis. However, serious bleeding is unpredictable and should temper the empiric use of full-dose heparin without adequate documentation of thromboembolic disease.

If bleeding occurs during heparin therapy, there are several therapeutic alternatives. First, the dosage can be lowered or the drug discontinued. If bleeding is life-threatening, anticoagulation can be reversed with protamine. Second, the source of bleeding should be investigated and, if possible, corrected.[32] For example, gastrointestinal bleeding from stress ulceration may be effectively treated with antacids and cimetidine. Other common bleeding sources are cutdown sites, surgical wounds, and recent fractures. It is often possible to control bleeding with transfusions and temporary discontinuation of heparin while the primary bleeding source is treated. Often, heparin can be carefully reinstituted in low doses within several days. Experienced investigators have suggested titrating the heparin dose slowly into the low therapeutic range.[32] Some authors have even suggested that achieving so-called therapeutic levels of anticoagulation may not be necessary. Heparin has several anticoagulant effects in low doses and may be adequate for preventing propagation of clot in patients with a high risk of bleeding.[32] Although this suggestion has some theoretical merit, it has never been studied. If severe and unremitting bleeding occurs, serious consideration should be given to venous interruption.

Oral anticoagulants are used for long-term treatment of thromboembolic disease. A common clinical practice is to use heparin for 7 to 10 days and then to continue anticoagulation with coumarin. This practice is based on animal studies that show that endothelialization of clot is complete after 10 days.[31,32] Oral anticoagulation should be started at maintenance doses; no loading dose is necessary. Heparin should be continued until the prothrombin time (PT) becomes prolonged, indicating coumarin effect, in about 3 to 5 days. The coumarin dosage should be adjusted to maintain the PT at 1.5 to 2 times control.

There is some evidence from uncontrolled studies that oral anticoagulation for at least 3 months prevents recurrence of venous thromboembolism.[36] Prophylaxis beyond this time is probably not necessary in most patients. However, an occasional patient experiences recurrence months or years after anticoagulation has been discontinued. Such a patient may be a candidate for long-term anticoagulation.

The use of oral anticoagulants can be risky. In two carefully designed prospective studies, serious hemorrhage occurred in 10% of patients placed on coumarin for DVT.[33,37] Bleeding is particularly likely in patients who are elderly or unreliable about taking their medications or in patients with a potential bleeding site such as a peptic ulcer. The PT must be monitored frequently, since the effect of coumarin is influenced by many common drugs.

Two recent investigations focus on the use of low-dose heparin for long-term anticoagulation in thromboembolism. One study showed that low-dose heparin was as effective as oral anticoagulants for preventing recurrence, wheras the other showed that it was not.[33,37] Both studies found that bleeding complications were significantly greater with coumarin than with low-dose heparin. The studies were not identical in design, and methodologic differences hinder comparison. However, for long-term anticoagulation, some clinicians favor the use of low-dose heparin in a dose of 5000 units subcutaneously every 12 hr. Since there are virtually no hemorrhagic complications, dosage adjustment is not necessary.

Venous Blockade

Some patients do not respond to anticoagulation therapy. They continue to have pulmonary emboli with adequate anticoagulation or serious bleeding, which necessitates stopping anticoagulation. In either case, some mechanical means can be used to block migration of clot to the lungs. Although venous blockade is widely accepted, no controlled studies have documented when or how such blockade should be performed.

The three methods of venous blockade are vena caval ligation, plication, and insertion of an umbrella filter.[38] Each method has complications. Both ligation and plication of the vena cava require abdominal surgery. Ligation rapidly produces lower extremity edema, which can become chronic and disabling. Furthermore, collaterals large enough to transmit clot can develop over weeks or months. Plication, either by clipping or by suturing of the vena cava, is designed to allow blood flow through fenestrations small enough to block clot. However, these fenestrations may become occluded with clot, and caval interruption can result.[38] The umbrella filter can be placed intravenously into the vena cava without surgery.[39] Reported experience with this method has vairied, but, in experienced hands, the filter can usually be inserted under fluoroscopic guidance. Initial problems with filter dislodgment seem to have been overcome by better design. The filter may also fill with clot and thereby occlude the cava.

The decision to use any of these three techniques should be based on several important facts. There must be evidence that the patient is experiencing ongoing thrombosis in his venous capacitance bed while on effective anticoagulation. A venogram is necessary to document the venous clot burden. If the clinician suspects recurrent pulmonary emboli on anticoagulation, a pulmonary angiogram may be required as well.

If recurrent emboli are suspected, several steps should be taken. Anticoagulation therapy should be reviewed, and, if it is inadequate, appropriate dosage adjustments should be made. A repeat perfusion lung scan should also be obtained. A scan with no new defects compared to the previous scan argues strongly against recurrence. If new defects are present and other disease processes are ruled out clinically, the degree of clot burden should be estimated from the perfusion scan. With obliteration of the pulmonary vasculature of 20% or less, the patient with no cardiopulmonary disease may tolerate further clots. Such a patient should be observed closely, particularly during the first several days of heparin therapy, and caval interruption should be considered only if new scan defects develop. Venography and pulmonary angiography should be performed. Evidence of clot in the lung on an angiogram, new perfusion defects on a scan, and the presence of clot in large capacitance veins on a venogram argue for venous blockade.

The patient with bleeding complications from anticoagulation presents a slightly different set of problems. As mentioned above, such patients may be treated with lower doses of heparin than non-bleeding patients and more attention to the primary bleeding site. If this fails, venous blockade should be considered, but only after radiographic documentation of venous clot has been obtained. If pulmonary embolism is present, the clinical decision for caval blockade is similar to that for recurrent emboli. If there is little clot in the lung, low-dose heparin should be used in the bleeding patient before caval blockade is embarked upon. Poor cardiopulmonary reserve makes caval blockade necessary. These strategies for venous blockade are summarized in Figure 26-2.

The best method of caval blockade depends on the experience of the institution and the underlying condition of the patient. Seriously ill patients are not good candidates for abdominal surgery to interrupt or clip the cava; for them, the vena cava umbrella is a better choice. However, for other patients, the choice may not be so clear. Inserting the umbrella requires experience, and some clinicians feel that the caval clip in selected patients gives sufficiently good results with minimal complications. Most surgeons tend to avoid caval plication because of the immediate increase it causes in lower extremity venous pressure and resultant edema.

Thrombolytic Agents and Embolectomy

The multicenter Urokinase Pulmonary Embolism Trial (UPET) generated much information about the natural history and treatment of pulmonary embolism. The trial showed that thrombolytic therapy with urokinase did not decrease mortality over heparin therapy.[40] The reason for these results was more apparent as the natural history of treated pulmonary embolism became clearer. Few patients die of pulmonary embolism when it is recognized and treated with heparin.[9] Sudden deaths occur when the disease is unrecognized and untreated. Rarely do patients present with massive pulmonary

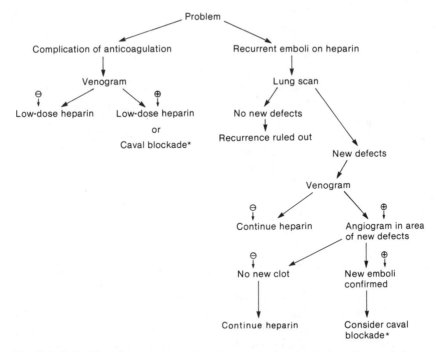

*A clinical decision depends on cardiopulmonary reserve and the volume of clot in venous capacitance vessels.

Fig. 26-2. Approach to caval blockade.

embolism on the brink of death. Because of pulmonary vascular reserve and fibrinolysis, even patients with massive emboli may respond well to anticoagulation and supportive therapy alone.

The thrombolytic drugs streptokinase and urokinase activate plasminogen and accelerate clot lysis. These agents can reduce clot burden in the pulmonary circulation and lower pulmonary artery pressure and right-heart strain.[32] However, since most patients do not present with right-heart failure, it is not surprising that thrombolytic therapy has not improved survival rates. Some authors have encouraged the liberal use of thrombolytic therapy, particularly when clot obliterates at least 40% of the pulmonary circulation, but this recommendation has not been supported by controlled study. There is some indirect evidence that the pulmonary microcirculation may be better restored with thrombolytics than with other therapy.[41]

Thrombolytic drugs are difficult to use without clinical experience.[32,42] Bleeding complications are high, and febrile and allergic reactions are common. These agents are contraindicated postoperatively and in patients who have an inflammatory site that is likely to bleed. In the surgical patient, these drugs should be considered only in the most desperate situations, when all other supportive measures have been unsuccessful. The details of thrombolytic therapy have been recently reviewed.[42]

Embolectomy to remove clot from the pulmonary artery has generally been unsuccessful in decreasing mortality. There have been some small, uncontrolled series of patients undergoing embolectomy, but none has shown improved survival.[43,44] Since embolectomy is reserved for only the most desperately ill patients, its mortality is high. However, it is likely that mortality with medical therapy in these patients would be equally high.

PROPHYLAXIS

Considerable research has been devoted to the prophylaxis of thromboebolic disease in surgical patients.[45] Most propective studies of prophylaxis have used radioactive fibrinogen scanning or venography to diagnose venous thrombosis. A small number of studies have also examined prophylaxis in pulmonary embolism and have based their diagnosis on the development of new lung scan defects or death from pulmonary embolism. The best approach to the many reported studies is examination of surgical subgroups, since each subgroup seems to behave differently with regard to prophylaxis.

The first and most widely studied population consists of patients undergoing thoracoabdominal surgery. There is substantial evidence from a variety of well-controlled double-blind studies that low-dose heparin reduces venous thrombosis from about 30% to less than 10%.[46,47] This effect may result from the ability of heparin even in low concentrations to accelerate the activity of antithrombin III. The latter is a potent inhibitor of activated clotting factor X.

The prevention of pulmonary embolism by low-dose heparin is less certain. The largest multicenter trial carried out showed a reduction in fatal pulmonary embolus with low-dose heparin. However, the reasons for this reduction were unclear. Overall mortality was no different in the control and prophylaxis groups.[10] Two other studies used perfusion scans supplemented by autopsy or embolectomy data to document pulmonary embolism. Both found a lower incidence of pulmonary embolism in heparin-treated than in control groups.[47,48]

Two independent investigations have cast some doubt on the usefulness of fibrinogen leg scanning in prophylaxis studies. In each of these studies, patients with venogram-proven femoral thrombosis or fatal pulmonary embolism had negative radioactive fibrinogen scans.[49,50] Therefore, although heparin may reduce calf vein thrombosis, its effect on thrombosis in more proximal, large veins, where most pulmonary emboli originate, is largely undocumented. However, the consensus is that low-dose heparin reduces venous thrombosis and fatal pulmonary embolism in the general surgical population.[10,34,45] Except in cases of pre-existing bleeding sited or platelet dysfunction, there have been few hemorrhagic complications of low-dose heparin in general surgical patients.

The American Heart Association currently recommends that all patients undergoing thoracoabdominal surgery receive low-dose heparin. The patient should not receive any antiplatelet drugs for 5 days before surgery, and all clotting studies should be normal. The recommended doses are 5000 units 2 hr before surgery and every 8 hr to 12 hr thereafter until the patient is ambulatory or discharged. Such prophylaxis in surgical patients could save an estimated 4000 to 8000 lives annually.

Low-dose heparin prophylaxis has been less effective in several other high-risk patient groups. Patients undergoing open prostatectomy do not clearly benefit from low-dose heparin prophylaxis. Two small series show opposite results, a third no beneficial effect, and a fourth reduction of venous thrombosis from 42% to 6% with low-dose heparin.[7,51–53] Therefore, low-dose heparin therapy in prostatectomy

and perhaps in other urologic procedures is probably not as effective in preventing venous thrombosis as it is in general surgery procedures.[2,19]

The question of prophylaxis against venous thrombosis is even more difficult in the case of patients who have had hip fractures or are undergoing hip surgery, because these patients have a high incidence of both venous thrombosis and fatal pulmonary embolism. The pathogenesis of venous thrombosis in these patients may be different from that in other patients, and direct trauma to the femoral vein may play a role. The area around the hip cannot be evaluated with fibrinogen scanning; accurate detection of proximal venous thrombosis is possible only with venography.[2,19] Unfortunately, although many reports focus on hip surgery, most have serious methodologic problems, including unblinded interpretations of scan and venogram data, reliance on fibrinogen scanning alone, and lack of adequate controls.[2,19]

The majority of studies show that low-dose heparin offers little protection from venous thrombosis in patients undergoing hip surgery.[2,19] Pooled data from a number of studies indicate that the incidence of venous thrombosis is 40% to 50% in control patients and 28% in those treated with low-dose heparin.[19,54] This modest reduction is hardly comparable to the substantial decrease that occurs among general surgical patients treated with this regimen. For this reason, alternative prophylaxis regimens have been examined for patients undergoing hip surgery.

Two antiplatelet drugs, aspirin and dextran, have been studied extensively in hip surgery. There is conflicting information about the efficacy of aspirin in preventing venous thrombosis. Using venography, one study documented the incidence of venous thrombosis to be 80% with aspirin.[55] Another revealed venous thrombosis in 80% of patients treated with low-dose heparin and in only 36% of those given aspirin.[6] Two other studies investigated the effect of aspirin prophylaxis on the incidence of pulmonary embolism in hip surgery. In one, aspirin decreased the incidence of nonfatal pulmonary emboli from 4% to 0.4%, and, in the second, a large, randomized, double-blind trial, aspirin decreased the incidence of fatal pulmonary emboli from 7% to 1%.[57] These results suggest that aspirin may have some effect in reducing the proximal-vein thrombosis that leads to pulmonary emboli.

The data regarding dextran are also unclear in the context of hip surgery. Studies using fibrinogen scanning alone have shown disappointing results.[2] However, in two studies in which venography was used for detection there was a reduction in the incidence of venous thrombosis from 40% to 10%.[58,59] The incidence of pulmonary embolism decreased from 10% to 2% when dextran was used.[2] The evidence therefore suggests that dextran is beneficial in cases of hip surgery.[2,19] However, it is expensive, requires daily intravenous dosing, and carries the risk of renal failure, anaphylaxis, and fluid overload.

Warfarin has consistently been shown to be effective in preventing venous thrombosis in high-risk patients undergoing hip surgery.[2,6,60,61] It also appears to cause a significant reduction in fatal pulmonary embolism, from 7% to less than 1%.[60] As with dextran, the major disadvantage of warfarin is bleeding, which can be particularly serious in hip surgery.

Aspirin, dextran, and warfarin have all been shown to be useful prophylactic agents in hip surgery. Dextran and warfarin are probably superior, but their benefits are counterbalanced by the increased risk of bleeding. Aspirin can be given in a dose of 650 mg twice daily after surgery. Dextran, 500 to 1000 ml, should be infused during anesthesia and is usually given for several days after surgery. Warfarin should be started before surgery but, in order for bleeding to be avoided, the PT should probably not be brought up to therapeutic levels until after surgery. The safety and efficacy of these drugs in hip surgery patients are not comparable to those of low-dose heparin in general surgical patients. A combination of drugs may ultimately prove more effective.[2,19]

Patients undergoing neurosurgical procedures pose a different problem. Although the incidence of venous thrombosis is this population is similar to that among general surgical patients, most neurosurgeons are unwilling to use drugs that increase the risk of bleeding. There have therefore been no controlled drug trials in neurosurgical patients. In one uncontrolled study in elective neurosurgery patients, low-dose heparin did not cause any adverse effects from bleeding.[62]

Physical measures designed to prevent venous stasis have been the treatment most widely studied in neurosurgical patients. The most effective of these is the pneumatic compression patients. The most effective of these is the pneumatic compression boot, an external device that compresses the lower extremities to promote venous blood flow. The boot can be applied during the surgical procedure, but, in most series, it is used after surgery. Two well-designed studies have shown a reduction in venous thrombosis in neurosurgery patients from 20% to 1.5% with the boot.[63,64] These results are comparable to the success of low-dose heparin in general surgical patients.

Physical measures have also been studied in other patient groups. The pneumatic compression boot has been used with apparently favorable results in patients undergoing hip surgery, but many studies suffer from suboptimal design.[2,19] The pneumatic boot does not appear to be beneficial in patients with malignancy undergoing surgery.[65] Other physical measures that have been evaluated include elastic stodkings and electrical muscle stimulation. Stockings that provide graded pressure up the entire leg can increase venous flow and may reduce venous thrombosis from 40% to 10% in general surgical patients, but these figures do not apply to older tube stockings.[66,67] Even the protection afforded by graded compression stockings is modest compared to that of low-dose heparin. Electrical stimulation of calf muscles increases venous flow and probably reduces venous thrombosis almost as well as low-dose heparin.[2,19] However, it is painful and has no practical role in the patient who is awake.

THE FAT EMBOLISM SYNDROME

Patients who have suffered serious trauma may develop neurologic and respiratory abnormalities attributed to the fat embolism syndrome (FES). Usually, the patient has sustained multiple fractures or a major fracture to a long bone. Less commonly, he has undergone complex orthopedic surgery, such as total hip replacement. Within 12 hr to 72 hr of such trauma, the patient develops fever, unexplained respiratory distress, mental confusion, and, often, a petechial rash. There may be progression to frank respiratory failure and coma, sometimes accompanied by renal failure.[68-70] The respiratory process resembles the adult respiratory distress syndrome (ARDS), with noncardiac pulmonary edema, a high al-

veolar–arterial oxygen gradient, and stiff lungs. The neurologic picture may begin with mild confusion and progress to stupor and coma without focal neurologic signs. This syndrome is seen in about 5% of trauma patients and carries an estimated mortality of 10% to 20%, usually from irreversible respiratory failure.[71] Its pathogenesis is incompletely understood, but, at autopsy, fat deposits are found in many organs, particularly in the lung and brain.[70]

The source of this fat deposition remains controversial.[68,69,72] An old and popular theory proposes that the fracture of long bones disrupts the adipose architecture of the marrow. Adipose tissue is extruded into the circulation and gives rise to fat emboli. A second theory hypothesizes that the stress of trauma induces biochemical changes in the circulation, causing the aggregation of circulating chylomicrons as fat droplets and their deposition in various organs. There are studies to support both theories, but, at the moment, neither pathogenetic theory offers practical information for treating or preventing FES.

Regardless of its origin, fat can derange organ function in several ways. Intravascular fat deposits may cause circulatory sludging and resultant ischemia. In the lung, the fat load may be sufficiently high to elevate pulmonary artery pressure and produce cor pulmonale. More commonly, however, diffuse alveolar capillary leak develops, similar to that seen in ARDS. ARDS occurs in many clinical settings, and its pathogenesis is usually obscure. However, in FES, the mechanism of ARDS may have a biochemical basis. Since the lung is rich in lipases, fat deposits may be readily degraded into free fatty acids. These compounds or other products may be toxic to the lung.[68]

Circulating fat may also cause platelet

aggregation, leading to the thrombocytopenia and petechiae often seen in patients with FES. Platelet collections may also release serotonin, which can exacerbate V/Q abnormalities in the lung.[68,69]

Clinical Features

The diagnosis of FES should be considered in any patient with fractures who develops respiratory distress, mental confusion, or petechial hemorrhage, particularly within the first 3 days of trauma. Respiratory distress may appear only as mild tachypnea or may be fulminant, with rapid progression to respiratory failure. Mental confusion may range from restlessness and mild disorientation to stupor and deep coma. The petechial rash occurs exclusively on the upper part of the body in the axillae, chest, flanks, conjunctiva, and, occasionally, soft palate. Sometimes fat can be seen in retinal vessels. Fever and tachycardia are common.

Laboratory data may reveal mild to severe thrombocytopenia and mild anemia. Elevations in serum lipase levels and lipiduria occur, but both can also be found in trauma patients without FES.[68,69] An ECG may show ischemia or right-heart strain with cor pulmonale. The chest roentgenogram early in the course may be normal, but a pattern suggesting pulmonary edema is usually seen if respiratory failure develops.[68,69,72] Arterial blood gases are useful for documentation of the progression of respiratory impairment.

Differential Diagnosis

The classic patient with confusion, respiratory distress, and petechiae poses little diagnostic problem. However, FES can present as isolated neurologic or pulmonary disease, and this may cause diagnostic confusion. The confused trauma patient may have suffered cerebral injury, such as an intracranial bleed, which may take hours or days to become manifest. The elderly patient, particularly if he is receiving analgesics, may become easily confused if metabolic changes such as hypoxia develop. Respiratory failure has multiple causes, including lung contusion, pneumonia, congestive heart failure, and pulmonary embolism.

There is no single laboratory test that confirms the diagnosis of FES. The clinician must therefore rely on a combination of clinical features and laboratory aids to make the diagnosis. However, certain facts are helpful. The development of FES is unlikely after the third day following trauma. Arterial hypoxemia is an invariable feature of FES regardless of whether it progresses to respiratory failure.[71] If respiratory failure supervenes, the pulmonary process most closely resembles noncardiac pulmonary edema. A petechial rash on the upper part of the body and fat in the retinal vessels are very suggestive of FES. Laboratory tests are nonspecific, but markedly elevated serum lipase levels or significant lipiduria may be helpful.[68] The patient with mental confusion or respiratory distress occurring within 3 days of a fracture should be carefully evaluated for the neurologic and pulmonary processes mentioned above. If no specific other diagnosis is clear, and particularly if a petechial rash develops, the diagnosis of FES can usually be made.

Treatment

The treatment of FES is supportive. Respiratory failure should be treated with supplemental oxygen and artificial ventilation if necessary. If percentages of oxygen greater than 50% are required, positive end-expiratory pressure may improve the alveolar–arterial oxygen gradient and reduce the oxygen requirement. Measurement of pulmonary capillary wedge pressure can be used to assess intravascular volume, since fluid overload can aggravate respiratory failure. The patient should be rigorously monitored for nosomial infection and barotrauma, both common complications of artificial ventilation.

A number of drugs have been used to treat fat embolism. There is agreement that massive doses of corticosteroids (e.g., methylprednisolone, 10 to 15 mg/kg/day for 4 to 5 days) are beneficial in FES.[68,69,72,73] Steroids may reduce inflammation, stabilize lyosomes, reverse bronchospasm, and decrease cerebral edema, but none of these actions has been proved in controlled studies. However, there is anecdotal evidence that steroids influence the clinical course of FES.[73,74] Two other drugs, heparin and intravenous alcohol, have fallen into disrepute since neither has been shown to be beneficial.[68,69,72] Lipolytic agents have also been tried without convincing success. Diuretics are often mentioned in the treatment of the respiratory failure of FES. If fluid overload occurs, they can lower left atrial pressure and minimize fluid leak into the lungs. However, their use must be guided by measurements of pulmonary capillary wedge pressure to prevent over-aggressive diuresis, which can seriously compromise cardiac output and oxygen delivery.

Prevention

Besides early immobilization of fractures, there are no known measures to prevent FES. Early recognition of FES may lead to prompt treatment with corticosteroids, but it is uncertain whether or not early intervention affects the clinical course. Patients undergoing elective orthopedic procedures, particularly those involving the hip, can develop FES.[68] Total hip replacement in particular significantly traumatizes the medulla of the femur when the femoral component of the prosthesis is inserted. Release of marrow fat occurs when unusual force is needed to seat the femoral prosthesis and can be decreased by venting of the femoral intramedullary canal during the procedure.

SUMMARY

1. **Pulmonary embolism should be considered in any surgical patient with dyspnea, pleuritic pain, or unexplained drop in blood pressure. Physical findings, short of signs of acute cor pulmonale or a pleural rub, are not helpful in the diagnosis pulmonary embolism.**

2. **Conventional laboratory tests are usually of little help in the diagnosis of pulmonary embolism. Normal arterial blood gas parameters are unusual in pulmonary embolism, but abnormal values are nonspecific. Acute right-heart strain on ECG strongly suggests pulmonary embolism but is rare. Chest x-ray often shows nonspecific findings of infiltrate, effusion, or atelectasis. Lung scanning provides probabilities of pulmonary embolism based on patterns of V/Q abnormalities. A low- or high-probability V/Q scan has an accuracy of 85% in experienced hands. This figure falls substantially for perfusion scanning alone, although a normal perfusion scan with no defects rules out pulmonary embolism. The angiogram is the most accurate but technically most**

complex study for diagnosis of pulmonary embolism; it should be employed if other laboratory tests are equivocal.

3. All patients with thromboembolic disease should be treated with anticoagulants unless there is danger of serious bleeding. Heparin should be used for 7 to 10 days to allow clot stabilization and lysis. Continuous infusion causes fewer bleeding complications than bolus therapy. Anticoagulant effect should be monitored to produce a PTT of 1.5 to 2 times control or a whole-blood clotting time of 2 to 3 times control. Bleeding complications should be treated with reduction of dose or cessation of therapy and correction of the underlying disorder. Frequently, heparin can be restarted in lower doses with no bleeding recurrence. Oral anticoagulation should commence in the second week of treatment and continue for 3 months. Low-dose heparin for long-term treatment is a potential alternative, though its effectiveness remains unproved.

4. Vena caval blockade may be indicated for (1) patients with recurrent pulmonary emboli on therapeutic doses of heparin and clot in their capacitance veins and (2) patients with thromboembolic disease who have serious bleeding complications on anticoagulation and still have clot in their capacitance veins. The choice of technique for venous interruption depends on the condition of the patient and local experience with these techniques.

5. Thrombolytic therapy may be dangerous in the surgical population because of the risk of bleeding. This therapy should be reserved for desperately ill patients who have not responded to conventional treatment. Pulmonary embolectomy has not been shown to improve survival and should rarely be attempted.

6. Low-dose heparin should be employed in patients undergoing thoracoabdominal surgery who have no prior bleeding tendency. Physical measures such as pneumatic compression may also be used as alternatives, but only boot compression yields results equal to those of low-dose heparin.

7. In patients undergoing hip surgery and open prostatectomy, there is a high risk of thrombosis, and low-dose heparin is ineffective. Aspirin, dextran, and warfarin have been demonstrated to be effective in patients undergoing hip surgery, but bleeding complications may supervene. Pneumatic boot compression has been modestly helpful. The most successful regimen for prophylaxis may be a combination of drugs and physical measures, but this possibility awaits the results of further studies.

8. FES should be considered in any patient with confusion, respiratory distress, and petechiae within 3 days of trauma. Corticosteroids such as methylprednisolone in doses of 10 to 15 mg/kg/day for 5 days appear to be beneficial. Heparin and intravenous alcohol should not be used.

REFERENCES

1. Rose SD: Prophylaxis of thromboembolic disease. Med Clin North Am 63:1205, 1979
2. Flanc C, Kakkar VV, Clarke MB: The detection of venous thrombosis of the legs using ¹²⁵I-labelled fibrinogen. Br J Surg 55:742, 1968
3. Kakkar VV, Howe CT, Nicolaides AN et al: Deep vein thrombosis of the leg. Is there a high risk group? Am J Surg 120:527, 1970
4. Gallus AS, Hirsh J, Tuttle RJ et al: Small

subcutaneous doses of heparin in prevention of postoperative deep vein thrombosis. N Engl J Med 293:1296, 1975

5. Gordon–Smith IC, LeQuesne LP, Grundy DJ, et al: Controlled trial of two regimens of subcutaneous heparin in prevention of postoperative deep vein thrombosis. Lancet 1:1133, 1972

6. Harris WH, Salzman LW, Athanasoulis C et al: Comparison of warfarin, low molecular weight dextran, aspirin and subcutaneous heparin in prevention of venous thromboembolism following total hip replacement. J Bone Joint Surg (Am) 56:1552, 1974

7. Kumowski M, Vandendris M, Steinberger R et al: Prevention of postoperative deep vein thrombosis by low dose heparin in urological surgery. Urol Res 5:123, 1977

8. Nicholaides AN, Field CS, Kakkar VV et al: Prostatectomy and deep vein thrombosis. Br J Surg 59:487, 1972

9. Dalen JE, Alpert JS: Natural history of pulmonary embolism. Prog Cardiovasc Dis 17:259, 1975

10. International Multi-centre Trial: Prevention of fatal postoperative pulmonary embolism by low doses of heparin. Lancet 2:45, 1975

11. Browse NC, Clemenson G, Croft DN: Fibrinogen detectable thrombosis in the legs and pulmonary embolism. Br Med J 1:603, 1974

12. Moser RM: State of the art—Pulmonary embolism. Am Rev Respir Dis 115:829, 1977

13. Heatley RV, Morgan A, Hughes LB et al: Preoperative or postoperative deep vein thrombosis? Lancet 1:437, 1976

14. Kakkar VV: The ^{125}I-labelled fibrinogen test and phlebography in the diagnosis of deep vein thrombosis. Milbank Mem Fund Q 50:206, 1972

15. Mansfield AO: Alteration in fibrinolysis associated with surgery and venous thrombosis. Br J Surg 59:754, 1972

16. Havig O: Deep vein thrombosis and pulmonary embolism. Acta Chir Scand Suppl 478:1, 1977

17. McIntyre KM, Sasahara AA: Hemodynamic and ventricular responses to pulmonary embolism. Prog Cardiovasc Dis 17:175, 1979

18. Kakkar VV, Corrigin TP: Detection of deep vein thrombosis: Surgery and current status. Prog Cardiovasc Dis 17:207, 1974

19. Sasahara AA, Sharma GVRK, Parisi AF: New developments in the detection and prevention of venous thromboembolism. Am J Cardiol 43:1214, 1979

20. Bell WR, Simon TL: The clinical features of submassive and massive pulmonary emboli. Am J Med 62:355, 1977

21. Bynum LJ, Crotty C, Wilson JE: Use of fibrinogen/fibrin degradation products and soluble fibrin complexes for differentiation of pulmonary embolism from nonthrombotic lung disease. Am Rev Respir Dis 114:285, 1976

22. Stein PD, Dalen J, McIntyre KM et al: The electrocardiogram in acute pulmonary embolism. Prog Cardiovasc Dis 17:247, 1975

23. Wilson JE, Pierce AK, Johnson RL Jr et al: Hypoxemia in pulmonary embolism. A clinical study. J Clin Invest 50:481, 1971

24. Bynum LJ, Wilson JE: Radiographic features of pleural effusions in pulmonary embolism. Am Rev Respir Dis 117:829, 1978

25. McNeil BJ: A diagnostic strategy using ventilation–perfusion studies in patients suspect for pulmonary embolism. J Nucl Med 17:613, 1976

26. Moses DC, Silver TM, Bookstein JJ: The complementary roles of chest radiography, lung scanning and selective pulmonary angiography in the diagnosis of pulmonary embolism. Circulation 49:179, 1974

27. Alderson PO, Rujanavech N, Secker–Walker RH et al: The role of 133 XE ventilation studies in the scientific detection of pulmonary embolism. Radiology 120:633, 1976

28. Bogren HG, Berman DS, Vismara LA et al: Lung ventilation–perfusion scintography in pulmonary embolism. Acta Radiol [Diagn] (Stockh) 19:933, 1978

29. Novelline RA, Baltavowich OH, Athanasoulis CA et al: The clinical course of pa-

tients with suspected pulmonary embolism and a negative pulmonary arteriogram. Radiology 126:561, 1978

30. Barrit DW, Jordan SC: Anticoagulant drugs in the treatment of pulmonary embolism. A controlled trial. Lancet 1:1309, 1960

31. Gallus AS, Hirsh J: Treatment of venous thromboembolic disease. Semin Thromb Hemostas 2:291, 1976

32. Genton E, Hirsh J: Observations in anticoagulant and thrombolytic therapy in pulmonary embolism. Prog Cardiovasc Dis 17:335, 1975

35. Hull R, Delmore T, Genton E et al: Warfarin sodium versus low-dose heparin in the long-term treatment of venous thrombosis. N Engl J Med 301:855, 1979

34. Sherry S: Low-dose heparin for the prophylaxis of pulmonary embolism. Am Rev Respir Dis 114:661, 1976

35. Salzman EW, Deykin D, Shapiro RM et al: Management of heparin therapy. Controlled prospective trial. N Engl J Med 292:1046, 1975

36. Coon WW, Willis PW: Recurrence of venous thromboembolism. Surgery 73:823, 1973

37. Bynum LJ, Wilson JE: Low-dose heparin therapy in the long-term management of venous thromboembolism. Am J Med 67:553, 1979

38. Crane C: Venous interruption for pulmonary embolism: Present status. Prog Cardiovasc Dis 17:329, 1975

39. Mobin-Uddin R, Utley JR, Bryant LR: The inferior vena cava umbrella filter. Prog Cardiovasc Dis 17:391, 1975

40. Urokinase–streptokinase embolism trial and phase 2 results. A cooperative study. JAMA 229:1606, 1974

41. Sharma GVK, Burleson VA, Sasahara AA: Effect of thrombolytic therapy on pulmonary capillary blood volume in patients with pulmonary embolism. N Engl J Med 303:842, 1980

42. Bell WR, Meek AG: Guidelines for the use of thrombolytic agents. N Engl J Med 301:1266, 1979

43. Alpert JS, Smith RE, Ockene IS et al: Treat-

ment of massive pulmonary embolism: The role of pulmonary embolectomy. Am Heart J 89:413, 1975

44. Miller GAH, Hall RJC, Paneth M: Pulmonary embolectomy, heparin and streptokinase: Their place in the treatment of acute massive pulmonary embolism. Am Heart J 93:568, 1977

45. Rose SD: Prophylaxis of thromboembolic disease. Med Clin North Am 63:1205, 1979

46. Kakkar VV, Spindler J, Plute PT et al: Efficacy of low doses of heparin in prevention of deep vein thrombosis after major surgery: A double-blind randomized trial. Lancet 2:101, 1972

47. Lahnborg G, Friman L, Bergstrom K et al: Effect of low-dose heparin on incidence of postoperative pulmonary embolism detected by photoscanning. Lancet 1:329, 1974

48. Kiil J, Kiil J, Axelsen P et al: Prophylaxis against postoperative pulmonary embolism and deep vein thrombosis by low dose heparin. Lancet 1:1115, 1978

49. Gruber UP, Pridrich R, Duckert F et al: Prevention of postoperative thromboembolism by dextran 40, low doses of heparin or xantinol nicotinate. Lancet 1:207, 1977

50. Groote Schurr Hospital Thromboembolus Study Group: Failure of low dose heparin to prevent significant thromboembolic complications in high risk surgical patients: Interim report of prospective trial. Br Med J 1:603, 1979

52. Browse NL, Negus D: Prevention of postoperative leg vein thrombosis by electrical muscle stimulation. An evaluation of [125]iodine-labelled fibrinogen. Br Med J 3:615, 1970

53. Coe NP, Collins RE, Klein L et al: Prevention of deep vein thrombosis in urological patients: A controlled, randomized trial of low-dose heparin and external pneumatic compression boots. Surgery 83:230, 1978

54. Venous Thrombosis Clinical Study Group: Small doses of subcutaneous sodium heparin in the prevention of deep vein thrombosis after elective hip operations. Br J Surg 62:348, 1975

55. Stamatakis JD, Kakkar VV, Lawrence D et al: Failure of aspirin to prevent postoperative deep vein thrombosis in patients undergoing total hip replacement. Br Med J 1:1031, 1978

56. Hume M, Turner RH, Kuriatiose T et al: Venous thrombosis after total hip replacement—Combined monitoring as a guide for prophylaxis and treatment. J Bone Joint Surg (Am) 58A:933, 1976

57. Zekert F, Kohn P: Eine randomisierte Studie über die postoperative Thromboseprophylaxe mit Acetylsalicylsaure. Med Welt 27:1372, 1976

58. Johnson SR, Bygdeman S, Eliasson R: Effect of dextran on postoperative thrombosis. Acta Clin Scand (Suppl) 387:80, 1968

59. Evarts CM, Peil CJ: Prevention of thromboembolic disease after elective surgery of the hip. J Bone Joint Surg (Am) 53A:1271, 1971

60. Morris GK, Mitchell JRA: Warfarin sodium in prevention of deep venous thrombosis and pulmonary embolism in patients with fractured neck of femur. Lancet 2:869, 1976

61. Hamilton HW, Crawford JS, Gardiner JH et al: Venous thrombosis in patients with fracture of the upper end of the femur: A phlebographic study of the effect of prophylactic anticoagulation. J Bone Joint Surg (Am) 52B:268, 1970

62. Barnett HG, Clifford JR, Llewellyn RC: Safety of mini-dose heparin administration for neurosurgical patients. J Neurosurg 47:27, 1977

63. Turpie AGG, Gallus AS, Beattie WS et al: Prevention of venous thrombosis in patients with intracranial disease by intermittent pneumatic compression of the calf. Neurology 27:435, 1977

64. Skellman JJ, Collins RCC, Coe NP et al: Prevention of deep venous thrombosis in neurosurgical patients: A controlled randomized trial of external pneumatic compression boots. Surgery 83:354, 1978

65. Hills NH, Pflug JJ, Jeyasingh K et al: Prevention of deep venous thrombosis by intermittent compression of calf. Br Med J 1:131, 1972

66. Schurr JH, Ibrahim SZ, Faber RG et al: The efficacy of graduated compression stockings in the prevention of deep vein thrombosis. Br J Surg 64:371, 1977

67. Holford CP: Graded compression for preventing deep venous thrombosis. Br Med J 2:969, 1976

68. Oh WH, Mital MA: Fat embolism: Current concepts of pathogenesis, diagnosis, and treatment. Orthop Clin North Am 9:769, 1978

69. Gossling HR, Donahue TA: The fat embolism syndrome. JAMA 241:2740, 1979

70. Dines DE, Burgher LW, Okazaki H: The clinical and pathologic correlation of fat embolism syndrome. Mayo Clin Proc 50:407, 1975

71. Peltier LF, Collins JA, Evants CM et al: Fat embolism. Arch Surg 109:12, 1974

72. Benatar SR, Ferguson AD, Goldschmidt RB: Fat embolism—Some clinical observations and a review of controversial aspects. QJ Med 41:85, 1972

73. Fischer JE, Turner RH, Herndon HH et al: Massive steroid therapy in severe fat embolism. Surg Gynecol Obstet 132:667, 1971

74. Ashbaugh DG, Petty TL: The use of corticosteroids in the treatment of respiratory failure associated with massive fat embolism. Surg Gynecol Obstet, 123:493, 1966

The Risks of Surgery in Patients with Asthma

PAUL C. ATKINS

Bronchial asthma is a chronic disease that affects 25 million Americans.[1,2] Airway obstruction due to asthma is totally reversible, unlike that occurring in congestive heart failure or chronic obstructive pulmonary disease. Often, middle-aged and elderly patients with histories of smoking have chronic cardiac or irreversible lung disease, making it impossible for the degree of reversible airway disease secondary to bronchial asthma *per se* to be defined precisely. Even in these circumstances, however, it is helpful to divide the disease processes into three categories: (1) irreversible fixed lung disease or chronic obstructive pulmonary disease; (2) reversible pulmonary dysfunction due to congestive heart failure or cardiac asthma; and (3) reversible respiratory disease due to asthma, which is by definition responsive to bronchodilators. The first two of these categories are discussed in other chapters. This chapter will focus on accurately characterizing asthma and its implications in the perioperative patient.

PATHOPHYSIOLOGY OF ASTHMA

The pathophysiology of asthma includes two basic abnormalities. The first is air-way hyperactivity, as demonstrated by increased sensitivity to nonspecific irritants (sulfur dioxide, nitrous oxide, citric acid), histamine, prostaglandin $F_{2\alpha}$, and cholinergic stimuli.[3] Whether this is secondary to an increased number of cholinergic receptors, a decreased number of beta-adrenergic receptors, or primary abnormalities in airway smooth muscle is unknown.[4] Second is edema of the bronchial wall and increased mucus secretion in the bronchial lumen.[5] Whether this is secondary to specific or nonspecific mast cell activation, release of mediators, or decreased beta-adrenergic and/or increased cholinergic activity is unclear.[6,7] Hyperirritability and mucus secretion lead to bronchial plugging, ventilation–perfusion imbalance, and clinical attacks of asthma. Therapy should be directed toward correction of both of these abnormalities.

SURGICAL RISK IN THE ASTHMATIC PATIENT

There are no controlled studies estimating surgical risk in asthmatic patients, partly because of the difficulty of defining asthma separately from chronic obstructive pulmonary disease. In some series, chronic bronchitis has been found to complicate asthma in 50% to 60% of patients.[8] Most authors consider the risk of surgery in asthma to be similar to that in chronic obstructive lung disease.[9]

Among patients with all types of pre-existing lung disease, 10% to 20% experience perioperative pulmonary complications. These complications, which include postoperative infection, atelectasis, and exacerbation of baseline disease sometimes leading to respiratory failure, are fully discussed in Chapters 23 and 24.[10] Perioperative factors that may exacerbate asthma include endotracheal intubation; anesthesia; dehydration with resulting increased sputum inspissation; and the patient's inability to clear secretions adequately because of pain, placement in the recumbent position, and the effects of various medications.[8,11-13] Endotracheal intubation, the major factor in asthmatic flares, probably irritates upper airway receptors.[14] Such irritation can be minimized by use of halothane, which allows for ease of induction and control of anesthesia and causes less postoperative secretion and bronchial hyperirritability than ether and other anesthetics.[14] However, ether can also be used safely in patients with asthma.[14] Premedications such as codeine, morphine, and cholinergic agonists can exacerbate asthma by nonspecific mediator release from mast cells or by aggravation of pre-existing abnormalities mentioned above. They should be avoided.[15]

EVALUATION OF THE ASTHMATIC PATIENT

Asthma is often a subclinical disease, and significant airway abnormalities may persist for 6 weeks after symptoms have subsided.[16] The patient may present with dyspnea, chest tightness, or chronic cough without wheezing.[17,18] Because significant impairment of pulmonary function can occur without symptoms, history and physical examination may not accurately indicate the severity of the asthma.[19]

Table 27-1 classifies patients with asthma according to severity. Preoperative evaluation of the asthmatic patient begins with verification of the diagnosis. Other conditions, such as congestive heart failure and chronic irreversible obstructive pulmonary disease, must be excluded. An atypical history deserves evaluation with pulmonary function tests before and after administration of bronchodilators to assess the presence of irreversible lung disease. Increases in total lung capacity and residual volume or decreases in vital capacity and carbon monoxide diffusion suggest chronic obstructive or restrictive pulmonary disease of nonasthmatic origin. Reversible lung disease is present when an increase of 200 ml or 10% or more in forced expiratory volume in 1 sec (FEV_1) occurs after administration of bronchodilators. In most instances, pulmonary function returns to at least 75% to 80% of predicted normal values.

A detailed preoperative physical examination is crucial. The presence of nasal polyps should preclude the use of aspirin and other prostaglandin inhibitors such as nonsteroidal anti-inflammatory agents. Accessory muscle use, dyspnea at rest, cyanosis, and pulsus paradoxus of more than 10 torr are signs of severe disease warranting immediate therapeutic intervention and contraindicating surgery until asthma is reversed. Laboratory evaluation should include at least screening spirometry to measure forced vital capacity, FEV_1, and maximum mid-expiratory flow rate at 25% to 75% of vital capacity.

Table 27-1. Staging of Asthma

Stage	History	Exam	FEV$_1$ (% predicted)	PO$_2$	P$_{CO_2}$	p*h*	Therapy	Operation
I	Asymptomatic or mild symptoms	Normal or slight wheezing	>75	Normal or slightly ↓	Normal or slightly ↓	Normal or slightly ↑	None or theophylline	Yes
II	Moderate symptoms	Wheezing or ↓ breathing sounds	50–75	↓	↓	↑	Theophylline	No
III	Severe symptoms	Wheezing or ↓ breathing sounds	<50	↓↓	Normal or ↑	Normal or ↓	Theophylline or corticosteroids	No
IV	Status asthmaticus	Wheezing or ↓ breathing sounds	Unobtainable	↓↓	↑	↓	Intubation steroids, theophylline	No

Abnormalities in any of these warrant more extensive pulmonary function tests with and without bronchodilators. In general, any patient with an FEV_1 of less than 75% of predicted values deserves arterial blood gas determinations.

Once historical information, including medication history and use of corticosteroids has been obtained and correlated with the physical examination and laboratory data, the clinical stage of the disease can be assessed and therapy instituted as needed (Table 27-1). All patients should stop smoking at least 1 week prior to surgery, avoid known or suspected irritant factors, and maintain adequate hydration.

TREATMENT OF ASTHMA

Patients in stage I of the disorder can undergo surgery safely. It is best to attempt to reverse any clinical or laboratory indication of even mild dysfunction before operation, but emergency surgery using bronchodilators usually presents no increased risk. Operation is contraindicated in patients in stage IV until respiratory failure is reversed. Patients in stages II and III should not undergo surgery until they are free of wheezing and their arterial blood gases and pulmonary function tests have returned to normal or stage I levels.

Therapy begins with theophylline derivatives for achievement of drug levels of 10 to 20 µg/ml. This usually requires maintenance doses of 1 to 2 g/day of aminophylline given as an intravenous loading dose of 6 mg/kg body weight over 30 min followed by 0.5 to 0.9 mg/kg/hr. For elderly patients, these doses should be cut in half. For obese patients, doses should be calculated on the basis of lean body weight. Tachycardia, palpitations, agita-

tion, nausea, and vomiting are signs of toxicity and warrant stopping the drug or reducing the dose until serum theophylline levels are determined. If this regimen does not lead to improvement to stage I levels, administration of steroids should be instituted.[20]

In patients previously treated with oral or inhalational steroids or in patients who have received parenteral steroids within 6 months of evaluation, replacement doses of hydrocortisone at 200 mg/day should be given in addition to current doses. If there is clinical evidence of active disease, combinations of bronchodilators and steroids should be administered. Inhalational steroids such as beclomethasone should be replaced with prednisone or its equivalent in doses of at least 20 mg/day for the period during which patients cannot use the inhaler. In addition, patients controlled with inhalational disodium chromoglycolate may need steroid coverage during this period.

During the operative procedure, adequate bronchodilation should be maintained with parenteral bronchodilators and steroids as determined by preoperative evaluation. Adequate hydration in the perioperative period remains the best expectorant for asthmatic patients. Postoperative chest physiotherapy, early mobilization, and minimization of anticholinergics and respiratory depressants will minimize the occurrence of bronchospasm, mucus impaction, and atelectasis. A recent study indicates that asthmatics on corticosteroids do not have a higher risk of postoperative complications than asthmatics not taking steroids.

SUMMARY

1. **Patients with asthma have a significant risk of perioperative complica-**

tion. **Risk increases with age, history of smoking, and type of surgery, and is highest for upper abdominal and thoracic procedures.**

2. **Factors increasing bronchial hyperirritability (cholinergic agents, betablockers and other irritants) and decreasing mobilization of secretions (dehydration and respiratory depressants) should be avoided.**

3. **Classification of asthmatics by history, physical examination, pulmonary function tests, and arterial blood gases is crucial in the evaluation of the need for specific therapy. Only asthmatics with stage I disease and with an FEV of less than 75% of predicted values can undergo surgical procedures without risk of complications.**

4. **Any asthmatic who has taken steroids within 6 months of operation or is receiving them in oral or inhalational form at the time of surgery needs adrenal coverage (hydrocortisone, 200 mg/day or its equivalent). Inhaled steroids should be replaced by prednisone in a dose of 20 mg/day or its equivalent.**

5. **Adequate bronchodilation and hydration, encouragement of expectoration, and minimization of exposure to irritants should reduce the risk of complications to normal in asthmatic patients undergoing surgery.**

REFERENCES

1. White WH: Social and economics aspects. NIAID Task Force Report: Asthma and Other Allergic Diseases, p 7. NIH Pub No 79-387, 1979
2. Scodding J: Asthma. Br Med J 63:12, 1963
3. Townley RG, Dennis M, Itkin IH: Comparative action of acetyl-beta-methylcholine, histamine and pollen antigens in subjects with hay fever and patients with bronchial asthma. J Allergy 36:121, 1965
4. Szentivanji A: The beta-adrenergic theory of the atopic abnormality in bronchial asthma. J Allergy 42:203, 1968
5. Terr AI: Bronchial asthma. In Baum AL (ed): Textbook of Pulmonary Diseases, 2nd ed, p 423. Boston, Little, Brown & Co, 1974
6. Orange RP: Immunopharmacological aspects of bronchial asthma. Clin. Allergy 3:521, 1973
7. Nadel SA: Neurophysiologic aspects of asthma. In Austen KF, Lichtenstein LM (eds): Asthma: Physiology, Immunopharmacology and Treatment, p 29. New York, Academic Press, 1973
8. Stein M, Abdel–Rassoul MI: Pre-operative and post-operative considerations in patients with bronchial asthma. In Weiss EB, Segal MS (eds): Bronchial Asthma, Mechanisms and Therapeutics, p 991. Boston, Little, Brown & Co, 1976
9. Thompson NB et al: Risk of surgery with obstructive lung disease. Br Med J 1:1093, 1958
10. Wightman JAK: A prospective survey of the incidence of post-operative pulmonary complications. Br J Surg 55:85, 1968
11. Schmider SM, Papper EM: Anesthesia for the asthmatic patient. Anesthesiology 22:886, 1961
12. Valentine MD: The asthmatic patient as a surgical risk. Surg Clin North Am 50:631, 1970
13. Rebuck AS, Pengelly LD: Development of pulsus paradoxus in the presence of airways obstruction. N Engl J Med 288:66, 1973
14. McFadden ER: Exertional dyspnea and cough as preludes to acute attacks of bronchial asthma. N Engl J Med 292:555, 1975
15. Corrao WM, Braman SS, Irwin RS: Chronic cough as the sole presenting manifestation of bronchial asthma. N Engl J Med 300:633, 1979
16. McFadden ER: The chronicity of acute attacks of asthma—Mechanical and therapeutic implications. J Allergy Clin Immunol 56:18, 1975
17. Oh SH, Patterson R: Surgery in corticosteroid-dependent asthmatics. J Allergy Clin Immunol 53:345, 1974

Complications of Transfusion in Surgical Patients

STANTON L. GERSON
ALAN D. SCHREIBER

Transfusion therapy provides a means of replacing whole blood or specific blood components. Although often routinely administered in the operative setting, transfusions carry the risk of significant side effects and can cause life-threatening emergencies. To provide appropriate transfusion therapy, the physician should understand the pathophysiology of the several possible types of transfusion reactions. This chapter discusses hemolytic transfusion reactions, complications, including non-A non-B hepatitis, problems peculiar to massive blood transfusions, and the danger of post-transfusion hemorrhage. The assistance of both the blood bank and the coagulation laboratory is often invaluable in the evaluation of a possible transfusion reaction and in the formulation of both diagnostic and management decisions.

TRANSFUSION REACTIONS

Hemolytic

Hemolytic transfusion reactions occur in approximately 1 of every 3000 transfu-sions.[1] They may occur soon after transfusion or after several days. Symptoms include fever and chills, shortness of breath, chest pain, tachycardia, nausea, vomiting, urticaria, hypotension, and signs and symptoms of anaphylaxis.[1-3] In one series from the Mayo Clinic, fever and chills occurred in over 40% of cases.[4] The majority of patients with an immediate transfusion reaction experience dyspnea, chest or back pain, hypotension, or sudden anxiety or nausea.

In a minority of cases, hemolytic transfusion reactions are due to nonimmune mechanisms in which hemolysis occurs because of poor storage techniques or exposure of blood to hypotonic solutions. However, most immediate hemolytic transfusion reactions are due to incorrectly cross-matched blood with incompatibility at the ABO locus or at the locus of a minor determinant.[5,6]

Incompatibility in the ABO system can cause intravascular hemolysis due to the presence of complement-fixing immunoglobulin M (IgM) anti-A or anti-B antibodies. In addition, some IgG anti-A or anti-B antibodies can activate the classic complement pathway and cause sufficient C8 and C9 deposition on the erythrocyte surface to cause intravascular hemolysis. Antibodies directed toward the minor Kell, Jk^a (Kidd), and Fy^a (Duffy) loci may also fix complement and cause significant intravascular hemolysis.[6,7] Prior exposure to blood products raises the likelihood that antibodies directed against the ABO, Kell, or Jk^a locus will develop. In addition, a prior pregnancy exposes a woman to foreign loci and probably explains the 3:1 female over male predominance of hemolytic transfusion reactions.[1,3,6,8]

The diagnosis of intravascular hemolysis can often be made by sedimentation of the blood and urine and the search for the presence of hemoglobin in the supernatant. Blood studies reveal a rise in serum levels of bilirubin and lactic dehydrogenase and, often, hemoglobinemia or hemoglobinuria. A Coombs' test is almost always positive, and careful crossmatching studies should confirm the presence in the patient's plasma of antibody that reacts with donor erythrocytes.[9] The antibody can often be eluted from the patient's red blood cells following transfusion, and the specificity of the antibody can be determined through the use of donor blood specimens. Future transfusions are safe, provided that both the crossmatch is compatible and the donor cells are negative for the antigen to which the patient has formed an antibody.

One-half of all transfusion fatalities involve a major hemolytic reaction.[5] The dangers of acute hemolytic transfusion reactions are acute renal failure and hemorrhage.[1,2] Acute tubular necrosis following a transfusion reaction carries a mortality as high as 50%, despite aggressive management and therapy.[1,2] Renal failure may be due to several factors, including renal tubular obstruction caused by precipitated hemoglobin, hypotension, renal vascular thrombosis due to disseminated intravascular coagulation, and the toxic effects of erythrocyte stroma on renal tubular cells. It appears that renal dysfunction accompanying transfusion of a large volume (200–500 ml) of incompatible blood is particularly serious, not often reversible, and associated with a poor prognosis.

Early and aggressive management to avoid renal failure may be successful. The steps of such management are the following:

I. Recognition
   A. Clinical signs: temperature of 101°F, chills, dyspnea, back or sternal pain
   B. Laboratory confirmation: hemoglobinemia, hemoglobinuria, falling hematocrit, newly positive Coombs' test, possibility of disseminated intravascular coagulation
   C. Altered renal function with reduced urine output
II. Initial therapy
   A. Stop transfusion
   B. Maintain blood pressure with normal saline at 500–1000 ml over 1–2 hr
   C. Institute osmotic diuresis with mannitol
   D. Institute diuresis with intravenous furosemide
III. Complications
   A. Renal failure
   B. Hemorrhage or thrombosis due to disseminated intravascular coagulation

As outlined above, the treatment of a hemolytic transfusion reaction depends upon stopping the transfusion, maintaining adequate blood pressure with a systolic pressure of greater than 100 torr and maintaining renal blood flow. To maintain urine output, mannitol and intravenous fluids followed by furosemide should be administered. If renal shutdown due to acute tubular necrosis occurs, an appropriate regimen for the treatment of acute renal failure, including fluid and protein restriction, should be instituted.[12]

Blood transfusions causing extravascular hemolysis are due to noncomplement-fixing antibodies or antibodies that are not efficient in activating the classic complement pathway. Commonly, this transfusion reaction is not as acute and occurs hours after the transfusion. Hemoglobinuria, hypotension, and renal failure are unusual.[1] Jaundice with increased serum levels of bilirubin and lactate dehydrogenase (LDH) and a falling hemoglobin may develop over a 1- to 4-day period. Antibodies, usually of the IgG class, are directed against a red-cell antigen such as one of the Rh loci (e.g., E, C, or D).[6,7] These IgG-coated red cells are then cleared by splenic macrophages that have Fc receptors on their surfaces. Such antibodies are present in previously transfused patients and are usually detected by cross-match.[9] Given sufficient time, a safe cross-match can usually be found.

Delayed

Delayed hemolytic transfusion reactions occur 2 to 10 days after blood transfusion.[10] An initially negative Coombs' test may become positive, with the indirect test more likely to be positive than the direct.[11] However, in some patients, it is difficult to demonstrate a positive Coombs' test even when the donor's red blood cells and the recipient's plasma are used. Under these circumstances, more sensitive

quantitative techniques than the standard Coombs' test will often detect the presence of circulating antibody. The presence of an isoantibody in the patient's plasma helps to distinguish a delayed transfusion reaction from autoimmune hemolytic anemia. In the latter case, usually only the direct Coombs' test is positive, and the antibody is directed against the host erythrocytes.

Laboratory findings of a delayed transfusion reaction may be subtle, with a mild fall in hematocrit, a rise in reticulocyte count, and an elevation of serum bilirubin or LDH levels.[12] The antibody is usually directed against the Rh or Kidd antigen, does not activate the classic complement pathway, and consequently does not cause intravascular hemolysis. Hemolysis is extravascular, and there is no threat of renal insufficiency. Rarely, intravascular hemolysis can occur in the presence of a potent complement-fixing antibody; under these circumstances, renal insufficiency and disseminated intravascular coagulation can supervene.

Delayed transfusion reactions can be difficult to diagnose, particularly when they are caused by an IgG antibody directed against a minor erythrocyte antigen. A history of previous exposure to blood products or prior pregnancy is suggestive. These reactions are most likely due to an accelerated immune response to a sensitizing erythrocyte antigen to which the patient has been previously exposed. Once documented, the antibody is typically present for 4 to 9 months but may still invoke another hemolytic event thereafter.[9] Hemolysis is generally not brisk and abates after all transfused red blood cells are cleared. Patients should be made aware of the specific antibody present so as to avoid subsequent transfusion reactions.

Hemolysis Secondary to Universal Donor Transfusions

In the case of severe trauma and blood loss, many units of whole blood may be needed. Under these circumstances, group-O, Rh-positive blood is often administered as universal donor blood with no further cross-matching. During the acute period, minor transfusion reactions such as febrile reactions, mild hemolysis, and some respiratory distress may occur. However, there may also be a delayed-onset hemolytic anemia.[2] This immune hemolysis is often associated with a positive Coombs' test and begins as the patient starts to produce his own red cells. Hemolysis is due to the transfusion of antibodies (often anti-A or anti-B) that are present in the donor blood and now react with the patient's cells. These antibodies may circulate in low concentrations for 10 to 60 days and can be identified by an alert blood bank.[13] Since hemolysis may be exacerbated by a subsequent cross-matched transfusion, only carefully cross-matched type-O blood should be used until the antibodies are cleared from the circulation.

Nonhemolytic

Febrile

Fever, shaking chills, pruritis, urticaria, and angioedema may occur during nonhemolytic complications of blood transfusions. Pyogenic material contaminating blood products are potent sources of fever and may be produced during preparation of blood products by their exposure to filters, glass, or changes in temperature. In addition, endotoxin may contaminate a blood product and precipitate severe shaking chills.[14,15] Often, fever can be managed with acetaminophen and chills with meperidine.

Management of febile transfusion reactions is outlined below.

Clinical setting
  Fever: acetaminophen, 650 mg per os
  Chills: meperidine, 25–50 mg IV
  Allergic reaction: antihistamines, epinephrine, hydrocortisone
  For white blood cell transfusions, premedicate with antihistamines and hydrocortisone
  For platelet transfusions, premedicate only after a previous reaction
Recommended modifications for future transfusions
  Allergic reactions: use different donor
  IgA deficiency: use washed, packed red cells
  Leukoagglutinin reaction: use washed, packed red cells
  White blood cell transfusion or platelet transfusion reactions: use a single donor who has no cross-reacting HL-A antibodies

Allergic

The transfusion of blood products can also produce signs and symptoms of a generalized allergic reaction. These include generalized pruritis, urticaria, angioedema, bronchospasm, and generalized anaphylaxis.[2,16,17] Sensitization to a plasma protein in transfused blood can provoke such allergic reactions and lead to a syndrome much like serum sickness. Atopic patients can react to minute amounts of foreign proteins in donor plasma, including pollen or food antigens, with subsequent manifestations of hypersensitivity. Some have been reported to react to small concentrations of transfused antibiotics.[15]

The signs and symptoms of these reactions suggest an immediate hypersensitivity mechanism involving IgE with release of histamine and SRS-A from mast cells. They are usually mild and respond readily to antihistamines and, if necessary, to corticosteroids.[17] However, when anaphylaxis occurs, prompt therapy with epinephrine, steroids, and a bronchodilator such as aminophylline is indicated.

IgA deficiency, which occurs in 1 in 700 persons, increases the risk of a severe hypersensitivity transfusion reaction.[18] Persons who have had previous exposure to IgA develop an anti-IgA antibody of the IgG type, and the reaction is caused by the interaction of this antibody with IgA in donor plasma. The resultant immune complex interacts with mast cells to release histamine.[18] IgA deficiency is one of the few causes of dramatic anaphylactic reactions, which occur after the transfusion of as little as 5 ml to 10 ml of plasma. Immediate measures to maintain an open airway and blood pressure are needed, and epinephrine and bronchodilators usually reverse the process. Diagnosis requires demonstration of circulating anti-IgA without IgA in the patient's plasma. Quantitative immunodiffusion is especially useful in establishing the diagnosis. Because the titer of anti-IgA antibody may be high, subsequent transfusions are hazardous unless they are from an IgA-deficient donor. Extensive washing of red blood cells removes donor IgA and reduces the chance of severe reactions.[7]

The pathogenesis of some clinical manifestations may involve activity of the kinin system initiated by activation of Hageman factor. Bronchospasm and hypotension after transfusion of blood products and intravascular hemolysis may be due to bradykinin release following Hageman factor activation by immune complexes, altered endothelium, or red-cell stroma.

Leukoagglutinin

When the primary manifestations of a transfusion reaction consist of dyspnea, bronchospasm, pulmonary infiltrates, and noncardiac pulmonary edema, a leukoagglutinin reaction should be suspected.[14] This reaction is often seen early in the course of the transfusion and is believed to be due to the transfusion of white blood cells contaminating the red-cell suspension. The white cells clump, or agglutinate, and are filtered by the pulmonary capillaries with subsequent release of vasoactive substances that cause bronchospasm, increased capillary permeability, and alveolar edema.[16] In severe cases, release of these substances can provoke disseminated intravascular coagulation (DIC) or anaphylaxis. The precise pathophysiology of the hypersensitivity reaction remains unclear. Platelet thrombi, which have been noted in some autopsy studies, may be a source of vasoactive substances.[14] Complement activation may also be involved, although its role remains speculative.

One precipitating factor is the presence of high-titer antileukocyte antibodies in recipient or donor plasma.[19] These antibodies develop after prior exposure to foreign HL-A antigens in previous transfusions or pregnancy.[7] The diagnosis is established by identification of anti-HL-A antibodies in a leukocyte cytotoxicity assay. Treatment consists of antihistamines or corticosteroids, which decrease the severity of the reaction and may modify the extent of pulmonary edema. Reactions may be prevented by use of frozen or unfrozen washed, packed red blood cells.

Reactions to White Blood Cell Transfusion

White blood cell transfusions are now recommended for severely granulocytopenic patients with fever secondary to documented bacterial infections that are unresponsive to antibiotics.[20] Immediate reactions to the white-cell transfusions consist of fever and chills and occur in about 75% of patients receiving white cells obtained by filtration leukopheresis and in about 40% of patients receiving white cells prepared by continuous flow centrifugation.[21] These minor reactions which may be due to the release of pyogenic products from leukocytes, can be successfully managed with acetaminophen, meperidine, antihistamines, or corticosteroids given prior to the transfusion. These reactions are not an indication for the transfusion to be stopped.

However, leukoagglutinin reactions as described above can also occur during white blood cell transfusions. These reactions may be profound and are clearly cause for the infusion to be stopped. Since single donors are used as a source of white cells, the blood bank should be notified when a leukoagglutinin reaction occurs so that the same donor will not undergo leukopheresis for the same recipient again. Subsequent donors should be screened for cross-reacting HL-A antibodies.

Graft-versus-host (GVH) disease is a rare complication following white-cell tranfusion of immunocompromised patients. To prevent GVH disease, some centers have suggested irradiating all blood products prior to transfusion to eliminate donor lymphocytes. However, because GVH reactions are uncommon after transfusion even in immunocompromised hosts, prophylactic irradiation of blood products is not a routine practice.

Reactions to Platelet Tranfusion

Surgical patients who require platelet transfusions are commonly thrombocytopenic because of bone marrow hypoplasia from recent chemotherapy or sequestration of platelets by a large spleen.[22] In addition, in patients who have been bleeding, transfusion of stored blood containing few platelets may produce thrombocytopenia severe enough to require supplementation. Most patients have not developed antiplatelet antibodies and can receive random donor platelets safely. However, some of those who have had multiple transfusions develop isoantibodies, alloantibodies that are commonly HL-A-specific. Following platelet transfusion, these patients may experience fever, chills, mild respiratory distress, and even bronchospasm. These symptoms may be due to release of serotonin and other vasoactive substances during the immune destruction of platelets. The platelet count usually fails to rise to its expected level. In order to avoid subsequent reactions, patients must undergo HL-A typing and screening for circulating anti-HL-A antibodies.[23]

Another common reaction to platelet transfusion is hypersensitivity to contaminating plasma proteins, small numbers of incompatible red blood cells, or pyrogens.[22] Under these circumstances, the patient may experience fever and rigors during transfusion, but the platelet count will rise over 2 to 6 hr with a normal platelet survival of 18 to 36 hr. This reaction can be controlled with hydrocortisone and antihistamines.

COMPLICATIONS

Infections

Bacterial

Significant morbidity accompanies infection transmitted through the transfusion of blood products that have been contaminated with organisms that can grow at the reduced temperatures at which blood is stored.[1,24] However, bacterial contamination of blood is uncommon, occurring in only 1% of blood products.[1,24] Although stored blood may contain *Staphylococcus epidermidis*, diphtheroids, enterococcus, *Bacillus subtilis*, and enterobacteriaciae, clinical sepsis is unusual because the inoculum infused is low.[14]

Since sepsis may mimic other types of acute transfusion reaction, persistent fever and rigors without apparent signs of hemolysis or hypersensitivity reaction should alert the physician to possible infection. Blood from the patient and transfusion bag should be cultured. Bacterial contamination can be prevented by maintenance of aseptic conditions and avoidance of additions of drugs to the infusion set or interruptions in the transfusion.[15,17] Because febrile transfusion reactions are significantly more common than bacterial septicemia, it is often reasonable to delay the administration of antibiotics until culture results are known.

Viral

Transmission of viral disease is a significant problem, particularly because expression of the disease may be latent.[14,24] Cytomegalovirus (CMV), Epstein–Barr virus (EBV), hepatitis B, and non-A non-B hepatitis are the major epidemiologic hazards (Table 28-1). Clinical evidence of infection includes seroconversion and the prodromal illness typical for each virus.

Transmitted CMV infection may be difficult to diagnosis.[25] A sudden rise in antibody titer and the appearance of the virus in the urine, blood, stool, or saliva are diagnostic but do not differentiate primary infection from reactivation. Identification of an IgM antibody suggests primary inoculation. A clinical syndrome similar to infectious mononucleosis develops 2 to 6 weeks after the transfusion. Patients complain of fever, malaise, and anorexia and manifest lymphadenopathy, mild hepatosplenomegaly, atypical lymphocytosis, and, occasionally, thrombocytopenia, granulocytopenia, hepatitis, and interstitial lung disease.[14,26] CMV infection is more likely to occur in immunosuppressed than in other patients.

CMV infection may be part of the postperfusion syndrome. Up to 21% of patients undergoing extracorporeal perfusion show seroconversion 2 to 6 weeks following the procedure.[26] Although only a minority of patients have clinically apparent disease, some have a protracted course. CMV is carried in a latent state by circulating lymphocytes. When transfused, these lymphocytes may undergo

Table 28-1. Diagnosis of Post-transfusion Viral Infections

Virus	Incidence (%)	Incubation Period [mean (range) in weeks]	Diagnosis	Outcome	Comments
CMV	3–5	4 (2–5)	Antibody, culture	May be protracted	Transmitted in WBCs, may be reactivation infection
EBV	1–3	2 (1–4)	Antibody	Favorable	Unusual in older age group
Hepatitis B	10	6 (4–30)	Antibody	Favorable	May be transmitted from HBcAg carrier
Hepatitis non-A non-B	85	7 (2–16)	Exclusion	Chronic liver disease in 23%	Variable clinical disease

WBCs = white blood cells; HBcAg = hepatitis B core antigen.

transformation, causing activation of the virus, infection of recipient cells, and clinical disease. In addition, donor lymphocytes may transform recipient cells, causing activation of latent virus in the host.[14] Therefore, CMV infection is also observed after granulocyte transfusions in immunosuppressed patients, such as those with acute leukemia.[27] Consequently, some centers deplete whole blood of lymphocytes to reduce the incidence of CMV seroconversion in high-risk patients.[25] Management of an established CMV infection is supportive; the disease is typically mild, except in the immunocompromised host. In the immunocompromised patient, withdrawal of immunosuppressive therapy should be considered.

EBV is a cause of postperfusion syndrome in some adults but is more common in children.[14] In this disease, a classic infectious mononucleosis prodrome may occur 2 to 6 weeks after transfusion. Since the infection is usually mild, patients are given supportive care, and seroconversion is documented.

Miscellaneous

Other nonbacterial, nonviral infections can also be transmitted through infusion of blood products. There have been reports of seroconversions indicating transmission of syphilis by this routine, although screening for syphilis is routinely performed prior to transfusion.[14] Toxoplasmosis has developed following leukocyte transfusions in the setting of both renal transplantation and acute leukemia.[28] Since toxoplasmosis can infect leukocytes and persist in an asymptomatic donor, it should be suspected in a recipient who develops lymphadenopathy, fever, rash, and hepatic dysfunction 1 to 3

weeks after a leukocyte transfusion. Transmission of Rocky Mountain spotted fever has also been documented after transfusion of blood from a donor who ultimately died of the disease.[29]

Transmission of malaria through transfusion has been reported and was commonly observed when blood products from returning servicemen were utilized during the Vietnam War.[30] This may again be a concern in view of the large number of refugees from Southeast Asia entering the United States. A history of exposure to malaria any time in the past should be a contraindication to blood donation, since transmission has been linked to exposure up to 20 years previously.[31] The clinical syndrome develops within 7 to 10 days of the transfusion and consists of fever, mild hemolysis, splenomegaly, and evidence of plasmodia on the peripheral blood smear. Once the diagnosis is established, treatment requires determination of the type of malaria and institution of effective therapy.

Post-transfusion Hepatitis

One of the most important complications of transfusion therapy is post-transfusion hepatitis (see Table 28-1). In 1973, icteric hepatitis occurred in 1.6% of recipients.[1] When blood donations were obtained at commercial centers, the incidence rose to 5% to 11%.[32,33] The development of screening procedures for hepatitis-associated antigen in the sera of prospective donors has been the most significant factor in decreasing this figure. In the past, hepatitis B virus was the cause of 30% to 50% of post-transfusion hepatitis, but now it accounts for less than 10% because carriers of hepatitis B surface antibodies are excluded from blood donation.[34] The persistent, low incidence of hepatitis B infection is most likely due to transfusions of blood containing either low-titer immune complexes that remain undetected or hepatitis B core antigen, for which screening is not usually performed.[35]

Non-A non-B hepatitis accounts for 85% to 90% of clinical post-transfusion hepatitis and occurs in 7% of patients who have received multiple transfusions.[36] Most episodes of hepatitis occur 6 to 8 weeks after exposure but can occur as early as 2 or as late as 16 weeks posttransfusion. Only 25% become symptomatic, with malaise, anorexia, fever, and jaundice, a syndrome analogous to hepatitis B disease occurring 1 to 4 weeks after the rise in serum transaminase concentrations.[33] The severity of the clinical syndrome is variable. Although symptoms and elevations in transaminase level usually resolve in 1 to 3 weeks, there may be a protracted illness and persistent liver function abnormalities.[37]

A major complication of infection with hepatitis is the development of chronic hepatitis. Serum transaminase levels may remain elevated for up to 6 months, and liver biopsy will reveal either chronic persistent or chronic active hepatitis in 23% of patients.[36,37] The majority of patients recover, and histologic changes resolve without development of postnecrotic cirrhosis.[37]

Prophylaxis for non-A non-B hepatitis in patients receiving multiple transfusions remains controversial. Immune serum globulin administration may decrease the incidence of infection to some extent; however, it proved ineffective in one well-controlled study.[32,38] Unfortunately, contaminated frozen or washed red-cell concentrates retain their infec-tious capacity.[39] Since there is no effective assay for non-A non-B hepatitis in donor blood, hepatitis will continue to be a major complication of blood transfusion.

Complications of Massive Blood Transfusions

The major complications of transfusion are hemolysis and hemorrhage. However, additional complications may be observed when massive blood transfusions are given (Table 28-2). Blood citrate levels can rise into the toxic range, and, in the presence of liver disease, subsequent alterations in citrate metabolism can lead to a significant depression in the serum concentration of ionized calcium.[1,40] Citrate metabolism is also depressed during prolonged periods of hypothermia, which often occur during cardiac surgery. When citrate levels exceed 100 mg/dl, muscle tremors, hypotension, and prolongation of the QT interval on the electrocardiogram can occur. They can be reversed in part by infusion of calcium gluconate. The mechanism of citrate toxicity remains controversial, since experimental prolonged citrate infusion has been shown to

Table 28-2. Massive Blood Transfusions

Complication	Prophylaxis
Citrate intoxication	Infusion of calcium gluconate
Hyperkalemia	Transfusion of fresh blood
Air embolus	Avoidance of air pockets in transfusion under pressure
Hypothermia	Use of prewarmed blood or IV tubing
Adult respiratory distress syndrome	Use of high-grade (Ultipor) 40-μ filter whenever more than 5 units are transfused

have little effect on cardiovascular function.[7,40] Citrate toxicity can be avoided during massive blood replacement by use of significant amounts of fresh whole blood and administration of calcium gluconate when more than 6 units of blood are transfused during a 1- to 3-day period.

Stored blood is often used when multiple blood transfusions are needed. The concentration of free potassium in such blood can be as high as 25 mg/dl, and the risk of hyperkalemia therefore becomes significant. Serum potassium levels should be monitored frequently, especially in patients with renal insufficiency. The concentration of free potassium in blood products correlates wth the duration of storage so hyperkalemia can be avoided by use of fresh whole blood or packed red blood cells when large volumes of blood are required.

Because of excessive bleeding in patients who have suffered trauma or are undergoing significant gastrointestinal hemorrhage, blood is often transfused rapidly. In this setting, air embolism is a major hazard, particularly when blood is transfused under pressure. Symptoms include cough, cyanosis, changes in mental status, and neurologic signs indistinguishable from those of acute hypoxia, including seizures. The diagnosis of air embolism is difficult to substantiate, and air pockets should be carefully avoided during massive blood transfusion under pressure.

Transfusion of large volumes of stored refrigerated blood through a central-line intravenous (IV) catheter can cause hypothermia. This increases the risk of cardiac arrhythmias, particularly ventricular fibrillation.[16] Hypothermia also increases oxygen consumption and metabolic rate as the body attempts to re-establish normal body temperature. If significant

amounts of refrigerated blood are transfused, steps should be taken either to warm the blood or to utilize extra IV tubing coiled in a warm-water bath to raise the temperature of the transfused blood.

A late consequence of repeated massive blood transfusions is the development of hemosiderosis. This is rarely of clinical consequence in otherwise healthy patients, but, in patients with such underlying disorders as sickle-cell anemia, thalassemia, congenital spherocytosis, and other chronic hemolytic anemias that in themselves cause accumulation of body iron, addition of more iron through transfusion can be significant. Iron in the form of hemosiderin can accumulate in the lung, liver, and kidney after transfusion of more than 50 units but rarely causes organ dysfunction except in patients with underlying chronic hemolytic disorders.

The adult respiratory distress syndrome (ARDS) is a major complication of massive blood transfusion. Although its etiology is unclear, it may be caused by microemboli of aggregated platelets, fibrin, and leukocytes present in stored blood. Vasoactive substances in platelets and leukocytes may be released and contribute to the syndrome. One report suggests that the use of an Ultipor filter, which has pores of 40 μ in diameter, rather than of a standard blood filter, the pores of which are 170 μ in diameter, significantly reduces the incidence of acute ARDS.[41] In this study, 50% of patients transfused with at least 19 units of blood through the standard filter developed pulmonary insufficiency, whereas only 17% of patients transfused through the Ultipor filter developed pulmonary decompensation. Other studies also suggest that there might be some benefit in using less porous filters.[14,42] High-grade 40-μ filters are relatively simple to use and are recommended when multiple transfusions are needed. The filter should be changed after administration of 10 units of whole blood.

Bleeding

Bleeding may occur after extensive blood transfusion and may be occult, pronounced, or life-threatening.[1,43,44] When bleeding occurs in this setting, several possibilities should be considered: an underlying bleeding diathesis, dilutional coagulation-factor deficiency, dilutional thrombocytopenia, disseminated intravascular coagulation, and post-transfusion purpura.[43] Each of these is managed differently and therefore requires accurate diagnosis (Table 28-3).

Diathesis, Coagulation-Factor Deficiency, and Thrombocytopenia

An underlying bleeding diathesis in the patient can be assessed by prothrombin time, partial thromboplastin time, platelet count, liver function tests, and nutritional status before transfusion. Even a mild bleeding disorder can be aggravated by multiple blood transfusions. An elevated prothrombin time and documented low levels of factor II, VII, IX, or X suggest underlying liver disease or nutritional deficiency. A low platelet count suggests either decreased production, as in disease of the bone marrow, or increased destruction or sequestration of platelets, as in immune thrombocytopenia, splenomegaly, or sepsis.

After massive blood transfusion, particularly with whole blood stored for more than 24 hr, significant deficiencies of factors V and VIII may result.[1,43,44] In addition, platelets survive poorly between 4°C and 10°C and are often deficient in stored whole blood. Therefore, the transfusion of large volumes of blood can dilute the in-

Table 28-3. Bleeding Diatheses Following Transfusion Therapy*

Disorder	Management
Coagulation-factor deficiency	Fresh frozen plasma, 2–4 units over 1 hr Repeat coagulation studies at 4- to 5-hour intervals Vitamin K, 10 mg subcutaneously × 3
Thrombocytopenia	10-unit platelet transfusion for a platelet count of <20,000/mm³ or for active bleeding with a platelet count of <100,000/mm³
Disseminated intravascular coagulation	Manage underlying disorder If factors are very low and bleeding serious, cautiously administer fresh frozen plasma ± platelets
Post-transfusion purpura	Plasmapheresis PL^{A1}-negative donors for future transfusions

*A full coagulation profile, including prothrombin time, partial thromboplastin time, platelet count, fibrinogen, and fibrin split products should be obtained to establish the diagnosis.

travascular compartment and produce bleeding because of relative thrombocytopenia and coagulation-factor deficiency. Postoperatively, patients may begin to bleed from the wound or venipuncture sites.

After determination that the prothrombin time or partial thromboplastin time is prolonged while the plasma concentrations of fibrinogen and fibrin split products are normal, 2 to 4 units of fresh frozen plasma should be administered over a period of 1 to 2 hr. If transfusion of large volumes is hazardous, cryoprecipitate can be substituted for fresh frozen plasma in many patients. Dilutional thrombocytopenia is usually transient and rarely a cause of significant clinical bleeding. If evidence of petechiae, mucosal bleeding, or retinal hemorrhage is evident, or if the platelet count is less than 20,000/mm^3, platelets should be infused in 10-unit increments.[22]

Disseminated Intravascular Coagulation

DIC may occur during or after transfusion. The mechanism, though not well understood, may involve the interaction of isoantibody with red blood cell antigen and the subsequent activation of Hageman factor and the intrinsic coagulation sequence. There is also evidence that lysed red-cell stroma can directly activate Hageman factor and initiate coagulation. Bleeding is often unsuspected and may become apparent, with diffuse oozing from the wound or venipuncture sites. A febrile or hemolytic transfusion reaction frequently precedes DIC in this setting.[6,9,17] DIC can be documented by the presence of elevated plasma levels of fibrin split products in conjunction with a fall in plasma fibrinogen concentration and platelet count. Management is discussed in Chapter 29.

DIC may also occur during major vascular surgery involving major trauma, resection of abdominal aortic aneurysms, or resection of vascular tumors. Patients undergoing these procedures may require large amounts of fresh frozen plasma to replace deficient clotting factors. If this precaution is taken, uncontrolled hemorrhage is unlikely to occur.[1,15]

Post-transfusion Purpura

Post-transfusion purpura is a delayed complication of transfusion therapy.[45] The patient develops purpura, petechiae, or frank blood loss 3 to 10 days after transfusion of any blood product containing platelets. A sudden drop in platelet count is observed, and bone marrow aspiration reveals adequate or abundant megakaryocytes. Post-transfusion purpura generally occurs in persons among the less than 5% of the population with platelets that lack the PL^{A1} antigen.[45,46] Patients develop antibodies after exposure to platelets that have this common platelet antigen. The syndrome is life-threatening because the decline in platelet count can be profound and the resultant bleeding extensive.

The pathogenesis of the thrombocytopenia is poorly understood, since autologous platelets are also destroyed, even though they lack the antigen against which the isoantibody is directed. It has been shown that host platelets of patients with post-transfusion purpura become coated with IgG and are destroyed by IgG antibody or an IgG-containing immune complex.[47] This process has also been suggested by the results of experiments in which transfusion of allogeneic A platelets into animals resulted in host platelet destruction.[48]

The most effective therapy for post-transfusion purpura is exchange transfusion or plasmapheresis with removal of the antiplatelet antibody. Prednisone may have some therapeutic effect, and PL^{A1} negative platelets, if available, can be effective if infused during active bleeding. Plasmapheresis has been shown to significantly decrease the duration of thrombocytopenia.[4] Patients should be transfused with washed red blood cells to reduce exposure to PL^{A1}-positive platelets. Ideally, PL^{A1}-negative platelets should be infused, but they are difficult to obtain, since they are present in only 5% of the population.

SUMMARY

1. **Hemolytic transfusion reactions may be sudden and life-threatening or subtle and mild. Each can be diagnosed**

by documentation of hemolysis and examination of blood for the presence of anti-erythrocyte antibodies. If intravascular hemolysis occurs, renal failure is a potential life-threatening complication, and immediate therapy to avoid renal shut-down is indicated.

2. **Fever during transfusion without hemolysis or evidence of a progressive hypersensitivity reaction is not an indication for the transfusion to be stopped. Fever can be treated with acetaminophen, chills with meperidine, and allergic reactions with antihistamines, sympathomimetics, and corticosteroids.**

3. **Post-transfusion infections are rare except for viral infections, which are predominantly non-A non-B hepatitis. The clinical syndrome is outlined in Table 28-1.**

4. **Massive blood transfusions cause a wide range of complications, as indicated in Table 28-2. Citrate toxicity can generally be avoided with the administration of calcium gluconate. Acute pulmonary insufficiency after multiple blood transfusions can be life-threatening, but its incidence may be reduced through the use of small-pore filters.**

5. **Post-transfusion hemorrhage, covered in Table 28-3, requires careful evaluation for accurate diagnosis. Once the type of bleeding diathesis and its cause are identified, appropriate treatment with fresh frozen plasma, platelets, or plasmapheresis can be undertaken.**

REFERENCES

1. Goldfinger D: Acute hemolytic transfusion reactions. Transfusion 17:85, 1977

2. Miller RD: Complications of massive blood transfusions. Anesthesiology 39:82, 1973

3. Lundberg WB, McGinniss MH: Hemolytic transfusion reaction due to Anti-A. Transfusion 15:1, 1975

4. Laursen B, Morling N, Rosenkuist J et al: Post-transfusion purpura treated with plasma exchange by Haemonetics cell separator. Acta Med Scand 203: 539, 1978

5. Cimo PL, Astar RH: Post-transfusion purpura. N Engl J Med 287:290, 1972

6. Pineda AA, Brzica SM, Taswell HF: Hemolytic transfusion reaction. Mayo Clin Proc 53:378, 1978

7. Issitt P, Issitt C: Transfusion reactions. In Issitt P, Issitt C: Applied Blood Group Serology, p 283. New York, Spectra Biologicals, 1979

8. Myhre BA: Fatalities from blood transfusion. JAMA 244:1333, 1980

9. Mollison PL: Blood Transfusion in Clinical Medicine, pp 557–616. London, Blackwell, 1979

10. Pineda AA, Taswell HF, Brzica SM Jr: Delayed hemolytic transfusion reaction. Transfusion 18:1, 1978

11. Croucher BE, Crookston MC, Crookston JA: Delayed hemolytic transfusion reaction simulating autoimmune hemolytic anemia. Vox Sang 12:32, 1967

12. Solanki D, McCurdy PR: Delayed hemolytic transfusion reaction. JAMA 239:729, 1978

13. Barnes A, Allen T: Transfusions subsequent to administration of universal donor blood in Vietnam. JAMA 204:695, 1968

14. Lang D, Valeri C: Hazards of blood transfusion. Adv Pediatr 24:311, 1977

15. Mollison PL: Blood Transfusion in Clinical Medicine, pp 617–660. London, Blackwell, 1979

16. Wolf CR, Carole VC: Fatal pulmonary hypersensitivity reaction to HL-A-incompatable blood transfusion. Transfusion 16:135, 1976

17. Baker RJ, Nyhus LM: Diagnosis and treatment of immediate transfusion reaction. Surg Gynecol Obstet 130:665, 1970

18. Schmidt AP, Taswell HF, Gleich GJ: Anaphylactic transfusion reactions associated with anti-IgA antibody. N Engl J Med 280:188, 1969

19. Ward H: Pulmonary infiltrates associated with leukoagglutinin transfusion reactions. Ann Intern Med 73:689, 1970

20. Alavi J, Root RK, Djerassi I et al: Clinical trial of granulocyte transfusions for infection in acute leukemia. N Engl J Med 296:706, 1977

21. Herzig R, Herzig G, Graw RG et al: Granulocyte transfusion therapy for gram negative septicemia. N Engl J Med 296:701, 1977

22. Slichter SJ: Controversies in platelet transfusion therapy. Ann Rev Med 31:509, 1980

23. Astar RH: Matching of blood platelets for transfusion. Am J Hematol 5: 373, 1978

24. Broude AI: Transfusion reactions from contaminated blood. N Engl J Med 258:1289, 1958

25. Lang D, Ebert P, Rodgers B et al: Reduction of post-perfusion cytomegalovirus infection following the use of leukocyte depleted blood transfusion. Transfusion 17:391, 1977

26. Prince AM, Szuness W, Millian JJ et al: A serologic study of cytomegalovirus infections associated with blood transfusions. N Engl J Med 284:1125, 1971

27. Winston DS, Ho WG, Howell CL et al: Cytomegalovirus infections associated with leukocyte transfusions. Ann Intern Med 93:671, 1980

28. Seigal S, Lunde M, Goldeman A et al: Transmission of toxoplasmosis by leukocyte transfusion. Blood 37:388, 1971

29. Wells G, Woodward T, Fisot P et al: Rocky Mountain spotted fever caused by blood transfusion. JAMA 239:2763, 1978

30. Garfield M, Ershle W, Mahi D: Malaria transmission by platelet concentrate transfusion. JAMA 240:2285, 1978

31. Najem G, Sulze A: Transfusion induced malaria from an asymptomatic carrier. Transfusion 16:473, 1976

32. Conrad ME, Knodell G, Bradley EL Jr et al: Risk factors in transmission of non-A, non-B post-transfusion hepatitis. Transfusion 17:579, 1977

33. Seeff LB, Wright ES, Zimmerman HJ et al: VA cooperative study of post-transfusion hepatitis. Am J Med Sci 270:355, 1975

34. Goche DJ, Greenberg HB, Rare NB: Correlation of Australia antigen with post-transfusion hepatitis. JAMA 212:877, 1970

35. Hoofnagle JH, Seeff LB, Bales AB et al: Type B hepatitis after transfusion with blood containing antibody to hepatitis B core antigen. N Engl J Med 298:1379, 1978

36. Aach RD, Kahn RA: Post-transfusion hepatitis: Comment and perspectives. Ann Intern Med 92:539, 1980

37. Aach RD, Shields HM, Lander JJ et al: Post-transfusion hepatitis leading to chronic hepatitis. Gastroenterology 75:732, 1978

38. Spellberg MA, Berman PM: The incidence of post-transfusion hepatitis and the lack of efficacy of gamma globulin in its prevention. Am J Gastroenterol 34:564, 1971

39. Haugen RR: Hepatitis after the transfusion of frozen red cells and washed red cells. N Engl J Med 301:393, 1979

40. Howland WS, Schweizer O, Carlan GC et al: The cardiovascular effects of low levels of ionized calcium during massive transfusion. Surg Gynecol Obstet 145:581, 1977

41. Reul G, Greenberg S, Lefrak E et al: Prevention of post-traumatic pulmonary insufficiency. Arch Surg 106:386, 1973

42. Duntschi M, Haisch C, Reynolds L et al: Effect of micropore filtration on pulmonary function after massive transfusion. Am J Surg 138:8, 1979

43. McKenna PJ, Scheinman HZ: Transient coagulation abnormalities after incompatible blood transfusion. Crit Care Med 3:8, 1975

44. Ingram GIC: The bleeding complications of blood transfusion. Transfusion 5:1, 1965

45. Shulman NR, Aster RH, Leitner A et al: Immunoreactions involving platelets. V. Post-transfusion purpura due to a complement fixing antibody against a genetically

controlled platelet antigen: A proposed mechanism for thrombocytopenia and its relevance in "autoimmunity." J Clin Invest 40:1597, 1961

46. Abramson N, Eisenberg PD, Aster RH: Post-transfusion purpura: Immunologic aspects and therapy. N Engl J Med 291:1163, 1974

47. Cines DB, Schreiber AD: Immune thrombocytopenia. N Engl J Med 300:106, 1979

48. Baldini M: Acute ITP in isoimmunized dogs. Ann NY Acad Sci 124:543, 1965

29

Clotting Abnormalities in the Surgical Patient

DAVID H. HENRY

Bleeding is a major concern in the surgical patient. This chapter addresses the evaluation of the patient with a known or suspected bleeding diathesis and the management of specific clotting abnormalities. The pathophysiology, diagnosis, and treatment of disseminated intravascular coagulation (DIC) in the surgical patient are also discussed.

PREOPERATIVE EVALUATION

The history is the most important element in the screening of a preoperative patient for hemostatic abnormalities. The patient should be questioned about inadequate hemostasis in prior trauma, surgery, or dental extractions as well as excessive bleeding during pregnancy or menses, familial bleeding, and aspirin use. Although any platelet or clotting-factor abnormality can underlie increased bleeding at surgery, patients with platelet abnormalities usually offer a history of easy bruising, heavy menses, or ecchymosis, whereas those with clotting-factor disorders more often experience muscle or retroperitoneal hematomas or bleeding into joints. Prolonged bleeding after dental extraction can be seen in either group. Platelet problems present with continuous oozing for more than 24 hr, whereas clotting-factor abnormalities cause bleeding to recur after initial hemostasis. In the latter case, the platelet plug stops initial bleeding, but the necessary fibrin meshwork needed for complete clotting cannot develop properly.

When the history and physical exam suggest a hemostatic abnormality, screening tests are indicated, including a platelet count, bleeding time, prothrombin time (PT), and activated partial thromboplastin time (PTT). One or more of these four tests will be abnormal in over 95% of clinically significant bleeding disorders when bleeding is present and will fail to detect only a few mild or very rare disorders. If abnormal, a clotting study should be repeated for verification.

Liver disease, use of anticoagulants, hemophilia, or malabsorption of vitamin K causing abnormal clotting can be readily detected by the patient's history.[1-3] In one survey of 97 preoperative patients with prolongation of the activated PTT, 37 were receiving anticoagulants, 27 had known liver disease, 4 had hemophilia, 4 had undergone intestinal bypass surgery, and 1 had malabsorption secondary to cystic fibrosis. In 10 patients, the abnormal results were due to laboratory error. The remaining 14 patients had an unexplained prolongation of less than 10 sec above control levels, and none of them had bleeding complications at surgery.[1] In another study, Eisenberg examined the usefulness of the routine admission PT as a screening test for bleeding.[2] In 97% of patients, a prolonged PT could have been predicted by history alone. Moreover, not only can hemostatic abnormalities be detected in most cases by history alone, but screening coagulation tests may be normal in patients with a clear-cut history of bleeding.[3,4]

However, despite the results described above, in a bleeding patient with a suspected or documented bleeding disorder, these four laboratory tests will be confirmatory in all but the most esoteric situations (e.g., factor XIII deficiency). The PT and PTT test the integrity of the extrinsic and intrinsic coagulation sequences, respectively. If the PTT is prolonged and the PT is normal, the defect lies in one or more of the intrinsic factors. Factor XII deficiency does not lead to bleeding. If both tests are abnormal, many factors may be deficient, but, more often, there is a major defect in the final common pathway involving factors X, V, II (prothrombin), or I (fibrinogen).

A platelet count is useful in evaluating the other arm of the coagulation system. If the count is decreased, the tendency to bleed correlates roughly with size of the decrement in platelet count below 100,000. If the platelet count is normal, platelet function may be abnormal and cause significant bleeding. A standard Ivy bleeding time, which provides a measure of platelet function, is less than 10 min if platelet count and function are normal. It is predictably abnormal when the platelet count is low and need not be done. Although a discussion of all abnormalities in PT, PTT, platelet count, and bleeding time underlying clinical bleeding is beyond the scope of this chapter, certain abnormalities are common, particularly in the perioperative setting.

PREOPERATIVE MANAGEMENT

Bleeding Due to Aspirin and Other Drugs

Aspirin causes an irreversible defect in platelet aggregation for the remainder of the life of the affected platelet, usually from 7 to 10 days. Aspirin acetylates the platelet enzyme cyclo-oxygenase, thereby inhibiting release of adenosine diphosphate (ADP) and preventing aggregation. Increased bleeding during or after surgery may occur despite a sometimes normal preoperative bleeding time. One or two aspirin tablets may alter platelet function for up to 10 days. Aspirin is the only drug with a prolonged effect on platelet function, but many other drugs also alter platelet function. These include nonsteroidal anti-inflammatory agents, tricyclic antidepressants, phenothiazines, steroids, some anesthetics, antiarrhythmics, antihistamines, and vitamin E. Clinical bleeding may also occur following administration of high doses of intravenous penicillin. Carbenicillin is the most common of any offender, since it is usually given in high doses.

Von Willebrand's Disease

Von Willebrand's disease is an autosomal dominant disorder in which platelet adhesion and factor VIII are abnormal.

The PTT and bleeding time may not be prolonged preoperatively but may become so during or after surgery. Therapy consists of preparations containing factor VIII, such as fresh frozen plasma or cryoprecipitate, both of which contain Von Willebrand's portion of the factor VIII molecule.[5] Patients should be followed by measurement of bleeding time and ristocetin aggregation. If these two tests correlate well, the bleeding time can be used alone.

Hemophilia

Hemophilia A or factor VIII deficiency and hemophilia B or factor IX deficiency are the most common inherited clotting-factor abnormalities. Hemophilia C, involving deficiency of factor XI, is less common but increasingly recognized. Hemophilias A and B are sex-linked recessive disorders, and hemophilia C exhibits autosomal recessive inheritance and is usually seen in Jews. In these three disorders, the bleeding time is normal but the PTT is usually prolonged. However, if the plasma concentration of the deficient factor is more than 25%, the test can be normal. Bleeding problems during surgery are associated with concentrations below this level. Treatment consists of factor replacement before and after surgery. The necessary quantity of cryoprecipitate or antihemophilic factor required to raise the factor VIII level to 80% of normal should be infused 2 hr prior to surgery, and half of the loading dose should be given every 12 hr for 10 to 14 days postoperatively to avoid delayed hemorrhage. The factor VIII level should be maintained above the 20% to 30% range; this can be monitored by either the factor VIII level or the activated PTT.

Bleeding Due to Acquired Anticoagulants

The lupus anticoagulant, an inhibitor of the prothrombin activator complex, is the most commonly acquired circulating anticoagulant. Although it is seen in approximately 10% of patients with systemic lupus erythematosus, one-half of patients with the anticoagulant have no evidence of the disease. The lupus anticoagulant is a rare cause of bleeding, and surgery can be performed without excessive bleeding.[6,7] Acquired antibodies to factor VIII may arise in the elderly and in women who have just delivered and cause clinical bleeding. Delineation of the course and treatment of bleeding disorders caused by other rare acquired inhibitors is beyond the scope of this chapter.

Other Clotting Abnormalities

Malnutrition, malabsorption, and bowel sterilization can all lead to deficiency of vitamin K and enough decrease in the hepatic activation of factors II, VII, IX, and X to cause bleeding. Vitamin K in a dose of 10 mg subcutaneously corrects the deficiency and normalizes the PT within 8 hr. Immediate control of bleeding requires fresh frozen plasma. Acquired coagulation abnormalities associated with liver disease are difficult to treat. Vitamin K can be given but is usually not effective. Prothrombin complex containing factors II, VII, IX, and X has been given to patients with advanced liver disease before liver biopsy, but the efficacy of this therapy has not been established. In advanced liver disease, the production of factor V may also be deficient; prothrombin complex does not provide all of the missing factors in this case. Low plasma fibrinogen levels may also be seen in patients with liver disease, DIC, or inherited dysfibrinogenemias and be associated with impaired hemostasis and wound healing. Factor X deficiency, reported in patients with systemic amyloidosis, may cause severe bleeding. Deficiency of factor XIII, which is rare, may lead to bleeding in patients with normal clotting studies.

THE PATIENT ON ANTICOAGULANTS

Patients who are undergoing surgery and taking anticoagulant medication fall into two categories: (1) those already on heparin or coumarinlike anticoagulants for a prior or concurrent condition; and (2) those placed on prophylactic low-dose heparin for the prevention of postoperative venous thrombosis and thromboembolism. In the latter case, the patient is usually given 5000 units of heparin subcutaneously 2 hr before surgery and 5000 units subcutaneously every 12 hr thereafter. Such a patient does not require monitoring of coagulation parameters, since the tests are not influenced by heparin at these low doses. There is general agreement that the use of low-dose heparin reduces the incidence of postoperative venous thrombosis and pulmonary embolism in otherwise hemostatically normal patients after all procedures except major orthopedic procedures and open prostatectomy (see Chap. 26).

Many studies have considered the question of whether low-dose heparin is associated with bleeding complications. These are summarized by Pachter and Riles, who noted in their series a 27% incidence of bleeding complications such as wound hematomas and hematuria.[8] They concluded that low-dose heparin should be used only in surgical patients with a high risk of developing venous thromboembolism. In contrast, Barnett and co-workers noted no bleeding complications in 150 patients who were given low-dose heparin before undergoing elective neurosurgical procedures.[9] Low-dose heparin is commonly used, and the consulting internist should be sure that the patient has not taken platelet-active agents such as aspirin within 5 days of surgery.

Patients taking anticoagulants for a prior or concurrent condition are usually fully anticoagulated with either coumarinlike agents or heparin. If the indication for anticoagulation appears to have been tenuous or the patient has had nearly a full course of the drug, anticoagulation can be stopped or reversed preoperatively. However, patients who have suffered prior thromboembolic events have a high risk of recurrent episodes during subsequent surgery. In this case, prophylaxis with low-dose heparin is indicated, and some authors advocate the use of full therapeutic doses. In patients requiring full therapeutic anticoagulation, most major surgical procedures can be safely performed except those involving the eye, central nervous system, or liver.[10] Because its onset of action is immediate and its effects can be rapidly reversed, heparin is preferred over coumarinlike agents for the patient requiring anticoagulation at the time of surgery. The effect of coumarin agents can be reversed by vitamin K and, more rapidly, by fresh plasma or fresh frozen plasma.

Heparin can be given either by intermittent bolus or by continuous infusion. Despite conflicting reports, it is generally felt that the continuous infusion method is associated with fewer bleeding episodes because it avoids the intermittently high serum levels that are achieved in the bolus method. However, a recent prospective study by Wilson and Lampman reports no difference in bleeding complications between patients receiving continuous heparin and patients receiving intermittent therapy.[11] As others, these investigators noted that bleeding complications are significantly more frequent in both treatment groups among patients with recent soft-tissue trauma or vascular damage and among patients with a Lee–White clotting time of greater than 35 min.

Patients who require anticoagulation in the perioperative period should be carefully controlled on heparin, with the activated PTT maintained well within the therapeutic range. Continuous infusion therapy is desirable to avoid intermittent periods of absolute anticoagulation. Some authors feel that continuation of coumarin derivatives does not cause increased bleeding during surgery, particularly minor surgery, and avoids problems of re-establishing anticoagulant control later.[12,13]

If postoperative bleeding in a patient on anticoagulants is life-threatening, the anticoagulant should be discontinued and reversed. Heparin is easily reversed by protamine. In less severe bleeding, the degree of anticoagulation should be determined and the dose of heparin lowered so as to decrease the PTT to the lower end of the therapeutic range. Local causes of bleeding should be corrected. Checks of the platelet count are useful, because heparin can cause thrombocytopenia with both hemorrhagic and thrombotic manifestations.[14] Platelet-active agents should be studiously avoided. Despite these measures, some patients with strong indications for anticoagulation will have significant postoperative bleeding and require

discontinuation or reversal of anticoagulants. The decision of whether to restart anticoagulation must be faced when the patient has been stabilized.

POSTOPERATIVE BLEEDING

Changes in coagulation occur in the postoperative period. Egan and associates studied coagulation parameters in 39 patients before and after surgery and found significant abnormalities in almost all of them.[15] The serum level of fibrin split products (FSP) was abnormally increased in 91% 24 hr after surgery, and values of over 46 µg/ml were found in 90% sometime in the postoperative period. Peak values were noted 3 to 4 days after surgery. The PT was abnormal sometime postoperatively in 82% but was never prolonged for more than 2 sec above the preoperative control time. Only 21% had a significant postoperative decline in platelet count, with no decrease to levels under 125,000. In 95% of the patients, the plasma fibrinogen level rose steadily postoperatively; no patient had a fibrinogen level of less than 375 mg/dl 3 to 4 days after surgery. All surgical procedures were elective, and no patient had a malignancy.

Any patient with a PT of greater than 2 sec above control time, a platelet count of less than 125,000, a decreased plasma fibrinogen level of less than 375 mg/dl 3 to 4 days after surgery, or a plasma level of FSP greater than 120 µg/ml falls outside the expected limits for postoperative changes in coagulation. In this case, DIC or other bleeding disorders should be suspected. These predictable postoperative changes themselves do not usually lead to clinical bleeding or thrombosis.

Postoperative bleeding or thrombosis is

commonly seen in certain clinical situations. Since the brain is rich in thromboplastic substance, head trauma and neurosurgery are two such instances. One study prospectively evaluated 26 patients with severe head trauma.[16] Half of these patients sustained injury that caused significant brain tissue destruction, whereas the other half did not. All patients in the first group exhibited a positive protamine test, suggesting active systemic fibrinolysis and lower than normal plasma fibrinogen levels. Platelet counts were significantly depressed in 4 of the 13. Several patients bled significantly from sites unrelated to their primary injury. In the second group, 12 of 13 had normal fibrinogen and platelet levels, only 3 had weakly positive protamine tests, and none had clinical bleeding. Serial tests after admission documented that the abnormal coagulation parameters returned to normal 24 hr without specific treatment. Unfortunately, no preinjury parameters were available, and all patients received dexamethasone. In a later series of 150 patients who were undergoing brain surgery or had sustained head trauma, 60 showed clinical or laboratory evidence of DIC.[17] Not all coagulation data in these patients were available, but many exceeded normal postoperative coagulation abnormalities. The changes appeared to be self-limited and returned to normal within the first postoperative day.

Heparin treatment is not indicated in the case of head trauma because of the potential for bleeding into the head. Coagulopathies are also reported following abdominal aortic replacement, many orthopedic procedures, prostatic surgery, and cardiopulmonary bypass.[18–21] Clinical DIC is uncommon in these situations.[22]

Insertion of a LeVeen shunt is another operative procedure that is associated with a postoperative coagulopathy.[23] One study examined the occurrence of DIC in 19 patients who had received such a shunt and found alterations in platelet count, PT, and plasma FSP indicative of DIC.[24] Moreover, these abnormalities correlated with good shunt function and disappeared with clotting of the shunt in 4 patients. Clinical bleeding or thrombosis did not occur. Typical abnormalities for patients with good shunt function and normal preoperative coagulation parameters included a platelet count of about 100,000, a prolonged PT of 4 sec above control time, and serum FSP of 200 µg/ml. Although no clinical bleeding or thrombosis occurred, these patients are categorized as having chronic, compensated DIC with a higher risk than normal of these complications. Heparin treatment has not been prospectively evaluated in these patients.

Postoperative coagulation problems are commonly seen by the consulting internist. One of the most frequent is suspected coagulopathy in a patient who is bleeding from the operative wound. The most common cause of wound bleeding is lack of adequate surgical hemostasis. Another cause of a bleeding diathesis in the postoperative patient is a coagulation abnormally overlooked preoperatively.

An internist may also be asked to evaluate an isolated coagulation abnormality noted in a postoperative patient. The platelet count can normally fall postoperatively to about 125,000. Drugs, posttransfusion purpura, DIC, hypothermia, infection, or severe bleeding should be considered as possible causes of significant thrombocytopenia. The PT normally does not exceed the control by more than 2 sec 3 to 6 days after surgery, and the

PTT remains normal. Significant postoperative abnormalities in these tests are usually due to vitamin K malabsorption, liver disease, or an unsuspected inherited factor deficiency.

The surgical patient frequently receives nothing by mouth and is usually given antibiotics. He thus receives no oral vitamin K, and antibiotic sterilization eliminates enough of the gut flora to decrease endogeneous bowel production. Decreased absorption of vitamin K, which is essential for hepatic clotting-factor activity, can become evident within several days to a week after surgery. Factor VII has the shortest half-life of all the clotting factors, and the deficiency is seen in a prolonged PT and bleeding. Treatment merely requires parenteral vitamin K replacement.

Despite a normal preoperative coagulation profile, a patient may have an occult bleeding disorder. The responsible coagulation factor may be decreased preoperatively, although not sufficiently to influence the test. During and after surgery, the factor is consumed and not replaced rapidly, producing an abnormal coagulation test with or without bleeding. If only the PT is prolonged, a factor VII deficiency is probably responsible. If only the PTT is prolonged, and it was normal preoperatively, a factor VIII, IX, or XI deficiency is likely. If both times are prolonged, a factor X, V, II, or I deficiency (or a qualitative abnormality such as dysfibrinogenemia) should be suspected. All of these factors can be analyzed individually so that an accurate diagnosis can be made and appropriate replacement treatment guided. If plasma factor VIII level is decreased, bleeding time prolonged, and platelet count normal, von Willebrand's disease is likely. A ristocetin aggregation test can be performed for confirmation.

DISSEMINATED INTRAVASCULAR COAGULATION

Pathophysiology

Any one of a number of pathologic processes can cause DIC:

Infection
    Gram-negative sepsis
    Gram-positive sepsis
    Rickettsial infection, especially Rocky Mountain spotted fever
    Viral infection
Obstetric
    Septic abortion
    Abruptio placentae
    Retained dead fetus
    Toxemia
Malignant
    Tumors, especially carcinoma of the lung, prostate, stomach, and pancreas, and promyelocytic leukemia
Shock of any cause
Miscellaneous
    Snake bite
    Heat stroke
    Burns
    Hemolytic transfusion reaction
    Vasculitis

All of the above causes share a common denominator that initiates the coagulation sequence (Fig. 29-1). Initiation may occur through damage to the vessel endothelium and exposure of underlying collagen or through release of thromboplastin from damaged or malignant tissue. The coagulation cascade is activated, and thrombin is formed. Thrombin cleaves fibrinopeptide A and fibrinopeptide B from fibrinogen to form fibrin. Fibrin can polymerize at the site of its formation to form a fibrin plug, or, if formed in excess, can diffuse away from its site of formation as a soluble fibrin monomer. Thrombin activates

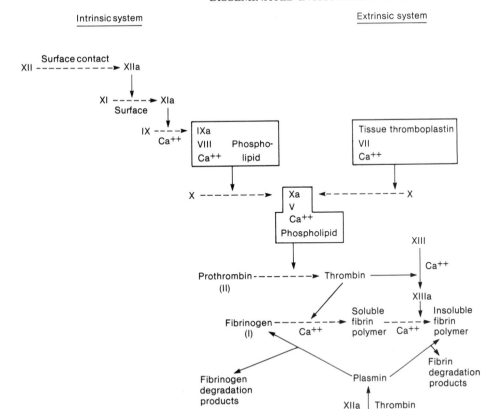

Fig. 29-1. Coagulation pathway.

factor XIII, which catalyzes the cross-linking of the fibrin polymer and makes it more stable. Thrombin amplifies its own production by further activating factors V and VIII. It also provides platelet factor III for the factor IX–factor VIII activation of factor X and the factor X–factor V conversion of prothrombin to thrombin. Thrombin causes platelets to release ADP and aggregate, and this may explain why platelets in DIC behave as if they have an intrinsic storage-pool defect. They behave like platelets that are depleted of ADP and do not aggregate, possibly because of repeated thrombin stimulation. As thrombin is generated, the fibrinolytic system is simultaneously activated by activated factor XII, thrombin, and the disrupted vascular endothelium. Plasmin is formed from plasminogen and cleaves fibrin or fibrinogen to form FSP. Excess FSP can interfere with fibrin polymerization and platelet function. As accelerated clotting and lysis proceed, platelets are consumed as they are caught in the microthrombi or aggregated by collagen and thrombin.

Acute Disseminated Intravascular Coagulation

In acute DIC, coagulation factors are depressed to abnormally low levels, fibrinolytic activity is increased, and platelets are widely consumed. There is no single laboratory test to confirm or exclude the diagnosis of DIC. Colman and co-workers retrospectively studied 60 patients with a pathologic diagnosis of DIC as evidenced by thrombi in the microcirculation.[25] They found that the PT was greater than 15 sec in 90% of patients, the plasma fibrinogen level less than 160 mg/dl in 70%, and the platelet count less than 150,000 in 90% (Table 29-1). If all three criteria were met in a given patient, the diagnosis of DIC was made. If two of the three were fulfilled, a confirmatory test, usually determination of the plasma FSP level, was performed. Plasma FSP concentrations were increased to greater than 5 μg/ml in 95% of the patients. Other confirmatory

tests are currently being developed. Fibrinopeptide A levels are increased in almost all cases, but this test may be too sensitive, producing many false-positive results.[26] Theoretically, antithrombin III levels should fall in DIC, and the concentration of antithrombin III–thrombin complexes should increase.

These laboratory tests for the diagnosis of DIC presuppose a normal underlying coagulation system. Clinicians have long recognized that patients with liver disease already exhibit abnormal baseline studies. All coagulation factors except factor VIII are made in the liver, and activated coagulation factors, fibrinolytic activators, and FSP are normally cleared by the liver. Chronic liver disease leads to portal hypertension, splenomegaly, and pooling of platelets. Colman and colleagues recognized this problem and analyzed patients with chronic liver disease described in the literature.[25] After establishing a "normal" range for PT, platelet count, fibri-

Table 29-1. Criteria for Diagnosis of DIC

Test	Normal Value (mean ± 1 SD)	Criteria for DIC*	DIC (% abnormal)	DIC Values (mean ± 2SD)
			Screening (60 patients, 69 episodes).‡	
Prothrombin time (sec)	12 ± 1	≥15	91	18 (14.5 − 48)†
Platelets (mg/μl)	250,000 ± 50,000	≤150,000	93	52,000 ± 48,000
Fibrinogen (mg/dl)	230 ± 35	≤160	77	131 ± 84
			Confirmatory (45 patients, 54 episodes)§	
Fi titer	<1:8	≥1:16	92	1:52 (1:11–1:256)†
Thrombin time (sec)	20 ± 1.6	≥25	59	27 (21–36)†
Euglobulin lysis time (min)	>120	≤120	42	

Abnormal Screening Tests	Confirmatory Test	Patients§
3/3	Not required	89%
2/3	Required	20%
0–1/3	Required + fibrin thrombi	9%

*Values greater than 2 SD from normal mean values.
†Range of ± 2 SD.
‡Prospective and retrospective studies combined.
§Prospective study.

Table 29-2. Criteria for Diagnosis of DIC when Liver Disease Is Present*

Test	Uncomplicated Cirrhosis† (mean ± SD)	Criteria for DIC‡	Mean Value for DIC (9 patients)
Screening			
Prothrombin time (sec)	14 ± 2	>25	29
Platelets (mg/μl)	176,000 ± 70,000	<50,000	35,000
Fibrinogen (mg/dl)	204 ± 55	<125	85
Confirmatory			
Fi titer	≤1:16	≥1:32	1:84
Thrombin time	92% Abnormal	Not used	86%
Euglobulin lysis time	67% Abnormal	Not used	57%

When liver disease is present, the diagnosis of DIC requires
1. 3/3 Screening criteria for liver disease, or
2. Response to heparin therapy and meeting of regular criteria.

*Patients were considered to have liver disease if any of the following features was manifest: jaundice (bilirubin < 3 mg/dl); cirrhosis suspected clinically (portal hypertension or esophageal varices), histologically, or at laparotomy; recent hepatitis; or centrilobular congestion (serum lactic dehydrogenase (LDH) > 1000 units and glutamic oxaloacetic transaminase (SGOT) > 800 Karmen units) due to congestive heart failure and confirmed by autopsy.

†Source of data: prothrombin time, platelet count, fibrinogen level, and Fi titer. The prothrombin time was originally expressed as the ratio of patient time to control time (average 1.16 ± 0.16). This was converted to seconds for the above comparison, with 12 sec as a control time. The average fibrinogen level was 316 ± 73 mg/dl.

‡Values greater than 2 sd from normal mean values.

nogen level, and FSP concentration for patients with uncomplicated cirrhosis, they choose values 2 standard deviations above the mean as indicative of DIC in these patients (Table 29-2). Application of these criteria to 18 patients with uncomplicated cirrhosis established two groups. Those in whom the diagnosis of DIC was made usually had a typical predisposing cause for DIC, such as infection, and bled from more than one site. Those in whom a diagnosis of DIC could not be made bled only from esophageal varices. In patients without liver disease, bleeding is a common manifestation of DIC and should be sought to support the diagnosis. Bleeding was the presenting manifestation in 78% of patients in one series, and bleeding from more than one site was seen in over 50%. Petechiae and purpura are usually counted as one site.

Any patient in whom a diagnosis of DIC is established preoperatively has higher than normal risk of bleeding at surgery.

Since DIC is always a secondary manifestation, surgery may be necessary to treat the underlying cause. The usual causes of DIC are sepsis, shock, obstetric complications, and malignancy. Once the decision to operate has been made, the question of whether heparin should be used before surgery to "buy time" often arises. Heparin presumably interferes with the coagulation cascade by inhibiting the actions of thrombin and factor X. Therefore, it should slow down fibrin production, decrease secondary fibrinolysis, and cause the rate of platelet consumption to fall.

The literature addresses the use of heparin only in the case of the obstetric patient with DIC. Gram-negative septic abortion with DIC in the pregnant patient leads to acute renal failure so often that some authors advocate the use of heparin in addition to antibiotics and surgical means to control infection.[27,28] Heparin has also been recommended prior to evacuation of a dead fetus from the uterus if the patient is not already in active labor.[29,30] In contrast, heparin is contraindicated in abruptio placenta because of an increased risk of placental bleeding.[31,32] Heparin has proved disappointing in toxemia of pregnancy even when there is laboratory evidence of DIC.[33,34] There have been no controlled studies of heparin treatment in DIC due to other causes.[35]

Careful attention to volume replacement and treatment of sepsis with antibiotics is crucial preoperatively, because both shock and sepsis themselves cause DIC. If heparin is used, it is usually given in a dose of 150 to 500 units/kg body weight per 24 hr by continuous intravenous infusion. The PT, platelet count, and plasma levels of fibrinogen and FSP should be titrated to normal, or the whole-blood clotting time should be arbitrarily maintained at 1½ to 2 times the normal control time.[36]

DIC may develop during surgery, with diffuse oozing in the surgical field or at venopuncture sites. Ecchymosis ultimately follows if the process is allowed to continue. If mismatched blood is responsible, clumped red blood cells may be observed on the scalpel.[37] Postoperative acute DIC must be differentiated from expected changes in coagulation parameters as discussed above. In DIC, the PT is more than 2 or 3 sec longer than the control time. The platelet count and plasma fibrinogen level fall to less than 150,000 and 160 mg/dl, respectively. The plasma FSP concentration level is variable postoperatively and can be elevated in many normal patients to the range seen in DIC. When the diagnosis of DIC is made, the most likely underlying cause is shock or sepsis.

As noted above, the literature is divided on the proper use of heparin in DIC.[25,36,38,39] Heparin can be administered while the primary underlying process is treated, but there are no clear guidelines for its use in the postoperative setting. Replacement of coagulation factors after heparin is started is theoretically feasible, but epsilon-aminocaproic acid alone to decrease fibrinolysis is always contraindicated and is only rarely used in conjunction with heparin and clotting factor replacement.

Chronic Disseminated Intravascular Coagulation

Low-grade or chronic DIC may be clinically inapparent. However, it is a real phenomenon that has been extensively studied in animal models. Cooper and associates infused thromboplastin at various rates into dogs and measured platelet and fibrinogen levels.[40] At high infusion rates, the typical picture of DIC developed with a significant fall in both platelet count and fibrinogen levels. At lower infusion rates, the platelet count fell, but fibrinogen concentrations rose. The authors postulated that thromboplastin at low infusion rates leads to an increase in fibrinogen turnover with a disproportionate rise in hepatic synthesis, resulting in an increased steady-state plasma concentration.

In order to document the presence of ongoing low-grade DIC in which synthesis of clotting factors is sufficient to keep up with consumption, Cooper and colleagues studied plasma levels of FSP and fibrinogen in 79 patients.[41] They assumed that a plasma FSP level above an arbitrarily chosen normal value defined intravascular fibrinolysis. They separated their 79 patients with increased plasma FSP levels into three groups on the basis of simultaneously drawn plasma fibrinogen concentrations. Increased plasma fibrinogen levels of greater than 370 mg/dl were found in 49, or 62%, of the patients. Within this group of patients with "overcompensated" fibrinogen production, platelet counts varied considerably between below and above normal. Assuming that none of the patients had liver disease with a decrease in clearance of FSP or the rare phenomenon of primary fibrinolysis, the postulate that low-grade DIC can occur with increased fibrinogen synthesis seems reasonable. Underlying diseases in this group of patients included vasculitis, primary renal disease, collagen vascular disease, and malignancy. No mention was made of clinical bleeding or clotting problems.

In contrast to the bleeding seen in typical acute DIC, thrombosis is more common in chronic, low-grade DIC. In the 19th century, Trousseau recognized an association between cancer and disseminated thrombosis.[42] Sack and co-workers extensively reviewed this relation in 192 cases of neoplasia associated with some form of arterial or venous coagulation abnormality.[43] The study underscores the variety of abnormalities in coagulation parameters that are seen in this patient population. Platelet counts and plasma fibrinogen levels were increased, decreased, or normal, but plasma FSP concentrations were usually elevated. The most common malignancies observed involved the pancreas (especially body or tail), lung, prostate, stomach, and acute leukemia. There was evidence of arterial emboli in 42 cases. In 31 of the 42, or 74%, nonbacterial thrombotic endocarditis involving the aortic and mitral valves with equal frequency served as the source of the emboli. Tricuspid valve endocarditis was uncommon.

Sun and associates underlined the frequency of coagulation abnormalities in patients with cancer.[44] Of their 61 patients with cancer, only 3 had no coagulation abnormalities; 82% had increased plasma FSP concentrations. Recent or current bleeding episodes were observed in 56%, and thrombophlebitis or thromboembolism was seen in 20%. Coagulation abnormalities were significantly more common in patients with metastatic disease. An increased frequency of clotting abnormalities in neoplasia was also reported by Hagedorn, who studied 50 patients with inoperable lung cancer.[45] Eleven patients had hemoptysis but only minimal mild coagulation abnormalities, suggesting underlying anatomic abnormalities of the bronchi. Only one patient had thrombosis of the subclavian vein. The entire subject of chronic DIC and neoplasia has recently been reviewed.[46]

The clinical significance of chronic DIC in the surgical patient is unclear. Mertens and colleagues studied 42 patients about to undergo transurethral resection of the prostate.[47] They measured plasma FSP levels and performed the qualitative ethanol gelation test, which, along with the protamine sulfate test, is a relatively crude paracoagulation test for measuring fibrin monomer in the plasma. The presence of fibrin monomer is thought to be evidence for systemic fibrinolysis.[48] About half of the 42 patients had benign disease, and the remainder had neoplasms. Those with malignancy bled more frequently, but the incidence of operative bleeding was higher in those patients who had preoperative abnormalities in either coagulation test regardless of the underlying disease. Intervention with preventive treatment such as heparin was not discussed, and no controlled therapeutic studies have been performed.[46]

SUMMARY

1. **When the history and physical examination suggest a hemostatic ab-**

normality, screening tests should include platelet count, bleeding time, PT, and activated PTT. If the patient is bleeding but the tests are normal, a bleeding diathesis is not the cause. If the patient is not bleeding and the tests are normal, a bleeding diathesis should still be suspected if the history of bleeding is strong.

2. One or two aspirin tablets may significantly alter platelet function for up to 10 days. Nonsteroidal anti-inflammatory agents, tricyclic antidepressants, phenothiazines, steroids, some anesthetics, antiarrhythmics, antihistamines, and vitamin E may reversibly affect platelet function for several hours. High doses of any intravenous penicillin may also cause clinical bleeding. Particular offenders are carbenicillin and high-dose penicillin.

3. Patients with Von Willebrand's disease should be followed with a bleeding time. Therapy consists of administration of preparations containing factor VIII, such as fresh frozen plasma or cryoprecipitate.

4. Bleeding during surgery in patients with hemophilia A, B, or C is associated with a plasma concentration of the deficient factor of less than 25% normal and a prolonged PTT. Treatment consists of factor replacement before and after surgery.

5. Surgery in patients with the lupus anticoagulant can be performed without risk of excessive bleeding.

6. Vitamin K deficiency secondary to malnutrition, malabsorption, and bowel sterilization prolongs the PT and can be corrected by vitamin K, 10 mg subcutaneously.

7. Patients on prophylactic heparin, 5000 units subcutaneously every 12 hr, do not require monitoring of coagulation parameters.

8. Patients on heparin who develop bleeding should have their platelet count checked as part of their evaluation, since heparin itself can cause thrombocytopenia.

9. In patients with a PT of greater than 2 sec above control, a platelet count of less than 125,000, a plasma fibrinogen of 375 mg/dl or less, or FSP of greater than 120 μg/ml 3 to 4 days after surgery, DIC should be suspected.

10. Heparin therapy for DIC is clearly indicated only in a septic abortion or evacuation of a dead fetus. The primary treatment of DIC is treatment of the underlying cause, which is usually shock or sepsis in postoperative patients.

REFERENCES

1. Robbins JA, Rose SD: PTT as a screening test. Ann Intern Med 90:796, 1979
2. Eisenberg JM, Goldfarb S: Clinical usefulness of measuring prothrombin time as a routine admission test. Clin Chem 22:1644, 1976
3. Owen CA, Bowie EJW, Thompson JH: The Diagnosis of Bleeding Disorders. Boston, Little, Brown & Co, 1975
4. Aggeler PM, Haag MS, Wallerstein RO et al: The mild hemophilias: Occult deficiencies of AHF, PTC and PTA frequently responsible for unexpected surgical bleeding. Am J Med 30:84, 1961
5. Chediak JR, Telfer MC, Green D: Platelet function and immunologic parameters in Von Willebrand's disease following cryoprecipitate and factor VIII concentrate infusion. Am J Med 62:369, 1977
6. Schleider MA, Nachman RL, Jaffe EA et al: A clinical study of the lupus anticoagulant. Blood 48:499, 1976

7. Boxer M, Ellman L, Carvalho A: The lupus anticoagulant. Arthritis Rheum 19:1244, 1976

8. Pachter HL, Riles TS: Low dose heparin: Bleeding and wound complications in the surgical patient. Ann Surg 186:669, 1977

9. Barnett HG, Clifford, JR, Llewellyn RC: Safety of mini-dose heparin administration for neurosurgical patients. J Neurosurg 47:27, 1977

10. Ellison N, Ominsky AJ: Clinical considerations for the anesthesiologist whose patient is oh anticoagulant therapy. Anesthesiology 39:328, 1973

11. Wilson JR, Lampman J: Heparin therapy: A randomized prospective study. Am Heart J 97:155, 1979

12. Wieberdink J: Safe preoperative anticoagulation. Thorax 22:567, 1967

13. Kloster FE, Briwtow JD, Seaman A: Cardiac catheterization during anticoagulant therapy. Am J Cardiol 28:67, 1971

14. Rhodes GR, Dixon RH, Silver D: Heparin induced thrombocytopenia with thrombotic and hemorrhagic manifestations. Surg Gynecol Obstet 136:409, 1973

15. Egan EL, Bowie EJW, Kazmier FJ et al: Effect of surgical operations on certain tests used to diagnose intravascular coagulation and fibrinolysis. Mayo Clin Proc 49:658, 1974

16. Goodnight SH, Kenoyer G, Rapaport S et al: Defibrination after brain tissue destruction. N Engl J Med 290:1043, 1974

17. Van der Sande JJ, Veltkamp JJ, Boekhout-Mussert RJ: Head injury and coagulation disorders. J Neurosurg 49:357, 365, 1978

18. Mulcare RJ, Royster TS, Phillips LL: Intravascular coagulation in surgical procedures on the abdominal aorta. Surg Gynecol Obstet 143:730, 1976

19. Demirjian Z, Sara M, Strulberg D et al: Disseminated intravascular coagulation in patients undergoing orthopedic surgery. Clin Orthop 102:174, 1974

20. Freidman NG, Hoag S, Robinson AJ et al: Hemorrhagic syndrome following transurethral prostatic resection for benign adenoma. Arch Intern Med 124:341, 1969

21. Muller N, Popou-Cenic S, Buttner W et al: Studies of fibrinolytic and coagulation factors during open heart surgery. II. Post-op bleeding tendency and changes in the coagulation system. Thromb Res 7:589, 1975

22. Doutremdeuich C: Letter: Haemostasis defects following cardiopulmonary bypass based on a study of 1350 patients. Thromb Haemost 39:539, 1978

23. LeVeen HH, Christoridian G, IpM et al: Peritoneovenous shunting for ascites. Ann Surg 180:580, 1974

24. Harman DC, Demirjian Z, Ellman Z et al: Disseminated intravascular coagulation with the peritoneovenous shunt. Ann Intern Med 90:774, 1979

25. Colman RW, Robboy SJ, Minna JD: Disseminated intravascular coagulation: A reappraisal. Ann Rev Med 30:359, 1979

26. Nossel HL, Younger LR, Wilner GB: Radioimmunoassay of human fibrinopeptide A. Proc Natl Acad Sci USA 68:2350, 1971

27. Clarkson AR, Sage RE, Lawrence JR: Causing coagulopathy and acute renal failure due to gram negative septicemia with abortion: Complete recovery with heparin therapy. Ann Intern Med 70:1191, 1969

28. Williams WJ (ed): Hematology, 2nd ed, p 1460. New York, McGraw-Hill, 1977

29. Lerner R, Margolin M, Slate WG et al: Heparin in the therapy of hypofibrinogenemia complicating fetal death in utero. Am J Obstet Gynecol 97:373, 1967

30. Gallup DG, Lucas WE: Heparin therapy of consumptive coagulopathy associated with intrauterine fetal death. Obstet Gynecol 35:690, 1970

31. Pritchard JA: Therapy of the defibrination syndrome of pregnancy. Mod Treatment 5:401, 1968

32. Pritchard JA, Beckken AG: Clinical and laboratory studies on severe abruptio placentae. Am J Obstet Gynecol 97:681, 1967

33. McKay DG: Hematologic evidence of disseminated intravascular coagulation in eclampsia. Obstet Gynecol Surv 27:399, 1972

34. Beecham JB, Watson WJ, Clapp JF III: Eclampsia, pre eclampsia and dissemi-

nated intravascular coagulation. Obstet Gynecol 43:576, 1974

35. Kazmier FJ, Bowie EJW, Hagedorn AB et al: Treatment of intravascular coagulation and fibrinolysis syndromes. Mayo Clin Proc 49:665, 1974

36. Heene L: DIC. Evaluation of therapeutic approaches. Semin Thromb Hemostas 3:291, 1977

37. Owen CA, Bowie EJW: Surgical hemostasis. J Neurosurg 51:137, 1979

38. Colman RW, Robboy SJ, Minna JD: Disseminated intravascular coagulation: A reappraisal. Annu Rev Med 30:359, 1979

39. Bowie EJW, Owen CA: Chronic intravascular coagulation and fibrinolysis syndromes. Semin Thromb Hemostas 3:268, 1977

40. Cooper HA, Bowie EJW, Didisheim P et al: Paradoxic changes in platelets and fibrinogen in chemically induced intravascular coagulation. Mayo Clin Proc 46:521, 1971

41. Cooper HA, Bowie EJW, Owen CA: Evaluation of patients with increased fibrinolytic split products (FSP) in their serum. Mayo Clin Proc 49:654, 1974.

42. Trousseau A: Phlegmasia alba dolens. Clinique Medicale de L'Hotel Diere de Paris. London, The New Sydenham Society, 3:94, 1865

43. Sack GH, Levin J, Bell WR: Trousseau's syndrome and other manifestations of chronic disseminated intravascular coagulation in patients with neoplasms: Clinical, pathophysiologic and therapeutic features. Medicine 56:1, 1977

44. Sun, NCJ, Bowie EJW, Kazmier FJ et al: Blood coagulation studies in patients with cancer. Mayo Clin Proc 49:636, 1974

45. Hagedorn AB, Bowie EJW, Elveback LR et al: Coagulation abnormalities in patients with inoperable lung cancer. Mayo Clin Proc 49:647, 1974

46. Weick JK: Intravascular coagulation in cancer. Semin Oncol 5:203, 1978

47. Mertens BF, Greene LF, Bowie EJW et al: Fibrinolytic split products and ethanol gelation test in preoperative evaluation of patients with prostatic disease. Mayo Clin Proc 49:642, 1974

48. Breen FA Jr, Tullis JL: Ethanol gelation test: A rapid screening test for intravascular coagulation. Ann Intern Med 69:1197, 1968

30

Surgery in Patients with Underlying Blood Disorders

BONNIE J. BLATT
ARTHUR P. STADDON

Patients with blood disorders commonly have superimposed illnesses requiring surgery. Although there is little data on the surgical risk or management of patients with these problems, this chapter reviews what is available and outlines an approach to patients with anemia, polycythemia, leukopenia, and platelet disorders in the surgical setting. Problems of hemostasis are covered in Chapter 29.

ANEMIA

It is commonly accepted that anemia increases the risk of surgery and anesthesia. A survey of over 1200 hospitals in the United States revealed that 88.1% required patients to have a hemoglobin level of greater than 9 g/dl before elective surgery.[1] However, the hypothesis that anemia increases risk by compromising the oxygen-carrying capacity of blood is poorly supported by often conflicting data in the literature. Lunn and Elwood, in a retrospective review of the association between preoperative hemoglobin levels and postoperative complications, found that men but not women with low hy-

moglobin levels were hospitalized longer and had more postoperative complications than average.[2] Mortality was higher than normal in both men and woman with anemia. Although the authors conclude that a relationship appears to exist between preoperative anemia and postoperative complications, their study does not establish causality, since anemia may be indicative of more severe disease. In contrast, Rawstron found that anemia was not associated with an increased number of postoperative complications.[3]

It is also generally accepted that anemia reduces tolerance to anesthesia. Rawstron found that a 45% reduction in hemoglobin was necessary before a definite decrease in tolerance to halothane anesthesia could be demonstrated in mice.[4] Cullen and Eger reduces hematocrits in animals to 10% of normal over a period of several days without significantly altering their anesthetic requirements.[5] The applicability of these studies to humans is as yet unknown.

Finally, it has been thought that anemia may also adversely affect wound healing. In one prospective study, however, Heughen and co-workers clearly showed that mild normovolemic anemia did not compromise healing.[6] This has also been documented in iron-deficiency anemia.[7]

Despite this controversy, it is generally accepted that anemia does increase surgical risk.[8,9] However, the lowest acceptable preoperative hemoglobin level is debated. A hemoglobin of 10 g/dl provides more oxygen to tissue than is needed for normal metabolic requirements.[8] Ventricular function decreases with levels of hematocrit between 24% and 31% but remains stable at levels between 32% and 42%, and coronary blood flow is maximal at a hematocrit of 32%.[8] At hemoglobin levels of 5 to 10 g/dl, blood flow to the left ventricle is evenly distributed, but, at lower levels, it is shunted away from the subendocardium with resultant ischemia.[11] There is some tentative evidence in dogs that anemia influences the amount of myocardium that is liable to necrosis.[12] Cardiac reserve is excellent when the hemoglobin level is 10 g/dl or more, but increases in cardiac output are inconsistent as hemoglobin decreases to 7 g/dl.[8]

It is difficult to establish preoperative hemoglobin requirements and the need for preoperative transfusions. The standard practice in preparing the anemic patient for elective surgery is to define the etiology of the anemia, if possible, to correct the anemia, and to operate only when the hemoglobin concentration is 9 to 10 g/dl or higher. Exceptions to this rule are sickle-cell disease and anemia associated with chronic renal disease, in which hemoglobin levels as low as 4 g/dl have been accepted in the perioperative setting.[8]

Once the decision to transfuse has been made, it is recommended that the procedure be done at least 24 hr before surgery for two reasons. First, it is easier to manage fluid status and avoid volume overload at this time than immediately preoperatively or during surgery. Secondly, levels of 2,3-DPG in transfused blood are low, causing a shift in the recipient's oxygen dissociation curve to the left, with decreased oxygen delivery to the tissues, and more than 24 hr are necessary to replete red-cell 2,3-DPG levels after large transfusions.[13,14]

Sickle-cell anemia is associated with high surgical morbidity and mortality.[15] Patients with SS, SC, and sickle B-thalassemia have the highest risk. Persons with sickle-cell disease and persistent fetal hemoglobin and persons with sickle trait do not share this risk, although the latter patients may develop symptoms in the face of severe hypoxia.[16,17] Conditions that precipitate sickle-cell crisis, including hypothermia, infection, acidosis, and dehydration, should be prevented.[18] Administration of oxygen for at least 24 hr to 48 hr before surgery has been recommended by some authors for patients with sickle-cell disease.[19]

Controversy surrounds the perioperative transfusion requirements of patients with hemoglobinopathies. Browne recommends that elective surgery be postponed until the hemoglobin level is 8 g/dl.[20] Other authors suggest that transfusions be avoided until the hemoglobin level falls to 5 to 7 g/dl.[21,22] Preoperative transfusion or partial exchange transfusion to reduce the concentration of hemoglobin S, even in patients with sickle-cell trait, is essential for open-heart surgery, angiography, and major thoracic, neurosurgical, and vascular operations.[19,23–25] For such cases, it has been suggested that the hemoglobin S concentration be reduced to less than 30% in this manner.[26] Although transfusions have been recommended prior to routine abdominal surgery, there are no data to support this practice.[26] Interestingly, the complication rate in one study was shown to be higher in patients who received preoperative transfusions (28%) than those who did not (13%), but this may reflect the fact that those who required transfusions were more seriously ill.[16] Some authors suggest that, after surgery, transfusion or exchange transfusion be continued to maintain a hemoglobin concentration of 10 g/dl or more for approximately 10 weeks. Surgical risk is not increased in patients with glucose-6-phosphate dehydrogenase (G6PD) as long as various drugs such as antimalarials, sulfonamides, para-aminosalicylic acid, chloramphenicol, and nitrofurantoin are avoided.

POLYCYTHEMIA

Surgical patients with polycythemia vera have a high risk of perioperative complications. Hemorrhage is most common, accounting for approximately 66% of complications and 69% of deaths in one series.[1] Venous and arterial thromboses are less common. Wasserman and Gilbert reviewed the course of 68 patients with polycythemia vera undergoing 81 operations.[27] The overall complication rate of 46% and the mortality rate of 16% were higher than in normals undergoing surgery. Patients with hematocrits of less than 52% prior to surgery had a morbidity rate of 28% and a mortality rate of 5%, compared to patients with uncontrolled disease, in whom the morbidity rate was 79% and the mortality rate 36%. Patients in whom levels of hemoglobin had been controlled for 4 months or more did better than those in whom control had been achieved less than 4 months before surgery.[28]

Patients with polycythemia vera have an increased red blood cell mass with resultant hypervolemia and increased blood viscosity, as reflected by the hematocrit. Increased blood viscosity leads to decreased cardiac ouput and peripheral blood flow, stasis and tissue hypoxia, decreased coronary blood flow, and increased coronary and peripheral resistance.[29] Increased blood viscosity predisposes patients to both thrombosis and hemorrhage.[27] Thrombocytosis is common and may exert an anticoagulant effect.[27,30] Abnormal clot retraction and qualitative platelet abnormalities, such as platelet factor III deficiencies and abnormal aggregation, have been clearly demonstrated.[19,27] There are also a slight prolongation in the prothrombin time and decreases in the plasma concentration of factors V and VII. The coexistence of these many abnormalities may lead to the increased postoperative hemorrhage seen in these patients.[27]

Elective surgery in patients with polycythemia vera should be delayed until the hematocrit has been less than 52% and the platelet count less than 500,000/mm^3 for several months. Phlebotomy and myelosuppressive agents are the treatments of choice.[31] In emergency surgery, phlebotomy should be performed immediately to decrease the hematocrit to 52%, the volume loss being replaced with plasma or plasma expanders. If bleeding occurs during or after surgery, fresh blood should be used for replacement, since it provides factor V and platelets as well as the other clotting factors that are found in stored blood.[27]

The issues of risk and perioperative management are not as straightforward in patients with secondary polycythemia. Many studies have shown extensive bleeding in secondary polycythemia, and thrombosis and hemorrhage are associated with the severe secondary polycythemia that is seen in congenital heart disease.[27] However, in mild or moderate secondary polycythemia, there is no evidence of increased operative risk and no need for phlebotomy. Patients with spurious polycythemia require no special perioperative measures, since their red-cell mass is normal.

LEUKEMIA AND LEUKOPENIA

With the advent of sophisticated supportive techniques, antibiotics, and platelet and granulocyte transfusions, surgery has become possible in leukemic patients.[32] Since these patients now live longer than they used to, complications requiring surgery occur more frequently.[33] These complications must be treated aggressively because of the mortality of 100% reported for leukemic patients who are treated conservatively without surgery.[32] In one report of 9 patients with acute myelocytic leukemia undergoing 10 major abdominal or thoracic procedures, 6, or 66%, survived for more than 1 month.[32] Another study showed similar results, with 8 of 11 patients surviving.[33] Successful surgical outcome is no longer felt to be dependent on hematologic remission.[33]

In the perioperative management of the leukemic patient, important measures include administration of specific antibiotics, when appropriate, platelet transfusions, if platelet counts are less than 50,000/mm³ even without bleeding, and careful monitoring and correction of coagulation parameters.[32] The role of granulocyte transfusions is not well defined but may reduce the risk of surgery in the leukopenic patient. Unless they are below 500/mm³, low granulocyte counts probably do not greatly affect wound healing or increase the risk of infection.[16] Bodey and co-workers have clearly demonstrated a quantitative relationship between the number of circulating white blood cells and the prevalence of infection.[34] The rate of infection increases somewhat when the absolute neutrophil count falls below 1000/mm³ but rises markedly with counts under 500/mm³. Granulocyte transfusions are efficacious in granulocytopenic patients who do not respond to antibiotics alone.[35] Some authors recommend that, if the marrow is hypoplastic and the granulocyte count is less than 200/mm³, granulocyte transfusions should be given for 10 days after surgery. If the marrow is not hypoplastic, transfusions should be withheld unless complications arise.[16]

Because a granulocytopenic patient cannot form pus, the only manifestation of infection may be fever. A significant fever of 101°F or higher should be aggressively evaluated and treated. If no source can be found, the patient should be treated with an appropriate antibiotic combination designed to be effective against pseudomonas.

PLATELETS

Bleeding may occur with thrombocytopenia or thrombocytosis or when platelets are functionally inadequate, as in dysproteinemias, scurvy, or collagen vascular disease. Surgical bleeding is rarely a problem when the platelet count exceeds 50,000/mm³, and spontaneous bleeding usually does not occur until the count falls below 10,000/mm³. The etiology of the thrombocytopenia dictates the management. In the patient with nonimmune-mediated thrombocytopenia requiring surgery, platelet transfusions with HL-A-unmatched platelets can be administered preoperatively for maintenance of a platelet count of 50,000/mm³. Multiple transfusions both during and after surgery may be required.[36] Transfusions should be given 24 hr before surgery, the bleeding time rechecked, and the platelet count maintained by small, frequent transfusions.[16] For every desired increment of 10,000/mm³ in platelet count, one needs the number of units equal to the patient's weight in kilograms divided by 70. Transfused platelets survive approximately 4 days. Possible transplant recipients or those sensitized to random donors should receive single-donor HL-A-matched platelets.[37,38]

In immune-mediated thrombocytopenia, transfused platelets are destroyed rapidly and are generally ineffective in raising the platelet count or decreasing bleeding. If splenectomy is required in patients with this disorder, platelets need not be given preoperatively unless the count is less than 10,000/mm³. When needed, transfusion should be done immediately before surgery.[16] Platelets should also be administered after the splenic pedicle is clamped.[19] In patients with immune-mediated thrombocytopenia who require both a splenectomy and other emergency surgery, the splenectomy should be done first and platelet transfusions given thereafter.

Platelet counts of greater than 1,000,000/mm³ are usually due to myeloproliferative disorders such as polycythemia vera, chronic myelogenous leukemia, myeloid metaplasia, or essential thrombocythemia and are associated with increased risk of hemorrhagic and thromboembolic events. The temporary thrombocytosis that is seen after splenectomy, trauma, or infection is not usually associated with bleeding.[39] The higher the platelet count, the more likely bleeding is to occur. The platelet count should therefore be lowered before surgery whenever possible.[16] If the procedure is elective, the platelet count can be lowered with myelosuppressive therapy. In emergency situations, plateletpheresis has been successfully employed to lower the platelet count to levels below 1,000,000/mm³ before surgery and may be performed postoperatively for maintenance.[40]

Qualitative platelet disorders may exist in themselves or accompany various systemic illnesses such as dysproteinemias, leukemia, and uremia. They may also be caused by drug therapy, most commonly with aspirin, other inflammatory agents, and high-dose penicillin. If a platelet abnormality is suspected, a bleeding time determination should be performed. Bleeding time, which is also affected by thrombocytopenia, is inversely related to the number of circulating platelets below 100,000/mm³.[41] Only rarely are more sophisticated tests of platelet function indicated. When platelet dysfunction has been identified, any contributing underlying process should be treated. Platelet transfusions should be administered preoperatively and the bleeding time repeated for determination of whether the platelets are effective.[19] Platelet transfusions are not useful in dysproteinemias or uremia. If the bleeding time is prolonged in uremia, the patient should undergo dialysis prior to surgery.[19]

A single 650-mg dose of aspirin can significantly prolong the bleeding time in normals for as long as 7 days.[19,42] One dose of 150 mg of acetylsalicylic acid inhibits platelet aggregation for as long as 7 days.[43] However, it is unknown whether the use of acetylsalicylic acid in surgical patients constitutes a major risk.[44] Interestingly, one study of platelet function during surgery in normal patients on no drugs documented progressive, although slight, inhibition and suggested that drugs known to cause platelet dysfunction be avoided because of their additive effect.[45]

In patients with pre-existing hemostatic abnormalities such as hemophilia and von Willebrand's disease, the effect of aspirin on platelets is potentiated.[46] Carbenicillin and other penicillins in high doses induce abnormal platelet aggregation lasting 2 to 4 days after the drug has been stopped and have been associated with bleeding complications.[47] It seems prudent to avoid these agents, to monitor the bleeding time, and to postpone surgery, if necessary. In emergency surgery, platelet transfusions should control perioperative bleeding.

SUMMARY

1. Patients with a hemoglobin concentration above 10 g/dl do not have higher than normal surgical risk.
2. Patients with hemoglobin SS, SC, and sickle-cell B-thalassemia do have increased operative risk. Inhaled gas should contain at least 50% oxygen, and oxygen administration should be continued for at least 24 hr postoperatively. Hemoglobin S concentration should be reduced to less than 30% before surgery.
3. Patients with G6PD deficiency do not have increased surgical risk, but drugs known to increase hemolysis should be avoided.
4. Patients with polycythemia vera are prone to thrombosis and hemorrhage. Elective surgery for these patients should be delayed until the hematocrit is less than 52% and the platelet count

less than 500,000/mm^3 for several months. Before emergency surgery, the hematocrit should be reduced to 52% by phlebotomy.
5. Patients with mild or moderate secondary polycythemia probably do not share the increased risk of those with polycythemia vera.
6. Surgery should not be withheld in the leukemic patient. Antibiotics, platelet transfusions, and granulocyte transfusions may be important.
7. In surgical patients with nonimmune thrombocytopenia, HL-A-unmatched platelets should be administered preoperatively for maintenance of a platelet count of 50,000/mm^3. In patients with immune thrombocytopenia requiring splenectomy, platelets should be given immediately before surgery if the count is less than 10,000/mm^3 and again after the splenic pedicle has been clamped.
8. Patients with platelet counts in excess of 1,000,000/mm^3 are prone to bleeding and thrombosis. Myelosuppressive therapy should be used before elective surgery and plateletpheresis before emergency surgery.
9. Aspirin prolongs the bleeding time and should be avoided if possible the week before surgery.

REFERENCES

1. Kowalshyn TJ, Prager D, Yong J: A review of the present status of preoperative hemoglobin requirements. Anesth Analg (Cleve) 51:75, 1972
2. Lunn JN, Elwood PC: Anaemia and surgery. Br Med J 3:71, 1970
3. Rawstron RE: Anemia and surgery: A retrospective clinical study. Aust NZ J Surg 39:425, 1970

4. Rawstron RE: Oxygen and anemia. Their effects in mice on induction time and survival time. Br J Anaesth 40:214, 1968

5. Cullen DJ, Eger EI: The effects of hypoxia and isovolemic anemia on the halothane requirements (M.A.C.) of dogs. III. The effects of acute isovolemic anemia. Anesthesiology 32:46, 1970

6. Heughen C, Grislis G, Hunt TK: The effect of anemia on wound healing. Ann Surg 179:163, 1974

7. Macon WL, Aries WJ: The effect of iron deficiency anemia on wound healing. Surgery 69:792, 1971

8. Rawstron RE: Preoperative haemoglobin levels. Anaesth Intensive Care 4:179, 1976

9. Moore F: Transcapillary refill, the unrepaired anemia and clinical hemodilution. Surg Gynecol Obstet 139:245, 1974

10. Case RB, Berglund E, Sarnoff SJ: Ventricular function. VII. Changes in coronary resistance and ventricular function resulting from acutely induced anemia and the effects thereof on coronary stenosis. Am J Med 18:397, 1955

11. Brazier J, Cooper N, Maloney JV et al: Acute normovolemic anemia. Effects on the adequacy and distribution of coronary blood flow. Surg Forum 24:203, 1973

12. Hofmann M, Hoffman M, Schaper W: Infarct size manipulation by alteration of hematocrit (abstr). Am J Cardiol 45:484, 1980

13. Valtis DJ, Kennedy AL: Defective gastransport function of stored red blood cells. Lancet 1:119, 1954

14. Beutler E, Wood L: The in vivo regeneration of red cell 2,3-diphosphoglycemic acid (DPG) after transfusion of stored blood. J Lab Clin Med 74:300, 1969

15. Spigelman A, Warden J: Surgery in patients with sickle cell disease. Arch Surg 104:761, 1972

16. Watson–Williams EJ: Hematologic and hemostatic considerations before surgery. Med Clin North Am 63:1178, 1978

17. Szentpetery S, Robertson L, Lower RR: Complete repair of tetralogy associated with sickle cell anemia and G-6PD deficiency. J Thorac Cardiovasc Surg 72:279, 1976

18. Oduro KA, Scarle JE: Anaesthesia in sickle-cell states: A plea for simplicity. Br Med J 4:596, 1972

19. Cooper BS, Churchill WH Jr: Hematology. In Vandam L(ed): To Make the Patient Ready for Anesthesia. Reading, MA, Addison-Wesley, 1980.

20. Browne RA: Anesthesia in patients with sickle cell anemia. Brit J Anaesth 37:181, 1965

21. Holzman L, Finn H, Lichtman HS et al: Anesthesia in patients with sickle cell disease. Curr Res Anesth Analg 48:566, 1969

22. Scarle JE: Anaesthesics in sickle cell states: A review. Anesthesia 28:48, 1973

23. Gilbertson AA: The management of anesthesia in sickle cell states. Proc Royal Soc Med 60:631, 1967

24. Yacoub MH, Baron J, Et-Etr A et al: Aortic homograft replacement of the mitral valve in sickle cell trait. J Thorac Cardiovasc Surg 59:571, 1970

25. Stockman JA, Nigro MA, Meshkin MM et al: Occlusion of large cerebral vessels in sickle cell anemia. N Engl J Med 287:846, 1972

26. Homi J, Reynolds J, Skinner A et al: General anaesthesia in sickle-cell disease. Br Med J 1:1600, 1979

27. Wasserman LR, Gilbert HS: Surgical bleeding in polycythemia vera. Ann NY Acad Sci 115:125, 1964

28. Cole WH: Operability in the young and aged. Ann Surg 138:145, 1953

29. Kemble, Hickman: Postoperative changes in blood viscosity and the influence of hematocrit and plasmafibrinogen. Br J Surg 59:629, 1972

30. Spaet TH, Bulleic S, Melamed S: Hemorrhagic thrombocythemia: A blood coagulation disorder. Arch Intern Med 98:377, 1956

31. Wasserman LR, Gilbert HS: The treatment of polycythemia vera. Semin Hematol 13:57, 1976

32. Bjornsson S, Yates JW, Mittelman A et al: Major surgery in acute leukemia. Cancer 34:1275, 1974

33. Seligman BR, Rosmer F, Ritz ND: Major surgery in patients with acute leukemia. Am J Surg 124:632, 1972

34. Bodey GP, Buckley M, Sathe YS et al: Quantitative relationship between circulating leukocytes and infection in patients with acute leukemia. Ann Intern Med 64:328, 1966

35. Alavi JB, Root R, Djerassi I et al : A randomized clinical trial of granulocyte transfusion for infection in acute leukemia. N Engl J Med 296:706, 1977

36. Bergin JJ, Zuck TF, Miller RE: Compelling splenectomy in medically compromised patients. Ann Surg 178:761, 1973

37. Kahan BD, Green D, Ruder A et al: Single donor, HLA-matched platelet transfusions for thrombocytopenic patients undergoing surgery. Surgery 77:247, 1975

38. McCredie KB: Platelet and granulocyte transfusion therapy. Postgrad Med 62:150, 1977

39. Silver D, McGregor FH Jr: Nonmechanical causes of surgical bleeding. Curr Probl Surg, Jan:1, 1970

40. Panlilio AL, Russ RF: Therapeutic plateletpheresis in thrombocythemia. Transfusion 19:147, 1979

41. Harken LA, Stichter SJ: The bleeding time as a screening test for evaluation of platelet function. N Engl J Med 287:155, 1972

42. Cohen LS: Clinical pharmacology and acetylsalicyclic acid. Semin Thromb Hemostas 2:146, 1976

43. O'Brien JR: Effects of salicylates on human platelets. Lancet 1:779, 1968

44. Merriman E, Bell W, Conlin M et al: Surgical postoperative bleeding associated with aspirin ingestion. Report of two cases. J Neurosurg 50:682, 1979

45. Kokores JA, Economopoulos TC, Alexopoulos C et al: Platelet function tests during major operation for gastrointestinal carcinoma. Br J Surg 64:149, 1977

46. O'Brien JR: Aspirin, haemostasis and thrombosis. Br J Haematol 29:524, 1975

47. Brown CH, Natelson EH, Bradshaw M et al: The hemostatic defect produced by carbenicillin. N Engl J Med 291:265, 1974

Prophylactic Antibiotics in Surgery

JAIME CARRIZOSA
ELIAS ABRUTYN

Prophylactic antibiotics have been used for years to prevent surgical infections, which contribute significantly to the morbidity and mortality of surgery. Despite extensive clinical experience and the existence of a large body of literature, their use in surgery has been controversial. However, in recent years, several excellent studies have aided in defining principles for the use of prophylactic antibiotics and identifying situations in which prophylaxis appears to be effective.[1–6] This chapter reviews the principles of prophylaxis and their applications.

GENERAL PRINCIPLES

The use of antibiotics in prophylaxis must be clearly distinguished from their role in the therapy of proved or suspected infection. Administration of antibiotics in cases of documented infection such as pneumonia or urinary tract infection is considered therapeutic usage, as it is in the context of surgery involving traumatic wounds, a gangrenous gallbladder, a ruptured appendix, or an ischemic bowel. In these and similar situations, bacterial contamination or infection is presumed to have already occurred, and antibiotics are given to treat an established infection. Antibiotics may also be given expectantly when infection is suspected but not yet proved by confirmatory studies. Therapeutic or expectant antibiotic use must be distinguished from prophylaxis because of differences in dosage schedule or duration of treatment.

Several principles have been established for the use of prophylactic antibiotics in surgery. The first principle rests on establishing the need for prophylaxis based on risk of infection. Prophylaxis should be considered in high-risk situations, but not in those of low risk unless the consequences of infection would be disastrous. Factors that modify the risk of wound infection after contamination include age, nutritional status, the nature of the underlying disease, the presence of necrotic tissue, and changes in blood supply.[7–10] Although important, these parameters are difficult to measure, but the standard classification of surgical procedures may permit a crude estimation of the risk of infection and need for prophylaxis.[11]

Clean operations are those in which aseptic technique is maintained, inflammation is not found, and the gastrointestinal, respiratory, or genitourinary tract is not entered. Such operations are usually elective, and wounds are nearly always closed by primary intention. The risk of infection in clean operations is less than 5%. Clean–contaminated operations are operations in which, despite entrance into the gastrointestinal, respiratory, or genitourinary tract, contamination by their contents is not significant. In these operations, the risk of infection is less than 10%. Contaminated operations are those in which acute inflammation but no inflammatory exudate is found and include operations in which there has been a major break in aseptic technique or spillage from a hollow viscus. Fresh open traumatic wounds fall into this category. The infection rate for contaminated operations approximated 20%. Dirty operations include those in which abscesses, purulent material, or a perforated viscus is found. Old traumatic wounds are also placed in this category, which carries an infection rate exceeding 30%.

Prophylaxis is generally not indicated for clean surgical procedures except in cases in which the consequences of infection would be catastrophic, as in infection complicating cardiac valve replacement. Prophylaxis is frequently considered in clean–contaminated operations and is almost always used in contaminated and dirty operations. In the latter two cases, the use of antibiotics is considered treatment of early or established infection rather than prophylaxis.

The second principle requires consideration of those organisms that commonly cause contamination and infection in a given setting, thereby guiding the choice of prophylactic antibiotic. For example, the possible role of *Staphylococcus aureus* in total hip replacement surgery and that of gram-negative organisms and anaerobes in colon surgery need to be taken into account.

The third principle states that antibiotics should be chosen on the basis of clinical and laboratory evidence of efficacy against the important, potentially infecting microorganisms.[12] All antibiotic regimens are selective, and no single antibiotic or combination is effective against all potential pathogens. Because of this, only common pathogens are covered by prophylaxis. Broad-spectrum coverage suppresses indigenous flora and selects for resistant organisms that may produce serious, difficult-to-treat infections.

The fourth principle requires the choice of nontoxic antibiotics with specific pharmacokinetic properties that make them especially effective in prophylaxis. Such properties will be discussed in more detail later in the text.

The fifth principle requires that the chosen antibiotic regimen be administered appropriately. Prophylaxis should be started before the procedure begins and, depending on the route of administration and the pharmacokinetic characteristics of the drug, at a frequency and dosage that will produce therapeutic serum drug levels when the incision is made. Prophylaxis started earlier is probably no more effective; long periods of prophylaxis preceding surgery lead to selection of resistant organisms. Serum and tissue drug levels must be maintained at therapeutic levels during the procedure. Since the serum half-lives of some antibiotics are short, additional doses may be required during long procedures.

After surgery, antibiotics should be continued only for a short time. This period is often no more than two or three days, and evidence suggests that shorter courses or even one dose may be equally effective.

Short-course therapy is effective in part because the bacteria load at the time of surgery when contamination occurs is small. In addition, fibrin, necrotic tissue, or compromise in blood supply, factors that make established infections difficult to treat, are usually not present when contamination occurs. Finally, prolonged prophylaxis may mask smoldering infection requiring different therapy.

The sixth principle dictates that the benefits of prophylaxis outweigh its dangers. Despite appropriate use, prophylactic antibiotics do not prevent all postoperative infections. Although prophylaxis is designed to prevent specific infections, such as those involving the wound or a prosthetic valve, it is not intended to combat infections in general. Pneumonia and urinary tract infection may occur even when wound infection has been successfully prevented. Prophylaxis is no substitute for meticulous surgical technique. The importance of strict aseptic technique, care in handling of tissues, closure of dead spaces, and elimination of necrotic debris cannot be over-emphasized.

ANTIBIOTIC SELECTION

The selection of antibiotics in prophylaxis is based on the type of surgical procedure being done, the species of common infecting organisms involved, and the characteristics of the drugs chosen. Prophylactic antimicrobial agents should ideally be nontoxic, inexpensive, and bactericidal in action. They should be available in parenteral form, preferably for intravenous use, and the serum drug concentration should reach therapeutic levels shortly after administration. The serum half-life of the drug should allow for maintenance of therapeutic levels throughout the procedure to obviate the need for additional doses intraoperatively and should distribute widely in tissues.[13] Although the clinical significance of protein binding remains controversial, it is thought that the level of free drug and its activity are inversely related to its affinity to serum proteins.

Even with adequate serum drug levels, several factors influence the effectiveness of prophylactic antibiotics. Drug concentrations are high in well-perfused tissues such as heart, lung, liver, and kidney and lower in relatively poorly perfused tissues such as muscle, skin, adipose tissues, bone, and ligaments.[13] Tissue hypoxia and acidosis may decrease the activity of some antibiotics. When bacteria are sequestered intracellularly, as in the case of S. aureus, the effectiveness of many antibiotics is decreased because they fail to penetrate phagocytes.

Among the various drugs used in prophylaxis, cephalosporins have clear advantages. They are bactericidal antibiotics with a broad spectrum of activity against organisms including S. aureus, all streptococci except enterococci, pneumococci, and some Enterobacteriaceae such as Escherichia coli, Klebsiella, and Proteus mirabilis. The newer cephalosporins, cefoxitin and cefamandole, have even wider activity against other organisms. Cefamandole is effective against Enterobacter species and cefoxitin against indole-positive Proteus, Serratia, and some types of Bacteroides fragilis. With the exception of cephaloridine, which is nephrotoxic at high doses, the cephalosporins have acceptably low toxicity, and relatively high serum levels can be achieved after intramuscular or intravenous administration. The half-lives of the different compounds vary, that of cefazolin being the longest at 100 min. Protein binding is also variable.

Penicillinase-resistant penicillins—methicillin, nafcillin, and oxacillin—have also been used successsfully. They are relatively inexpensive, nontoxic, bactericidal agents with excellent activity against gram-positive cocci, in particular against S. aureus.

ORTHOPEDIC SURGERY

The risk of infection in orthopedic surgery is variable, depending in part on the nature of the procedure. Most orthopedic operations can be classified as clean, with a risk of infection of less than 5%. However, prophylaxis is generally given before clean procedures involving prosthetic devices because the consequences of infection in this setting would be especially serious. Surgical treatment of open fractures, thought to be a clean–contaminated procedure, usually includes antibiotics. In this case, contamination is considered to have already occurred, and the use of antibiotics is viewed as therapeutic rather than prophylactic.

Many measures other than administration of systemic antimicrobials have been used to prevent infection in orthopedic surgery. These include the use of ultraviolet light, incorporation of antibiotics into bone cement, perfusion of wounds with antimicrobics by way of ingress and egress tubes, and measures to purify the air in the surgical suite, including laminar flow. Success has been reported with each of these methods, but the data are not entirely convincing.

Hip Fractures

Repair of hip fractures may carry a higher incidence of infection than other clean orthopedic procedures because it involves manipulation of previously traumatized tissues and insertion of a prosthetic device. However, the benefit of prophylaxis in reducing the rate of infection is unclear. Boyd and Burke reported a reduction in deep infections among patients undergoing hip repair by methods other than total hip replacement.[14] The rate of infection was 0.8% in the group receiving prophylactic nafcillin and 4.8% in the control group, with no difference in the incidence of infected hematoma. Other less well-designed studies evaluating prophylactic cloxacillin in the repair of intratrochanteric fractures and in the insertion of Austin–Moore prostheses do not demonstrate such differences.[15–17] Until definitive studies are performed, prophylaxis appears to be indicated in hip repair because of poor functional results after removal of an infected prosthesis.

Total Joint Replacement

The rate of infection after surgical replacement of a joint may be higher than normal because of the presence of foreign bodies, including cement, or because of the length and difficulty of the procedure. Infections after such surgery may be classified as early or late. Early infections occur within 2 months of surgery and are commonly caused by S. aureus and S. epidermidis; late infections occur thereafter and are frequently caused by S. aureus, E. coli, and P. aeruginosa. Early infections are thought to result from contamination of the wound during surgery and late infections from bacteremic episodes unrelated to the operation. One controlled study has shown that 2 weeks of prophylactic therapy with cloxacillin reduces the frequency of late infections.[18] This suggests that some late infections may also be the result of contamination during surgery and that prophylaxis against S. aureus and *S. epidermidis* may be effective in preventing some infections; however, confirmation is required. Other studies have indicated that short-course antibiotic prophylaxis is beneficial.[19-21]

Acceptable short-course prophylaxis regimens include cephalothin, 2 g, nafcillin, 500 mg, or cefazolin, 1 g given intravenously 1 hr before surgery and every 4 hr to 6 hr therafter for 24 to 48 hr. These agents are likely to be effective against most staphylococci. On the basis of studies of prophylaxis in other clean surgical procedures, there is reason to believe, but no firm data to confirm, that a single dose of antibiotic may be effective. The benefits of long-course prophylaxis require further evaluation. Prophylactic antibiotics are often used in patients who have a prosthesis in place when they undergo any operative procedure or instrumentation thought to be associated with a high incidence of bacteremia, but there are no studied evaluating their value.

Other Clean Orthopedic Procedures

The use of antibiotics in clean orthopedic procedures is probably not indicated. Pavel and colleagues demonstrated a significant reduction in the rate of wound infection in all such orthopedic procedures from 5% in his control group to 2.8% among patients receiving cephaloridine before and during the operation.[22,23] However, when the results were classified according to anatomic site of surgery, the number of patients in each group was small and the differences not significant. Because the risk of infection is low and the benefit of prophylaxis minimal, the use of antibiotics in clean procedures does not appear to be justified. However, a case can be made for prophylaxis in some spinal surgery, such as that for cor-

rection of scoliosis. This operation is long and difficult, and postoperative infection has disastrous consequences.

SURGERY OF COLON AND RECTUM

Elective colorectal surgery is considered to be clean–contaminated. It is performed in areas of heavy bacterial colonization, with a high probability of contamination of the peritoneal surface. In such cases, the rate of postoperative infection ranges between 10% and 50%. Proposed prophylactic antibiotic regimens fall into three major categories: intestinal antisepsis, systemic prophylaxis, and irrigation with topical antibiotics.[24] Innumerable regimens involving different antimicrobial agents and combinations of different prophylactic modalities have been proposed.

Intestinal Antisepsis

Mechanical cleansing and preoperative oral administration of antibiotics have been used to reduce the intraluminal mass of aerobic and anaerobic bacteria. Thorough mechanical cleansing transiently reduces the bacterial load by removing large amounts of feces from the colon, but it does not sterilize the colon. Mechanical cleansing alone reduces the incidence of wound infection and sepsis after colorectal surgery. The most commonly used regimen requires 48 hr to 72 hr and includes a low-residue diet for the first 24 hr to 48 hr followed by a liquid diet for 24 hr, cathartics, and enemas usually composed of saline solutions to reduce electrolyte losses.

Mechanical cleansing has been combined with administration of oral antibiotics to reduce the bacterial load further, and the combination appears to be more effective than mechanical cleansing alone. Several studies have shown that mechanical cleansing and either neomycin and erythromycin, neomycin and tetracycline, neomycin and metronidazole, or kanamycin and metronidazole given for 1 or 2 days before surgery reduce the infection rate from approximately 30% to 40% in the group given mechanical cleansing alone to 8% to 10% among patients who are receiving antibiotics as well.[25-36] Other regimens include the use of neomycin with sulfathalidine and erythromycin with kanamycin.[30,37,38] One popular regimen consists of 1 g of oral neomycin and 1 g of oral erythromycin base given during the afternoon and evening of the day before surgery. Doses are administered 19 hr, 18 hr, and 9 hr before the scheduled procedure. No enemas are given the evening before surgery, but the patient evacuates 3 hr before going to the operating room. Another regimen consists of 500 mg of neomycin and 250 mg of tetracycline given orally 4 times daily in the 48 hr before the procedure.[31,32]

Single agents have been studied in multiple trials. In one study, doxycycline in a dose of 200 mg orally every 4 hr to 6 hr with mechanical cleansing reduced infection rates from 45% to 12% when compared to mechanical cleansing alone.[39] Drugs like doxycycline, tetracycline, erythromycin, and metronidazole are absorbed, and their effectiveness may lie not only in their intraluminal activities but also in their systemic effects. Other drugs that have been tried as single agents include neomycin, streptomycin, kanamycin, gentamicin, tetracycline, lincomycin, metronidazole, and several sulfonamide derivatives.[40,41] The activity of these single agents against bowel flora is limited, and selection of resistant flora frequently occurs. In the absence of well-controlled studies demonstrating their efficacy, single drugs are not recommended. Potentially toxic drugs should be avoided. In addition to their potential for allowing the emergence of resistant aerobic and anaerobic bacteria, oral agents may encourage overgrowth with organisms like staphylococci or produce pseudomembranous colitis. The latter complication has occurred after administration of any of several antibiotics by the oral or parenteral route.

Systemic Antibiotics

Since it has been demonstrated that prophylactic antibiotics must be given before or at the time of bacterial challenge in order to be effective, several studies have evaluated the benefit of prophylactic systemic without oral antimicrobials.[42-47] In their prospective study, Polk and Lopez–Mayor demonstrated that 1 g of cephaloridine administered just before surgery and 5 hr and 12 hr later reduced the rates of wound and intra-abdominal infections from 30% in the control group to 7% in those treated.[42] Patients in both groups received mechanical bowel preparation. Similarly, Stone and co-workers showed that systemic cefazolin was effective in reducing the incidence of wound infection from 16% to 4%.[43] Penicillin alone and gentamicin with lincomycin or clindamycin have been shown to be effective in other studies.[44]

The results of studies comparing regimens of mechanical cleansing with oral antibiotics to those of mechanical cleansing with systemic antibiotics are conflicting. In one study, patients receiving metronidazole and kanamycin parenterally had a lower infection rate than patients given the same drugs orally. The oral regimen was associated with a higher incidence of bacterial overgrowth and pseudomembranous colitis. Lewis and associated found no difference in rate of would infection between preoperative parenteral cephaloridine and oral neomycin and erythromycin.[45] The well-designed Veterans' Administration Cooperative Study demonstrated the infection rate to be 39% in patients given parenteral cephalothin and 6% in patients given oral neomycin and erythromycin with or without cephalothin.[46] Additional studies are in progress.

Topical Antibiotics

A third modality of prophylaxis in colorectal surgery consists of irrigation with antibiotic solutions. The benefit of such antibiotics has not been evaluated in rigorous well-controlled studies, and firm conclusions cannot be drawn.[48] Adsorption of these agents can occur, and toxic compounds such as neomycin should be avoided.

To summarize, it appears that mechanical preparation with an oral antibiotic or a systemic antibiotic that produces therapeutic levels at the time of surgery is effective in reducing infectious complications of colorectal surgery. The neomycin and erythromycin regimen outlined above can be used orally, and cefazolin can be employed systemically. The efficacy of oral neomycin and erythromycin alone compared to neomycin and erythromycin with a parenteral cephalosporin is currently under investigation.

GASTRODUODENAL SURGERY

Gastroduodenal procedures fall within the category of clean–contaminated surgery. The overall rate of infectious complications is variable, ranging from 3% to 28% and averaging approximately 10%. The benefit of prophylaxis is difficult to assess, but one study showed that a 3-dose course of cephaloridine effectively reduces the infection rate.[42]

Currently, there is a trend to place patients undergoing gastroduodenal surgery into low- and high-risk groups.[49] Low-risk patients are those without impairments in normal host defenses (e.g., bowel motility or gastric acid production) undergoing primarily elective operation (e.g., surgery for duodenal ulcer that is unresponsive to medical treatment or that bleeds repeatedly). Risk may be low because of the protective effect of the relatively sterile acid environment of the stomach. Organisms found in the stomach include streptococci, lactobacilli, staphylococci, in low numbers, and, occasionally, anaerobic bacteria or enterobacteriaceae. In contrast, high-risk procedures are those in which host defenses are compromised and include surgery for gastric carcinoma, peptic ulcer disease with obstrucion, and acute hemorrhage from gastric or duodenal ulcer.

Using this classification, Lewis and colleagues studied 109 patients undergoing gastroduodenal surgery.[50,51] No organisms or only gram-positive cocci were isolated from the gastric contents of patients in the low-risk group. Gram-positive cocci, gram-negative rods, Candida, and anaerobic streptococci were isolated from the stomachs of high-risk patients. Identification of isolated organisms allowed prediction of both the risk and the etiology of infection.

Reported infection rates for various conditions requiring gastroduodenal surgery also support the separation of patients into low- and high-risk groups. Infection rates of 3% to 10% have been reported for duodenal ulcer surgery and of 16% to 48% for procedures involving a perforated gastric ulcer, gastric tumor, and gastrointestinal hemorrhage. In a well-designed trial of prophylactic antibiotics, Nichols and co-workers determined the incidence of postoperative sepsis in high-risk patients undergoing gastroduodenal surgery.[52] Patients who had received 3 doses of cefamandole beginning 1 hr before surgery had an infection rate of 5%, whereas patients given a placebo agent had a rate of 35%. At present, it seems advisable to consider prophylaxis only in patients with a high risk of infection. The choice of cephalosporin is reasonable.

BILIARY TRACT SURGERY

The role of prophylactic antibiotics in biliary surgery is unclear. Several studies have evaluated prophylaxis primarily in elective biliary surgery and found it to be beneficial.[53–61] In separate studies, gentamicin, tobramycin with lincomycin, intravenous trimethoprim–sulfamethoxazole, and cefazolin, even in a single dose, were shown to be effective. However, the risk of infection in otherwise healthy patients undergoing biliary surgery with or without incidental cholelithiasis is low.

As in gastroduodenal surgery, it appears useful to classify patients undergoing biliary tract surgery into low- and high-risk groups. The risk of infection is high if bacteria are present in the bile. Infected bile contains 10^4 to 10^8 organisms, including E. coli, enterococci, S. aureus, and others, and these frequently cause infection after biliary surgery. In contrast, the rate of infection in patients with uncontaminated bile is about 2%. The need

for prophylaxis can be based on an intraoperative Gram stain of the bile, and cultures of bile can be performed during surgery to guide therapy if infection develops.[57] High-risk patients to be considered for prophylaxis are those with acute cholecystitis, obstructive jaundice, or common-duct stones without jaundice, patients over the age of 70, and patients with a recent history of fever and chills.

Antibiotics used in the prophylaxis of biliary surgery are often chosen on the basis of their hepatic excretion. However, when obstruction is present, drug levels in bile are undetectable. A reasonable prophylactic regimen in high-risk patients consists of cefazolin, 500 mg before surgery and every 6 hr to 8 hr theraffter for a total of 24 hr. Gentamicin and other nephrotoxic antibiotics are not recommended for routine use.

GYNECOLOGIC SURGERY

Abdominal Hysterectomy

The use of prophylactic antibiotics in abdominal hysterectomy remains controversial. The rates of infection following this procedure vary, depending on definitions of morbidity used in different studies. For example, the frequency of wound and deep pelvic infection is about 10% to 15%, but the rate of complication approaches 40% when febrile or operative morbidity and other infections such as urinary tract infections or pneumonia are included. Febrile or operative morbidity is often defined as temperature elevation in excesss of 38°C on two separate occasions at least 6 hr apart during a defined period after surgery excluding the first 24 hr. Since the definition of febrile morbidity varies among studies, comparisons are difficult. Because proven infections are relatively uncommon, most studies of prophylaxis rely on evaluation of this variably defined parameter. An additional problem in the study of infection in abdominal hysterectomy is the difficulty of defining the precise nature of an infection e.g., wound infection or pelvic cellulitis) even when it is clearly present.

Several studies using primarily cephalosporin support the use of this agent in prophylaxis.[62–65] In a prospective study using cephalothin, Allen and co-workers reported a decrease in febrile morbidiy from 41% to 14% with a decreased hospital stay in the treated group.[63] In another study of cephaloridine on the day of surgery followed by cephalexin for 4 days after surgery, Ohm and Galask showed that antibiotics reduced operative morbidity from 39% to 15%.[64] However, the groups studies were small, and the differences were not statistically significant. Duration of hospitalization was not decreased, and resistant organisms were recovered from patients receiving antibiotics. Cefazolin given preoperatively followed by cefalexin postoperatively until removal of the urinary catheter and carbenicillin have also been shown to reduce the complication rate. Grossman and his colleagues compared penicillin and cefazolin prophylaxis in abdominal and vaginal hysterectomy.[65] There were fewer infections among the antibiotic-treated patients undergoing abdominal hysterectomy, but there were no differences in febrile morbidity or duration of hospital stay.

Although these studies suggest that prophylaxis is beneficial, the data are not entirely convincing. The low frequency and mild severity of infection after abdominal hysterectomy suggest that routine prophylaxis is not justified. Short-course prophylaxis consisting of a single dose of antibiotics should be evaluated.

Vaginal Hysterectomy

The incidence of complications following vaginal hysterectomy varies, depending on the definition of complications used, the type of operation carried out, and perhaps the age of the patient. In vaginal hysterectomy, as in total abdominal hysterectomy, the presence of infection is often difficult to document, and a reduction in febrile or operative morbidity is frequently used as a measure of success. If febrile morbidity is excluded, the incidence of wound infections, including those of the vaginal cuff, pelvic cellulitis, or adnexal abscesses, is high, ranging from 12% to 64%, and justifies evaluation of the benefits of prophylaxis.

Initial studies of antibiotic prophylaxis using intramuscular chloramphenicol alone or a combination of penicillin and streptomycin showed a reduction in febrile morbidity. The combination was more effective than the chloramphenicol alone. The introduction of cephalosporins resulted in a wide evaluation of their prophylactic benefit with generally good results. Allen and colleagues showed that cephalothin given on the day of surgery and for 3 days thereafter reduced febrile morbidity.[63] Studying the efficacy of cefazolin given just before surgery and 6 hr and 12 hr postoperatively, Polk documented a reduction in rates of pelvic infection from 21% in the placebo group to 2% in the treated group. Febrile morbidity and length of hospital stay were reduced in patients given cefazolin. Grossman and co-workers showed that cefazolin given before surgery and every 6 hr thereafter for a total of 48 hr was also effective.[65]

Several studies have evaluated the efficacy of short courses of prophylactic antibiotics.[66–75] Ledger and associates showed that cephaloridine given only on the day of surgery was as effective as a regimen of preoperative cephaloridine and postoperative cephalexin for 5 days.[66] Mendelson and co-workers found that a single 2-g dose of cephradine was as effective a regimen as 1 g given preoperatively and every 6 hr after surgery for 24 hr.[67] Lett and colleagues obtained comparable results with a single dose of 1 g of cefazolin just prior to surgery or a regimen of 3 preoperative doses of cephaloridine 10 hr apart.[68]

Many other regimens have been evaluated. Jennings administered cefazolin before operation and cephalexin postoperatively until the urinary catheter was removed.[69] Biven and associates and Ohm and Galask used combined cephalothin–cephalexin regimens for 5 days.[70,71] Roberts and Homesley used carbenicillin in a dose of 2 g intravenously just prior to surgery followed by 2 g every 6 hr for 5 days.[72] Bolling and Plunkett used either ampicillin or tetracycline for 7 days.[74] More complicated regimens designed to provide broader coverage including anaerobic flora use gentamicin and clindamicin or metronidazole. However, these regimens do not appear to be more efficacious. Further comparative trials are required.

Two recent comprehensive reviews conclude that prophylaxis is useful and can be accomplished with a single preoperative dose of cephalosporin.[3,73] We recommend 1 g of cefazolin given intramuscularly or intravenously 1 hr before surgery.

The use of prophylactic antibiotics has been evaluated in obstetric procedures including cesarean section and will not be discussed here. The reader is referred to several recent studies.[76–87]

UROLOGIC SURGERY

The effects of prophylactic antibiotics on the frequency of postoperative fever, urinary tract infection, gram-negative bacteremia, and epididymitis, as well as the duration of hospitalization, have been evaluated in the setting of prostatectomy. Various studies have evaluated several potentially useful agents, including cephalosporins, gentamicin, kanamycin, trimethoprim–sulfamethoxazole, nitrofurantoin, and a combined regimen of kanamycin and trimethoprim–sulfamethoxazole.[87–96] The role of prophylaxis, however, remains unclear. One review of the literature found that: (1) some trials included patients undergoing both open and transurethral prostatectomy; (2) some studies included patients both with and without sterile urine; (3) criteria used for evaluating morbidity or defining parameters such as postoperative fever and significant bacteriuria differed; and (4) the duration of postoperative catheterization was not consistently specified. Moreover, most regimens were administered for more than 5 days and some for 10 days. None evaluated short-course regimens. The results of the various studies suggest that there is no consistent clinical benefit to be derived from prophylaxis in patients with sterile urine undergoing transurethral prostatectomy. Benefit in other subgroups is unclear.

Despite the absence of data, a reasonable approach can be adopted. Patients with bacteriuria are given antibiotics to sterilize the urine by the time of surgery and reduce the risk of gram-negative bacteremia. To do this, 24 or 48 hr of therapy is usually sufficient, and longer periods of treatment may predispose to the selection of resistant organisms. Patients with sterile urine are not treated but are followed closely postoperatively. Subsequent culture-proven infections are treated. Closed drainage systems prevent or delay development of infection, but irrigation with neomycin–polymyxin solutions is not recommended. The same approach is used in other urologic procedures such as that involving removal of infected stones.

NEUROSURGICAL PROCEDURES

Neurosurgical procedures are classified as clean surgery and have low infection rates. Postoperative infections commonly involve organisms such as S. aureus, S. Epidermidis, and P. aeruginosa. Unfortunately, no conclusive studies of prophylaxis have been published, and even tentative conclusions cannot be drawn from the available data.[97–99] Savitz and Malis used 2 doses of clindamycin intraoperatively and reported reduced rates of infection in patients undergoing craniotomy with microsurgical techniques but not in patients undergoing laminectomy.[97] However, the number of patients included in these studies is too small for the results to be reliable. Wyler and Kelly studied the effect of ampicillin in external ventriculostomies and reported a reduction in infection rates from 27% among patients in the control group to 9% among patients receiving antibiotics.[99] However, other prospective controlled studies are not available. Theoretically, antibiotics for prophylaxis should be bactericidal, able to penetrate the blood-brain barrier, thus producing high cerebrospinal fluid and brain levels, and active against the common infecting organisms. No data are available to permit us to recommend prophylaxis in neurosurgical procedures.

VASCULAR SURGERY

Vascular surgery is clean but often involves implantation of foreign materials. Possible catastrophic consequences of graft infections have been cited to justify prophylaxis. S. aureus is the most common infecting organism complicating vascular procedures, and some experimental data support the use of prophylactic antibiotics. Wilson and co-workers showed that preoperative cephalothin prevented graft infection in dogs when S. aureus was injected at the time of graft implantation.[100] Lane and Abrutyn showed that oxacillin and vancomycin reduced the frequency of S. aureus infection on newly created arteriovenous fistulas in rabbits.[101]

In one large study in humans, Kaiser and associates evaluated the use of 1 g of cefazolin given preoperatively and then every 6 hr for 4 doses after surgery.[102] Rates of infection varied for different surgical procedures. No infections were noted among 103 patients undergoing brachial or carotid artery surgery or among 56 patients undergoing femoral artery surgery. In patients undergoing femoral–lower leg bypass procedures or abdominal aortic resection, infection rates were lower with prophylaxis, but the differences were not significant. Skin preparations with povidine–iodine rather than hexachlorophene–ethanol also appeared to be associated with a lower rate of infection.

Although prophylaxis appears to be of some benefit in vascular procedures performed on the abdominal aorta and the vessels of the lower extremity, it remains controversial in other procedures.[103] In practice, prophylactic antibiotics are used widely in vascular surgery. The regimen proposed by Kayser may be used, but individual surgeons approach the issue of prophylaxis differently.[102] Additional studies with single-dose antibiotics are needed.

SUMMARY

1. Clean operations are those in which (1) the gastrointestinal, respiratory, or genitourinary tract is not entered; (2) aseptic technique is maintained; and (3) inflammation is not found. Antibiotic prophylaxis is generally not necessary in clean procedures but is often considered when prosthetic devices are implanted, since the consequences of infection can be catastrophic.
2. Clean–contaminated operations are those in which the gastrointestinal, respiratory, or genitourinary tract is entered but in which contamination is not significant. Prophylaxis should be considered.
3. Infection rates for contaminated and dirty operations exceed 20% and 30%, respectively. Antibiotics are used as treatment of established infection.
4. Prophylactic antibiotics are not recommended for most clean orthopedic procedures.
5. Colorectal surgery requires prophylaxis consisting of mechanical cleansing plus oral or systemic antibiotics or both. Oral neomycin and erythromycin or a systemic cephalosporin should be used.
6. Patients undergoing gastroduodenal or biliary tract surgery may have either a high or a low risk of infection. Prophylaxis with a cephalosporin is recommended only for high-risk patients.
7. The low frequency and mild severity of infections encountered after abdominal hysterectomy suggest that routine prophylaxis is not justified.
8. Prophylaxis with a single preoperative dose of a cephalosporin is recommended in vaginal hysterectomy.
9. Patients undergoing prostatectomy with bacteriuria should be given antibiotics for 24 hr to 48 hr preoperatively. Those with sterile urine should not be given antibiotics. Closed drainage systems should be used when possible; irrigation with neomycin–polymyxin solutions is not recommended.
10. Prophylaxis is recommended in vascular procedures involving the abdominal aorta or vasculature of the lower extremities.

REFERENCES

1. Kunin C M: Veterams Administration *Ad hoc* Interdisciplinary Advisory Committee on Antimicrobial Drug Usage. I. Prophylaxis in surgery. JAMA 237:1003, 1977
2. Hurley DL, Howard P, Hahn HH: Perioperative prophylactic antibiotics in abdominal surgery. Surg Clin North Am 59:919, 1979
3. Hirshmann JV. Inui TS: Antimicrobial prophylaxis: A critique of recent trials. Rev Infect Dis 2:1, 1980

4. Chodak GW, Plaut ME: Use of systemic antibiotics for prophylaxis in surgery. Arch Surg 112:326, 1977

5. DiPiro JT, Record KE, Schanzenbach KS et al: Antimicrobial prophylaxis in surgery. Part I. Am J Hosp Pharm 38:320, 1981

6. Nichols RE: Use of prophylactic antibiotics in surgical practice. Am J Med 70:686, 1981

7. Miles AA, Miles EM, Burke J: The value and duration of defense reactions of the skin to the primary lodgment of bacteria. Br J Exp Pathol 38:79, 1957

8. Polk HC: Prevention of surgical wound infection. Ann Intern Med 89:770, 1978

9. Nahai R, Lamb JM, Havican RG et al: Factors involved in disruption of intestinal anastomoses. Am Surg 43:45, 1977

10. Cruse P: Infection surveillance: Identifying the problems and the high-risk patient South Med J 70:4, 1977

11. National Academy of Sciences, National Research Council, Division of Medical Sciences: *Ad hoc* Committee of the Committee on Trauma and Post-operative Wound Infection: The use of ultraviolet radiation of the operating room and of various other factors. Ann Surg (Suppl) 160:1, 1964

12. Moellering RC Jr, Kunz LV Poitras JW et al: Microbiologic basis for the rational use of prophylactic antibiotics. South Med J (Suppl) 70:8, 1977

13. Neu HC: Clinical pharmacokinetics in preventive antimicrobial therapy. South Med J (Suppl) 70:14, 1977

14. Boyd RF Burke JF Colton T: A double blind clinical trial of prophylactic antibiotics in hip fractures. J Bone Joint Surg (Am) 55A:1251, 1973

15. Tengve B, Kjellander J: Antibiotic prophylaxis in operations on trochanteric femoral fractures. J Bone Joint Surg (Am) 60A:97, 1978

16. Fogelberg EV, Zitzman EK, Stinchfield FE: Prophylactic penicillin in orthopedic surgery. J Bone Joint Surg (Am) 52A:95, 1970

17. Ericson C, Lidgren L, Lindberg L: Cloxacillin in prophylaxis of postoperative infection of the hip. J Bone Joint Surg (Am) 55A:808, 1973

18. Carlsson AS, Lidgren L, Lindberg L: Prophylactic antibiotics against early and late deep infections after total hip replacement. Acta Orthop Scand 48:405, 1977

19. Wilson PD Jr: Joint replacement. South Med J (Suppl) 70:55, 1977

20. Visuri T, Antila P, Laurent LE: A comparison of dicloxacillin and ampicillin in the antibiotic prophylaxis of total hip replacement. Ann Chir Gynaecol 65:58, 1976

21. Pollard JP, Hughes SPF, Scott JE et al: Antibiotic prophylaxis in total hip replacement. Br Med J 1:707, 1979

22. Pavel A., Smith R.L., Ballard A. et al Prophylactic antibiotics in clean orthopedic surgery. J Bone Joint Surg (Am) 56A:777, 1974

23. Pavel A, Smith RL, Ballard A et al: Prophylactic antibiotics in elective orthopedic surgery: A prospective study of 1591 cases. South Med J 70:50, 1977

24. Polk HC Jr: Antibiotic prophylaxis in surgery of the colon. South Med J (Suppl) 70:27, 1977

25. Nichols RL Condon RE: Preoperative preparation of the colon. Surg Gynecol Obstet 132:323, 1971

26. Nichols RL, Condon RE, Gorbach SL et al: Efficacy of preoperative antimicrobial preparation of the bowel. Ann Surg 176:227, 1972

27. Nichols RL, Broido P, Condon RE et al: Effect of preoperative neomycin–erythromycin intestinal preparation on the incidence of infectious complication following colon surgery. Ann Surg 178:453, 1973

28. Clarke JS, Condon RE, Bartlett JG et al: Preoperative oral antibiotics reduce septic complications of colorectal operations: Results of prospective, randomized double blind clinical study. Ann Surg 186:251, 1977

29. Bartlett JG, Condon RE, Gorbach SL et al: Veterans' Administration cooperative study on bowel preparation for elective colorectal operations: Impact of oral antibiotic regimen on colonic flora, wound Irrigation cultures and bacteriology of septic complications. Ann Surg 188:249, 1978

30. Vargish T, Crawford LC, Stallings RA et al: Randomized prospective evaluation of orally administered antibiotics in operations on the colon. Surg Gynecol Obstet 146:193, 1978

31. Washington JA II Dearing WH, Judd ES et al: Effect of preoperative antibiotic regimen on development of infection after intestinal surgery: Prospective, randomized, double blind study. Ann Surg 180:562, 1974

32. Judd ES: Preoperative neomycin-tetracycline preparation of the colon for elective operations. Surg Clin North Am 55:1325, 1975

33. Matheson DM, Arabi L, Baxter–Smith D et al: Randomized multicentre trial of oral bower preparation and antimicrobials for elective colorectal operations. Br J Surg 65:597, 1978

34. Arabi Y, Dimock R, Burdon DW et al: Influence of bowel preparation and antimicrobials on colonic flora. Br J Surg 65:555, 1978

35. Goldring J, McNaught W, Scott A et al: Prophylactic oral antimicrobial agents in elective colonic surgery. Lancet 2:997, 1975

36. Gillespie E, McNaught W: Prophylactic oral metronidazole intestinal surgery. J Antimicrob Chemother (Suppl) 4:29, 1978

37. Rosenberg IL, Graham NG, Donibal FT et al: Preparation of the intestine in patients undergoing major large bowel surgery, mainly for neoplasms of the colon and rectum. Br J Surg 58:266, 1971

38. Wapnick S, Guinto R, Reizis I, et al: Reduction of postoperative infection in elective colon surgery with preoperative administration of kanamycin and erythromycin. Surgery 85:315, 1979

39. Hoyer H, Wetterfors J: Systemic prophylaxis with doxycycline in surgery of the colon and rectum. Ann Surg 187:362, 1978

40. Willis AI, Ferguson IR, Jones PH et al: Metronidazole in prevention and treatment of bacteroides infections in elective colonic surgery. Br. Med. J 1:607, 1977

41. Brass C, Richards GK, Ruedy J et al: The effect of metronidazole on the incidence of postoperative wound infection in elective colon surgery. Am J Surg 135:91, 1978

42. Polk LC, Lopez–Mayor JF: Postoperative wound infection: A prospective study of determinant factors and prevention. Surgery 66:97, 1969

43. Stone HH, Hooper CA, Kolb LD et al: Antibiotic prophylaxis in gastric, biliary and colonic surgery. Ann Surg 184:443, 1976

44. Stokes EJ, Waterworth PM, Franks V et al: Short-term routine antibiotic prophylaxis in surgery. Br J Surg 61:739, 1974

45. Lewis RT, Allan CM, Goodall RG et al: Antibiotics in surgery of the colon. Can J Surg 21:339, 1978

46. Condon RE, Bartlett JG, Nichols RL et al: Preoperative prophylactic cephalothin fails to control septic complications of colorectal operations: Results of controlled clinical trial. A Veterans' Administration Cooperative Study. Am J Surg 137:68, 1979

47. Crenshaw CA, Gaugles E, Webber CE et al: Cephalothin–tobramycin as a preventive antibiotic combination. Surg Gynecol Obstet 147:713, 1978

48. Pollack AV, Froome K, Evans M: The bacteriology of primary wound sepsis in potentially contaminated abdominal operations: The effect of irrigation, povidone–iodine and cephaloridine on the sepsis rate assesed in a clinical trial. Br J Surg 65:76, 1978

49. Stone HH: Gastric surgery. South Med J (Suppl) 70:35, 1977

50. Lewis RT: Wound infection after gastro-duodenal operations: A ten-year review. Can J Surg 20:435, 1977

51. Lewis RT, Allan CM, Goodall RG et al: The discriminate use of antibiotic prophylaxis in gastroduodenal surgery. Am J Surg 138:640, 1979

52. Vichols RL, Smith JW, Webb WR: Efficacy of antibiotic prophylaxis in high risk gastroduodenal operations. Abstract #627. 20th Interscience Conference in Antimicrobial Agents and Chemotherapy, New Oleans, LA, October 1980

53. Chetlin SH, Elliott DW: Biliary bacteremia. Arch Surg 102:303, 1971

54. Chetlin SH, Elliott DW: Preoperative antibiotics in biliary surgery. Arch Surg 107:319, 1973

55. Keighley MRB, Baddeley RM, Burdon DW et al: A controlled trial of parenteral prophylactic therapy in biliary surgery. Br J Surg 62:275, 1975

56. Keighley MRB: Prevention of wound sepsis in gastrointestinal surgery. Br J Surg 2:462, 1978

57. McLeish AR, Keighley MRB, Bishop HM et al: Selecting patients requiring antibiotics in biliary surgery by immediate Gram stains of bile at operation. Surgery 81:473, 1977

58. Elliott DW: Biliary tract surgery. South Med J 70:31, 1977

59. Strachan CJL, Black J, Powis SJA et al: Prophylactic use of cefazolin against wound sepsis after cholecystectomy. Br Med J 1:1254, 1977

60. Morran C, McNaught W, McArdle CS: Prophylactic co-trimoxazole in biliary surgery. Br Med J 2:462, 1974

61. Griffiths DA, Shorey BA, Simpson RA et al: Single dose preoperative antibiotic prophylaxis in gastrointestinal surgery. Lancet 2:325, 1976

62. Goosenberg J, Ernich JP, Schwarz RH: Prophylactic antibiotics in vaginal hysterectomy. Am J Obstet Gynecol 105:503, 1969

63. Allen JL, Rampone JF, Wheeless CR: Use of a prophylactic antibiotic in elective major gynecologic surgery. South Med J 71:251, 1978

64. Ohm MJ, Galask RP: The effect of antibiotic prophylaxis on patients undergoing total abdominal hysterectomy. I. Effect on morbidity. Am J Obstet Gynecol 125:442, 1976

65. Grossman JH III, Greco TP, Minkin JP et al: Prophylactic antibiotics in gynecologic surgery. Obstet Gynecol 53:537, 1979

66. Ledger WJ, Sweet RL, Headington JT: Prophylactic cephaloridine in the prevention of postoperative pelvic infections in premenopausal women undergoing vaginal hysterectomy. Am J Obstet Gynecol 115:776, 1973

67. Mendelson J, Portnoy J, DeSaint VJR et al: Effect of single and multidose cepharadine prophylaxis on infectious morbidity of vaginal hysterectomy. Obstet Gynecol 53:31, 1979

68. Lett WJ, Ansbacher R, Davison BL et al: Prophylactic antibiotic for women undergoing vaginal hysterectomy. J Reprod Med 19:51, 1977

69. Jennings RH: Prophylactic antibiotics in vaginal and abdominal hysterectomy. South Med J 71:251, 1978

70. Biven MD, Neufeld J McCarty WD: The prophylactic use of Keflex and Keflin in vaginal hysterectomy morbidity. Am J Obstet Gynecol 122(2):169, 1975

71. Ohm MJ, Galask RP: The effect of antibiotic prophylaxis on patients undergoing vaginal operations and the effect on morbidity. Am J Obstet Gynecol 123:590, 1975

72. Roberts JM, Homesley HD: Low dose carbenicillin prophylaxis for vaginal and abdominal hysterectomy. Obstet Gynecol 52:83, 1978

73. Holman JF, McGowan JE, Thompson JD: Perioperative antibiotics in major elective gynecologic surgery. South Med J 71:417, 1978

74. Bolling DR, Plunkett GD: Prophylactic

antibiotics for vaginal hysterectomies. Obstet Gynecol 41:689, 1973

75. Matthews DD, Agarwal V, Gordon AM, et al: A double blind trial of single-dose chemoprophylaxis with co-trimoxazole during vaginal hysterectomy and repair. Br J Obstet Gynecol 86:737, 1979

76. Weissberg SM, Edwardo ML, O'Leary JA: Prophylactic antibiotics in cesarean section. Obstet Gynecol 38:290, 1971

77. Morrison JC, Coxwell WL, Kennedy BS et al: The use of prophylactic antibiotics undergoing cesarean section. Surg Gynecol Obstet 36:425, 1973

78. Gibbs RS, DeCherney AH, Schwarz RH: Prophylactic antibiotics in cesarean section: A double blind study. Am J Obstet Gynecol 114:1048, 1972

79. Gibbs RS, Hunt JE, Schwarz RH: A follow-up study on prophylactic antibiotics in cesarean section. Am J Obstet Gynecol 117:419, 1973

80. Moro M, Andrews M: Prophylactic antibiotics in cesarean section. Obstet Gynecol 44:688, 1972

81. Kreutner AK, Del Bene VE, Delamar D et al: Perioperative antibiotic prophylaxis in cesarean section. Obstet Gynecol 52:279, 1978

82. Kreutner AK, Del Bene VE, Delamar D et al: Perioperative cephalosporin prophylaxis in cesarean section: Effect on endometritis in high-risk patients. Am J Obstet Gynecol 134:925, 1979

83. Green SL, Sarubbi FA, Bishop EH: Prophylactic antibiotics in high risk cesarean section. Obstet Gynecol 51:569, 1978

84. Work BA: Role of preventive antibiotics in patients undergoing cesarean section. South Med J 70:44, 1977

85. Bibbs RS, Weinstein AJ: Bacteriologic effects of prophylactic antibiotics in cesarean section. Am J Obstet Gynecol 126:226, 1976

86. Gibbs RS, Jones PM, Wilder CJY: Internal fetal monitoring and maternal infection following cesarean section. A prospective study. Obstet Gynecol 52:193, 1978

87. Phelan JP, Pruyn SC: Prophylactic antibiotics in cesarean section: A double blind study of cefazolin. Am J Obstet Gynecol 52:193, 1978

88. Gonzalez R, Wright R, Blackard CE: Prophylactic antibiotics in transurethral prostatectomy. J Urol 116:203, 1976

89. Morris MJ, Golavski D, Guinnesa MDG, et al: The value of prophylactic antibiotics in transurethral prostatic resection: A controlled trial with observations on the origin of postoperative infection. Br J Urol 48:479, 1976

90. Hills NH, Bultitude MI, Eykyn S: Co-trimoxazole in prevention of bacteriuria after prostatectomy. Br Med J 2:498, 1976

91. Gibbons RP, Stark RA, Correa RJ et al: The prophylactic use of misuse of antibiotics in transurethral prostatectomy. J Urol 119:381, 1978

92. Herr HW: Use of prophylactic antibiotics in the high-risk patient undergoing prostatectomy: Effect on morbidity. J Urol 109:686, 1973

93. Berger SA, Nagar H: Antimicrobial prophylaxis in urology. J Urol 120:319, 1978

94. Chodak GW, Plaut ME: Systemic antibiotics in urologic surgery: A critical review. J Urol 121:695, 1979

95. Ruebush TK II, McConville JH, Calia FH: A double blind study of trimethoprin–sulfamethoxazole prophylaxis in patients having transrectal needle biopsy of the prostate. J Urol 122:492, 1976

96. Korbel EI, Maher PO: Use of prophylactic antibiotics in urethral instrumentation. J Urol 116:744, 1976

97. Savitz MH, Malis LI: Prophylactic clindamycin for neurosurgical patients. NY State J Med 76:64, 1976

98. Horwitz NH, Curtin JA: Prophylactic antibiotics and wound infections following laminectomy for lumbar disc herniation. J Neurosurg 43:727, 1975

99. Wyler AR, Kelly WA: Use of antibiotics with external ventriculostomies. J Neurosurg 37:185, 1972

100. Wilson SE, Wang S, Gordon HE: Periop-

erative antibiotic prophylaxis against vascular graft infection. South Med J 70:68, 1977

101. Lane T, Abrutyn E: Induction and prevention of experimental arterio-venous fistula infections. Antimicrob Agents Chemother (Suppl) 16:638, 1979

102. Kaiser AB, Clayson KR, Mulherin JL et al: Antibiotic prophylaxis in vascular surgery. Ann Surg 188:283, 1978

103. Pitt HA, Postier RG, MacGowan WAL et al: Prophylactic antibiotics in vascular surgery: Topical, systemic, or both. Ann Surg 192(3):356, 1980

Approach to the Patient with Postoperative Fever

32

GEORGE HARRISON TALBOT
STEPHEN J. GLUCKMAN

The internist is routinely called upon to evaluate patients with postoperative fever. This situation can present a difficult diagnostic challenge and demands a great deal of skill and perseverance. This chapter presents a fundamental approach to this often complex but frequent problem.

Fever may occur after almost any type of operation and is virtually universal after extensive procedures such as cardiac surgery.[1] However, often no etiology for the fever is identified. In Klimeck's and co-workers' review of postoperative patients with temperatures over 101°F, 18% were found to be febrile due to infection, and 82% were thought to be febrile for reasons unrelated to infection. Among the former, wound, urinary tract, and pulmonary infections were the most prevalent at 40%, 25%, and 20%, respectively. In the latter group, fever was attributed only to the effects of surgery in 90%, and a more specific diagnosis was not made.[2]

The etiologies of postoperative pyrexia fall into one of three broad categories. The first consists of general causes, which should be considered in any febrile, postoperative patient regardless of the specific surgical procedure involved. Examples include intravenous catheter phlebitis, drug fever, and deep venous thrombosis. The second category comprises causes related to the specific operative procedure, such as sternal wound infection after open-heart surgery or bacterial meningitis following craniotomy. The etiologies comprising the third group are entirely independent of the given surgical problem and occur with the same frequency in a similar, nonsurgical population. Most postoperative fevers fall into the first two categories. It is generally reasonable to consider problems relating to the surgery before evaluating the patient for an unrelated illness.

GENERAL CAUSES OF POSTOPERATIVE FEVER

General causes of postoperative fever include both infectious and noninfectious processes. A standard approach is to define febrile complications by their temporal onset in relation to the operative procedure. Though certain complications are indeed more likely to occur at one particular time than another, this is not always the case. Since overdependence on such schemata may potentially lead to misdiagnosis, it is preferable to approach each patient individually, keeping the following processes in mind.

Wound Infection

Wound infection, whether superficial or deep, continues to head the list of proven causes of postoperative fever, despite its decreased incidence with improvement in surgical technique and appropriate use of prophylactic antibiotics. Several recent reviews deal with the mechanisms of inflammation and the localization of infection.[3–5] A number of systemic and local abnormalities contribute to decreased host resistance and subsequent wound infection. Systemic abnormalities include: (1) extremes of age; (2) abnormalities of nutrition, including obesity and malnutrition; (3) defective glucose metabolism; (4) adrenocorticosteroid excess or deficiency; (5) shock and decreased perfusion; (6) certain malignancies and their treatment with irradiation and chemotherapy; and (7) aberrations in reticuloendothelial system function, immunoglobulin production, and cell-mediated immunity. Local factors, which are even more important, include the presence of necrotic tissue, decreased local wound perfusion, hematoma formation, tissue dead space, and foreign bodies.[3]

These local and systemic factors predispose to colonization by bacteria from either exogenous or endogenous sources.[6] Environmental sources of bacteria include the air, equipment and personnel in the operating room, the patient's own skin, and the patient's postoperative surroundings. Current technology and technique have diminished the danger of these sources, and a major concern now is acquisition of infection from endogenous sites by direct contact or by way of the bloodstream.

It may be difficult to decide whether a wound is infected. The criteria outlined by Robson and associates are helpful.[3] A wound is not infected if it heals primarily without discharge. If there is purulent discharge, even if it is culture-negative, a wound should be considered infected. Quantitative wound cultures have proved helpful to some authors.[7] Finally, wounds properly labeled as possibly infected include inflamed but nondraining wounds or culture-positive wounds without purulent drainage. Stitch abscesses are placed in a separate category if inflammation and drainage are minimal and are confined to the suture sites, if the wound itself heals primarily, and if the suture sites clear spontaneously within 72 hr after removal of the sutures.[3]

The risk of developing wound infection is directly related to the degree of contamination at surgery. In one series of over 15,000 operative wounds, there was an increasing rate of infection from 3.3% in clean wounds to 28.6% in dirty ones, with an overall rate of 7.8%.[3] Other authors have noted similar results.[8] Factors identified as contributing to a higher infection rate include long duration of surgery, increased length of preoperative hospitalization, and the presence of infection at a remote site.[2,3,8–10]

When wound infection is suspected, a Gram stain and culture of the drainage or of aspirated material are crucial.[11] Polymorphonuclear leukocytes and organisms on a Gram-stained preparation suggest the presence of infection. Staphylococci and streptococci remain major offenders, although antibiotic-induced ecologic pressures have resulted in the emergence of previously uncommon organisms such as gram-negative rods and, in selected instances mycobacteria and fungi.[10,12,13]

Hematoma Formation

Hematoma formation may complicate almost any surgical intervention, especially one involving vascular and orthopedic procedures. The distinction between hematoma formation and wound abscess may be difficult, in that both may appear as localized areas of inflammation. Furthermore, an originally bland hematoma may evolve into an overt suppurative process after bacterial superinfection. When profuse but occult bleeding complicates intra-abdominal or intrathoracic surgery, the diagnosis may be even harder to establish but should be suspected when fever is acompanied by falling hemoglobin and hyperbilirubinemia levels and elevated lactate dehydrogenase levels without external blood loss or abnormal hepatic function. Careful aseptic needle aspiration of accessible hematomas may aid in the differentiation of a hematoma from a seroma or wound abscess. However, violation of a closed space may itself induce septic complications and should not be done without careful consideration of its risks.

Pulmonary Disorders

Pulmonary disorders, including atelectasis, aspiration pneumonia, and empyema are among the most common causes of postoperative fever. They are discussed fully in Chapter 24.

Deep Venous Thrombosis and Pulmonary Embolism

Deep venous thrombosis and pulmonary embolism should always be considered in the febrile postoperative patient.[14] Physi-

cal examination has limited sensitivity in diagnosing thrombophlebitis in the lower extremities.[15] Moreover, when prostatic or other pelvic veins are involved, examination is often totally unrevealing. Similarly, pulmonary embolism may occur without the classic signs and symptoms, and ventilation–perfusion scanning, venography, and pulmonary arteriography may be required to confirm the diagnosis.[14] Physicians should not dismiss the possibility of thrombosis or embolism either because of the presence of a hectic fever curve suggestive of sepsis or because of the absence of overt signs and symptoms.[16]

Intravenous Catheters

Intravenous catheters may induce fever by either infectious or noninfectious mechanisms. The latter is more common and can be the result of irritation by the catheter itself or by the infused fluids, including certain antibiotics and hypertonic nutritional solutions.[17] Irritation occurs most prominently with peripherally placed lines and is usually readily diagnosed through inspection of the catheter site. Pyogenic infection, including overt suppurative thrombophlebitis, may complicate a pre-existent chemical phlebitis or may arise de novo.[17–19] Despite assiduous attention from special catheter-care teams, hyperalimentation lines placed in large central veins are still major offenders. The factors primarily responsible for pyogenic infection include the frequently prolonged duration of catheterization and the composition of the infusates.[20–23] The diagnosis may not be evident on inspection of the site; local signs and symptoms may be absent.[20,24]

When pyogenic complications develop, a variety of pathogens may be responsible. *Staphylococcus aureus* should always be suspected, but coagulase-negative staphylococci and gram-negative rods may be isolated.[17,22,25,26] Various fungi, including *Candida albicans* and *Torulopsis glabrata*, may colonize central lines and subsequently cause septicemia and disseminated infection.[17,27–35] Documentation of invasive fungal disease may be difficult; persistently positive blood cultures after removal of the catheter and evidence of fungal endophthalmitis are most specific. A rare complication of intravenous therapy may occur when bacteria are introduced directly into the patient as a result of contamination of the plastic administration sets or of the solution itself.[17] This diagnosis is difficult to establish in an individual patient but should be considered if an outbreak of septicemia due to a single species of organism develops in the hospital setting. Hydrophilic gram-negative rods and yeasts are the pathogens most frequently isolated in such situations.[17] In-dwellng arterial catheters may also be a source of infection.[36] Quantitative and semiquantitative cultures of venous and arterial catheter tips have been useful in determination of the source of bacteremia when a catheter is in use.[36–38]

Urinary Tract Infection

Urinary tract infection must always be considered a potential source of fever in postoperative patients, particularly in those requiring prolonged urethral catheterization. Despite strict catheter care and maintenance of a closed drainage system, the incidence of infection increases with the length of time the catheter remains in place.[39] Prophylactic antibiotics decrease infection rates in the short term but increase the risk of antimicrobial resistance among those pathogens that do arise; they are therefore not recommended.[39,40] After 3 weeks of catheterization, virtually all patients become colonized regardless of whether or not antibiotics have been given. The presence of fever usually suggests upper tract involvement. Males may also develop fever from catheter-associated prostatitis or epididymitis. Examination of the urinary sediment with culture and sensitivity testing are first-line diagnostic procedures in most febrile postoperative patients.

Drug-Related Causes

Drug fever is another diagnostic possibility in the febrile postoperative patient.[41,42] Although almost every drug has at one time been implicated as the cause of fever, some agents are more likely to cause elevations in temperature than others. Some commonly used drugs that cause fever, which may be the only manifestation of a drug reaction, are listed below:[41,42]

Antimicrobials
    Penicillins
    Cephalosporins
    Sulfonamides
    Nitrofurantoin
    Isoniazid
    Amphotericin B
    Rifampin
Cardiovascular agents
    Hydralazine HCL
    Alpha-methyldopa
    Quinidine
    Procainamide
    Diphenylhydantoin
    Thiazides
    Furosemide
Other agents
    Allopurinol
    Iodides
    Prophylthiouracil
    Salicylates

Patients with drug fever often feel and look better than their spiking temperature curves suggest they should. This clue may be helpful in the diagnosis of drug-induced fever when the classical skin rash and eosinophilia are absent.

Whenever the diagnosis of drug fever is entertained, suspected medications should be discontinued. When an indispensable medication is likely to be at fault, the physician must decide whether the risks of continued administration outweigh those of withdrawal or substitution with another agent. In the absence of severe cutaneous or visceral complications such as erythema multiforme, hepatitis, or interstitial nephritis, continuation of an offending but indispensable drug may be the safer course. Under special circumstances, careful rechallenge with a medication that has previously been discontinued may be helpful in substantiating the diagnosis of drug fever.

Endocrinologic Causes

Endocrinologic causes of fever, which are rare but correctable, are occasionally precipitated by the stress of surgery and anesthesia.[43] Acute adrenal insufficiency may present as refractory hypotension, occasionally with concomitant eosinophilia and acid–base disturbances. Signs of Addison's disease, such as hyperpigmentation, may not be present to aid the diagnosis. Conversely, the adrenal medullary over-activity of a pheochromocytoma may present as postoperative fever, labile hypertension, flushing, nausea, vomiting, and tachycardia. Finally, thyroid storm may occur postoperatively with extreme pyrexia and other manifestations of hypermetabolism. As alluded to above, these causes of postoperative fever, though uncommon, are especially important because they are life-threatening if untreated and often remediable if prompt and appropriate therapy is instituted.

Malignant Hyperthermia

Malignant hyperthermia is a rare disorder of skeletal muscle that can cause postoperative fever.[44–46] This genetically transmitted disease of abnormal sarcoplasmic calcium release is classically induced by muscle relaxants such as succinylcholine, though inhalation anesthetics such as halothane, cyclopropane, and methoxyflurane and other factors including high ambient temperatures, emotional excitement, injury, infection, and exercise have also been implicated. Although hyperthermia usually begins 10 min to 30 min after induction of anesthesia, it may be delayed for several hours postoperatively.

Temperatures in hyperthermia are usually in the range of 39°C to 42°C but may reach 44°C to 46°C. The anesthesiologist may first note the patient's failure to achieve complete relaxation with more than the normal degree of muscle fasciculation; tachypnea, tachycardia, other tachyarrhythmias, and cyanosis soon follow. Skeletal muscle rigidity is seen in 80% of patients, and acidosis, hypoxemia, hyperglycemia, hyperphosphatemia, hypocalcemia, and hyperkalemia may occur. Myoglobinemia and subsequent myoglobinuric acute renal failure often supervene. Rapid recognition of this dramatic syndrome may result in salvage of the patient if drastic cooling procedures and dantrolene are instituted immediately, but mortality remains 30% to 40%.[47]

Transfusion Reactions

Transfusion reactions may be incriminated as a cause of postoperative fever.[48] Most febrile reactions can be attributed to antibodies directed towards white blood cells, platelets, or plasma antigens present in transfused whole blood. Fever may be the only clinical manifestation. Individual blood products such as white cells given to neutropenic patients may also cause fever. Acute intravascular hemolysis, a rare cause of transfusion-related fever, is most often due to ABO incompatibilities and tends to be more catastrophic than extravascular hemolysis due to antibody incompatibilities. The former may progress to shock, renal failure, and disseminated intravascular coagulation; in the latter, these are uncommon. Nonimmune febrile reactions after blood transfusions may also occur. If blood becomes infected during storage and handling, fever and shock may result from infusion of preformed endotoxin as well as from infusion of viable bacteria. When fever occurs during a transfusion, the product should be cultured and returned to the blood bank for repeat cross-matching. In rare instances, assaying the material for endotoxin has proved helpful.

Other infections may be transmitted by transfused blood. Viral hepatitis is most common. This may be hepatitis B, but non-A non-B hepatitis is more often implicated, as discussed below. Cytomegalovirus (CMV), syphilis, malaria, and brucellosis may also be transmitted through transfusion. Febrile syndromes due to those organisms tend to occur well after the immediate postoperative period.

Liver Disease

Liver disease may result in postoperative fever. Drugs, infectious agents, tissue hypoxia due to hypotension, passive congestion, direct trauma, biliary obstruction, and chronic malnutrition with refeeding by hyperalimentation have all been associated with abnormal hepatic function following surgery.

A drug classically implicated in postoperative hepatitis is the anesthetic halothane.[49] Fever typically appears at the end of the first week following surgery but may occasionally be delayed for several weeks and, in second episodes, may occur after only 1 or 2 days. Nausea and vomiting often accompany the fever, and hepatic enlargement and tenderness are usually noted. Leukocytosis, eosinophilia, and enzyme elevations consistent with hepatocellular injury are found on laboratory evaluation.

The frequency of halothane-related liver injury has probably been overestimated because of difficulty in distinguishing it from the myriad other possible causes of hepatic dysfunction that can arise in the postoperative period. Best estimates of the incidence of true halothane hepatitis range from 1 in 2,500 to 1 in 9,000, with an overall mortality figure of 1 in 20,000.[49] Major factors associated with the development of hepatocellular dysfunction following exposure to halothane include closely spaced multiple exposures and pre-existing hepatic disease.[49] Patients who are elderly, female, and obese, who have a history of other allergy, or who are undergoing major abdominal surgery may be predisposed to its development.

Nonanesthetic medications should also be suspect in any case of postoperative hepatitis. Sulfonamides, salicylates, phenothiazines, phenylbutazone, indomethacin, nitrofurantoin, isoniazid, methyldopa, and erythromycin estolate have been implicated in such reactions.[42] One notable example is oxacillin, which may induce leukopenia and eosinophilia in addition to fever and hepatitis.[50]

Fever and hepatitis due to infectious agents may occur in the postoperative period. As noted above, non-A non-B hepatitis and hepatitis B are the most common and are generally secondary to blood transfusions.[51-53] Hepatitis B has a relatively long incubation time and generally need not be considered in the immediate postoperative period. Non-A non-B hepatitis may be caused by at least two separate viruses, and one of these may have an incubation period as short as 2 weeks. Therefore, fever due to hepatitis induced by the latter kind of virus may be a consideration in some postoperative settings, especially if multiple transfusions have been administered. Of 388 patients followed prospectively after open-heart surgery, 30 (7.7%) developed viral hepatitis; of these, 26 (6.7%) were thought to have non-A non-B hepatitis, and 3 (0.8%) were thought to have hepatitis B.[54]

Members of the Herpes virus family, especially CMV, may rarely cause postoperative hepatitis.[55]

CAUSES OF FEVER IN SPECIFIC TYPES OF SURGERY

Cardiac Surgery

Cardiac surgery, including coronary artery bypass grafting and insertion of prosthetic heart valves, is almost uniformly associated with the development of postoperative fever lasting several days.[1] Fever persisting for longer than 1 week causes concern, but the literature suggests that this may occur in as many as 36% to 73% of patients.[1,56] Many of these fevers remain unexplained and are self-limited. In one series, all patients with unexplained fever after 1 week had become afebrile by the 19th postoperative day.[1]

Infection is a feared complication of cardiac surgery. Its incidence ranges from 2% to 15%, including both cardiac and extracardiac sites.[57] In addition to the usual infections seen after any surgery, major infectious complications peculiar to cardiac surgery include endocarditis, sternal wound infection, mediastinitis, and purulent pericarditis.

Prosthetic valve endocarditis (PVE) can be divided into early and late forms on the basis of onset before or after 60 days following surgery.[58–63] Late PVE resembles natural valve endocarditis in its course and microbiology.[61,62] Early PVE, more often fulminant than late PVE, is commonly due to staphylococci, gram-negative rods, or fungi.[63,64] In addition to fever, chills, and new or changing murmurs, patients may demonstrate shock, uncontrollable septicemia, refractory congestive heart failure, and manifestations of major systemic emboli. Signs of long-standing endocarditis such as Roth's spots, splenomegaly, and clubbing are absent. Conjunctival petechiae may be observed in noninfected patients after cardiac surgery, making this finding nonspecific. Mortality with either medical therapy or combined medical and surgical intervention is in the range of 50% to 90%.

Sande and colleagues have pointed out that not all patients with sustained bacteremia in the early postoperative period have PVE.[65] In a series of 22 such patients, the group without valvular involvement had early bacteremia (median of 12 days) caused by gram-negative rods in 70%. Almost all had obvious extracardiac sources of bacteremia, and none developed a changing murmur. This subgroup of bacteremic patients has a relatively favorable prognosis.

Sternal wound infection has a variable presentation that depends mostly on the virulence of the infecting organism.[66,67] Some of the less aggressive pathogens such as coagulase-negative staphylococci and atypical mycobacteria may not cause clinical illness for months or even years. However, infection may develop quickly with wound dehiscence and extrusion of overt pus when more virulent pathogens are involved. Since the sternal incision is in continuity with the sternum itself, osteomyelitis and even mediastinal infection may supervene. In febrile postoperative patients with sternal wound purulence, infection of deeper tissue sites must be suspected. Successful management may require surgical exploration to delineate and drain involved areas.

On occasion, mediastinitis or purulent pericarditis complicates open-heart surgery, typically appearing 1 to 3 weeks postoperatively.[68,69] Bor and associates reported a 3.4% incidence of infectious mediastinitis among 616 cardiac procedures performed through median sternotomy incisions from 1975 to 1979.[68] The incubation period averaged 11.5 days, with a range of 3 to 36 days. Fever and bacteremia often antedated obvious local wound infection. The diagnosis may be difficult if there is no evidence of purulence from within the wound or drainage tubes. Purulent pericarditis may also present a diagnostic challenge. Pericardial tamponade, a physical sign that often leads to the diagnosis of purulent pericarditis in nonsurgical patients, is understandably absent, because the pericardium is usually not closed after cardiac surgery. The patient with purulent pericarditis or mediastinitis frequently has a tumultuous postoperative course and may require re-exploration for bleeding with placement of pericardial or mediastinal drains. Purulent pericarditis in this setting is usually fatal.[69]

In addition to these infectious causes of fever, one noninfectious syndrome is also important, if only because it is so often diagnosed. The terms "postcardiotomy" and "postpericardiectomy syndrome" have been used to describe a particular group of clinical and laboratory findings that commonly occur 2 or 3 weeks postoperatively but sometimes as early as 1 week or as late as 5 to 10 months after surgery.[1,55,56] These include fever, substernal pain, pericardial and pleural friction rubs, and a variety of nonspecific laboratory abnormalities consisting of leukocytosis, elevated sedimentation rate, chest x-ray evidence of cardiac enlargement, and electrocardiographic manifestations of pericarditis. Many possible causes have been discussed, including starch-induced pericarditis, virus reactivation, and an immunologic phenomenon involving antibodies to heart tissue.[70]

Although early reports suggested an incidence as high as 40%, more recent papers have applied more stringent criteria for the diagnosis and have noted a consequent drop in incidence.[1,55,56] Currently accepted clinical criteria require that patients have persistent or recurrent fever beyond the seventh postoperative day in association with a pericardial friction rub. Defined in this way, the syndrome has been observed in only 6.2% of patients.[56] Livelli and his colleagues noted that leukocytosis, pleuritic chest pain, pericardial rubs, pleural effusion, or mediastinal widening on chest x-ray were as common in afebrile as in febrile patients.[1] The presence or absence of any of these features was thus not predictive of which patients would develop recurrent pericarditis after discharge. The authors therefore suggested that the term "postpericardiotomy syndrome" be reserved for those few patients with late illness. This strict definition gives an incidence of about 5% and denies many febrile postoperative patients a convenient explanation of their fever. This may be beneficial if it results in closer attention to febrile episodes and lessens the chance that a significant complication will be missed.

What about the patient whose fever persists without a diagnosis? Hospitalization need not be extended if all else is going well and no source of infection is localized by clinical or laboratory examination.[1] Exactly what is the cause of unexplained postoperative fever in this and other settings remains obscure. It probably includes varying combinations of operative trauma, hematoma formation, and ongoing reactions to a variety of drainage tubes in the mediastinum and chest.

A later febrile complication of cardiac surgery is the postperfusion syndrome, which occurs in about 3% to 10% of patients undergoing cardiopulmonary bypass, with onset in the second postoperative month.[55] Features include fever and hepatosplenomegaly with lymphocytosis, atypical lymphocytes on peripheral blood smear, and abnormalities in hepatic function. Current data implicate CMV infection. The course of the disease is rarely serious, and spontaneous resolution occurs over a period of several weeks. Its importance lies in its potential to mislead the physician and the consequent complications of an extensive diagnostic evaluation.

Neurosurgery

Although patients on neurosurgical services are subject to the general causes of fever already discussed, central nervous system infections are of particular concern. Patients with penetrating or nonpenetrating major craniospinal trauma have a higher than normal risk of developing bacterial meningitis.[71,72] Patients with nonpenetrating injury and meningitis may have an overt external communication with the subarachnoid space and leakage of cerebrospinal fluid (CSF) from the ears or nose. In such cases, the route of bacterial spread is obvious. At other times, the communication is occult. Such CSF fistulas occur in 3% to 50% of all cases of nonpenetrating head trauma.[72]

In patients with closed head injury, meningitis may occur within the first 72 hr of the injury. The pneumococcus is the usual pathogen, although infections due to other organisms such as *Hemophilus influenzae* do occur.[71,73] Infection develops in 17% of patients with CSF rhinorrhea, as compared to 4% of patients with otorrhea.[72] This is presumably because potential pathogens such as *S. aureus, H. influenzae*, and pneumococci are more common in the nasopharynx than in the external auditory canal. When the injury is penetrating or has required surgical intervention, meningitis, often caused by gram-negative rods or *S. aureus*, may occur after a delay of at least several days.[71] The use of prophylactic antibiotics in the patient with opened or closed head trauma might be expected to affect the incidence and type of infectious sequelae, but data from controlled studies are lacking.

Patients undergoing neurosurgical procedures for indications other than trauma also have a high risk of developing bacterial meningitis. In one study, 20% of all patients with meningitis were neurosurgical patients.[74] The most frequent pathogens were nonpneumococcal, gram-positive organisms, including *S. aureus*, coagulase-negative staphylococci, and enterococcal species. Gram-negative rods accounted for 8.5% of the entire group. Staphylococcal species accounted for 19% of all neurosurgery-associated meningitis in another series, but gram-negative rods were more common, being responsible for 69% of proven cases of postoperative meningitis.[75] The most frequent isolates were *Escherichia coli* and

Klebsiella species; *Pseudomonas* and *Proteus* species were less common.

Fever is usually present, but classic signs of meningitis such as headache, nuchal rigidity, and decreased level of consciousness may be absent or, if present, difficult to interpret because of the underlying illness. Seizures and focal signs correlate with a poor prognosis. Most patients have a peripheral leukocytosis with a leftward shift. The only way to confirm the diagnosis is by examining the CSF. A high opening pressure as well as elevation of the protein concentration and leukocyte count are often found. Since both of these findings can occur after routine neurosurgery, hypoglycorrhachia is an important finding. This disorder was present in 85% of patients in the above-mentioned study but is only rarely observed in noninfected patients.[75]

Patients with any of the several varieties of ventricular shunts that exist may develop infection with one of a wide spectrum of organisms. Though this problem most commonly affects young children, one-fifth of shunt-infected patients in one study were above the age of 16.[76] Estimates of the frequency of CSF shunt infections have ranged from 7% to 29%; two large series describe an overall rate of about 13% in patients of all ages with all types of shunts.[76–78]

The presentation of shunt infection is variable. Although patients with infected shunts often appear acutely ill with fever, lethargy, meningismus, and evidence of local wound infection, they may not exhibit aberrations in mental status, nuchal rigidity, or high fever. Tenderness over the valve and tubing is a frequent finding. Patients often present with symptoms and signs of shunt malfunction rather than infection and occasionally demonstrate no clinical findings despite persistently positive cultures drawn from the tubing or valve.[79] Finally, a rare presentation in patients with ventriculoatrial shunts is hypocomplementemic glomerulonephritis and a syndrome that mimicks bacterial endocarditis with low-grade fever and splenomegaly.

Symptomatic infection usually becomes apparent within the first month or two after surgery: 60% of patients presented within 30 days in one series and 70% within 60 days in another.[76,78] Of all infections, 35% occur while the patients are still in the hsopital after surgery. Factors that predispose to infection include extremes of age, performance of more than two shunting procedures, congenital malformations, normal-pressure hydrocephalus, and a high personal infection rate of the operating surgeon.[76] The type of shunt, whether ventriculoatrial or ventriculoperitoneal, and the use of prophylactic antibiotics do not appear to affect the incidence of infection. Fever immediately after surgery is common and does not predict subsequent infection.

Examination of CSF obtained from the shunt itself or from the lumbar subarachnoid space is critical. The opening pressure and protein concentration are usually elevated. White blood cell counts and glucose concentration are usually abnormal in patients with shunt infection, although less so than in patients with bacterial infection of the CSF. Culture is extremely helpful, revealing a staphylococcal species in well over 50% of cases. Gram-negative rods, followed in frequency by occasional streptococci and other species, are also found. George and co-workers found no difference in specific bacteria seen between early (≤30 days postoperatively) and late (≥30 days postoperatively) infection.[76] It is important to remember that organisms such as anaerobic diphtheroids may be pathogens rather than contaminants in the setting of a prosthetic implant.[80] Mixed aerobic and anaerobic enteric flora, when cultured from a ventriculoperitoneal shunt, suggest the presence of bowel perforation by the distal tip of the tubing.[81]

Several authors have documented significant infectious complications, specifically meningitis, occurring with external ventriculostomies.[82,83] Smith and Alksne encountered 3 such infections in a series of 65 cases, giving a rate of 4.6%.[83] A snug fit between the tubing and the dura to minimize leakage of CSF and strict maintenance of a closed system are crucial if infection is to be avoided. Both the duration of catheter placement and the use of prophylactic antibiotics may play a role in the development of infection, but prospectively acquired data have not been accumulated to answer this question.

Vascular Grafts

Vascular grafts, like other prosthetic devices, may become infected. Major infections in grafts occur at an average rate of 1% to 2%, with a range of 0.25% to 6%.[84–88] Presentation is variable and includes (1) fever, chills, sweats, or bacteremic shock; (2) local inflammation and wound drainage; (3) alterations in flow through the graft with either overt thrombosis and distal ischemia or petechiae distal to the graft; and (4) breakdown of the suture line with false aneurysm formation and external or internal hemorrhage. A well-described example of internal hemorrhage is acute gastrointestinal bleeding secondary to aortoenteric fistula formation between the proximal end of an abdominal aortic graft and the bowel. Goldstone and Moore have pointed out that infections of vascular grafts are analogous to infections of prosthetic heart valves.[85] They also fall into early and late groups, in this instance defined as before and after 3.5 months postoperatively. S. aureus and gram-negative organisms predominate in the early group, whereas coagulase-negative staphylococci occur in the later group.

Graft infection develops as a consequence either of direct contamination during surgery or of bacterial seeding from a distant site some time after surgery. Grafts are experimentally most susceptible to bacterial infection in the immediate postoperative period, when formation of a neointimal lining has not been completed. Other clinically and experimentally important factors include the type of graft, the location of the graft, the suture material, and the use of prophylactic antibiotics. The highest infection rates are noted in grafts in the femoral and inguinal regions. The presence of remote infection at the time of surgery or the development of extraprosthetic infection postoperatively are additional risk factors.

When graft infection is suspected, blood cultures, wound cultures, arteriography, ultrasonography, and sinography may be helpful in confirming the diagnosis. Management usually involves removal of the graft, but, occasionally, a combination of aggressive local therapy and long-term antibiotic treatment may succeed in suppressing, though rarely eradicating, the infection.

Obstetric Procedures and Gynecologic Surgery

With postpartum fever in the obstetric patient raises the possibility of infectious complications, especially endometritis. In one study, postpartum endometritis was found in almost 4% of nearly 2700 women undergoing delivery.[89] The patient develops fever and lower abdominal pain and tenderness shortly after the appearance of a foul-smelling, purulent vaginal discharge. Often there is a history of premature rupture of the membranes, difficult delivery, or amnionitis. Bacteremia, septic shock, and death may supervene. In one series, 8% of more seriously ill patients had positive blood cultures.[90] Endometritis is a common cause of bacteremia on obstetric and gynecologic services, and one study reports that approximately 50% of septic episodes in obstetric patients in a 1-year period were due to postpartum endometritis.[91]

Bacteria isolated from the blood are the same as those isolated from the endometrium.[91,92] The most commonly recovered aerobes are *E. coli*, enterococci, and beta-hemolytic streptococci, and the most frequently isolated anaerobic pathogens are peptococci, peptostreptococci, and *Bacteroides fragilis*. Because of the difficulty involved in obtaining endometrial cultures that have not been contaminated with cervical flora, antibiotic therapy must often be empiric; in critically ill patients, it should include coverage for all of these bacteria. In addition, staphylococci and *Mycoplasma hominis* have occasionally been implicated.[93,94]

Compared to vaginal delivery, cesarean section is more frequently associated with postoperative febrile morbidity (defined as a temperature of 38°C or greater on 2 or more readings, excluding those in the first 24 hr).[95–97] In one study, 19.7% of patients who had undergone primary cesarean section developed this complication; in a control group of women who had delivered vaginally, the incidence was 2.4%.[96] Endometritis accounted for almost half of the febrile morbidity in each group. Wound infection occurs in 1% to 5% of

all patients operated upon; urinary tract infection is also extremely common.[93,96,98,99] These two processes, as well as occasional lower respiratory tract infections, cause the bulk of febrile complications not related to endometritis. Conditions predisposing to post-cesarean-section febrile morbidity are not universally agreed upon. Among those implicated include antepartum risk factors (high parity or age, concurrent medical problems) as well as intrapartum ones (significant bleeding, prolonged rupture of membranes before delivery, internal monitoring).[95–97]

Occasionally, the postpartum patient develops a pelvic abscess, but this complication occurs more commonly after gynecologic procedures.[99] Subgluteal and retropsoas abscesses after paracervical and pudendal nerve block anesthesia have been described, as have epidural infections following spinal anesthesia.[93] Finally, mastitis may be the cause of fever in some patients.[93]

Septic abortion has been encountered less frequently since abortion laws have been liberalized. However, infection following therapeutic abortion still occurs, and the same vaginal microflora are usually at fault.[89] Though extremely uncommon, the most dramatic form of this type of infection is clostridial myonecrosis of the uterus, which is characterized by acute toxemia, shock, disseminated intravascular coagulation, and hemolysis.[89] A Gram stain suggestive of *Clostridium* species or a culture positive for *Clostridium perfringens* must be interpreted with caution, since these organisms may normally colonize the female genital tract. Only in the proper clinical setting do these findings require aggressive surgical and medical therapy.

Gynecologic procedures are frequently

complicated by fever and overt infection. Incidence rates increase with the extent of the procedure carried out and are lowest after laparotomy and abdominal hysterectomy and highest after operations such as radical vulvectomy and pelvic exenteration.[100] Urinary tract and wound infections are common. Pelvic cellulitis and abscess formation, more serious complications, may lead to bacteremia and death. Hevron and Llorens described 49 cases of postoperative abscesses in 1600 major pelvic procedures.[101] Abscesses are more frequent following vaginal than abdominal surgery.[100–102] Purulent collections may be found on physical examination and by ultrasonography in the vaginal cuff, cul-de-sac, or adnexal areas.[99,103]

Ovarian abscesses are especially common after vaginal hysterectomy but may follow other types of pelvic surgery or develop in the puerperium.[99] Vaginal cuff abscess usually presents early in the postoperative period, at a mean of 8 days after surgery, whereas deeper pelvic abscesses, whether ovarian or tubal or in the cul-de-sac, tend to become clinically apparent later, at a mean of 18 to 20 days.[101] Abscesses characteristically produce fever and pain. Intraperitoneal collections, however, may produce a progressive mass effect or present with catastrophic rupture, peritonitis, and sepsis.[103]

Patients with fever, pelvic symptoms, or bacteremia in whom an abscess cannot be found by repeated internal examination and ultrasonography are described as having pelvic cellulitis. Antibiotic therapy alone is curative in this group, whereas a drainage procedure is often necessary in patients with true abscess formation. In either instance, one may expect to recover a mixture of aerobic and anaerobic bacterial pathogens.

Septic pelvic thrombophlebitis must be considered in the postoperative patient who has no identifiable abscess or extragenital source and who remains febrile despite administration of broad-spectrum antimicrobials known to be active against pelvic flora.[93,99,103–105] Though this diagnosis is extremely difficult to confirm, there is a group of persistently febrile patients, often with a paucity of pelvic or extrapelvic signs and symptoms, who defervesce and improve clinically after treatment with heparin.[105] Such a trial of anticoagulation may thus be diagnostic as well as therapeutic. Unless a patient has a documented pulmonary embolism or the thrombosed pelvic veins are visualized at laparotomy, the diagnosis can only be inferred from the response to heparin. Since these patients are also thought to be infected, antibiotics are generally continued along with the heparin. Improvement in the temperature curve should occur within 48 hr to 72 hr; absence of a response should lead the physician to consider other diagnoses.

Urologic Surgery

Procedures involving the urinary tract may cause both local and systemic complications associated with fever. Although hematomas and thromboembolism may occur, many postoperative fevers are found to be infectious in origin. Urologic patients often require in-dwelling urethral catheters after surgery. This predisposes them to bacteriuria, occasionally with accompanying fever. However, bacteriuria does not necessarily mean symptomatic infection, and, furthermore, not all symptomatic urinary tract infections produce fever. A positive urine culture, especially without pyuria, may not elucidate the cause of postoperative fever in such patients.

Bacteremia with or without septic

shock is particularly common after surgery of the prostate, with an incidence ranging from 2% to 66%.[106,107] Factors predisposing to bacteremia include preoperative catheterization, the presence of a urinary tract infection before surgery, and pathologically proven prostatitis.[106] Cystoscopy and urethral dilitation have been associated with bacteremia in some series but not in others.[106,107] Operations on the bladder and upper tracts are less likely to induce bacteremia with one important exception: patients undergoing diversionary procedures involving ileal conduit construction are subject to bacteremia, acute pyelonephritis, pelvic abscess, and peritonitis.[108,109] It is important to remember that preoperatively sterile urine does not guarantee that postoperative septicemia originating in the urinary tract will not occur, though it does decrease the likelihood of this complication.

Other complications in patients undergoing lower urinary tract surgery or placement of in-dwelling urethral catheters include acute bacterial prostatitis, prostatic abscess, epididymitis, and orchitis. Characteristic findings are usually evident on physical examination. A less common complication that may occur more than 2 weeks postoperatively is osteomyelitis of the pubic symphysis.[110] This must be distinguished from osteitis pubis, a noninfectious process, which may also present with low-grade fever, pubic pain, leukocytosis, and radiographic evidence of bone destruction. Sinus tract formation with purulent drainage or isolation of a pathogenic bacterium from a bone biopsy with histopathologic changes of osteomyelitis confirms the presence of infection. Osteomyelitis may also develop at other sites following urologic surgery. Batson's plexus and arterial dissemination have both been implicated in the spread of infection to lumbar vertebrae.[111] Arterial spread is more likely when other noncontiguous osseous structures are involved. Persistent local pain and fever are the cardinal manifestations of osteomyelitis.

The bacteria associated with infections following urinary tract surgery are usually enteric organisms such as E. coli. However, when therapy is contemplated, consideration must be given to hospital-acquired pathogens such as Pseudomonas and Serratia. A particular association of Staphylococcus aureus with prostatic abscess should be noted.

Patients undergoing renal transplantation have their own unique set of febrile complications, but discussion of this special group is beyond the scope of this chapter. The interested reader is referred to several recent reviews.[112-114]

Orthopedic Surgery

Although the etiology of fever in the postoperative orthopedic patient may include any of the processes discussed in the first section of this chapter, the consultant should particularly consider local wound disorders and venous thrombosis with or without pulmonary embolism.

Many orthopedic procedures entail considerable tissue trauma with resultant local bleeding. Hematoma formation is therefore particularly common and may cause fever. The affected patient may be uncomfortable but does not appear toxemic. In the obvious case, a tense, warm, erythematous, and painful swelling is discovered at the incision, perhaps accompanied by local edema and purpura. At times, it may be difficult to distinguish hematoma from local wound infection, and bacterial superinfection may complicate an initially aseptic process. Despite the possibility of introducing infection, needle aspiration of the collection may be indispensable, because documentation of the presence of infection may necessitate further surgery. Occasionally, the collection of blood may be deep and the presence of hematoma not appreciated on examination. Suspicions should be raised if the postoperative hematocrit is disproportionately low for estimated blood loss, especially if the patient has been excessively anticoagulated.

Open wounds requiring surgery are particularly prone to infection. In one series, 15% of open fractures became infected, as did 22% of open joint wounds and 50% of open soft tissue injuries.[115] Many of these wounds were already infected at the time of hospital admission. Although some authors have not found such a high rate of overt infection, they have confirmed the high incidence of bacterial contamination, providing a rationale for the use of prophylactic antibiotics.

The overall incidence of postoperative infection in cases not involving trauma is considerably less. Incidence rates in published series range from 0.7% to 11%, with most falling between 2% and 5%.[116–118] Half of these infections are major, necessitating further surgery or resulting in functional disability. Staphylococci, both coagulase-positive and coagulase-negative, are major pathogens causing many types of infections ranging from wound infection to osteomyelitis.

Total hip replacement is being performed with increasing frequency. Fever in the first few postoperative days is nearly universal and is not a predictor of subsequent complications. However, persistent or late fever is worrisome, because deep infection carries an ominous prognosis for the prosthesis. The incidence of deep infection after hip replacement ranges from 0 to 11%, with most series reporting rates between 0.5% and 2%.[116]

Previous hip surgery with or without infection increases risk; the use of prophylactic antibiotics and a clean operating room with laminar air flow appear to decrease it.[119] Bladder catheterization, urinary tract infection, culture-positive wound drainage, or remote infection may also be associated with higher than normal rates of infection.[120] As noted above, hematoma formation and drainage may also predispose patients to infection, but, of course, spontaneous drainage may itself be the result of infection.

Deep hip infection should be suspected when the patient continues to experience pain after the immediate postoperative period. The presence of wound drainage, prolonged fever, or dislocation of the prosthesis supports the diagnosis. Deep hip sepsis in the first 3 months after surgery is likely to present with typical signs and symptoms of infection, whereas late infection thereafter may be manifested only by persistent and worsening pain. Any patient with a hip prosthesis who has unremitting or recurrent pain without obvious cause or radiologic evidence of dislocation must be suspected of having an infected joint even without fever, local signs of inflammation, drainage, or an elevated erythrocyte sedimentation rate. Approximately 40% to 50% of all infections present early; presentation of late infection may be delayed for months or even years.[116]

The etiologic pathogens, specifically *Staphylococcus aureus* and coagulase-negative staphylococci, are predominantly gram-positive.[116,121] The latter classically cause a more indolent process, but the former can also cause smoldering infection. Wilson and associates have noted that the incidence of gram-negative bacterial infection of hip prostheses has increased in recent years.[122] *Pseudomonas,*

Proteus, Serratia, E. coli and *Klebsiella* have all been isolated in this context.

Abnormal laboratory parameters are few in number and nonspecific. The sedimentation rate may be the most sensitive test, especially in the early group, but interpretation is complicated by the routine elevation found in almost all patients in the early postoperative period.[116] Radiographic changes such as periosteal reaction in the femoral shaft, cortical bone resorption, and dislocation of the prosthesis may require several weeks to become evident and are unlikely to be helpful in the immediate postoperative period.[123] Arthrography, bone scanning, and tomography may be useful, but, ultimately, needle aspiration for Gram stain and culture or direct visual inspection at surgery with microbiologic evaluation may be necessary for the diagnosis to be made.[123]

Infection of total knee arthroplasty is similar to infection of total hip replacement.[124]

Abdominal Surgery

Fever is common following abdominal, in particular gastrointestinal, surgery. Infection is a major cause of the fever, with wound infection predominating. Its incidence is affected by many factors, including the use of prophylactic antibiotics and the performance of incidental appendectomy.

The risk of wound infection after gastroduodenal surgery has been directly related to the bacterial count in the gastric contents, which, in turn, is dependent on the underlying pathology. In one study, total viable gastric bacterial counts per milliliter were 3.8×10^1 with duodenal ulcer, 6.95×10^4 with gastric ulcer, and 1.9×10^7 with gastric carcinoma. Wound infection rates for the three groups were 17%, 38%, and 56%, respectively.[125] Other authors have noted a similar relationship between risk of infection and underlying pathology.[126,127]

The risk of wound infection with cholecystectomy is increased by concomitant choledochotomy and by the presence of infected bile.[98,128,129] Its incidence has been variably reported as higher than or no different from that of incidental appendectomy.[128,129] Rates of wound infection with appendectomy range from 2% to 9% with nonperforated organs and from 8.3% to 25% when perforation has occurred. They are about 35% with overt appendiceal abscess formation.[130] Wound infection rates after colorectal surgery vary from 2.1% to over 60%.[131,132]

Multiple studies have documented the preponderance of native gut flora isolated from established wound infection following gastrointestinal tract surgery.[89,133–136] Enteric gram-negative rods, enterococci, and anaerobes including *Bacteroides* are common, suggesting that endogenous intraoperative contamination plays a major role in the pathogenesis of this complication.[134]

Postoperative peritonitis after abdominal surgery occurs with a frequency of 1.5% to 8.0% with an attendant mortality rate of 50% to 90%.[137] Its pathogenesis is variable. When contamination has already taken place before surgery, as in appendiceal perforation, postoperative peritonitis may simple be a continuation of the pre-existing process, which cannot be adequately controlled by surgical intervention. Intraoperative contamination may derive either from an external source, such as a member of the surgical team or the operating room environment itself, or from an internal source, such as the opening of a nonsterile viscus. Finally, postoperative contamination may result from an unrelated secondary disease, such as acute cholecystitis, or from a variety of postoperative complications, including breakdown of an anastamotic site.

When infection becomes localized within the abdomen, an intraperitoneal, retroperitoneal, or visceral abscess results.[138,139] Like peritonitis, this may be a consequence of the primary disease process requiring surgery, the surgical procedure itself, or an intercurrent illness. Visceral abscesses usually form in the liver but may occur in the pancreas, spleen, or kidneys. Retroperitoneal abscesses are less commonly associated with surgery but may develop anteriorly in the retroperitoneal space when surgery is undertaken in the presence of established infection.

Of all intraperitoneal abscesses, subphrenic abscesses are the best described.[140–146] The use of antibiotics has tended to transform their once fulminant presentation into a more insidious, chronically debilitating, and often occult process. In addition, common causes have changed from perforated gastric ulcer and appendicitis at the turn of the century to biliary and gastric surgical procedures today. Responsible microorganisms are derived endogenously from the gastrointestinal tract. Fever, chills, and pain are frequent but not invariable findings. There is a high incidence of symptoms and signs related to the chest in addition to those referable to the abdomen; together, they constitute the so-called thoracoabdominal complex.[141,146] Similarly, radiographs may reveal abnormalities above the diaphragm, such as atelectasis, pneumonitis, effusion, or empyema, as well as abnormalities below it such as air-fluid levels, limited diaphragmatic motion, and hepatic displacement. Ultraso-

nography, gallium and liver–lung scanning, and computerized tomography comprise available modalities for noninvasive diagnosis, though abscesses can escape detection for prolonged periods of time.

Postsurgical febrile complications relating to the pancreas may arise from both infectious and noninfectious processes.[147] Acute postoperative pancreatitis usually results from intraoperative trauma to the pancreas itself or to surrounding structures such as the biliary tree and stomach. Injury may be so slight as to be inapparent except in retrospect. The incidence of pancreatitis following gastric resection has been reported to be as high as 3%. Pancreatitis may also result from surgery at distant, even extra-abdominal, sites, but its pathogenesis in this instance is unclear. In either event, the patient may present with minimal findings suggesting pancreatitis or may demonstrate the full-blown syndrome with fever, abdominal pain and tenderness, and ileus as well as extra-abdominal findings including adult respiratory distress syndrome, arthritis, and rash. Intraoperative trauma to the pancreas may also result in structural abnormalities, particularly pseudocyst formation. Pseudocysts themselves may be associated with fever, but a persistently febrile course in a toxemic patient should suggest the possibility of bacterial superinfection of a cyst or of the pancreas itself with overt abscess formation.[148]

Starch peritonitis is an additional cause of fever after abdominal surgery.[149–153] Most cases occur in the third postoperative week, but onset may occur from 5 to 42 days postsurgery. Signs and symptoms besides fever include diffuse abdominal pain and distention. Findings often suggest intestinal obstruction. Several authors have emphasized the distinct absence of toxemia, despite high fever, and a worrisome abdominal examination. Routine laboratory evaluation is usually not helpful. Although absence of a leukocytosis is typical, cases have been reported with peripheral blood counts over 20,000.[153] Polarizing microscopy can establish a diagnosis by allowing identification of starch granules in aspirated ascitic fluid.[154] The disease is self-limited but can last several weeks. Therapy with either corticosteroids or indomethacin has been reported to give dramatic relief.

THERAPY

It is impossible to provide specific recommendations about empiric antimicrobial therapy for all febrile postoperative patients, since such a wide variety of clinical situations is encompassed. Nonetheless, the following generalizations may be kept in mind.

1. Fever alone is not an indication for immediate antimicrobial therapy. If the patient is not at all toxemic, and if no source of infection is clinically identified, antibiotics may be withheld pending further data. If a source is found on initial evaluation, therapy may be instituted at once, with antibiotic selection determined by an understanding of the pathogens likely to be at fault in that specific situation.
2. The sicker the patient, the more likely it is that empiric therapy is justified, and the broader antimicrobial coverage should be. If a patient is desperately ill, coverage should be extended to include all reasonably possible organisms.
3. Whenever possible, empiric therapy should be based on the results of a

Table 32-1. Antibiotic Regimens for Empiric Therapy of Suspected Sepsis

A	B
Penicillinase-resistant penicillin (e.g., nafcillin or oxacillin)	Gentamicin or tobramycin
Cephalosporin (e.g., cefazolin)	Amikacin

Gram-stained specimen from the infected site.
4. Infections that develop in the hospital are more likely to be caused by relatively resistant pathogens than infections that occur outside the hospital.
5. Table 32-1 gives some examples of broad-spectrum coverage. Any of the drugs in column A may be combined with any of the drugs in column B.
6. If a gastrointestinal or gynecologic source is likely, coverage for B. fragilis should be included by the addition of clindamycin.
7. If enterococcus is a likely pathogen, ampicillin or carbenicillin should be included.
8. Although the combination of ampicillin, clindamycin, and an aminoglycoside is a standard regimen for patients with abdominal infection, some authorities feel that cefoxitin alone is acceptable if the patient has a low probability of being colonized with resistant, aerobic, gram-negative rods.

Once an initial regimen has been initiated, further therapeutic and diagnostic decisions will depend not only on accumulated laboratory data, but also on the patient's response to therapy. Persistent, undefined fever should prompt repeated, thorough physical examinations and judicious repetition of basic laboratory tests. As mentioned above, change in or, if possible, removal of in-dwelling lines or monitoring devices may be a rewarding and life-saving maneuver. Finally, discussions with the attending surgeons and other consulting physicians are crucial when more invasive diagnostic or therapeutic interventions are considered.

SUMMARY

Fever in the postoperative patient may arise from a number of possible sources, both infectious and noninfectious. Though the approach may vary in different situations, there are certain generalizations that are applicable to the evaluation of most patients. It is helpful to approach postoperative fever in a rational, stepwise fashion, as outlined below, in order to avoid overlooking any possible sources.

1. Thorough history and chart review, with particular attention to
   a. Preoperative course and pre-existing medical and surgical problems
   b. Medications received, including anesthetics and antibiotics
   c. Nature of the surgical procedure, including whether performed under elective or emergency conditions
   d. Intraoperative and postoperative complications
   e. Presence and time of placement of vascular and urinary catheters as well as other tubes and monitoring devices
   f. Timing of blood product transfusions
   g. History of allergies
2. Physical examination with particular attention to
   a. The operative site and areas contiguous to it
   b. The presence of catheters and indwelling monitoring devices, as well as to areas around their entry points
   c. Signs suggestive of deep vein thrombosis
   d. Decubiti secondary to pressure necrosis or sterile abscesses from intramuscular injections
   e. The lower respiratory tract
3. Initial laboratory evaluation, including
   a. Urinalysis, urine Gram stain, and culture
   b. Sputum Gram stain and culture
   c. Gram stain and culture of wound exudate or of drainage from closed systems such as pleural or mediastinal tubes; anaerobic culture, when the specimen can be properly obtained
   d. Blood cultures
   e. Complete blood count with differential
   f. Chest x-ray
4. If no diagnosis is apparent, one should then consider
   a. Changing and culturing all intravascular catheters
   b. Withdrawing medications suspected of causing fever
5. Depending upon the specific clinical situation and the information accrued, more extensive tests may often be helpful and are occasionally crucial. These may include liver function tests, radiographic contrast studies, radionuclide scanning, venography, arteriography, and computerized tomography.
6. When appropriate, antimicrobial therapy may be instituted according to the guidelines outlined above.

REFERENCES

1. Livelli FD Jr, Johnson RA, McEnany MT et al: Unexplained in-hospital fever following cardiac surgery. Natural history, relationship to the postpericardiotomy

syndrome, and a prospective study of therapy with indomethacin versus placebo. Circulation 57:968, 1978

2. Klimeck JJ, Ajemian ER, Gracewski JG et al: A prospective analysis of fever in hospitalized patients. Presented at the Second International Conference on Nosocomial Infections, Atlanta, Georgia, August 5–8, 1980

3. Robson MC, Krizek TJ, Heggers JP: Biology of surgical infection. Curr Probl Surg, March:1, 1973

4. Polk HC, Fry D, Flint LM: Dissemination and causes of infection. Surg Clin North Am 56:817, 1976

5. Ryan GB: Inflammation and localization of infection. Surg Clin North Am 56:831, 1976

6. Pollack AV: Surgical wound sepsis. Lancet 1:1283, 1969

7. Krizek TJ, Robson MC: Evolution of quantitative bacteriology in wound management. Am J Surg 130:579, 1975

8. Cruse PJE, Foord R: The epidemiology of wound infection: A prospective 10-year study of 62,939 wounds. Surg Clin North Am 60:27, 1980

9. Davidson AIG, Clark C, Smith G: Postoperative wound infection: A computer analysis. Br J Surg 58:333, 1971

10. Edwards LD: The epidemiology of 2056 remote site infections and 1966 surgical wound infections in 1865 patients: A four-year study of 40,923 operations at the Rush–Presbyterian–St. Luke's Hospital, Chicago. Ann Surg 184:758, 1976

11. Nichols RL: A technique for specimen collection of postsurgical exudate of wounds. Surg Gynecol Obstet 144:91, 1977

12. Altemeier WA, Hummel RP, Hill EO et al: Changing patterns in surgical infections. Ann Surg 178:436, 1975

13. Johnstone FRC: Infection on a surgical service. Present incidence compared with that of 1957. Am J Surg 120:192, 1970

14. Bell WR, Simon TL, DeMets DL: The clinical features of submassive and massive pulmonary emboli. Am J Med 62:355, 1977

15. Sasahama AA, Sharma GVRK, Parisi AF: New developments in the detection and prevention of venous thromboembolism. Am J Cardiol 43:1214, 1979

16. Murray HW, Ellis GC, Blumenthal DS et al: Fever and pulmonary thromboembolism. Am J Med 67:232, 1979

17. Maki DG, Goldmann DA, Rhame FS: Infection control in intravenous therapy. Ann Intern Med 79:867, 1973

18. Stein JM, Pruitt BA: Suppurative thrombophlebitis. A lethal iatrogenic disease. N Engl J Med 282:1453, 1970

19. Muenster AM: Septic thrombophlebitis. A surgical disorder. JAMA 230:1010, 1974

20. Hoshal VL: Intravenous catheters and infection. Surg Clin North Am 52:1407, 1972

21. Ryan JA, Abel RM, Abbott WM et al: Catheter complications in total parenteral nutrition. N Engl J Med 290:757, 1974

22. Sanders RA, Sheldon GE: Septic complications of total parenteral nutrition. A five-year experience. Am J Surg 132:214, 1976

23. Freeman JB, Lemire A, MacLean D: Intravenous alimentation and septicemia. Surg Gynecol Obstet 135:708, 1972

24. Freeman R, King B: Recognition of infection associated with intravenous catheters. Br J Surg 62:404, 1975

25. Freeman JB, Litton AA: Preponderance of gram-positive infections during parenteral alimentation. Surg Gynecol Obstet 139:905, 1974

26. Weakley S, Hopkins WE, Mays ET: Epidemic gram-negative septicemia in surgical patients. Am J Surg 124:363, 1972

27. Richards KE, Pierson CL, Bucciarelli L et al: Monilial sepsis in the surgical patient. Surg Clin North Am 52:1399, 1972

28. Rodrigues RJ, Wolff WI: Fungal septicemia in surgical patients. Ann Surg 180:741, 1974

29. Ashcraft KW, Leape LL: Candida sepsis complicating parenteral feeding. JAMA 212:454, 1970

30. Curry CR, Quie PG: Fungal septicemia in patients receiving parenteral hyperali-

mentation. N Engl J Med 285:1221, 1971

31. Rose HD: Venous catheter-associated candidemia. Am J Med Sci 275:265, 1978

32. Rodrigues RJ, Shinya H, Wolff WI et al: *Torulopsis glabrata* fungemia during prolonged intravenous alimentation therapy. N Engl J Med 284:540, 1971

33. Berkowitz ID, Robboy SJ, Karchmer AW et al: *Torulopsis glabrata* fungemia—A clinical pathologic study. Medicine (Baltimore) 58:430, 1979

34. Gaines JD, Remington JS: Disseminated candidiasis in the surgical patient. Surgery 72:730, 1972

35. Bernhardt HE, Orlando JC, Benfield JR: Disseminated candidiasis in surgical patients. Surg Gynecol Obstet 134:189, 1972

36. Band JD, Maki DG: Infections caused by arterial catheters used for hemodynamic monitoring. Am J Med 67:735, 1979

37. Cleri DJ, Corrado ML, Seligman SJ: Quantitative culture of intravenous catheters and other intravascular inserts. J Infect Dis 141:781, 1980

38. Maki D, Weise CE, Sarafin HW: A semi-quantitative culture method for identifying intravenous catheter-related infection. N Engl J Med 296:1305, 1977

39. Garibaldi RA, Burke JP, Dickman ML et al: Factors predisposing to bacteriuria during in-dwelling urethral catheterization. N Engl J Med 291:215, 1974

40. Shapiro SR, Santamarina A, Harrison JH: Catheter-associated urinary tract infections: Incidence and a new approach to prevention. J Urol 112:659, 1974

41. Lipsky BA, Hirschmann JV: Drug fever. JAMA 245:851, 1981

42. Parker CW: Drug allergy. N Engl J Med 292:511, 1975

43. Simon HB, Daniels GH: Hormonal hyperthermia. Endocrinologic causes of fever. Am J Med 66:257, 1979

44. Stephen CR: Malignant hyperpyrexia. Ann Rev Med 28:153, 1977

45. Britt BA: Etiology and pathophysiology of malignant hyperthermia. Fed Proc 38:44, 1979

46. Britt BA: Malignant hyperthermia: A pharmacogenetic disease of skeletal and cardiac muscle. N Engl J Med 290:1140, 1974

47. Dantrolene for malignant hyperthermia during anesthesia. Med Lett Drugs Ther 22:61, 1980

48. Pineda AA, Brzica SM, Taswell HF: Hemolytic transfusion reaction. Recent experience in a large blood bank. Mayo Clin Proc 53:378, 1978

49. Carney FMT, Van Dyke RA: Halothane hepatitis: A critical review. Anesth Analg (Cleve) 51:135, 1972

50. Onorato IM, Axelrod JL: Hepatitis from intravenous high-dose oxacillin therapy. Findings in an adult in-patient population. Ann Intern Med 89:497, 1978

51. Feinstone SM, Purcell RH: Non-A, non-B hepatitis. Ann Rev Med 29:359, 1978

52. Robinson WS, Lutwick LI: The virus of hepatitis, type B. N Engl J Med 295:1168, 1976

53. Aach RD, Kahn RA: Post-transfusion hepatitis: Current perspectives. Ann Intern Med 92:539, 1980

54. Berman M, Alter HJ, Ishak KG et al: The chronic sequelae of non-A, non-B hepatitis. Ann Intern Med 91:1, 1979

55. Koster FE: Diagnosis and management of complications of prosthetic heart valves. Am J Cardiol 35:872, 1975

56. Roses DR, Rose MR, Rapaport FT: Febrile responses associated with cardiac surgery. Relationships to the postpericardiotomy syndrome and to altered host immunologic reactivity. J Thorac Cardiovasc Surg 67:251, 1974

57. Baffes TG, Blazek WV, Fridman JL et al: Postoperative infections in 1136 consecutive cardiac operations. Surgery 68:791, 1970

58. Madison J, Wang K, Gobel FL et al: Prosthetic aortic valvular endocarditis. Circulation 50:940, 1975

59. Wilson WR, Jaumin PM, Danielson GK et al: Prosthetic valve endocarditis. Ann Intern Med 82:751, 1975

60. Slaughter L, Morris JE, Starr A: Prosthetic

valvular endocarditis. Circulation 47:1319, 1973

61. Dismukes WE, Karchmer AW, Buckley MJ et al: Prosthetic valve endocarditis. Analysis of 38 cases. Circulation 48:365, 1973

62. Karchmer AW, Dismukes WE, Buckley J et al: Late prosthetic valve endocarditis. Clinical features influencing therapy. Am J Med 64:199, 1978

63. Seelig MS, Speth CP, Kozinn PJ et al: *Candida* endocarditis after cardiac surgery. J Thor Cardiovasc Surg 65:583, 1973

64. Rubinstein E, Noriega ER, Simberkoff MS et al: Fungal endocarditis: Analysis of 24 cases and review of the literature. Medicine (Baltimore) 54:331, 1975

65. Sande MA, Johnson WD, Hook EW et al: Sustained bacteremia in patients with prosthetic cardiac valves. N Engl J Med 286:1067, 1972

66. Culliford AT, Cunningham JN Jr, Zeff RH et al: Sternal and costochondral infections following open heart surgery. J Thor Cardiovasc Surg 72:714, 1976

67. Ein ME, Bradshaw MW, Williams TW: Median sternotomy infections. Presented at the 20th Interscience Conference on Antimicrobial Agents and Chemotherapy, New Orleans, Louisiana, September 22–24, 1980

68. Bor D, Rose R, Modlin J et al: Infectious mediastinitis—A common complication of cardiac surgery. Presented at the 20th Interscience Conference on Antimicrobial Agents and Chemotherapy, New Orleans, Louisiana, September 22–24, 1980

69. Rubin RH, Moellering RC Jr: Clinical microbiologic and therapeutic aspects of purulent pericarditis. Am J Med 59:68, 1973

70. Engle MA, McCabe JC, Ebert P et al: The postpericardiotomy syndrome and anti-heart antibodies. Circulation 49:401, 1974

71. Jones SR, Luby JP, Sanford JP: Bacterial meningitis complicating cranial–spinal trauma. J Trauma 13:895, 1973

72. MacGee EE, Cauthen JC, Brackett CE: Meningitis following acute traumatic cerebrospinal fluid fistula. J Neurosurg 33:312, 1970

73. Bryan CS, Jernigan FE: Post-traumatic meningitis due to ampicillin-resistant *Hemophilus influenzae*. J Neurosurg 51:240, 1979

74. Weinstein MP, LaForce FM, Mangi RJ et al: Non-pneumococcal gram-positive coccal meningitis related to neurosurgery. J Neurosurg 47:236, 1977

75. Mangi RJ, Quintiliani R, Andriole VT: Gram-negative bacillary meningitis. Am J Med 59:829, 1975

76. George R, Leibrock L, Epstein M: Long-term analysis of cerebrospinal fluid shunt infections. A 25-year experience. J Neurosurg 51:804, 1979

77. Venes JL: Control of shunt infection. Report of 150 consecutive cases. J Neurosurg 45:311, 1976

78. Schoenbaum SC, Gardner P, Shillito J: Infections of cerebrospinal fluid shunts: Epidemiology, clinical manifestations and therapy. J Infect Dis 131:543, 1975

79. Fokes EC: Occult infections of ventriculoatrial shunts. J Neurosurg 33:517, 1970

80. Everett ED, Eickhoff TC, Simon RH: Cerebrospinal fluid shunt infections with anaerobic diphtheroids (*Propionibacterium* species). J Neurosurg 44:580, 1976

81. Brook I, Johnson N, Overturf GD et al: Mixed bacterial meningitis: A complication of ventriculo and lumboperitoneal shunts. J Neurosurg 47:961, 1977

82. Buckwold FJ, Hand R, Hansebout RR: Hospital-acquired bacterial meningitis in neurosurgical patients. J Neurosurg 46:494, 1977

83. Smith RW, Alksne JF: Infections complicating the use of external ventriculostomy. J Neurosurg 44:567, 1976

84. Willwerth BM, Waldhausen JA: Infection of arterial prostheses. Surg Gynecol Obstet 139:446, 1974

85. Goldstone J, Moore WS: Infection in vascular prostheses. Clinical manifestations

and surgical management. Am J Surg 128:225, 1974

86. Fry WJ: Vascular prosthesis infections. Surg Clin North Am 52:1419, 1972

87. Bernhard VM: Management of infected vascular prostheses. Surg Clin North Am 55:1411, 1975

88. Szilagyi DE, Smith RF, Elliott JP et al: Infection in arterial reconstruction with synthetic grafts. Ann Surg 176:321, 1972

89. Sweet RL, Ledger WJ: Puerperal infectious morbidity—a two-year review. Am J Obstet Gynecol 117:1093, 1973

90. Finegold SM, Bartlett JG, Chow AE et al: Management of anaerobic infections. Ann Intern Med 83:375, 1975

91. Ledger WJ, Norman, McGee C et al: Bacteremia on an obstetric–gynecologic service. Obstetrics 121:205, 1975

92. Gibbs RS, O'Dell TN, MacGregor RR et al: Puerperal endometritis: A prospective microbiologic study. Obstetrics 121:919, 1975

93. Gibbs RS: Treatment of refractory postpartum fever. Clin Obstet Gynecol 19:83, 1976

94. Wallace RJ, Alpert S, Browne K: Isolation of *Mycoplasma hominis* from blood cultures in patients with postpartum fever. Obstet Gynecol 51:181, 1978

95. Hagen D: Maternal febrile morbidity associated with fetal monitoring and cesarean section. Obstet Gynecol 46:260, 1975

96. Ott WJ: Primary cesarean section: Factors related to post-partum infection. Obstet Gynecol 57:171, 1981

97. Green SL, Sarubbi FA: Risk factors associated with post-cesarian section febrile morbidity. Obstet Gynecol 49:686, 1977

98. Wenzel RP, Hunting KF, Osterman CA: Postoperative wound infection rates. Surg Gynecol Obstet 144:749, 1977

99. Schwarz RH: Management of postoperative infections in obstetrics and gynecology. Clin Obstet Gynecol 19:97, 1976

100. Ledger WJ, Reite A, Headington JT: The surveillance of infection on an in-patient gynecology service. Am J Obstet Gynecol 113:662, 1972

101. Hevron JE, Llorens AS: Management of postoperative abscess following gynecologic surgery. Obstet Gynecol 47:553, 1976

102. Swartz RH: Prophylaxis of minor febrile and major infectious morbidity following hysterectomy. Obstet Gynecol 54:284, 1979

103. Gorbach SL: Antibiotic therapy of obstetric and gynecologic infections. Surg Clin North Am 55:1373, 1975

104. Ledger WJ: Infections in obstetrics and gynecology. New developments in treatment. Surg Clin North Am 52:1447, 1972

105. Josey WE, Staggers SR: Heparin therapy in septic pelvic thrombophlebitis: A study of 46 cases. Am J Obstet Gynecol 120:228, 1974

106. Sullivan NM, Sutter VL, Mims MM et al: Clinical aspects of bacteremia after manipulation of the genitourinary tract. J Infect Dis 127:49, 1973

107. Ives JCJ, Browne AK, Jones WW et al: Bacteraemia following urologic surgery. Br J Surg 58:32, 1971

108. Schmidt JD, Hawtrey CE, Flocks RH et al: Complications, results and problems of ileal conduit diversions. J Urol 109:210, 1973

109. Harbach LB, Hall RC, Hockett ATK et al: Ileal loop cutaneous urinary diversion: A critical review. J Urol 105:511, 1971

110. Burns JR, Gregory JG: Osteomyelitis of the pubic symphysis after urologic surgery. J Urol 118:803, 1977

111. Hale JE, Aichroth P: Vertebral osteomyelitis: A complication of urological surgery. Br J Surg 61:867, 1974

112. Simmons RL, Balfour HH, Lopez C et al: Infection in immunosuppressd transplant recipients. Surg Clin North Amer 55:1419, 1975

113. Eickhoff TC: Infectious complications in renal transplant recipients. Transplant Proc 5:1233, 1973

114. Ramsey PG, Rubin RH, Tolkhoff–Rubin NE et al: The renal transplant patient with fever and pulmonary infiltrates: Etiology, clinical manifestations and management. Medicine (Baltimore) 59:206, 1980

115. Lidgren L, Lindberg L: Orthopaedic infections during a five-year period. Analysis of patient material from an orthopaedic clinic, 1963–1967. Acta Orthop Scand 43:325, 1972

116. Hunter G, Dandy D: The natural history of the patient with an infected total hip replacement. J Bone Joint Surg (Br) 59:293, 1977

117. Lidgren L, Lindberg L: Postoperative wound infections in clean orthopaedic surgery. Review of five-year material. Acta Orthop Scand 45:161, 1974

118. Raahave D: Postoperative wound infection after implant and removal of osteosynthetic material. Acta Orthop Scand 47:28, 1976

119. Fitzgerald RH: Reduction of deep sepsis following total hip arthroplasty. Ann NY Acad Sci 353:262, 1980

120. Anstutz HC, Kass V: Management of the septic total hip replacement. In The Hip. Proceedings of the 5th Open Scientific Meeting of the Hip Society. St. Louis, CV Mosby, 1977

121. Nelson JP: The operating room environment and its influence on deep wound infection. In The Hip. Proceedings of the 5th Open Scientific Meeting of the Hip Society. St. Louis, CV Mosby, 1977

122. Wilson PD, Salvati EA, Blumenfield EL: The problem of infection in total prosthetic arthroplasty of the hip. Surg Clin North Am 55:1431, 1973

123. Hunter GGA, Dandy D: Diagnosis and natural history of the infected total hip replacement. In The Hip. Proceedings of the 5th Open Scientific Meeting of the Hip Society. St. Louis, CV Mosby, 1977

124. Pety W, Bryan RS, Coventry MB et al: Infection after total knee arthroplasty. Orthop Clin N Am 6:1005, 1975

125. Gatehouse D, Dimoch F, Furdon DW et al: Prediction of wound sepsis following gastric operations. Br J Surg 65:551, 1978

126. Lewis RT: Wound infection after gastroduodenal operations: A 10-year review. Can J Surg 20:435, 1977

127. Nichols RL, Miller B. Smith JW: Septic complications following gastric surgery: Relationship to the endogenous gastric microflora. Surg Clin North Am 55:1367, 1975

128. Pollack, Evans M: Wound sepsis after cholecystectomy: Effect of incidental appendectomy. Br Med J 1:20, 1977

129. Wolloch Y, Feigenberg Z, Zer M et al: The influence of biliary infection on the postoperative course after biliary tract surgery. Am J Gastroenterol 67:456, 1977

130. Simonowitz DA, White TT: Postoperative complications of appendectomy (including adhesions). Clin Gastroenterol 8:429, 1979

131. Fikri E, McAdams AJ: Wound infection in colonic surgery. Ann Surg 182:724, 1975

132. Burton RC: Postoperative wound infection in colonic and rectal surgery. Br J Surg 60:363, 1973

133. Lorber B, Swenson RM: The bacteriology of intra-abdominal infections. Surg Clin North Am 55:1349, 1975

134. Leigh DA: Wound infections due to *Bacteroides fragilis* following intestinal surgery. Br J Surg 62:375, 1975

135. Anderson CB, Marr JJ, Ballinger WF: Anaerobic infections in surgery. A clinical review. Surgery 79:313, 1976

136. Thadepalli H, Gorbach SL, Broido PW et al: Abdominal trauma, anaerobes and antibiotics. Surg Gynecol Obstet 137:270, 1973

137. Pichlmayr R, Lohlein D: Acute postsurgical syndromes. Clin Gastroenterol 8:249, 1979

138. Nichols RL: Infections following gastrointestinal surgery: Intra-abdominal abscess. Surg Clin North Am 60:197, 1980

139. Nichols RL: Intra-abdominal sepsis: Characterization and treatment. J Infect Dis (Suppl) 135:54, 1977

140. Sanders RC: The changing epidemiology of subphrenic abscess and its clinical and radiological consequences. Br J Surg 57:449, 1970

141. Konvolinka CW, Olearczyk A: Subphrenic abscess. Curr Probl Surg, Jan:3, 1972

142. DeCosse JJ, Poulin TL, Fox PS et al: Subphrenic abscess. Surg Gynecol Obstet 138:841, 1974

143. Bonfils–Roberts EA, Barone JE, Nealon TF Jr: Treatment of subphrenic abscess. Surg Clin North Am 55:1361, 1975

144. Wang SMS, Wilson SE: Subphrenic abscess. The new epidemiology. Arch Surg 112:934, 1977

145. Halliday P, Halliday JH: Subphrenic abscess: A study of 241 patients at the Royal Prince Edward Hospital, 1950–73. Br J Surg 63:352, 1976

146. Carter R, Brewer LA: Subphrenic abscess: A thoracoabdominal complex: The changing picture with antibiotics. Am J Surg 108:165, 1964

147. Malagelada JR, Go VLW, Remine WH et al: Postsurgical complications involving the pancreas. Clin Gastroenterol 8:455, 1979

148. Warshaw AL: Pancreatic abscesses. N Engl J Med 287:1234, 1972

149. Ignatius JA, Hartmann WH: The glove starch peritonitis syndrome. Ann Surg 175:388, 1972

150. Soderberg CH, Lou Y, Randall HT: Glove starch granulomatous peritonitis. Am J Surg 125:455, 1973

151. Bates B: Granulomatous peritonitis secondary to corn starch. Ann Intern Med 62:335, 1965

152. Sugerbaker PH, McReynolds RA, Brooks JR: Glove starch granulomatous disease. Am J Surg 128:3, 1974

153. Holmes EC, Eggleston JC: Starch granulomatous peritonitis. Surgery 71:85, 1977

154. Warshaw AL: Diagnosis of starch peritonitis by paracentesis. Lancet 2:1054, 1972

Anaphylactic Reactions to Radiographic Contrast Media

PAUL C. ATKINS

The administration of radiographic contrast media (RCM) has become commonplace in the preparation of patients for surgery. The growing use of selective arteriography, coronary angiography, and computerized tomography exposes an increasing number of patients to contrast media. Of all patients undergoing such procedures, 5% to 8% will have a reaction, 1% to 2% of which will be life-threatening.[1,2] This chapter will discuss different types of reaction, their pathogenesis, relative risks, and methods of prevention and treatment. Special emphasis is placed on anaphylaxis. Reactions following the administration of contrast media that cause renal failure, uricosuria, and hyperviscosity are discussed elsewhere.

CLASSIFICATION

Zweiman and co-workers have developed a useful classification of reactions to RCM administered to the intravascular space.[3] The first group consists of *vasomotor* reactions, including nausea, vomiting, flushing, transient dizziness, and dysesthesias resulting in tingling and numbness of the lips, arms, and extremities.

These transient symptoms occur almost immediately after intravascular administration of RCM, last from 1 min to 5 min, and rarely prove severe or persistent enough to require treatment. More important, some of these symptoms occur almost universally in patients receiving rapid intravascular administration of RCM. Undue anxiety or an exaggerated vasomotor response to RCM may be erroneously labled as anaphylaxis.

A second type of reaction is manifested by *dermal* signs and symptoms not of an urticarial nature. These include generalized itching and a variety of morbilliform and papular eruptions. Although often bothersome, they are not life-threatening and ordinarily need not concern the physician regarding future studies. However, one dermal eruption, urticaria–angioedema, although usually self-limited, may be part of a more severe generalized reaction and should therefore be considered a *forme fruste* of an anaphylactic reaction.

The *anaphylactic* type of reaction, the most severe, consists of any of the following: dyspnea, wheezing, hypotension, syncope, and urticaria or angioedema. Anaphylaxis occurs in 1% to 2% of all patients exposed to RCM and accounts for fatalities in 1 in 10,000 to 1 in 40,000 procedures.[2,3] Most of these reactions begin within 5 min of administration and persist for 30 min to 24 hr. In general, the earlier the onset of symptoms, the more severe the reaction. Fatal sequelae occur within 30 min in 95% of patients. Skin reactions alone, which develop hours after administration of RCM, are rare and usually not life-threatening and can generally be treated symptomatically. Any reaction occuring after 24 hr is not anaphylactic and may be unrelated to the administration of dye.[4]

Several groups have published prophylactic regimens thought to decrease the risk and severity of anaphylactic reactions in susceptible patients receiving RCM.[3,5] Therefore, distinguishing between these reaction types has important clinical implications.

RISK FACTORS

Assessment of the risk of developing a reaction to RCM has been inadequately studied. Most studies assessing risk factors do not separate anaphylactic from other reactions. Some have not even separated modes of RCM administration. All have been misled by the fact that many patients known to have had prior reactions either refuse or are excluded from subsequent challenge with RCM.

Most contrast agents are water-soluble, iodinated, aromatic compounds with basic or polar side-chains. Consequently, several large surveys implicate iodine and shellfish allergies as significant risk factors for developing RCM reactions, but there is no good evidence to support this.[1] There does seem to be higher than normal risk in allergic patients, particularly those with a history of bronchospasm. Elderly persons and patients with significant cardiorespiratory disease have higher mortality from anaphylactic reactions.[5] A history of previous anaphylactic reactions increases the risk of experiencing them again to 23% to 30% (a fivefold increase).[6]

Anaphylactic reactions are extremely uncommon after administration of RCM orally or into nonvascular spaces. Although there have been single reports of chronic urticaria persisting after myelography and of systemic anaphylaxis after salpingography, these are rare.[7,8] In the latter case, and occasionally in retrograde pyelography, forceful RCM administration with significant vascular penetration can be implicated. However, these cases are so unusual that even susceptible patients are at minimal risk if contrast medium is not forcibly extruded during these procedures. Intravascular or lymphatic administration of RCM carries a higher risk for the development of anaphylactic reactions. The risk is highest and the reactions most severe after intravenous cholangiography, but it is also increased with other intravascular studies, including intravenous pyelography, coronary and cerebral angiography, and computerized tomography with contrast.[1,2,6] Risk factors are summarized below.

Clinical condition of patient
    Age
    Atopic and asthmatic history
    Significant cardiorespiratory disease
    Past history of anaphylactic RCM reactions
Type of study
    Intravascular administration of RCM, including computerized tomography
    Intravenous cholangiography
    Lymphatic administration of RCM

PATHOPHYSIOLOGY

Rapid intravascular introduction of a hyperosmolar substance such as RCM may cause nonspecific tissue destruction and increase local hyperosmolality.[9] These factors may be responsible for transient aggregation of formed elements in the circulation, perhaps leading to some deaths during cardioangiography.[10] RCM may also interact with basophils, mast cells, the complement system, and the coagulation system. Mechanisms of RCM reactions are outlined below.

Hyperosmolar effects
Aggregation of formed elements
Basophil and mast-cell degranulation
    By direct hyperosmolar effect
    Through activation of complement
    (C3a, C5a)
    Through immunoglobulin E (IgE) interaction (very rare)
Complement activation
Coagulation pathway activation

In vitro incubation of RCM with basophils can cause degranulation and mediator release, which may account for in vivo histamine elevation in the blood after RCM administration.[7,11,12] RCM infusions have been shown in both in vivo and in vitro studies to activate the complement and coagulation systems.[11–13] Given that hyperosmolar stimuli, activated components of the complement system (C3a, C5a), or IgE antibody–antigen interactions may activate basophils and mast cells, it seems logical that RCM interacts with mediator-rich cells through all of these systems (Table 33-1). However, it has not been possible to demonstrate heightened response of basophils and mast cells in RCM-reactive subjects, and only one study has implicated IgE antibodies.[7,11–13] Table 33-1 and the above list summarize putative mechanisms underlying RCM reactions and the products of mast-cell or basophil activation. Therapeutic intervention and premedication regimens are predicated upon the prevention or counteraction of the effects of mast-cell or basophil degranulation.

Table 33-1. Products of Mast-Cell and Basophil Activation

Product	Effect
Vasoactive Amines	
Histamine	Vasodilation,
Serotonin	hypotension, bronchospasm, itching
Kininogens	
Basophil and lung kallikreins of anaphylaxis	Vasodilation, bronchospasm, skin lesions, coagulation
Arachidonic Acid Metabolites	
Prostaglandins; slow-reacting substance of anaphylaxis	Hypotension, bronchospasm
Other Factors	
Eosinophil and neutrophil chemotactic factors; superoxide radicals	Increased tissue destruction, inflammatory cell infiltration

PROPHYLAXIS AND TREATMENT

Only patients receiving intravascular or lymphatic administration of RCM should be viewed as having an increased risk for serious reactions. If the patient has not been previously exposed or does not have a history of reactions to RCM, the risk of any reaction is 5% to 8%, and that of a serious reaction is 1% to 2%. The physician cannot make recommendations based upon a history of atopy or reactions to iodides or shellfish. In our experience, no undue precautions or preparations are necessary in this setting.[3,6]

In patients with a history of previous reactions, evaluation and pretreatment are essential. Details of the prior reaction should be categorized as vasomotor, dermal, or anaphylactic as described at the beginning of this chapter. Patients with histories of vasomotor and skin reactions, except urticaria and angioedema, do not have an increased risk of serious RCM reactions. They should be reassured and not premedicated. However, because of inadequate data, the radiologist should be notified and remain available throughout the study.

Patients who have had previous anaphylactic or urticarial reactions carry a high risk of repeated reaction. The study should be deferred if not absolutely necessary, or studies involving nonvascular administration of RCM may suffice. If an intravascular study must be performed, informed consent should be received, and pretreatment with prednisone in a dose of 40 mg every 6 hr for 24 hr before and 18 hr after RCM administration is indicated. In addition, diphenhydramine hydrochloride (Benadryl), 50 mg, is given 30 min before the procedure. These premedications clearly reduce the incidence and severity of severe RCM reactions in susceptible patients.[3,5] An intravenous line should be inserted; epinephrine, Benadryl, intubation apparatus, and the physician must be immediately available throughout the procedure.

If an RCM reaction occurs, the following steps should be taken. Vasomotor and skin reactions need be treated only by reassurance, fluid replacement, or administration of antipruritic therapy. Anaphylactic or urticarial–angioedematous reactions should be treated with fluid replacement, maintenance of the airway, and immediate subcutaneous administration of 0.3 ml to 0.5 ml of 1:1000 epi-

nephrine. The epinephrine may be repeated every 15 min to 30 min as needed. Oxygen and intravenous aminophylline should be administered for bronchospasm. Blood pressure and pulse should be continuously monitored. Persistent or severe hypotension calls for more fluids with appropriate central venous catheter monitoring and may require intravenous epinephrine (1 ml of a 1:10,000 dilution) with subsequent monitoring for developing hypertension and supraventricular tachycardia.[14] This dose may be repeated every 5 min to 15 min. In addition, as much as 2 hr to 2½ hr may be necessary for replacement of the effective volume deficit caused by peripheral vasodilation. Because this may be followed by fluid overload when vasoconstriction occurs, intensive care unit monitoring is essential.[14] Finally, Benadryl in a dose of 50 mg to 100 mg should be given to block further mediator release. Therapy is summarized below.

Vasomotor
    Reassurance
    Volume repletion
Dermal
    Antipruritics
Anaphylactic
    Epinephrine—0.3 ml to 0.5 ml subcutaneously every 15 min to 30 min
    Volume repletion—may need up to 24 hr to prevent hypotension
    Bronchospasm—epinephrine or aminophylline
    Benadryl—50 mg to 100 mg
    Monitoring of respiratory function and electrocardiogram
Severe or persistent hypotension—epinephrine, 1 ml 1:10,000 intravenously every 5 min to 15 min; massive fluid replacement in intensive care unit setting

SUMMARY

1. RCM reactions can be classified as vasomotor, dermal, or urticarial–anaphylactic.
2. Vasomotor and skin reactions require no prophylaxis or treatment.
3. Anaphylactic reactions occur after intravascular RCM. Patients who have had previous RCM reactions require prophylaxis as outlined in (5) below.
4. Treatment of RCM reactions is outlined above.
5. Evaluation and management of patients with a prior history of RCM reaction may be summarized as follows: Classify reaction as vasomotor, dermal, or anaphylactic. Vasomotor and nonurticarial skin reactions carry no increased risk and require no premedication. For urticarial or anaphylactic reactions:
   a. Establish the need for intravascular study.
   b. Obtain the patient's informed consent.
   c. Administer premedication.
      —Prednisone, 40 mg every 6 hr for 24 hr before and 18 hr after RCM administration
      —Benadryl, 50 mg 30 min before study
   d. Put intravenous line in place.
   e. Make sure that the intubation apparatus, epinephrine, Benadryl, and the physician are immediately available.

REFERENCES

1. Shehadu W: Adverse reactions to intravascularly administered contrast media. Am J Roentgenol Radium Ther Nucl Med 124:145, 1975
2. Schatz M: Adverse reactions to radiographic contrast media: A practical approach. Immunology and Allergy Practice. 1:44, 1979
3. Zweiman B, Mishlin MM, Hilbreth EA: An approach to the performance of contrast studies in contrast material reactive persons. Ann Intern Med 83:159, 1975
4. Delage C, Irey NS: Anaphylactic deaths. A clinicopathologic study of 43 cases. J Forensic Sci 23:525, 1970
5. Kelly JF, Patterson R, Lieberman P et al: Radiographic contrast media studies in high-risk patients. J Allergy Clin Immunol 62:181, 1978
6. Cogen FC, Zweiman B: Adverse radiographic contrast media reactions. Compr Ther 4:50, 1978
7. Lieberman R, Siegle RL, Taylor WW: Anaphylactoid reactions to iodinated contrast material. J Allergy Clin Immunol 62:174, 1978
8. Elias J: Anaphylactic reaction after salpingography. J Allergy Clin Immunol 66:242, 1980
9. Bernstein E, Palmer J, Aaberg T et al: Studies of toxicity by hypaque—90% following rapid intravenous injections. Radiology 76:88, 1961
10. Reed R: Cause of death in cardioangiography. J Thorac Cardiovasc Surg 38:685, 1959
11. Cogen FC, Norman ME, Dunsky E et al: Histamine release and complement changes following injection of contrast media in humans. J Allergy Clin Immunol 64:299, 1979
12. Simon RA, Schatz M, Stevenson DD et al: Radiographic contrast media infusions. J Allergy Clin Immunol 63:281, 1979
13. Arroyave CM, Schatz M, Simon RA: Activation of the complement system by radiographic contrast media: Studies in vivo and in vitro. J Allergy Clin Immunol 63:276, 1979
14. Obeid AI, Johnson L, Potts J et al: Fluid therapy in severe systemic reaction to radiopaque dye. Ann Intern Med 83:317, 1975

Management of the Surgical Patient with Cerebrovascular Disease

FRANCISCO GONZALEZ–SCARANO
HOWARD I. HURTIG

The patient with atherosclerosis of the cerebral blood vessels maintains a precarious and potentially unstable balance between blood flow to the brain and the brain's metabolic needs. The stress of surgery can upset this balance, especially if hypotension, anoxia, and increased serum viscosity develop. The purpose of this chapter is to review problems peculiar to the patient with cerebrovascular disease (CVD) or stroke who is facing surgery and to propose guidelines for preoperative management.

TYPES OF CEREBROVASCULAR DISEASE

Patients with CVD usually fall into one of three categories: (1) those with completed stroke; (2) those with transient cerebral ischemia (TIA); or (3) those with asymptomatic cervical bruit(s).

A completed stroke produces neurologic deficit lasting longer than 24 hr. Stroke-induced disability may be permanent or may resolve completely.[1] Functional outcome is generally proportional to the severity of the initial deficit but is often unpredictable. The time interval between a past stroke and surgery is important because of the increased risk of neurologic complications known to accompany operative intervention the first few weeks after the onset of stroke symptoms.[2] The recovering brain is more susceptible to stress during this critical interval.

TIA causes acute neurologic symptoms that resolve within 24 hr. These episodes are probably caused by hemodynamic compromise in the territory of a tightly stenotic vessel or by artery-to-artery embolization from an ulcerated extracranial carotid artery.[3,4] Transient ischemic episodes lasting more than 24 hr are labeled reversible ischemic neurologic deficits (RIND) and are managed as TIAs.[5] It is essential to distinguish between symptoms that reflect disease of the anterior or internal carotid system and symptoms that reflect disorder of the posterior or vertebrobasilar circulations, because surgical therapy is in most instances possible only in the former case. A comprehensive discussion of differential symptomatology and theories of pathogenesis is beyond the scope of this chapter.

An asymptomatic cervical bruit may arise from the carotid, subclavian, or other major artery and serves as a general indicator of arteriosclerosis rather than as a specific predictor of stroke. Fields has defined three groups of patients with asymptomatic carotid bruits: (1) those who are asymptomatic; (2) those with neurologic symptoms that cannot be anatomically localized to the arterial territory supplied by the noisy vessel; and (3) those in whom a carotid bruit is discovered incidentally before noncarotid surgery.[6] Asymptomatic patients with carotid bruits or other evidence of extracranial carotid disease documented by noninvasive testing or angiography may have an increased risk of stroke, although the natural histories of these abnormalities have not been well defined.[6–8]

Patients in each of these groups have different risks or stroke during surgery and require individualized management. Unfortunately, published reports do not always distinguish among patients with different types of CVD when determining the risks of general surgery of the success of particular management strategies.

The goal of preoperative evaluation in these patients should be a careful effort to estimate the absolute need for the contemplated surgical procedure. Does the risk of neurologic complications outweigh the presumed benefit of the planned operation? Operative risk itself may be subdivided into two major components, that of general anesthesia and that associated with specific surgical procedures. Procedures that may produce hypotension or require carotid manipulation such as carotid endarterectomy are of special concern. Other problems, especially cardiac disease, may compound the operative risk of stroke for the patient with CVD.

Estimating overall surgical risk is only the beginning. The next important step is decreasing risk before surgery; however, the number of therapeutic maneuvers available to do so is limited. Surgery can be delayed for the patient with a healing cerebral infarct. In contrast, the patient with mild, fixed deficits remains disabled or may worsen with time, and indefinite postponement of necessary elective surgery will only complicate matters. Patients with TIA and RIND may need specific treatment of extracranial carotid disease by carotid endarterectomy before other surgery is performed, or they may need medical therapy with anticoagulants or agents that inhibit platelet aggregation. If the risk of perioperative stroke is unacceptably high and not likely to be decreased by specific preoperative treatment, surgery should be postponed indefinitely.

RISKS OF STROKE

Cardiac Surgery

The large number of operations currently performed in the treatment of coronary artery disease has allowed detailed study of neurologic complications in patients with this disorder (Table 34-1).[9] Patients undergoing coronary artery bypass grafting (CABG) are probably susceptible to ischemic complications because of diffuse atherosclerotic disease. Reul and co-workers retrospectively studied 1287 patients who had had CABG surgery, 65 of whom had had other concurrent cardiac procedures between 1968 and 1971.[10] Major neurologic complications were reported to occur in 1% of these patients, but de-

Table 34-1. Neurologic Complications of Coronary Artery Bypass Grafting

Study	No. Patients	Neurologic Complication Rate (%)	Stroke Rate (%)
Reul[10]	1287	1	
Ashor[11]	100*	4	2
Breuer[12]	400	16†	
Lee[13]	943		0.7
Gonzalez–Scarano[14]	1427	1.3	0.8
Urschel[15]	17	0	0

*65 years and older.
†1.8% of functional significance.

tails of type and severity were not provided. Ashor and associates reported on 100 consecutive patients aged 65 and over undergoing surgery for coronary artery disease and ventricular aneurysms between 1969 and 1972.[11] Strokes occurred in 2 patients, and 4 others had episodes of confusion. Breuer and colleagues found major functional central nervous system deficits in 1.8% of 400 patients undergoing CABG at the Cleveland Clinic.[12] The total incidence of neurologic complications was 16%. Many of these complications were focal deficits, suggesting a cerebrovascular etiology. In a group of 943 patients studied retrospectively by Lee and co-workers, 0.7% had cerebrovascular complications following CABG.[13] Five of the patients in the group had a prior history of CVD but suffered no complications. Similarly, 0.8% incidence of stroke following CABG was found among 1427 consecutive patients studied retrospectively at the Hospital of the University of Pennsylvania from 1974 to 1978.[14]

Urschel and colleagues reported a series of 17 patients with both CVD and coronary artery disease undergoing CABG. None developed stroke during CABG, but 1 patient did so during a subsequent carotid endarterectomy.[15] These 17 patients were part of a larger population of patients with TIAs who were treated with combined or staged carotid endarterectomy and CABG. Barnes and associates screened 120 patients scheduled for CABG or peripheral arterial reconstruction for extracranial carotid disease with ocular plethysmography and Doppler ultrasonography.[16] Of the entire group, 19 asymptomatic patients, or 16%, had evidence of flow-reducing stenosis of 50% in at least one carotid artery. Only 10 of the 19 had a cervical bruit. None of the 19 had prophylactic carotid endarterectomy, and none had a cerebrovascular complication.

Cardiac valvular surgery imposes a risk of cerebral ischemia and anoxia that has been well recognized since Gilman's classic study.[17] More recent studies generally support the impression that operative and postoperative neurologic complications in cardiac valvular surgery are due either to operative hypotension or to particulate emboli associated with the use of cardiopulmonary bypass.[18–22] Bypass filtration devices are probably responsible for the declining incidence of central nervous system complications in valvular surgery.[22] In addition, most of the population with rheumatic valvular disease is relatively young and not necessarily prone to stroke. It is therefore unlikely that reports on the neurologic morbidity of open-heart surgery would be helpful in the study of the risk of surgery in general in patients with CVD.

Arterial Reconstructive Surgery

Aortic and aortoiliac reconstructive surgery is theoretically hazardous to perfusion of the brain because of the risk of hypotension during the process of clamping and unclamping of the aorta. Baker and co-workers studied patients undergoing abdominal aortic aneurysmectomy at the Hospital of the University of Pennsylvania between 1962 and 1969.[23] There were 11 patients with known CVD among the group of 390; 6 had TIAs and 5 had a history of stroke. There were no deaths among these 11 patients and no worsening in those with a history of stroke. No mention was made of change in neurologic status in those with TIA. Of 150 patients without a history of CVD operated on between 1966 and 1969, 1 had a new stroke, yielding an incidence of 0.7%. The authors recommended postponement of elective surgery for 6 weeks following a cerebral infarct.

Treiman and associates published two reports on a continuing series of patients with CVD undergoing elective abdominal aortic surgery.[24,25] The first was a retrospective study of 200 patients who had undergone aortoiliac bypass or aneurysmectomy between 1963 and 1972.[24] Of these patients, 31, or 15.5%, had asymptomatic cervical bruits, and 23, or 11.5%, had a history of cerebral infarction or TIA. None of the 54 in the two groups had a postoperative stroke. Of the patients with neither symptoms nor bruit, 2 developed strokes following aneurysmectomy. Of 28 patients who survived emergency aneurysmectomy during the same period, 1 developed a brainstem infarction. In Treiman's second report, the number of patients in the series increased to 511.[25] Of these, 97 patients had carotid bruits, 70 of which were asymptomatic, and 68 had a history of cerebral ischemia with or without bruit. Eighteen of these patients had had prior carotid endarterectomy. The remainder, including 5 patients with angiographically proved carotid stenosis, had abdominal vascular operations without specific precautions. One of the patients with proven bilateral carotid stenoses developed postoperative hemiplegia. Three patients without known CVD developed cerebral infarcts. The overall incidence of postoperative stroke in the population with CVD in this study was 0.8%, a figure that can be contested because a number of the patients underwent endarterectomy prior to aortic surgery. A similar fraction of patients without preoperative evidence of CVD had postoperative strokes.

A retrospective series published by Carney and co-workers considered the carotid bruit a risk factor in aortoiliac reconstructive surgery.[26] This series included some of the patients studied by Baker.[23] Of 248 patients, 35, or 14%, had carotid bruits. Of these 35, 2 had undergone carotid endarterectomy. None of the 33 patients with bruits and no prior endarterectomy suffered postoperative stroke. Fourteen patients had experienced TIAs before surgery, and 1 of this group had undergone prophylactic carotid endarterectomy. Among the 13 remaining, 2, or 15%, had strokes. Of 206 patients without suspected CVD, 2 had strokes. The total stroke incidence in the series was 1.6%. With one exception, other studies of abdominal aortic surgery have reported an incidence of stroke in an unselected population of less than 2%.[26,27] Neurologic complications of extracardiac surgery are listed in Table 34-2.

Carotid Endarterectomy

The morbidity and mortality of carotid endarterectomy have decreased with improved surgical technique and more rational selection of patients.[28] Sundt and colleagues reviewed 331 patients and grouped them according to neurologic and medical risk. Neurologically stable

Table 34-2. Neurologic Complications of Extracardiac Vascular Surgery

Study	Type of Surgery	No. Patients	Type of CVD	Morbidity and Mortality from CVD (%)
Barnes[16]	CABG and peripheral arterial reconstruction	19	>50% Stenosis of carotid	0
Baker[23]	Aortic aneurysmectomy	11	TIA and stroke	0
Treiman[24]	Abdominal aortic	54	Mixed	0
Treiman[25]	Abdominal aortic	97	Mixed	0.8
Carney[26]	Aortoiliac	33	Cervical bruit	0
Carney[26]	Aortoiliac	13	TIA	15
Takaki[33]	Mixed*	12	24% stenosis of carotid	8.3

*Mixed—includes patients with asymptomatic bruits.

patients with no major medical risks had a total morbidity and mortality of 2% following carotid endarterectomy.[29] For patients who had coronary artery disease, severe hypertension, severe obesity, chronic obstructive pulmonary disease, or age over 70 years, the combined risk rose to 7%. The primary cause for increased morbidity in this group was myocardial infarction. This figure probably underestimated risk in seriously ill patients, because Sundt's patients had been screened and accepted as reasonable candidates for elective surgery.

Ennix and associates reported on 1238 patients undergoing carotid endarterectomy, 212 of whom or 17%, had had cardiac symptoms.[30] Of these, 77 underwent endarterectomy without prior CABG, and the mortality in this group was 18.2%. The remaining patients, who had combined carotid–coronary procedures or staged procedures with CABG performed first, had a mortality of 3%. Electrocardiographic changes or a history of myocardial infarction were not as predictive of a poor outcome after carotid surgery as the presence of symptoms. Previously, Rubio and Guinn had found a mortality rate of 16% after carotid endarterectomy in patients

with any history or electrocardiographic evidence of coronary artery disease.[31]

Summary of Risk

Available data regarding patients with CVD undergoing surgery is incomplete and frequently inconclusive or contradictory. Recommendations for management can therefore be only tentative. Unfortunately, management strategies may become established despite inadequate trials, hindering future efforts to acquire more information.

The risk of surgery has not been determined with confidence for any of the three major categories of patients with CVD. Table 34-1 summarizes information from published studies. In CABG, the number of patients reported thus far who have CVD and have not been subjected to prior carotid surgery is too small for any conclusion to be reached. Available figures suggest that the risk of stroke is not high. This is confirmed by the low risk of neurologic complications in the population undergoing CABG, a patient group with known atherosclerotic disease. Studies in patients with abdominal aortic surgery have been more extensive and are therefore more useful. Patients with a history of TIAs form a high-risk group for cerebrovascular complications following this type of surgery. The cervical bruit itself is not a good predictor of neurologic morbidity. Published series do not identify patients with a history of cerebral infarction well enough for conclusions to be drawn about this group.

The role of preoperative noninvasive studies remains controversial.[32] Barnes and co-workers studied 19 patients undergoing CABG and peripheral arterial reconstruction and found no correlation between abnormal tests and neurologic outcome.[16] In contrast, Takaki and associates reported one stroke in 12 patients with abnormal noninvasive tests undergoing different surgical procedures.[33] Their one complication occurred in a patient who had both abnormal noninvasive studies and history of TIA.

The risk of complications following carotid endarterectomy in patients with medical problems is well defined, and Sundt's study shows an increase above normal to 7% in the presence of serious systemic disease.[29] As reported by Ennix and colleagues, the risk of carotid endarterectomy in cardiac patients is even higher, at 18.2%.[30] Rubio and Guinn found a similarly high rate of complications in patients with heart disease.[31]

CAROTID REPAIR BEFORE SURGERY

Most studies dealing with the management of patients with CVD undergoing noncarotid surgery are uncontrolled surveys of patients with coronary artery disease. Bernhard and co-workers studied 31 patients with CVD, 24 of whom had had two TIAs with past stroke and 5 of whom had asymptomatic cervical bruits.[34] All

had carotid and coronary surgery, but the operative sequence was changed as experience was accumulated. Fifteen patients had carotid repair before CABG. Of these patients, 3, or 20%, died of heart disease following endarterectomy, and 2 other patients died following CABG, yielding a total mortality of 33%. Fifteen patients had simultaneous carotid endarterectomy and myocardial revascularization. In this group, there was 1 postoperative stroke but no deaths. Only 1 patient had CABG before carotid surgery. The authors concluded that simultaneous repair was preferable to staged procedures.

A different conclusion was reached by Urschel and colleagues in their nonrandomized series of 32 patients with concomitant carotid and coronary disease.[15] Their patients were subjected to combined or staged surgery, depending on the severity of their disease.[8,25] High-risk cardiac patients, those with preinfarction angina or disease of the left main arteries, had a simultaneous procedure. There were no deaths and only negligible complications among 8 patients. Eight patients had carotid endarterectomy first, and 1 developed a postoperative myocardial infarction. Of 17 patients who had CABG initially, 1 developed a stroke. The authors suggested that combined CABG and carotid surgery be performed in a sequence determined by the system that is more seriously involved.

A study from Stanford is more systematic in its approach to the patient with generalized vascular disease.[35] Of 874 patients referred to that center for coronary surgery, 105, or 12%, had a history of TIAs, stroke, or bruits. Forty-nine had abnormal carotid arteriograms. The candidates for both CABG and carotid surgery were then subdivided according to cardiac status. High-risk patients had simultaneous surgery, whereas patients considered stable underwent staged repair. Of the 29 patients undergoing combined procedures, 4 died and 1 had postoperative RIND. Of the deaths, 2 were due to stroke. Carotid endarterectomy was performed first in 23 cases, with no operative deaths and one instance of transient neurologic deficit. Two patients developed persistent angina following carotid surgery and required emergency CABG. Results were classified according to the site of the extracranial vascular lesion, but the numbers are too small for adequate comparison. The authors concluded that sequential surgery was optimal in patients with stable disease. However, they admitted that their two groups were not comparable, since high-risk patients underwent simultaneous procedures.

Okies and associates reported on 16 patients with arteriographically proven carotid and coronary artery disease who had combined repair procedures.[36] These patients had been referred because of cardiac disease, and the CVD of some was asymptomatic. Of the 16, 2 patients developed neurologic deficits postoperatively, and 1 suffered a cardiac death. The study suggested that the combined surgical approach to carotic–coronary surgery is safe but should be considered primarily for patients with severe disease of both systems.

In another large coronary–carotid series by Hertzer and co-workers, 174 patients with either TIAs or asymptomatic bruits underwent repair of both systems.[37] Between 1969 and 1973, the staged procedures were carried out on 59 patients. After 1973, simultaneous surgery was performed in most of the 115 patients. Of the patients undergoing staged procedures, 86% were asymptomatic. There was a 3% incidence of stroke, and 5% of the patients

had myocardial infarctions while awaiting CABG. Two patients had TIAs. The simultaneous surgery group consisted of 80 patients who were asymptomatic and 35 patients with TIA or stroke. Of these, 10 patients, or 8.7%, had postoperative neurologic deficits appropriate to the site of the vascular lesion. Another 3 patients, or 2.6%, suffered neurologic deficit that was inappropriate to the site of extracranial disease. The incidence of neurologic morbidity was greater among the patients with TIA (12%) than among the patients with asymptomatic lesions (2.5%). The patients in the combined surgery group had more severe heart disease and a higher incidence of contralateral carotid occlusion. The authors recommended a staged approach for patients with stable heart disease or frequent TIAs and simultaneous repair for patients with severe heart disease, including those with left main coronary artery obstruction or unstable angina.

Two studies have explored the use of carotid surgery prior to other noncoronary operations. Crawford, Palamara, and Kasparian reported on 130 patients submitted to carotid endarterectomy and various other vascular and nonvascular procedures excluding CABG.[38] The patient population is too diverse for any firm conclusions to be drawn about the ultimate benefit of surgery, but simultaneous carotid and noncarotid surgery resulted in 1 postoperative stroke among 42 patients (2.4%). Lefrak and Guinn performed prophylactic carotid surgery in 34 patients with asymptomatic carotid bruits requiring another vascular operation.[39] Two patients developed complications following the carotid procedure, one having myocardial infarction and the other suffering a hemispheric stroke. There were no neurologic complications among the 32 patients who had their second operation, although 5 patients died from other thrombotic events.

MANAGEMENT

Stroke

Cerebral blood flow immediately after stroke is unstable, and brain metabolism is generally depressed, often in regions outside the immediately ischemic territory.[40] Large cerebral infarcts may take 6 to 8 weeks to resolve. Elective operations should not be done during this critical recovery phase, and emergency procedures should be attended by careful maintenance of adequate intravascular volume and "normal" or high blood pressure.

Cerebral arteries and arterioles have the unique property of autoregulation, an intrinsic feedback mechanism that ensures stability of blood flow independent of fluctuations of blood pressure. Arteriosclerosis and acute stroke upset autoregulation and may expose the brain to the dangers of blood pressure dependency.[41] High blood pressure may produce increased intracranial pressure, and low pressure may lead to brain ischemia.

Patients who have survived a hypertensive intracerebral hemorrhage need equally careful management. Small dilatations of end-arterioles in the basal ganglia, cerebellum, and brainstem—Charcot–Bouchard aneurysms—are the result of chronic uncontrolled hypertension and tend to rupture into the parenchyma of the brain. Although such hemorrhages are often lethal, the routine use of computerized tomography (CT) has demonstrated that many intraparenchymal hematomas are small slit-like collections of blood that merely stretch rather than destroy brain tissue. Consequently, neurologic deficits in these patients are often mild or reversible. The use of sequential CT scanning is helpful in determination of the time at which complete resolution of the clot has occurred. In the absence of any relevant studies, it is wise to wait for dissolution of the intracerebral hematoma before performing any elective surgery. A minimum of 6 weeks is recommended.

Transient Cerebral Ischemia

Most studies do not distinguish between patients with TIAs indicating ischemia in the anterior circulation and patients whose symptoms suggest compromise of the posterior circulation. Carotid endarterectomy is generally only feasible in disease of the extracranial carotid system, but, frequently, carotid repair is done for symptoms that are either nonspecific or suggest occlusion in the vertebrobasilar system. In any case, among patients with CVD, the subgroup of those with TIAs requires some form of therapeutic intervention; if untreated, a significant proportion will develop permanent neurologic deficit.[42]

The Canadian Cooperative Study Group provided evidence that aspirin in a dose of 1300 mg/day can reduce the frequency of TIAs and the incidence of completed stroke in men.[43] An American study also showed a beneficial effect from aspirin.[44] Nonrandomized trials had previously suggested that anticoagulants such as heparin and dicumarol also diminish the frequency of TIAs in susceptible patients.[45] A recent study found no difference between the degree of reduction in the number of TIAs achieved by antiplatelet agents and that achieved by anticoagulants.[46] However, the efficacy of carotid endarterectomy in reducing TIAs and stroke has not been compared with that of aspirin or anticoagulant treatment in a randomized study.

The method of therapy is often chosen largely on the basis of factors such as estimation of surgical risk, local surgical experience, likelihood of compliance with chronic medication regimens, and physician or patient preference. Even with limited data, in view of the few studies that suggest an increase in surgical morbidity among patients with TIAs, we would argue that such patients should be treated prior to systemic surgery. This is most important if TIAs have occurred within the preceding 12 months, since the incidence of stroke is highest during that period of time.[47]

Although it is possible to keep patients on oral anticoagulants in cases in which local hemostasis can be readily achieved, treatment with dicumarol and derivatives is inappropriate immediately before major surgery. In this case, oral anticoagulant can be stopped and heparin begun preoperatively. Aspirin may be tolerable in the perioperative period; however, it has been shown to increase the number of bleeding complications following CABG when administered within 7 days of surgery.[48] If aspirin is used for prophylaxis in TIAs it should be continued up to the time of surgery and restarted as soon as possible after the procedure.

The literature on the performance of carotid endarterectomy for TIAs prior to other surgery is extensive. However, the conclusions reached by most authors are seriously compromised by the lack of randomized studies. The morbidity of angiography, reported to be approximately 13%, is often neglected.[49] The sequential, or staged, approach in which carotid repair is performed first is the preferred approach for patients with stable systemic disease and TIAs with extracranial vascular disease. It is important to remember that the mortality rate in this group is greater than that among unselected patients undergoing carotid endarterectomy.[29]

Simultaneous carotid–coronary surgery can be performed at medical centers using a two-team approach. When feasible, this method is best for patients who have a high risk of occlusion in either the cerebral or the cardiac circulation. Patients with frequent TIAs, tight bilateral carotid stenoses, or contralateral occlusion with ipsilateral stenosis should be considered high-risk cases. Even with simultaneous procedures, the morbidity and mortality in this group is substantial, having been estimated at 17% in one series.[37]

A substantial number of patients with TIAs suggesting disease in the carotid system do not have angiographically definable extracranial vascular disease.[50] Some of these patients may suffer from emboli from the endocardium or cardiac valves. Other patients have atherosclerotic narrowing or arteries that are inaccessible by an extracranial surgical approach. Anastomosis of the superficial temporal artery to the middle cerebral artery has recently become a feasible alternative for these patients, but indications for this operation have not been clearly determined.[51] A collaborative study is currently in progress to test the efficacy of this procedure in preventing recurrent stroke.[52] We would expect the operative morbidity among patients with medical problems to be greater than that associated with the comparatively simple endarterectomy procedures. We would therefore recommend that patients in this category be treated with aspirin.

Patients with vertebrobasilar ischemic episodes appear to have a lower stroke rate than patients with carotid ischemic episodes.[53] This may be due to the inclusion of patients with light-headedness and other nonspecific symptoms in the study populations. The primary mode of therapy for these patients is administration of antiplatelet drugs. The value of surgical repair of the vertebral arteries, including the removal of compressing osteophytic spurs, has not been tested in a controlled study. The syndrome of subclavian steal provides the single exception in which surgical treatment is accepted, although the choice of specific procedures is still debated.[54,55] The preoperative patient with ischemia in the posterior circulation should be treated with aspirin throughout the perioperative period. Any necessary maneuvering of the neck should be done with extreme caution, and hemodynamic stability should be maintained.

Asymptomatic Cervical Bruits

Bruits are often misleading indicators of arterial disease.[56] Heyman and co-workers recently found a poor correlation between the location of an asymptomatic bruit and the site of eventual brain infarction and suggested that a bruit is no more than a general index of atherosclerotic disease.[8] The influence of cervical bruits on the neurologic morbidity of systemic surgical procedures appears to be negligible. The aforementioned relevant studies are those of Treiman and colleagues and Carney and associates, both of which deal with abdominal aortic surgery.[24-26] In these small groups, there was no correlation between the presence of a bruit and postoperative stroke. The reports by Barnes and co-workers and Takaki and associates added that oculoplethysmography and phonoangiography are equally poor pre-

dictors of neurologic complications of surgery.[16,33] Unfortunately, the numbers of asymptomatic patients with cervical bruits or positive noninvasive tests in these four studies are small, and it is possible that significant associations between bruits or abnormal noninvasive tests and neurologic complications were missed because of an inadequate sample size. Nevertheless, we must conclude that investigation and surgical treatment of patients with asymptomatic cervical bruits will not alter central nervous system morbidity following systemic surgery.

SUMMARY

1. **Most studies report a low risk of neurologic complications following both cardiac and extracardiac surgery.**
2. **Elective surgery should be postponed for a minimum of 6 weeks following a completed stroke.**
3. **Elective surgery should be postponed following intracerebral hemorrhage until the hematoma has resolved.**
4. **The risk of carotid endarterectomy in patients with serious cardiac disease is high.**
5. **Patients who have had TIAs, especially within the last 12 months, should be evaluated prior to surgery. Patients with posterior TIAs should be treated with aspirin. Patients with inoperable anterior TIAs should be treated with aspirin.**
6. **Patients with frequent TIAs or tight bilateral stenoses have a high risk of stroke and should undergo endarterectomy before or with systemic surgery. If endarterectomy is not done, these patients should receive aspirin. If atrial fibrillation is present or aspi-**

rin fails, warfarin (Coumadin) should be used.

7. An asymptomatic cervical bruit probably does not increase the neurologic morbidity of systemic surgery; therefore, no preoperative treatment is required.

REFERENCES

1. Gresham GE, Fitzpatrick TE, Wolf PA et al: Residual disability in survivors of stroke—The Framingham Study. N Engl J Med 293:954, 1975

2. Blaisdell WF, Clauss RH, Galbraith JG et al: Joint Study of Extracranial Arterial Occlusion. IV. JAMA 209:1889, 1969

3. Denny–Brown D: Treatment of recurrent cerebrovascular symptoms and the question of vasospasm. Med Clin North Am 35:1457, 1951

4. Genton E, Barnett HJM, Fields WS: Cerebral ischemia: The role of thrombosis and of antithrombotic therapy. Stroke 8:150, 1977

5. Report of the National Institute of Neurological and Communicative Disorders and Stroke. Ad hoc Committee on Cerebrovascular Disease: A classification and outline of cerebrovascular diseases. II. Stroke 6:565, 1975

6. Fields WS: The asymptomatic carotid bruit—Operate or not? Stroke 9:269,1978

7. Ackerman RH: A perspective on non-invasive diagnosis of carotid disease. Neurology 29:615, 1979

8. Heyman A, Wilkinson WE, Heyden S et al: Risk of stroke in asymptomatic persons with cervical arterial bruits. N Engl J Med 302:838, 1980

9. Braunwald E: Coronary artery surgery at the crossroads. N Engl J Med 297:661, 1977

10. Reul GJ, Morris GC, Howell JF et al: Current concepts in coronary artery surgery—A critical analysis of 1,287 patients. Ann Thorac Surg 14:243, 1972

11. Ashor GW, Meyer BW, Lindesmith GG et al: Coronary artery disease surgery in 100 patients 65 years of age and older. Arch Surg 107:30, 1973

12. Breuer AL, Hanson MR, Furlan AJ et al: Central nervous system complications of myocardial revascularization. A prospective analysis of 400 patients (abstr). Stroke 11:136, 1980

13. Lee MC, Geiger J, Nicoloff D et al: Cerebrovascular complications associated with coronary artery bypass procedure (abstr). Stroke 10:107, 1979

14. Gonzalez–Scarano F, Hurtig HI: Neurologic complications of coronary artery bypass grafting: A case-control study. Neurology (in press)

15. Urschel HC, Razzuk MA, Gardner MA: Management of concomitant occlusive disease of the carotid and coronary arteries. J Thorac Cardiovasc Surg 72:829, 1976

16. Barnes RW, Marszalek PB, Rittgers SE: Asymptomatic carotid disease in preoperative patients (abstr). Stroke 11:136, 1980

17. Gilman S: Cerebral disorders after open heart operations. N Engl J Med 272:489, 1965

18. Tufo HM, Osterfeld AM, Shekeuf R: Central nervous system dysfunction following open heart surgery. JAMA 212:1333, 1970

19. Sotanemi K: Brain damage and neurological outcome after open heart surgery. J Neurol Neurosurg Psychiatry 43:127, 1980

20. Brierly JB: Neuropathological findings in patients dying after open heart surgery. Thorax 18:291, 1963

21. Bass RM, Longmore DB: Cerebral damage during open heart surgery. Nature 222:30, 1969

22. Branthwaite MA: Prevention of neurological damage during open heart surgery. Thorax 30:258, 1975

23. Baker AG, Roberts B, Berkowitz HD et al: Risk of excision of abdominal aortic aneurysms. Surgery 68:1129, 1970

24. Treiman RL, Foran RF, Shore EH et al: Carotid bruit. Significance in patients undergoing an abdominal aortic operation. Arch Surg 106:803, 1973

25. Treiman RL, Foran RF, Cohen JL et al: Ca-

rotid bruit: A follow-up report on its significance in patients undergoing an abdominal aortic operation. Arch. Surg. 114:1138, 1979

26. Carney WI, Stewart WB, DePinto DJ et al: Carotid bruit as a risk factor in aortoiliac reconstruction. Surgery 81:567, 1977

27. Gomes MMR, Bernatz PE: Aorto-iliac occlusive disease. Arch Surg 101:161, 1970

28. Thompson JE, Talkington CM: Carotid endarterectomy. Ann Surg 32:5, 1975

29. Sundt TM, Sandok BA, Whisnant JP: Carotid endarterectomy complications and preoperative assessment of risk. Mayo Clin Proc 50:301, 1975

30. Ennix CL, Lawrie GM, Morris GC et al: Improved results of carotid endarterectomy in patients with symptomatic coronary disease. An analysis of 1,546 consecutive carotid operations. Stroke 10:122, 1979

31. Rubio PA, Guinn GA: Myocardial infarction following carotid endarterectomy. Cardiovascular diseases. Bull Texas Heart Inst 3:404, 1973

32. Kartchner MM, McRae LP: Non-invasive assessment of the progression of extra-cranial carotid occlusive disease. In Diethrich EB (ed): Non-invasive Cardiovascular Diagnosis, p 19. Baltimore, University Park Press, 1978

33. Takaki HS, McNawan MF, Yao JST et al: Influence of non-invasive screening on care of patients with carotid stenosis. In Diethrich EB (ed): Non-invasive Cardiovascular Diagnosis, p 3. Baltimore, University Park Press, 1978

34. Bernhard VM, Johnson WD, Peterson JJ: Carotid artery stenosis association with surgery for coronary artery disease. Arch Surg 105:837, 1972

35. Mehigan JT, Buch WS, Pipkin RD et al: A planned approach to coexistent cerebrovascular disease in coronary artery bypass candidates. Arch Surg 112:1403, 1977

36. Okies JE, MacManus Q, Starr A: Myocardial revascularization and carotid endarterectomy: A combined approach. Ann Thorac Surg 26:560, 1977

37. Hertzer NR, Loop FD, Taylor PC et al: Staged and combined surgical approach to simultaneous carotid and coronary vascular disease. Surgery 84:803, 1978

38. Crawford ED, Palamara AE, Kasparian AS: Carotid and non-coronary operations: Simultaneous, staged and delayed. Surgery 87:1, 1980

39. Lefrak EA, Guinn GE: Prophylactic carotid artery surgery in patients requiring a second operation. South Med J 67:185, 1974

40. Slater R, Reivich M, Goldberg H, et al: Diaschisis with cerebral infarctions. Stroke 8:684, 1977

41. Scheinberg P, Meyer JS, Reivich M et al: Cerebral circulation and metabolism in stroke. Stroke 7:212, 1976

42. Goldner JC, Whisnant JP, Taylor WF: Long-term prognosis of TIA. Stroke 2:160, 1971

43. Barnett HJM: Canadian Cooperative Study Group. A randomized trial of aspirin and sulfinpyrazone in threatened stroke. N Engl J Med 299:53, 1978

44. Fields WS, Lemak NA, Frankowski RF et al: Controlled trial of aspirin in cerebral ischemia. Stroke 8:301, 1977

45. Millikan CH, McDowell FH: Treatment of transient ischemic attacks. Stroke 9:299, 1978

46. Olson NE, Brechter C, Backlund H et al: Anticoagulant vs. anti-platelet therapy as prophylactic against cerebral infarction in transient ischemic attacks. Stroke 11:4, 1980

47. Cartlidge NE, Whisnant JP, Elveback LR: Carotid and vertebral–basilar transient cerebral ischemic attacks. A community study, Rochester, Minnesota. Mayo Clin Proc 52:117, 1977

48. Torosian M, Michaelson EL, Morganroth J et al: Aspirin and coumadin-related bleeding after coronary-artery bypass graft surgery. Ann Intern Med 89:325, 1978

49. Toole JF, Yvson CP, Janewan R et al: Transient ischemic attacks: A prospective study of 225 patients. Neurology 28:746, 1978

50. Marshall J, Wilkinson IMS: The prognosis of carotid transient ischemic attacks in patients with normal angiograms. Brain 94:395, 1971

51. Sundt TM, Siekert RG, Piepgras DG et al: Bypass surgery for vascular disease of the carotid system. Mayo Clin Proc 51:677, 1976

52. Reinmuth OM: Intracranial bypass surgery for cerebral disease and the responsibility of the practicing physician. Stroke 10:344, 1979

53. Marshall J: The natural history of transient ischemic cerebrovascular attacks. Q J Med 33:309, 1964

54. Reivich M, Holling HE, Roberts B et al: Reversal of blood flow through the vertebral artery and its effects on cerebral circulation. N Engl J Med 265:878, 1961

55. Fields WS, Lemak NA: Joint study of extracranial occlusion. VII. Subclavian steal: A review of 168 cases. JAMA 22:1139, 1972

56. Zeigler DK, Zileli T, Dick A et al: Correlation of bruits over the carotid artery with angiographically demonstrated lesions. Neurology 221:860, 1971

35

Postoperative Delirium

JAMES L. STINNETT
STEVEN A. SILBER

The medical consultant is often asked to evaluate patients who manifest changes in affect, behavior, and thinking after surgery. The physiologic, behavioral, and autonomic changes that accompany delirium complicate the postoperative course and may increase morbidity significantly. In order to establish the correct etiology and institute appropriate therapy, it is necessary to distinguish between functional and organic disturbances. Delirium may well be the first manifestation of a systemic disorder unmasked by the stress of surgery. This chapter will focus on the recognition, causes, and treatment of postoperative delirium.

INCIDENCE AND DEFINITION

The incidence of postoperative delirium varies with the type of surgery performed and the presence of various risk factors. In a group of 57,600 surgical patients, Knox noted the incidence of severe postoperative mental changes to be 1 in 1,600.[1] Of 36 cases of severe psychiatric disturbance, 12% to 33% were classified as "confusional states." Significant mental status changes, including delirium, have been observed in patients following cardiac, ophthalmologic, orthopedic, abdominal, and gynecologic surgery.

Specific operative procedures are associated with an especially high incidence of postoperative delirium. Whereas the incidence of delirium among general surgical patients is less than 0.19%, the rate in early postcardiotomy patients was 38% to 59%.[2] This decreased to 24% as operative techniques improved.[3] Blachy and Starr coined the term "postcardiotomy delirium" to describe mental changes in these patients.[2] Patients undergoing aortic valve or multiple valve replacement have a higher incidence of delirium than patients undergoing mitral valve replacement.[3] Valvular surgery of any type, however, is more likely to result in postoperative psychosis than coronary artery bypass procedures.[4]

The recent Diagnostic and Statistical Manual of Mental Disorders (DSM-III) of the American Psychiatric Association lists five specific criteria that are necessary for the diagnosis of delirium.[5] These criteria are listed below:[1]

1. Clouding of consciousness (reduced clarity of awareness of the environment)
2. At least two of the following:

a. Perceptual disturbance (misinterpretations, illusions, or hallucinations)
b. Speech that is at times incoherent
c. Disturbance of the sleep–wakefulness cycle with insomnia or daytime drowsiness
d. Increased or decreased psychomotor activity
3. Disorientation and memory impairment (if testable)
4. Clinical features that develop over a short period of time (usually hours or days) and tend to fluctuate over the course of the day
5. Evidence from the history, physical examination, or laboratory tests of a specific organic factor judged to be etiologically related to the disturbance

The DSM-III criteria comprise a rather narrow definition of delirium in comparison with others that include psychologic rather than purely organic factors in establishing the diagnosis of delirium. We therefore distinguish delirium clinically from functional or psychogenic psychosis by the presence in delirium of (1) deficits in high cortical functioning, such as decreased memory, disorders of consciousness, and disorientation, and (2) alterations in normal metabolic and physiologic processes that, if corrected, result in return to baseline mental status.

The central feature of delirium is a clouded state of consciousness or change in level of awareness. Clinically, delirium is characterized by changes in the ability to shift, focus, and sustain attention, and difficulty in screening out irrelevant and distracting stimuli. One can test distractibility and inability to focus on cognitive tasks by asking the patient to pick out a certain letter in a group of randomly presented letters, subtract serial sevens, or repeat a series of digits forward and backward.

The most common variant of psychomotor abnormality in delirium is the type characterized by aroused, agitated, or poorly organized, non-goal-directed behavior. Occasionally, patients demonstrate purposeless stereotyped movement such as repetitive picking at bedclothes. In some cases, agitation progresses to destructive behavior such as jumping out of bed and pulling out intravenous lines. Delirium tremens following abstinence from alcohol is the prototype of hyperactive delirium.

Hypoactive delirium, characterized by stupor and apathy, is referred to as "quiet delirium." This state is often overlooked because the patient volunteers little spontaneous speech and rarely manifests overtly abnormal behavior. On a busy surgical ward or intensive care unit, the quiet, "good" patient is assumed to have normal cerebral function; however, one need only ask a few questions to realize that the patient is actually delirious.[6,7]

Altered perceptions in delirium may take the form of illusions or hallucinations. A shadow on the wall, for example, may be interpreted as an attacking animal (illusion), or the patient may "see" threatening people in his room when in fact no one is present (hallucination). The delusional conviction of the reality of the hallucination may lead to an emotional (e.g., fear) and a behavioral (e.g., flight) response consistent with the altered perception. Hallucinations are usually visual but may also be auditory, tactile, gustatory, olfactory, or proprioceptive. The clinician should specifically ask whether the patient is experiencing any unusual perceptions such as hearing voices or seeing things. Sometimes a patient will deny these experiences because he is frightened or confused by them. However, his behavior may indicate that he is hallucinating even if he verbally denies it. For example, his eyes may dart around the room or he may turn his head from side to side in response to perceived voices.

The delirious patient may show disorganized and tangential thinking and difficulty in grasping relationships to the environment. He may be disoriented and have loss of both short- and long-term memory. If the patient's concentration and attention are seriously impaired, testing of orientation or memory may be impossible. If he can understand and respond, the patient may be disoriented to time, place, or purpose. Short-term memory loss is common and can be tested by asking the patient independently verifiable questions such as what he had for breakfast that morning or how long he has been in the hospital. Delirious patients occasionally manifest a reversal of the sleep–wakefulness cycle with nighttime insomnia and daytime drowsiness.

One of the cardinal manifestations of delirium is its development over a short period of time and its fluctuation in severity. Rapid changes in mental status may cause the patient to appear lucid with minimal abnormalities at one point during the day and disoriented several hours later. If the consultant arrives during a lucid interval, he may conclude that the referring physician has over-reacted or that the process that caused the initial mental status change has been corrected. Since the usual course of a delirium is one of fluctuation from hour to hour and from day to day, the consultant should attempt to see the patient at various times during the day.

One well-organized clinical manifestation of the fluctuating nature of delirium is the "sundowning syndrome." In the evening, patients who have been lucid during the day suddenly become confused and agitated because of sensory deprivation. This same reaction can be precipitated by drugs, particularly central nervous system (CNS) depressants that alter sensory input or interfere with cognitive integration.

BIOLOGIC CAUSES

Postoperative delirium results from the interaction of various biologic, psychologic, and socioenvironmental factors. It is rarely caused by one factor alone and often becomes manifest when a number of these factors operate together to reach a threshold level.

The differential diagnosis of organic postoperative delirium includes several major categories of etiologic factors. Although any of these factors can alter mental status in any setting, some occur more commonly after surgery as an occult but compensated pathophysiologic process is exacerbated by the stress of the operation. The physician should approach the delirious postoperative patient as he would any other patient with acute alterations in mental status, with special attention to factors specific to the preoperative setting and intraoperative events.

Preoperative Factors

Any pathophysiologic process that directly or indirectly affects brain function preoperatively can predispose a patient to postoperative delirium. Age alone is a critical factor. The incidence of postoperative delirium increases markedly in patients over the age of 45.[2,3,8] Organic brain syndrome is the most common antecedent medical condition in patients who manifest postoperative changes in mental status. The etiologies of organic brain syndrome include (1) presenile dementia (Alzheimer's or Pick's disease); (2) senile dementia (diffuse cerebrovascular disease, strokes, normal pressure hydrocephalus); (3) space-occupying lesions (metastatic and primary brain tumors, aneurysms, arteriovenous malformations, subdural hematomas); (4) infections (previous meningitis, brain abscess, tertiary syphilis, "slow virus"); and (5) miscellaneous disorders (CNS vasculitis, chronic alcohol abuse, head trauma, sarcoidosis). Many patients with organic brain disease who manifest only minimal impairment in cognitive functions preoperatively decompensate and become delirious after surgery.

Many other chronic diseases predispose the patient to the development of postoperative mental status changes. If the stability of patients with chronic heart or pulmonary disease is upset by surgery, profound secondary changes in neurologic function may result.

Uremic patients demonstrate altered mental status probably because of the accumulation of toxic metabolites and accelerated cerebrovascular disease. Dementia associated with chronic dialysis has also been described. In patients with acute or chronic renal disease, problems with blood pressure, acid–base equilibrium, volume status, and osmolality contribute to disordered brain physiology. Altered mental status in patients with portal-systemic encephalopathy is caused by the accumulation of metabolites that function as false neurotransmitters. Florid hepatic encephalopathy is obvious, but its more subtle presentation may be missed until the patient deteriorates after surgery. Unexpected postoperative mental status changes may suggest endocrine abnormalities, including hypo- and hyperthyroidism, hyperparathyroidism, Cushing's disease, and adrenal insufficiency. These may not have been considered during the routine preoperative evaluation.

Hematologic diseases affecting the CNS, including profound anemia, leukemia, thrombocytosis, and the hyperviscosity syndrome seen in plasma cell dyscrasias, rarely escape detection before surgery. Vitamin B_{12} deficiency, however, which can cause neurologic sequelae without anemia, must be considered. In the chronic alcoholic or malnourished patient suffering from thiamine deficiency, the intravenous infusion of glucose during surgery may precipitate or worsen Wernicke–Korsakoff psychosis. Patients with chronic psychiatric disorders are likely to experience postoperative alterations in mental status. A prior history of depression or a previous episode of postoperative delirium increases the likelihood of similar changes recurring after surgery.[8] Postoperative delirium is particularly common in patients with antecedent chronic alcohol or drug abuse.

Intraoperative Factors

Several intraoperative factors play a role in the development of postoperative delirium. Unexpected hypotension or hypoxemia can cause decreased cerebral anoxia, which may lead to postoperative changes in mental status. Intraoperative hemodynamic and oxygenation difficulties may be transient and go unheeded by the surgeon or anesthesiologist. When the etiology of postoperative mental changes is unclear, a thorough review of the surgical record in consultation with the anesthesiologist may be rewarding.

Certain drugs administered in the perioperative period can lead to mental status changes. In patients with underlying cardiac, renal, or hepatic disease, the metabolism and excretion of sedatives, narcotics, and barbiturates may be impaired, leading to high serum levels and prolonged effects in the postoperative period. These drugs have all been associated with dose-dependent paradoxic reactions, especially in elderly patients with intrinsic brain disease.

As noted above, the type of procedure carried out may alert the physician to the possible development of delirium. Postcardiotomy delirium is one case that has been extensively studied. Obvious factors, such as the overall length of the procedure and the degree of hypothermia, have been ruled out as predisposing factors.[4,9] The effect of the length of time of cardiopulmonary bypass has been debated, and a positive correlation with the development of postcardiotomy delirium has been noted in some studies but not in others.[3,4,8,10,11] Children under the age of 14 rarely develop postcardiotomy delirium, whereas older patients and men have an increased risk of doing so, leading to the hypothesis that occult cerebrovascular disease with intraoperative cerebral ischemia contributes to the development of the syndrome.[3,9,11] The severity of preoperative illness and the presence of antecedent organic brain disease or chronic psychiatric illness are contributing factors.[3,12]

Tufo and co-workers performed autopsies on patients who had undergone cardiac surgery and had developed inappropriate behavior or abnormal neurologic changes postoperatively.[10] Definite lesions in the CNS were found in 90%, the most common being anoxic changes in the hippocampus, diffuse foci of infarction in gray matter, and areas of perivascular tissue damage in white matter. Tufo concluded that the presence of neurologic

dysfunction strongly correlated with age and the degree and duration of intraoperative hypotension while the patient was on bypass. Inadequate cerebral perfusion during bypass may also result from microemboli that form during the passage of blood through oxygenators. In animal studies, this "microembolic encephalopathy" has been shown to be avoided by blood filtration.[13] Emboli generated during intracardiac manipulations in valvular heart surgery may explain the increased incidence of postoperative psychosis in these patients when compared to that of patients undergoing coronary artery bypass procedures.

Other specific surgical procedures have been linked to the development of postoperative psychiatric syndromes. "Black patch delirium" following ophthalmologic surgery may be due to sensory deprivation in elderly patients with underlying organic brain syndrome and in some cases to toxicity from anticholinergic agents.[14,15] Particularly mutilating surgery, such as that involving extensive head and neck dissection, or surgery perceived as altering sexual function, such as hysterectomy, mastectomy, or orchiectomy, is associated with an increased incidence of postoperative depression.[16,17]

Postoperative Factors

Several important factors in the development of delirium after surgery require special attention. An assessment of hemodynamic and respiratory function is mandatory. Myocardial depression and inappropriate volume replacement during surgery may lead to congestive heart failure and inadequate cerebral perfusion. Even without peripheral manifestations, severe hypoxemia or hypercarbia may develop because of central hypoventilation, upper airway obstruction, atelectasis, aspiration, pulmonary embolism, or splinting. A detailed neurologic exam must be performed to exclude the possibility of a perioperative cerebrovascular accident. The absence of focal neurologic deficits combined with abnormal mental status necessitates further investigation into possible organic causes of brain dysfunction.

Altered metabolism of drugs that affect the CNS may result in prolonged effects after surgery. Therefore, a careful review of the medication record is important. Drug withdrawal syndromes with dramatic mental status changes are seen in patients who chronically ingest alcohol, barbiturates, benzodiazapines, narcotics, or hypnotics. Often, the physician is unaware of the extent of preoperative drug use either because the patient withholds information or because an adequate drug and alcohol history is not obtained in an emergency setting. When a drug withdrawal syndrome is suspected, it is imperative that the patient's drug history be reviewed with family or friends. Many drugs used in the perioperative period cause or exacerbate delirium. Lidocaine, cimetidine, xanthine derivatives, atropine, alpha-methyldopa, propranolol, L-dopa, steroids, and digoxin have all been associated with toxic delirium. Obtaining serum drug level is often useful, but some drugs such as digoxin and propranolol may cause toxicity even at therapeutic levels. The patient may infrequently obtain illicit drugs from outside the hospital, and, in such cases, serum and urine screens may be useful.

Many metabolic abnormalities arising in the postoperative period alter CNS function. Hyponatremia may be due to edematous states, adrenal insufficiency unmasked by the stress of surgery, or the injudicious use of hypotonic fluids when the patient's level of antidiuretic hormone (ADH) is high. The syndrome of inappropriate ADH secretion (SIADH) has been described in an increasing number of clinical settings. After surgery, pain alone stimulates the secretion of antidiuretic hormone (ADH) from the hypothalamus. Drugs shown to induce SIADH include morphine, chlorpropamide, vincristine, carbamazepine, and amitriptyline. The type and severity of neurology dysfunction vary with both the degree of hyponatremia and the rapidity with which it develops. Lethargy, confusion, and coma occur with gradually progressive hyponatremia, whereas agitation, irritability, and seizures accompany more rapid changes. Symptoms should not be ascribed to hyponatremia unless the serum sodium concentration is below 125 mEq/liter.

Hyperosmolar states also lead to alterations in brain metabolism. Hypernatremia can result from excessive free water losses and salt administration in patients who do not have access to water. This is seen in patients receiving prolonged tube feeding or intravenous hyperalimentation who cannot drink or have an impaired thirst mechanism. Hyperosmolar nonketotic coma may occur in volume-depleted patients with maturity-onset diabetes in the setting of a physiologic stress such as surgery. The CNS signs of hyperosmolar states are similar to the signs of hyponatremia, ranging from agitation with confusion and a clouded sensorium to seizure and coma.

Hypoglycemia, with its attendant alterations in mental status, may be a problem for the insulin-requiring diabetic in the perioperative period, when exogenous insulin requirements vary markedly. Hypoglycemia is otherwise unlikely to occur except in patients with advanced renal or hepatic failure or in those patients with large retroperitoneal tumors in whom it is unmasked by decreased oral intake after surgery.

Other miscellaneous metabolic abnormalities must also be considered. Hypercalcemia for any reason, including hyperparathyroidism, multiple myeloma, occult neoplasm, or immobilization, may worsen with mild volume depletion in the perioperative period and lead to a variety of psychiatric syndromes. Severe hypophosphatemia with serum phosphate concentrations of less than 1 mg/dl in malnourished or debilitated patients causes weakness, lethargy, confusion, and sometimes even coma. Finally, acid–base disturbances from a variety of causes may contribute to changes in mental status after surgery.

Delirium may be the first sign of impending sepsis. Fever and leukocytosis may be absent in the elderly, debilitated, or catabolic surgical patient. Postoperative CNS infections are uncommon except following specific neurosurgical or head and neck procedures; however, an altered mental status and other signs of systemic infection without an identifiable source often necessitates a lumbar puncture.

PSYCHOLOGIC AND ENVIRONMENTAL CAUSES

There is controversy concerning the role of anxiety in the pathogenesis of postoperative psychologic changes. One point of view contends that anxiety generated by the realistic appraisal of what is involved in surgery is associated with good psychologic adaptation in the postoperative period. Alternatively, when denial is the dominant mechanism for coping, anxiety levels are low and the postoperative course is smooth.[8,11]

The patient's perception of the real and symbolic meanings of the organ or part of the body involved in surgery is important to consider. Patients undergoing heart surgery often speak of the anxiety generated by surgery on an organ considered to be the basis for life. Patients having brain surgery are anxious about injury to the organ that constitutes the biologic substrate of all that is special and unique to them. A woman undergoing a mastectomy or hysterectomy may feel that surgery will directly affect her body image and identity as a woman. A man undergoing orchiectomy or other genital–urinary procedure may feel that his manhood will be irrevocably altered. A person receiving an organ transplant may feel that his body has been invaded. Some patients with ostomies believe that their bodies have been changed in a way that may seriously affect their self-esteem and sense of body integrity. Each of these reactions is highly individual, and there is a wide spectrum of responses to any one operation.

The ability of the patient to adjust to the sick role is another factor that contributes to the development of postoperative psychiatric illness. Relinquishing autonomy and becoming dependent on others for help with basic biologic functions such as eating, bathing, and toilet needs is extremely stressful for some persons. Postoperative pain contributes to the overall psychologic burden of the patient. Inadequate amounts of analgesics are often prescribed.[18] By increasing anxiety and sapping necessary psychologic reserves, chronic unrelieved pain in the immediate postoperative period may lead to delirium.

Sleep deprivation may be the most important psychologic factor in the genesis of postoperative delirium. Although relieved that they have survived the operation, many patients experience a sense of heightened vigilance and anxiety and are afraid to fall asleep. The constant high noise and activity levels and lack of light–dark cycles in intensive care units prevent patients from sleeping adequately. Studies of normal volunteers have shown that definite psychologic changes begin to occur after 2 to 3 days of total sleep deprivation.[19] In many types of postoperative delirium, particularly postcardiotomy delirium, there is an initial lucid interval in the immediate postoperative period that lasts 2 to 3 days. During this period, there is progressive sleep deprivation, with the subsequent development of delirium. The similarity of the clinical course in postoperative patients and normal persons who are sleep-deprived lends support to the notion that sleep deprivation is an important determinant of postoperative delirium.[3,20,21]

The patient's environment is another important factor in the development of postoperative delirium. Most recovery rooms and intensive care units are frightening places in which the sensory experience is markedly different from normal. The sensory experience is affected by monotony, deprivation, and bombardment of stimuli. Monitors and ventilators emit a constant, monotonous sound. Usual time-orienting cues are absent, and lights are on around the clock. For normal psychologic functioning, it is necessary to ensure modulated sensory input and avoid extremes of sensory deprivation and overload. Patients who exhibit signs of postoperative delirium often improve when they are transferred out of the intensive care unit to a regular hospital floor.

MANAGEMENT

Early recognition and treatment of the patient with postoperative delirium is aimed at controlling behavior that might significantly interfere with postoperative care and increase morbidity and mortality and at uncovering and correcting underlying pathophysiologic processes that are detrimental to the patient's overall condition. Preventive steps before surgery significantly decrease the incidence of postoperative delirium. Lazarus and Hagens showed that preoperative counseling by nurses and psychiatrists significantly decreases postoperative psychiatric complications.[22] Most surgical centers involved in open-heart surgery provide preoperative counseling to orient patients to the environment of the recovery room and intensive care unit as well as to the monitoring life-support systems and therapeutic procedures that will be used.

Once signs of delirium appear, the standard treatment consists of neurologic drugs such as chlorpromazine or haloperidol. Haloperidol, a butyrophenone, is the drug of choice because, unlike chlorpromazine, it has little effect on blood pressure. The drug is given in doses of 1 mg to 5 mg intramuscularly, and the frequency of administration is titrated by the patient's response. For delirium, haloperidol should not be prescribed on a straight-order basis, since individual responses are difficult to predict. The patient should be re-evaluated every 30 min and the medication repeated with appropriate dosage adjustments until adequate behavioral control has been obtained. The target symptoms of most concern are psychomotor agitation, hallucinations, and confused thinking. The therapeutic endpoint should be adequately controlled behavior conducive to good postoperative care. The medication should be continued until hallucinations have ceased and thought processes are normal. Care should be taken to avoid neuroleptic-induced stupor. In a series of postcardiotomy patients in a surgical intensive care unit, Cassem and Sos administered intravenous doses of haloperidol ranging from 5 mg to 185 mg over a 24-hr period.[23] The drug had no significant effect on blood pressure, heart rate, or ventilation. Neurologic side-effects such as extrapyramidal signs were infrequent and mild. Dudley and associates used intravenous haloperidol in doses of up to 20 mg and achieved resolution of severe psychomotor agitation without significant cardiovascular or CNS toxic effects.[24] Intravenous haloperidol acts rapidly in acute delirium, usually within 2 min to 5 min, and avoids the pain and inconvenience of repeated intramuscular injections.

Extrapyramidal signs, including acute dystonic reactions, the parkinsonism–bradykinesia syndrome and akathisia are documented side-effects of haloperidol. Acute dystonia, also known as oculogyric crisis, is more frequently seen in men than in women and occurs more often than parkinsonism. Usually limited to muscle spasm of the face, tongue, jaw, or neck, it occasionally affects the limbs and causes painful flexion. Dystonic reactions are rapidly reversed by parenteral administration of an anticholinergic drug such as benztropine in a dose of 1 mg to 3 mg. The parkinsonism–bradykinesia syndrome, which consists of decreased spontaneous movement, cog-wheel rigidity, and increased salivation with drooling, can also be reversed by anticholinergic agents.

Akathisia is one of the most common and troubling side-effects of the neuroleptic drugs. It is difficult to document because its manifestations consist of a primarily subjective sense of anxiety, restlessness, tension, and an irresistible urge to move. The discomfort of these sensations is heightened in patients who must remain immobile postoperatively. This side-effect also responds to anticholinergic drugs, although less readily than acute dystonic reactions and parkinsonism.

Drug withdrawal states in the postoperative period may be life-threatening. If possible, the responsible drug should be identified and restarted. This is especially true for barbiturate withdrawal, which, after 48 hr to 96 hr, leads to agitation, delirium, weakness, hypotension, and seizures. For alcohol or other drug withdrawal syndromes, benzodiazepenes such as diazepam, chlordiazapoxide, or oxazepam are the drugs of choice. Phenothiazines should be avoided because they lower the seizure threshold. When given intramuscularly, benzodiazepenes are poorly absorbed and produce unpredictable plasma levels.[25] These drugs should therefore be given orally or intravenously. In patients with liver disease, who cannot metabolize drugs normally, oxazepam is best because it has no pharmacologically active metabolites and a relatively short half-life. Unlike other benzodiazepene drugs such as diazepam or chlordiazepoxide, it is directly conjugated with glucuronide. This step is more readily carried out by an impaired liver than demethylation, deamination, and hydroxylation, which are necessary for the metabolism of longer-acting benzodiazepenes.[26]

Attempts should be made to enable postoperative patients to get uninterrupted sleep. Nursing procedures at night should be deferred if they are not critical for patient care. If the patient is in an intensive care unit, curtains should be drawn around his bed and lights dimmed at night to decrease sensory stimulation.

Varying and controlling sensory input is important. Sometimes even the simplest of interventions, such as allowing the patient to have a radio or television, can have a salutary therapeutic effect. Placing a calendar within the patient's visual field and marking off the days helps him to orient himself in time. Familiar objects such as pictures of family and friends are comforting. Nursing personnel and family should be encouraged to keep the patient oriented frequently to time and place. Seeing the same nurses regularly helps the patient to develop a sense of trust and familiarity with the staff.

Nurses and physicians should reassure the patient that his confusing experience is temporary and does not mean that he is mentally ill. The staff should not assume that the delirious patient has no insight or awareness. After recovery from delirium, some patients reveal that they were aware of their confusion and were extremely frightened. If the experience is not acknowledged and explained by the staff, apprehension may increase and delirium worsen.

SUMMARY

1. **Delirium is a syndrome of deficits in high cortical function characterized by an acute onset and a fluctuating course. The major clinical features of delirium are alterations in consciousness, perception, attention, memory, orientation, and psychomotor behavior.**

2. **Advancing age, underlying intrinsic neurologic deficits, many acute or chronic medical illnesses, and chronic psychiatric syndromes are predictors of the possible development of postoperative delirium. The stress of surgery in patients with these conditions may be enough to produce delirium.**

3. **Hypoxemia, hypercarbia, hypotension, electrolyte abnormalities, sepsis, and acute cerebrovascular accident must be excluded in patients with postoperative delirium.**

4. **Drug withdrawal must always be considered as a cause of postoperative delirium.**

5. **Haloperidol in appropriate dose is the drug of choice for the treatment of delirium.**

REFERENCES

1. Knox SJ: Severe psychiatric disturbances in the postoperative period—A five-year survey of Belfast Hospital. J Ment Sci 107:1078, 1961
2. Blachy PH, Starr A: Post-cardiotomy delirium. Am J Psychiatry 121:371, 1964
3. Heller SS, Frank KA, Malm JR et al: Psychiatric complications of open-heart surgery. N Engl J Med 283:1015, 1970
4. Rabiner CJ, Wallner AE, Fishman J et al: Psychiatric complications following coronary bypass surgery. J Nerv Ment Dis 160:342, 1975
5. Diagnostic and Statistical Manual of Mental Disorders, 3rd ed. Washington DC, American Psychiatric Association, 1980
6. Lipowski ZJ: Delirium, clouding of consciousness and confusion. J Nerv Ment Dis 145:227, 1967

7. Engel GL, Romano J: Delirium: A syndrome of cerebral insufficiency. J Chronic Dis 9:260, 1959

8. Morse RM, Litin E: Post-operative delirium: A study of etiologic factors. Am J Psychiatry 126:388, 1969

9. Kornfeld DS, Zimberg S, Malm JR et al: Psychiatric complications of open-heart surgery. N Engl J Med 273:287, 1965

10. Tufo HM, Ostfeld AM, Shekelle R: Central nervous system dysfunction following open-heart surgery. JAMA 212:1333, 1970

11. Layne OL, Yudofsky SC: Post-operative psychosis in cardiotomy patients. N Engl J Med 284:518, 1971

12. Rubenstein D, Thomas K: Psychiatric findings in cardiotomy patients. Am J Psychiatry 126:360, 1969

13. Brennan RW, Patterson RH, Kessler J: Cerebral blood flow and metabolism during cardiopulmonary bypass: Evidence of microembolic encephalopathy. Neurology 21:665, 1971

14. Summers WK, Reich TC: Delirium after cataract surgery: Review and 2 cases. Am J Psychiatry 136:386, 1979

15. Ziskind E, Jones H, Folante W: Observations on mental symptoms in eye patched patients: Hypnagogic symptoms in sensory deprivation. Am J Psychiatry 116:893, 1960

16. Anath J: Hysterectomy and depression. Obstet Gynecol 52:724, 1978

17. Lindemann E: Observations on psychiatric sequelae to surgical operations in women. Am J Psychiatry 98:132, 1941

18. Marks RM, Sacher EJ: Undertreatment of medical in-patients with narcotic analgesics. Ann Intern Med 78:173, 1973

19. Johnson LC: Psychological and physiological changes following total sleep deprivation. In Kales A (ed): Sleep Physiology and Pathology: A Symposium, p 206. Philadelphia, JB Lippincott, 1969

20. Johns W, Large AA, Masterson JP et al: Sleep and delirium after open heart surgery. Br J Surg 61:377, 1974

21. Sveinsson I: Post-operative psychosis after heart surgery. J Thorac Cardiovasc Surg 70:717, 1975

22. Lazarus HR, Hagens JH: Prevention of psychosis following open heart surgery. Am J Psychiatry 124:1190, 1968

23. Cassem NH, Sos J: Intravenous use of haloperidol for acute delirium in intensive care settings (abstr). Presented at the 131st Annual Meeting of the American Psychiatric Association, Atlantic, GA, May 8–12, 1978

24. Dudley DL, Rowlett DB, Loebel PJ: Emergency use of intravenous haloperidol. Gen Hosp Psychiatry 1:240, 1979

25. Greenblatt DJ, Shader RI, Koch–Weser J et al: Slow absorption of intramuscular chlordiazepoxide. N Engl J Med 291:1116, 1974

26. Greenblatt DJ, Shader RI: Pharmacokinetic understanding of anti-anxiety drug therapy. South Med J 71 (Suppl):2, 1978

Drug Reactions and Interactions in the Surgical Patient

BERNADETTE MARIE PASTEWSKI
PHILIP P. GERBINO

Most patients receive an average of 7 to 10 medications during hospitalization.[1,2] Surgical patients may receive an additional 5 to 10 agents related to an operative procedure. The risk of drug reactions and interactions increases with the quantity and number of medications administered. For example, a patient who receives a theophylline preparation and is subsequently given erythromycin may exhibit theophylline toxicity.[3,4] During surgery, this interaction may be compounded by an anesthetic, such as halothane, which may potentiate the arrhythmogenicity of theophylline.[5]

Most drug-related problems in surgical patients can be avoided. Obvious medication hazards can be detected by a comprehensive medication history and a careful evaluation of the patient's current medications and diseases. This chapter begins with a brief discussion of the important aspects of the medication history. The remainder of the chapter emphasizes drug–drug and drug–disease reactions and interactions in surgical patients. Descriptions of drug–drug and drug–disease reactions and interactions in nonsurgical patients can be found in general reviews.[6–9]

MEDICATION HISTORY

The medication history is a vital tool in the management of the surgical patient. A recommended approach to obtaining a drug history is the following:[10]

Allergic history
   Ask patient about known reactions to drugs, food, cosmetics
   Identify allergen (trade vs. generic name)
   Get detailed description of reaction
      Onset and duration
      Route of contact with allergen
      Method by which reaction resolved
Medication history
   Identify current medication
   Identify dosage of medication
   Determine frequency of dosing schedule
   Determine length of time medication has been taken
   Determine reason for medication

A determination of whether a patient is prone to adverse effects, drug toxicities, hypersensitivity reactions, idiosyncrasies, or drug fever will enable early identification of potential problems. Drug allergies must be documented. Determining the exact nature of a reaction is important in the determination of whether it is truly immunologic. Most "allergies" are not true immunologic reactions. Many are extensions of pharmacologic effects of the drug or toxicities due to improper dosing. They can be avoided by alteration of the dose or substitution of a drug of different chemical structure with similar pharmacologic effects.

In drug allergy, cross-reactivity between a true drug allergen and its structural congener is likely. Congeners must be avoided if a serious reaction such as anaphylaxis to the original drug has occurred. Mild dermatologic reactions do not always constitute a contraindication to the administration of structurally similar agents. For example, dermatologic cross-reactivity between penicillins and cephalosporins is minimal despite the presence of cross-reacting antibodies in the serum.[11,12] Only about 8% of patients who develop an erythematous maculopapular rash to penicillins exhibit dermatologic cross-reactivity with cephalosporins.[12]

Precision in determining all of the patient's current medications, including over-the-counter preparations, is mandatory, because chronic, stable regimens can be altered during surgery. For example, the use of high-dose daily steroids for a period of 2 weeks or more prior to surgery may diminish adrenal reserve.[13–15] The stress of surgery may precipitate an adrenal crisis in patients who do not continue to receive these steroids. Abrupt withdrawal of antihypertensive agents has been associated with episodes of rebound hypertension and anginal attacks.[6,17] Pharmacokinetics of drugs may be altered during surgery, presenting unforeseen problems. Drugs with long half-lives, such as digoxin, or agents that undergo significant enterohepatic circulation, such as tricyclic antidepressants, are eliminated slowly. A drug reaction or interaction may consequently persist for an extended period of time.

Over-the-counter preparations are quite capable of precipitating drug reactions and interactions. Laxatives, antidiarrheals, antacids, cold and cough preparations, and pain medications such as aspirin are frequent sources of problems. Aspirin-containing products prolong bleeding time and can produce oozing in surgical patients because of their effect on platelet adhesion and aggregation.[18] Failure of the physician to recognize that many over-the-counter products contain aspirin will compromise the accuracy of the patient's medication history.[19]

Social habits influence drug reactions and interactions through alterations in drug metabolism. Induction of cytochrome P-450 enzymes in the liver occurs in both cigarette smokers and chronic alcohol abusers. Greater than normal theophylline clearance with subsequently greater dose requirement has been demonstrated in such patients. However, alcohol abusers with hepatitis and cirrhosis may exhibit less than normal clearance of this agent.[20]

TYPES OF DRUG REACTIONS

Drug reactions may be adverse, toxic, idiosyncratic, or allergic. Adverse reactions are undesirable but are known and expected. Toxicity is merely an extension of a desired pharmacologic effect to an intensity that may be harmful to the patient. Idiosyncratic reactions are infrequent and unexpected. Because of their unpredictability, they are also difficult to manage. Other reactions include temperature alterations such as drug fever.

Allergic or hypersensitivity reactions may be either immediate or delayed.[21] Both are encountered in surgical patients. Fisher reported the incidence of hypersensitivity reactions to all anesthetic agents to be 1 in 5,000.[22] Hypersensitivity reactions range from simple dermatologic manifestations to potentially fatal anaphylaxis. Nonimmune anaphylactoid reactions are caused by drugs that affect histamine release directly or through activation of complement (C_3), leading to histamine release.[22] Such reactions can occur on first exposure to a drug, and subsequent exposure may be safe. In contrast, initial administration of a drug may result in a minor reaction such as fever, whereas a second exposure may produce a complete and possibly fatal true anaphylactic reaction. Anaphylaxis is an immunoglobulin E (IgE)-mediated reaction that requires prior sensitization and exposure to the drug.[21] Use of agents and structural congeners that have previously produced such reactions is absolutely contraindicated.

Drug fever usually occurs within 7 to 10 days of surgery.[23,24] Clinical manifestations that distinguish drug fever from infectious fever include urticaria, lymphadenopathy, and eosinophilia.[23] Discontinuation of the offending agent usually results in resolution of symptoms in 2 to 7 days. Drugs with substantial enterohepatic recycling, such as sulfonamides and tricyclic antidepressants, may produce fever and associated symptoms for several weeks despite discontinuation of therapy.

The pathologic mechanism of drug fever can be classified into three major categories. The first and most common type is fever associated with drug administration. Caustic drug solutions such as tetracycline, cephalosporin, vancomycin, amphotericin B, diazepam, and thiopental can produce thrombophlebitis and resulting fever.[25] Utilization of 0.5-μ filters can minimize drug fever associated with drug particulates.[25] Sterile abscesses following multiple intramuscular injections of certain drugs, including pentazocine, amobarbital, and penicillin, are associated with drug fever.[23,24,26]

Second, hypersensitivity and idiosyncratic reactions account for approximately 25% of drug fevers.[23] If the patient has been sensitized to the drug, fever associated with hypersensitivity reactions may occur within hours of the agent's administration.[23] The "goal-post" fever pattern in hypersensitivity is seen when a drug administered for a febrile condition itself causes fever after several days of normal temperature.[27,28] Drug fever due to hypersensitivity reactions has been reported with ketamine, methoxyflurane, thiopental, halothane, d-tubocurarine, and scopolamine.[23,24] Cross-sensitization between anesthetics causing drug fever has not been reported.

Febrile response due to the pharmacologic effect of a drug, the third mechanism of drug fever, is rare. However, agents with anticholinergic effects such as phenothiazines, antihistamines, and belladonna alkaloids can prevent heat loss centrally by anhidrosis, whereas vasoconstrictors such as epinephrine may do so peripherally. In addition, amphetamines stimulate thermoregulatory centers in the central nervous system (CNS). Finally, even placebos have been noted to cause drug fever.[29]

Local Anesthetics

Local anesthetics have both local and systemic activity. The local effect consists of pharmacologic blockade of sodium- and potassium-mediated nerve impulse generation and conduction.[30] There are relatively few local adverse reactions associated with local anesthetics. Systemic toxicity is more frequent, accounting for the majority of complications and deaths associated with local anesthetics.[31]

Local anesthetics administered parenterally may cause swelling at the injection site owing to local irritation, faulty injection technique, or concomitant local vasoconstrictor use.[31-33] When applied topically, some of the agents may produce local irritation. A nonimmunologic reaction may result from direct irritation of the mucosal cell by the drug, appearing after one or several applications. Mucous membranes may become inflamed, edematous, and ulcerated. Some drugs produce topical sensitization such as the localized angioedema that is seen with procaine during dental procedures.[34,35] Prolonged or repeated local contact causes immunologic sensitization, probably mediated by IgE.

Vasoconstrictors, such as epinephrine, may be used with local anesthetics to prolong their effect. Necrosis and gangrene, particularly in fingertips and toes, have been associated with the use of epinephrine in patients with peripheral vascular disease.[30,31,36]

Most systemic reactions to local anesthetics are due to high concentrations in the plasma. For example, 20 ml of 1.5% lidocaine (300 mg) without epinephrine is commonly used in lumbar epidural anesthesia.[30] Peak plasma concentrations of 3 µg/ml rarely cause toxicity. Dizziness, tinnitus, nausea, and vomiting occur when plasma concentrations are within the range of 3 to 5 µg/ml.[32] Plasma concentrations in excess of 5 µg/ml are associated with generalized tonic–clonic seizures and subsequent CNS depression. This may occur if a large single dose is injected rapidly. CNS toxicity after administration of ester-type local anesthetics is usually of short duration because of rapid hydrolysis by plasma esterases. Because local anesthetics of the amide-type must undergo hepatic degradation, CNS toxicity and convulsions after administration of these agents are usually of longer duration.[30,32] A general classification of local anesthetics may be seen below:

Ester-type
   Cocaine
   Benzocaine
   Procaine (Novocaine)
   Chloroprocaine (Nesacaine)
   Butethamine (Monocaine)
   Meprylcaine (Oracaine)
   Tetracaine (Pontocaine)
   Butacaine (Butyn)
   Butyl Aminobenzoate (Butesin)
   Naepaine (Amylsine)
Amide-type
   Dibucaine (Nupercaine)
   Lidocaine (Xylocaine)
   Mepivacaine (Carbocaine)
   Prilocaine (Citanest)
   Bupivacaine (Marcaine)

Bradycardia and hypotension resulting from local anesthetic administration may be delayed or immediate and present as syncope or asystole.[32] Tetracaine has been reported to cause cardiovascular collapse without CNS excitation.[37]

The use of epinephrine with local anesthetics has both advantages and shortcomings. In theory, vasoconstriction reduces systemic toxicity by maintaining high local concentrations of the anesthetic and prevents high anesthetic plasma concentrations. Epinephrine, however, has systemic effects even when used locally. Aellig and co-workers studied normal subjects given epinephrine in doses of 2.5 ml to 8 ml of a 1:80,000 dilution and noted increases in heart rate up to 40 beats/min above baseline with minimal changes in blood pressure.[38] When less than 2 ml of this dilution was administered to 40 patients with documented atherosclerotic disease, no significant changes were noted in blood pressure or pulse rate.[39] Patients with angina or hyperthyroidism do not tolerate catecholamines well. In these patients, epinephrine concentrations should not exceed 1:250,000.[36] Norepinephrine and vasopressin have also been used as local vasoconstrictors. Vasopressin produces less intense vasoconstriction than epinephrine or norepinephrine and rarely affects heart rate or blood pressure when given in a concentration of 0.03 IU/ml.[36]

The incidence of hypersensitivity reactions to local anesthetics is less than 1%.[32] Ester-type anesthetics are more frequently associated with hypersensitivity reactions than amide-type agents. When patients experience anaphylactoid or other symptoms thought to be due to hypersensitivity to the ester-type anesthetic, substitution with an amide-type agent is recommended.[40] Several but not all ester-type local anesthetics cross-react by providing the same antigenic determinants for recognition by antibody.[30,31] For example, the esters aminobenzoic acid and ethylaminobenzoic acid (benzocaine) do not exhibit cross-reactivity, but the ester para-aminobenzoic acid does cross-react with other ester-type agents.[41] Amide-type agents do not cross-react with one another. If there is sufficient question about a patient's allergic history, provocative

dosing testing (PDT) may be necessary. Incaudo and colleagues have outlined detailed methods for PDT serial dilutions.[42]

Idiosyncratic reactions to local anesthetics are rare. Hallucinations and disorientation have occurred after small intra-arterial doses of local anesthetics.[43] Methemoglobinemia and cyanosis have been reported with prilocaine, benzocaine, and Cetacaine.[44]

General Anesthetics

The cornerstones of anesthetic therapy are the inhalational and intravenous general anesthetic agents. Inhalational anesthetics include both the gaseous agents (e.g., cyclopropane, ethylene, and nitrous oxide) and the volatile liquids (e.g., chloroform, ether, fluoroxene, halothane, methoxyflurane, enflurane, and isoflurane). Chloroform and ether are no longer used in contemporary practice because of flammability, hepatotoxicity, and nephrotoxicity. Intravenous anesthetic agents include ketamine, thiopental, fentanyl, droperidol, morphine, diazepam, propanidid, and alphoxalone.

Depth of anesthesia is usually dependent on and proportional to the concentration of the general anesthetic in the CNS.[45] Concentration gradients in alveoli, blood, and CNS tissue determine the level of anesthesia when inhalational anesthetics are administered. Rapid primary distribution of intravenous agents into the CNS with subsequent distribution into muscle and fat provide the anesthetic effect. General anesthetics also depress myocardial and respiratory function, in addition to producing CNS anesthesia.[45] Altering the hepatic metabolism or renal elimination of general anesthetics may prolong CNS and systemic depressant effects and produce adverse effects and toxicity.

All inhalational anesthetics depress myocardial function by altering excitation–contraction coupling through inhibition of the enzyme actinomycin-ATPase.[45,46] Nitrous oxide in a 40% concentration depresses myocardial function only minimally.[46] Concomitant use of nitrous oxide with other inhalational anesthetics is popular, since it allows for a reduction in the concentration of cardiac depressant anesthetics. The myocardial depressant effects of halothane, enflurane, isoflurane, and methoxyflurane on contractility and cardiac index are dose-dependent.[46–50] These agents produce minimal changes in peripheral vascular resistance and heart rate. The combination of nitrous oxide and enflurane causes less cardiac depression than enflurane alone at equipotent anesthetic doses.[48,50,51] However, in the presence of narcotics, nitrous oxide decreases cardiac index and increases peripheral vascular resistance.[52,53] Intravenous doses of 1 to 2 mg of morphine per kilogram of body weight decreases cardiac output by causing venodilation with only minimal myocardial depression.[54] The cardiovascular effects of fentanyl are similar to those of morphine. Cardiovascular studies have confirmed the direct negative inotropic effect of ketamine with an initial increase in blood pressure die to a decreased baroreceptor response.[55] Diazepam in doses of 5 mg to 25 mg does not produce significant myocardial depression, but doses of greater than 60 mg are associated with decreased blood pressure and cardiac output.[56]

The degree of respiratory depression caused by general anesthetics is directly related to the concentration of anesthetic in the blood and the level of anesthesia achieved. Naloxone, a direct narcotic antagonist, reverses the effects of meperidine and of opiates such as morphine.[57,58]

Naloxone does not reverse respiratory depression produced by inhalational anesthetics.[59] Thiopental, ether, and cyclopropane should be avoided in asthmatics because of their propensity to produce bronchial irritation and bronchospasm. Halothane, methoxyflurane, enflurane, fluoroxene, isoflurane, and ketamine are frequently used in asthmatic patients because they produce little or no bronchial irritation and do not increase bronchial secretions.

All inhalational anesthetics cause some degree of neuromuscular blockade. They do so in the following decreasing order: ether = methoxyflurane = enflurane = isoflurane > cyclopropane > halothane = fluoroxene = nitrous oxide. Potentiation of neuromuscular blockade by antibiotics such as aminoglycosides and neuromuscular blocking agents such as d-tubocurarine is most evident with ether, methoxyflurane, enflurane, isoflurane, cyclopropane, and halothane.[60–64] Nitrous oxide, ethylene, and thiopental cause only minimal, if any, neuromuscular blockade.

All halogenated anesthetics and barbiturates undergo biotransformation in the liver. The halogenated agents, primarily halothane and methoxyflurane, decrease splanchnic blood flow, and this may compromise hepatic function and elevate serum transaminase enzymes transiently following surgery.[65] Barbiturates, benzodiazepines, and all halogenated anesthetics except nitrous oxide and cyclopropane have been reported to activate microsomal enzymes.[66,67] Potential drug–drug interactions and hepatotoxicity may occur because of altered hepatic metabolism of drugs given before and after surgery.

Degradation of inhalational anesthetics occurs in the liver by oxidation, dehalogenation, and conjugation. With the exception of inorganic fluoride, the metabolites are generally considered nontoxic. The hepatotoxicity of halothane, enflurane, and isoflurane is controversial. Halogenated anesthetics such as halothane, enflurane, chloroform, and methoxyflurane have been associated with hepatotoxicity.[68–76] Two mechanisms have been proposed: (1) immune-hypersensitivity reactions, in which the anesthetics or their metabolites serve as haptens; and (2) toxicity due to metabolites acting as direct hepatotoxins.[68,77] Recent studies suggest that the incidence of severe hepatic necrosis due to halothane is 1 in 7,000 to 10,000 and the incidence of minor liver dysfunction is much higher.[69] Work in animals has confirmed that structural and functional hepatic damage after administration of halothane occurs only when enzyme induction and hypoxia produce large concentrations of reductive metabolites.[71] Hypoxia appears to increase the covalent binding of halothane metabolites to hepatic microsomal lipid.[78] Clinical data showing that 95% of halothane hepatitis occurs after repeat exposure support the notion of a hypersensitivity mechanism.[75] Moreover, in 55% of the cases, repeat exposure to anesthesia occurred within 4 weeks.[75] Definitive comparative trails of the hepatic effects of halothane, enflurane, and isoflurane are required to clarify the incidence and mechanisms of their hepatotoxicity.

Renal toxicity following methoxyflurane anesthesia has been correlated with increased blood levels of inorganic fluoride (>50 μg-mol/liter) released by biotransformation in the liver.[79–81] Inorganic fluoride interferes with the tubular reabsorption of water and produces vasopressin-resistant polyuria. Degradation of enflurane also produces inorganic fluoride to a lesser extent.[82–84] Although no obvious renal dysfunction has been observed with enflurane, urine osmolarity and response to vasopressin decrease within 24 hr of exposure.[84] Drug–drug interactions with methoxyflurane have been implicated in the production of nephrotoxicity.[85,86] Both methoxyflurane and enflurane should be avoided in patients with renal dysfunction.

Adverse hematologic reactions due to inhalational anesthetics have been reported only after prolonged exposure to nitrous oxide.[87–89] These reactions include a suppression of all bone marrow elements after 48 hr. No bone marrow suppression has been noted after only 24 hr.[89]

When hypersensitivity reactions to general anesthetics occur, barbiturates are frequently implicated.[90,91] The incidence of thiopental-induced hypersensitivity reactions is about 1 in 14,000 to 29,000.[90] Althesin, a recent addition to the class of general anesthetics, appears to have a slightly higher incidence of hypersensitivity reactions, estimated by Watkins and co-workers to be 1 in 11,000 to 19,000 and by others to be as frequent as 1 in 1,900.[92,93] Idiosyncratic reactions to general anesthetics are rare. One case of local skin depigmentation has been reported following the administration of althesin, but no previous reports of skin changes due to other general anesthetics appear in the literature.[94]

Neuromuscular Blocking Agents

Neuromuscular blocking agents (NMBAs) supplement general anesthesia by inducing flaccid paralysis of skeletal muscle through the selective inhibition of neurochemical transmission at the neuromuscular junction.[60,61] Nondepolarizing agents such as d-tubocurarine, metocurarine, pancuronium, alcuronium, and gallamine competitively inhibit acetylcholine binding at postjunctional membrane receptors.[95,96] Depolarizing agents such as succinylcholine and decamethonium bind to postjunctional membranes and produce persistent depolarization and desensitization of the receptors to acetylcholine.[60,61]

Although the sequence of muscle relaxation and paralysis is similar for the two types of NMBA there is considerable variability in dosage response. In addition, repeated doses of nondepolarizing agents produce a cumulative effect, whereas depolarizing agents produce partial tachyphylaxis. For example, when 0.04 mg/kg of pancuronium is given to normal subjects, the magnitude of muscle depression ranges from 50% to 100% of baseline. Recovery time to 50% of baseline activity varies from 0 to 81 min with a mean of 37 min.[96] The nondepolarizing agent pancuronium produces complete paralysis for only 10 min, but partial blockade and end-plate sensitivity continue for an additional 30 min to 40 min.[61] Because of this lingering sensitivity, supplemental doses of pancuronium should be reduced by 30% to 50% for prevention of prolonged postoperative paralysis and apnea. There is less intense paralysis following a second dose of the depolarizing agent succinylcholine, but the duration of the transmission block becomes progressively longer and may extend apnea in sensitive patients.[60,61]

In view of this variability, identification of patients with unusual sensitivities to average doses of these muscle relaxants becomes important. Factors that contribute to prolonged paralysis and apnea include concomitant administration of drugs with neuromuscular blockade activity (e.g., aminoglyosides), altered electrolyte balance, and complicating diseases.[97-101] The clinically important drug–drug and drug–disease interactions with muscle relaxants are outlined in Tables 36-2 through 36-6 and will be discussed later in this chapter.

The adverse effects of NMBAs are an extension of their pharmacologic activity. There are predictably profound effects on the cardiovascular system and the eye. Effects on the heart and peripheral circulation are mediated by stimulation or inhibition of either nicotinic receptors in autonomic ganglia or muscarinic receptors in the sinus node or by systemic histamine release by the relaxants.[60,61] Generally maximal cardiovascular effects are observed within 1 min to 5 min of an intravenous injection. When circulatory changes occur after more than 5 min, other etiologic factors such as the concomitantly administered anesthetic agents or altered serum electrolytes should be considered.

Gallamine, pancuronium, and alcuronium increase heart rate, especially in patients with baseline heart rates in the range of 60 to 70.[102-105] Gallamine-induced tachycardia is dose-dependent, with increases of up to 100% of baseline at doses of 1 mg/kg.[102] Heart rates of 90 to 120 are not uncommon with doses of 0.3 to 0.5 mg/kg. Pancuronium-induced tachycardia may also be dose-dependent, with increases of 15% to 25% in heart rate following administration of 0.02 to 0.03 mg/kg.[96] Lower doses may increase heart rate to the range of 70 to 90 through weak vagolytic activity. In patients receiving pancuronium with either morphine or halothane, marked tachycardia of 120 to 140 has been reported.[103,104] Alcuronium has very weak vagolytic activity and rarely produces tachycardia.[105] In the absence of histamine release, d-tubocurarine and metocurarine generally do not produce substantial changes in heart rate.[95,105] Tachycardia may be observed only after rapid intravenous injection of high dose d-tubocurarine (>0.7 mg/kg) and metocurarine (>0.4 mg/kg).[95,105] Succinylcholine may produce either bradycardia or tachycardia.[106] Tachycardia is most common in patients receiving atropine preoperatively. Severe sinus bradycardia, nodal rhythms, and asystole are more common in patients who are not being treated with atropine or who are receiving repetitive doses of succinylcholine.[106]

Ventricular arrhythmias may occur after administration of gallamine or pancuronium in conjunction with halothane or cyclopropane. In this setting, the anesthetic lowers the threshold for ventricular excitability.[107] Ventricular tachycardia was reported following pancuronium administration in a patient on chronic imipramine therapy; however, halothane was used concurrently.[108] Alcuronium, d-tubocurarine, and metocurarine rarely cause cardiac arrhythmias. In fact, d-tubocurarine has been shown to increase the threshold for arrhythmias induced by epinephrine.

Hypotension following administration of d-tubocurarine is severe in patients receiving beta-blockers and halogenated anesthetics.[105] Tubocurarine produces hypotension through ganglionic blockade and systemic histamine release. Metocurarine is a weaker vasodilator than d-tubocurarine, producing only a 7% fall in mean arterial pressure following rapid, high-dose intravenous injection.[95] Few cardiovascular changes occur with low-dose, slow administration. Alcuronium, gallamine, and pancuronium produce minimal cardiovascular depression. As a result, these muscle relaxants are advantageously used in hypovolemic patients or with concomitant vasodilating anesthetics such as halothane.[109] Although pancuronium may elevate arterial pressure by 10 torr to 20 torr, only one case of severe hypertension has been reported.[110] The hypertension was reversed with diazepam, supporting the hypothesis that the blood pressure elevation is mediated by anxiety-stimulated catecholamine release rather than by a specific sympathomimetic activity of pancuronium.

Increased intraocular pressure has been observed after succinylcholine administration in patients with detached retinas and glaucoma.[61] This effect is produced by sustained cholinergic-mediated contraction of the extraocular muscles and is potentiated by long-acting anticholinesterases such as echothiophate.[111] No changes in intraocular pressure have been reported with nondepolarizing agents.

Anaphylactoid type hypersensitivity reactions are related to the neuromuscular blocking agents' release of histamine in the following order of decreasing activity: d-tubocurarine > metocurarine > decamethonium > succinylcholine > alcuronium = gallamine = pancuronium.[60,95,96] Most anaphylactoid reactions occur with high-dose, rapid, intravenous injection of d-tubocurarine in susceptible patients.[61] In patients with allergic histories, Mongar and Whelan observed only minimal histamine release and no clinical manifestations after slow administration of therapeutic doses of d-tubocurarine.[112] Succinylcholine, pancuronium, gallamine, and alcuronium have also been shown to release little or no histamine.[60,96]

Severe anaphylactic reactions have been reported in patients with histories of allergies or asthma.[113–116] This suggests the possibility of IgE-mediated hypersensitivity. Although pancuronium is still considered the muscle relaxant of choice for the asthmatic patient, preanesthetic sensitivity testing in susceptible patients may decrease the risk of life-threatening hypersensitivity reactions.[96] Idiosyncratic reactions to muscle relaxants are rare. One case of myoglobinuria has been reported after administration of succinylcholine.[117]

Antiocholinergics

Anticholinergic agents have been traditionally used preoperatively to reduce bronchial secretions stimulated by irritating anesthetics such as ether.[118] Less irritating anesthetics such as halothane have largely eliminated this problem. Some investigators omit routine preoperative anticholinergics with no adverse consequences.[119] However, surveys indicate that over 50% of anesthesiologists still use anticholinergics preoperatively, most commonly atropine, scopolamine, and glycopyrrolate.[120]

Most adverse effects of the anticholinergics are dose-related extensions of their pharmacologic activity and primarily involve the cardiovascular system, gastrointestinal tract, and the eye as outlined in Table 36-1. However, some cardiovascular effects may not be dose-related, depending on concomitant anesthetic administration. With doses of atropine alone of 0.2 mg to 0.4 mg, paradoxical bradycardia occurs, whereas with doses of 0.4 mg to 0.6 mg, heart rate returns to baseline.[121] At doses exceeding 0.6 mg, heart rate proportionally increases with increasing doses. However, no further increase in heart rate above 130 to 150 occurs at doses greater than 3 mg.[122]

The arrhythmogenic potential of an anticholinergic is difficult to predict at any given dose. Arrhythmogenicity seems to be dependent on the choice of anesthetic.

Table 36-1. Dose-Related Effects of Atropine

Dose (mg)	Effect
0.2–0.4	Parodoxical bradycardia
0.4–0.6	30% Reduction in bronchial secretions Inhibition of salivation and sweating Baseline heart rate
1.0	65% Reduction in bronchial secretions Dry mouth, dry skin, tachycardia Decreased peristalsis
2.0	Above symptoms more pronounced Difficulty in micturition Decreased gastric secretions
5.0	Above symptoms more pronounced Urinary retention
> 10.0	Anticholinergic toxicity—ataxia, hallucinations, delirium, seizures, dysrhythmias, coma

Atrioventricular dissociation, nodal rhythms, and ventricular extrasystoles are frequently reported with atropine and scopolamine. The frequency of arrhythmias with atropine at doses of 0.4 mg is 17% with halothane anesthesia and 54% with cyclopropane.[123,124]

Glycopyrrolate inhibits salivation and sweating at a dose of 0.2 mg.[125] At this same dose, cardiovascular effects are minimal. Mirakhur and co-workers observed for changes in pulse rate or arrhythmias in patients given atropine (1.0 mg), glycopyrrolate (0.2 mg), or no anticholinergic premedication.[126] Only atropine produced substantial tachycardia prior to induction of anesthesia with thiopental and nitrous oxide. After induction of this anesthesia, a minimal increase in heart rate was noted in each group. Neither atropine nor glycopyrrolate influenced the pressor response evoked by tracheal intubation. With thiopental and nitrous oxide anesthesia, arrhythmias were observed in 35%

of patients who had been given atropine and in 10% of patients who had received glycopyrrolate. No arrhythmias occured in the non-premedicated group.

The gastrointestinal effects of these three anticholinergic agents are decreasing peristalsis, delayed gastric emptying, and a reduction in the opening pressure of the cardioesophageal sphincter.[118,121,127] Intragastric pH and cardioesophageal sphincter pressure are important considerations, because surgical patients are prone to aspiration. Since the effect of glycopyrrolate on increasing gastric pH is unclear, antacids or cimetidine are frequently used as prophlaxis against aspiration.[125,128]

Anticholinergics should be avoided in patients with glaucoma, who are at risk for increased intraocular pressure.[118] Two case reports of transient blindness have been associated with intramuscular administration of atropine. In one patient, blindness developed after atropine was used as a premedication for spinal anesthesia for transurethral resection of the prostrate.[129] Gooding and Holcomb reported that atropine-induced transient blindness was reversed by pilocarpine.[130]

The CNS effects of anticholinergics are considered to be manifestations of toxicity rather than adverse reactions. Both atropine and scopolamine are tertiary ammonium compounds that penetrate the blood-brain barrier.[118,121] Anticholinergics administered in recommended preanesthetic doses usually produce little or no CNS effects, but in elderly patients, doses of atropine as low as 0.4 mg can cause prolonged postoperative sedation.[131] Scopolamine is 8 times more potent than atropine in producing central effects; as a result, the recommended preanesthetic dose of scopolamine may produce confusion, lethargy, and prolonged sleep even in normal patients.[118]

Anticholinergic psychosis is characterized by excitation and hyperactivity alternating with depression and somnolence.[132] Other accompanying signs of anticholinergic toxicity include intense vasoconstriction, hot, dry skin, opthalmologic signs, hallucinations, delirium, generalized tonic–clonic convulsions, and sometimes coma.[132] Deaths have rarely resulted from anticholinergic intoxication. CNS effects occur with cumulative doses exceeding 5 mg to 10 mg of atropine. No central effects are seen with glycopyrrolate, because the highly polar quarternary ammonium structure of this agent does not allow penetration of the blood-brain barrier.[125]

Only one case of possible anaphylaxis has been reported to occur with atropine.[133] In this situation, the patient was also concurrently given propanidid and suxamethonium, both of which have been reported to cause anaphylaxis. In vitro data support the possibility that atropine and propanidid can produce an anaphylactoid reaction through the release of histamine.[133] Idiosyncratic reactions to atropine are rare.

DRUG–DRUG INTERACTIONS

Pharmacokinetics include the absorption, distribution, biotransformation, and elimination of drugs.[134] Alterations in pharmacokinetics by the interaction of two or more drugs may adversely affect the pharmacologic activity of one or more of the agents as well as alter their durations of action. Drug–drug interactions may be additive, synergistic, or antagonistic.[6–8] Additive effects occur when the combined effect of drugs are equal to the sum of the individual effect on each drug. When the combined effect of the drugs is greater than the sum of the effects of each drug, the total effect is termed synergistic. Antagonism occurs when the combined effect of the drugs results in less pharmacologic activity than that produced by the sum of the effects of each.

The mechanisms of drug–drug interactions provide a basis for an understanding of their pharmacologic effects. These mechanisms can be broadly categorized into six groups:[6–8]

1. Physical/chemical incompatibilities
2. Alterations in absorption and receptor site uptake
3. Alterations in protein binding
4. Modification of drug activity at the receptor site
5. Acceleration or retardation of metabolism
6. Alterations in elimination

Incompatibilities

Physical incompatibilities among drugs cause visible alterations such as discoloration in solutions or formation of precipitates. Chemical incompatibilities involve inactivation of pharmacologic activity without visible changes.[135] Barbiturates commonly produce both physical and chemical incompatibilities because of their low pKa and high pH.[6–8,135,136] For example, when thiopental at pH 10.8 is mixed with the narcotic meperidine at pH 3.5, a precipitate appears.[8,135] Mixing barbiturates with calcium or magnesium solutions results in precipitation of insoluble carbonate and magnesium salts. An example of chemical incompatibility is the rapid inactivation of succi-

nylcholine or pancuronium when administered together with thiopental.[8,135,136] These muscle relaxants, which are amine salts, liberate insoluble free base in the highly alkaline solution of thiopental.

Diazepam, chlordiazepoxide, and phenytoin are both physically and chemically incompatible with all other intravenous medications.[6–8,135–137] In addition to avoiding concomitant administration or physical mixture of these drugs with other medications, the physician should flush the intravenous line with a drug-free solution before and after their administration.

Absorption

The rate of absorption or receptor site uptake of a drug may be altered by another drug.[6–8] Drugs administered subcutaneously or intramuscularly depend on the vascularity of the site of injection for absorption. Epinephrine-induced vasoconstriction decreases systemic absorption of local anesthetics.[6] Use of more than one inhalational anesthetic may alter diffusion capacity and receptor site uptake of one of the agents by the alveoli, producing the so-called "second gas effect."[138] The addition of nitrous oxide to an inspired anesthetic mixture containing halothane and oxygen accelerates the rate of alveolar uptake of halothane. High concentrations of halothane in the alveoli increase the risk of halothane toxicity.

Protein Binding

Binding of drugs to proteins in the serum determines the quantity of free drug available for binding to receptor sites.[6–8] Displacement of one drug from protein-binding by another because of greater affinity is important for highly protein-bound drugs such as oral anticoagulants.[139] Barbiturates are frequently involved in displacement interactions. For example, pentobarbital anesthesia can be prolonged or deepened by displacement of the anesthetic by highly protein-bound x-ray contrast medium.[140]

Receptor Activity

Modification of receptor activity occurs when two or more drugs possess similar capacities to bind to the same receptor site, as in the case of naloxone, which antagonizes the CNS depressant effects of opiate narcotics.[6–8,57] Potentiation of neuromuscular blockade may occur when aminoglycosides are administered to patients receiving d-tubocurarine.[141]

Drug Metabolism

Interacting drugs may alter drug metabolism.[6–8] Changes in microsomal enzymatic oxidation affect the biotransformation of some anesthetic agents in the liver. Barbiturates, alcohol, and halogenated anesthetics are potent enzyme inducers.[6–8,66,67] Inhibition of plasma enzymes may decrease drug metabolism. Patients with glaucoma taking the anticholinesterase echothiopate may experience prolonged apnea when given succinylcholine. This is due to depletion of plasma pseudocholinesterase by ecothiopate.[111]

Elimination

Drug elimination by the kidney may be affected by changes in systemic pH and alterations in pulmonary ventilation. Renal excretion of phenobarbital is enhanced when urine pH is greater than 7.5.[142] If ventilation is depressed by narcotics, elimination of nitrous oxide is delayed, and the anesthetic effect is prolonged.[45]

A summary of the specific drug–drug interactions that are associated with anesthetic agents is listed in Tables 36-2 through 36-5. Table 36-2 identifies clinically verified drug incompatibilities and categorizes drug combinations as either compatible or incompatible. The term compatibility means that no alteration in the pharmacologic activity of either drug in a given combination, whether mixed or administered simultaneously, occurs. The term incompatibility indicates that there is a physical or chemical interaction between the drugs leading to the pharmacologic inactivation of one or both of the drugs.[6–8,135,136]

Tables 36-3, 36-4, and 36-5 are organized according to drug–drug interactions with various types of anesthetic agents. Each table lists the interacting agent(s) in alphabetical order with the pharmacologic mechanism of the interaction and its anesthetic implication. Mechanisms are categorized into one of the six groups previously described. Each interaction is referenced and noted as either clinically significant or possibly clinically significant.

The anesthetic agents most frequently involved in drug–drug interactions are the NMBAs, especially with antibiotics. Aminoglycosides, polymyxin, and colistin are clinically important in potentiating the neuromuscular blockade of the muscle relaxants.[60,61,141,143–146] The relative potencies of the aminoglycosides in producing neuromuscular blockade can be ranked in decreasing order: neomycin > streptomycin > netilmicin > kanamycin = amikacin > gentamicin = tobramycin.[97,141,143–146] Lincomycin and tetracycline are infrequently implicated in the prolongation of postoperative respiratory depression.[60,61]

Text continued on page 557

Table 36-2.
Anesthetic Agent Combinations

— = no documentation available; I = incompatible; C = compatible

(Hansten DH (ed): Drug Interactions. 4th ed. Philadelphia, Lea & Febiger, 1979; American Pharmaceutical Association (eds): Evaluation of Drug Interactions, 2nd ed. Washington DC, American Pharmaceutical Association, 1976; Hartshorn E: Handbook of Drug Interactions. 3rd ed. Hamilton, IL, Drug Intelligence Publications, 1976; Hull CJ: Br J Anaesth 51:579, 1979; Kramer W et al: Drug Intell Clin Pharmacol 5:211, 1971)

	Amobarbital	Atropine	Benzquinamide	Chlorpromazine	Dimenhydrinate	Diphenhydrinate	Droperidol	Fentanyl	Fentanyl & Droperidol	Glycopyrrolate	Hydrocortisone	Hydroxazine	Kentamine	Levorphanol	Meperidine	Morphine	Pancuronium	Pentazocine	Pentobarbital	Phenobarbital	Prochlorperazine	Promethazine	Scopolamine	Secobarbital	Succinylcholine	Thiopental	d-Tubocurarine
d-Tubocurarine	I	C	C	C	I	C	C	C	C	I	I	I	I	I	C	C	I	C	C	C	C	C	C	C	I	C	I
Thiopental	I	I	I	I	I	I	I	I	I	I	C	I	I	I	I	C	C	C	I	I	C	C	I	I	C	I	C
Succinylcholine	I	I	I	I	I	I	I	I	I	I	I	I	I	I	I	I	I	I	I	I	I	I	I	I	I	I	I
Secobarbital	I	I	I	I	I	I	I	I	I	I	I	I	I	I	I	I	I	I	I	I	I	I	I	C	I	C	C
Scopolamine	I	C	C	C	C	C	C	C	C	I	I	C	I	I	C	C	I	C	C	C	C	C	C	I	C	C	C
Promethazine	I	C	C	I	I	C	C	C	C	I	I	I	I	I	C	C	I	I	I	I	C	C	I	I	C	C	C
Prochlorperazine	I	C	C	I	C	I	C	I	I	I	C	C	I	I	C	C	I	I	C	C	C	I	C	I	C	C	C
Phenobarbital	I	I	I	I	I	I	I	I	I	I	I	I	I	I	I	I	I	I	I	I	I	I	C	C	I	C	C
Pentobarbital	I	C	C	I	I	I	I	I	I	I	I	I	I	I	I	I	I	I	I	I	I	I	C	C	I	C	C
Pentazocine	I	C	C	C	I	I	I	I	I	I	I	C	I	I	I	I	I	I	C	C	C	C	I	C	C	I	C
Pancuronium	I	I	I	I	I	I	I	I	I	I	I	I	I	I	I	I	I	I	I	I	I	I	I	I	I	I	I
Morphine	I	C	C	C	I	C	I	I	I	C	I	C	I	I	C	C	I	I	C	C	C	C	I	I	I	I	C
Meperidine	I	C	C	C	C	C	I	I	I	C	I	C	I	I	C	C	I	I	C	C	C	C	I	I	I	I	C
Levorphanol	I	I	I	I	I	I	I	I	I	I	I	I	I	I	I	I	I	I	C	C	C	I	I	I	I	I	C
Kentamine	I	I	I	I	I	I	I	I	I	I	I	I	I	I	I	I	I	I	I	I	I	I	I	I	I	I	I
Hydroxazine	I	C	C	I	C	I	I	I	I	C	I	C	I	I	C	C	I	C	I	I	C	C	C	I	I	I	C
Hydrocortisone	I	I	I	I	I	I	I	I	I	I	I	I	I	I	I	I	I	I	I	I	I	I	I	C	I	C	C
Glycopyrrolate	I	I	I	C	I	I	C	C	C	I	I	C	I	I	C	C	I	I	I	I	I	I	C	I	I	I	I
Fentanyl & Droperidol	I	C	I	I	I	I	I	I	I	C	I	I	I	I	I	I	I	I	I	I	I	I	C	I	I	I	C
Fentanyl	I	C	C	I	I	I	I	I	I	C	C	I	I	I	I	I	I	I	I	I	I	I	C	I	I	I	C
Droperidol	I	C	C	I	I	I	I	I	I	C	C	I	I	I	I	I	I	I	I	I	C	I	C	C	C	C	C
Diphenhydrinate	I	C	C	I	I	I	I	C	C	I	I	I	I	I	I	I	I	I	I	I	C	I	C	C	I	C	C
Dimenhydrinate	I	I	I	I	I	I	I	I	I	I	C	C	C	I	I	I	I	I	I	I	C	I	C	C	C	C	C
Chlorpromazine	I	C	C	I	I	C	I	I	I	I	I	C	I	I	C	C	I	C	I	I	C	C	C	C	I	C	C
Benzquinamide	I	C	C	I	I	I	I	I	I	I	I	I	I	C	C	C	I	C	C	I	I	I	C	C	C	I	C
Atropine	I	I	C	C	I	C	C	C	C	I	I	C	I	I	C	C	I	C	C	I	C	C	C	I	I	I	C
Amobarbital	I	I	I	I	I	I	I	I	I	I	I	I	I	I	I	I	I	I	I	I	I	I	I	I	I	I	I

[549]

Table 36-3. Drug Interactions with Nondepolarizing Neuromuscular Blocking Agents

Interacting Agent(s)	Pharmacologic Mechanism (Group)*	Dose Recommendation
Antibiotics—aminoglycosides, colistin, polymyxin, lincomycin, tetracycline	Neuromuscular blockade is possible with antibiotics alone. Concomitant use potentiates neuromuscular blockade. (4)	Reduce dose of NMBA.†[61,97,143–146]
Diuretics—thiazides, furosemide, ethacrynic acid, metolazone, acetazolamide	Diuretic-induced hypokalemia, hyponatremia, hypochloremia, metabolic acidosis or alkalosis produces alterations in ions and pH, increasing the sensitivity to muscle relaxants. (4)	Caution—Hypokalemia may prolong neuromuscular blockade.‡[147,148]
Ganglionic-Blocking Agents—trimethaphan, hexamethonium	Compete with acetylcholine at neuromuscular junction, potentiating neuromuscular blockade. (4)	Caution—May prolong neuromuscular blockade.‡[149]
Hydrocortisone	Reported to partially antagonize the neuromuscular blockade of pancuronium in patients with adrenal insufficiency. (4)	Caution—Partially antagonizes neuromuscular blockade.‡[150]
Inhalational Anesthetics—halothane	More pronounced hypotension with d-tubucurarine. (4)	Caution—Concomitant use may potentiate hypotensive effect.‡[63]
ether, enflurane, isoflurane, methoxyflurane, fluroxene	Neuromuscular blockade is possible with inhalational anesthetic alone. Concomitant use potentiates neuromuscular blockade. (4)	Reduce dose of NMBA.†[62–64,151,152]
Intravenous Anesthetics—ketamine	Decreases presynaptic release of acetylcholine, prolonging the neuromuscular blockade effect. (4)	Caution—May prolong neuromuscular blockade.‡[154]
Lithium Carbonate	Selective pancuronium–lithium interaction: lithium may affect acetylcholine synthesis or release, increasing neurotransmitter at neuromuscular junctions. (4)	Reduce dose of NMBA.†[155]
Magnesium Sulfate	Hypermagnesemia (> 7.0 mEq/liter) decreases acetylcholine release at neuromuscular junction, increasing sensitivity to muscle relaxants. (4)	Reduce dose of NMBA in hypermagnesemia.†[99]
Neostigmine	Inhibits cholinesterase, thereby increasing tissue levels of acetylcholine and reversing the competitive blockade. (5)	Used to reverse neuromuscular blockade.†[144]

Nitrates—nitroglycerin (IV)	Selective pancuronium–nitroglycerin interaction, possibly due to involvement of metabolite accumulation prolonging the neuromuscular blockade. (5)	Prolongs neuromuscular blockade. (Note: IV nitroglycerin > 0.5 µg/kg/min must be started prior to pancuronium injection for blockade to be prolonged)†[156,157]
Quinidine	Quinidine (IV) produces neuromuscular blockade alone; concomitant use potentiates the neuromuscular blockade. (4)	Caution—May prolong neuromuscular blockade.‡[158]
Succinylcholine	Selective pancuronium–succinylcholine interaction inhibits plasma cholinesterase, thereby increasing acetylcholine levels. (5)	Delays onset of neuromuscular blockade by direct antagonism and prolongs action of succinylcholine.†[159]
Thiopental	Agent's alkaline solution liberates free base from muscle relaxants, inactivating relaxants. (1)	Avoid mixture—incompatible.†[8,135,136]
Theophylline	Constant aminophylline infusion producing high levels (> 35 mg/liter) antagonizes neuromuscular blockade effect due to increased release of acetylcholine via cAMP. (4)	Excessive levels antagonize neuromuscular blockade. Therapeutic levels do not antagonize neuromuscular blockade.†[160]
Tricyclic Antidepressant imipramine	Selective pancuronium–imipramine interaction: pancuronium-induced tachyarrhythmias observed in patients on imipramine and halothane. (4)	Caution—Avoid combination of pancuronium–imipramine–halothane.‡[161]
amitriptyline	Neostigmine—amitriptyline: increased ST and T-wave abnormalities observed, with a greater tendency than normal to arrhythmias. (4)	Caution—Avoid combination of amitriptyline and neostigmine.‡[162]

*Group 1: Physical/chemical incompatibilities
Group 2: Alterations in absorption and receptor site uptake
Group 3: Alterations in protein binding
Group 4: Modification of drug activity at the receptor site
Group 5: Acceleration or retardation of metabolism
Group 6: Alterations in elimination

†Clinically significant

‡Possibly clinically significant

IV = intravenous; CAMP = adenozine 3′:5′ = cyclic phospate

Table 36-4. Drug Interactions with Depolarizing Neuromuscular Blocking Agents

Interacting Agent(s)	Pharmacologic Mechanism (Group)*	Dose Recommendation
Antibiotics—aminoglycosides, colistin, polymyxins (lincomycin, tetracycline)	Neuromuscular blockade is possible with antibiotic alone; concomitant use potentiates neuromuscular blockade. (4)	Reduce dose of NMBA.†[61,97,143-146]
Cytotoxic Agents—alkylating agents, nitrogen mustards, cyclophosphamide, chlorambucil, mechlorethamine	Inhibition of plasma cholinesterase by cytotoxic agents prolongs succinylcholine activity. (5)	Caution—May prolong neuromuscular blockade.‡[163]
Dantrolene	Centrally acting muscle relaxant reduces muscle fasiculation. (4)	Reduces the incidence of postoperative myalgia.[164]
Diazepam	Centrally acting muscle relaxant reduces (1) muscle fasiculations, (2) increased serum potassium, and (3) increased CPK. (4)	Reduces the incidence of postoperative myalgia.†[165]
Digitalis—digoxin, digitoxin	Digitalis toxicity enhanced due to increased sensitivity of myocardium to arrhythmias.	Caution—Avoid use of succinylcholine in patients on digitalis.‡[166]
Diethylstilbestrol	Decreases plasma cholinesterase, increasing succinylcholine levels. (5)	Caution—May prolong neuromuscular blockade.‡[167]
Diuretics—spironolactone, triamterene	Diuretic-induced hyperkalemia potentiates succinylcholine-induced hyperkalemia. (4)	Caution—Avoid concomitant use of potassium-sparing diuretics and succinylcholine.‡[168]
Echothiophate—phospholine iodide eye drops	Long-acting anticholinesterase reduces cholinesterase serum levels, prolonging succinylcholine activity. (5)	Concomitant use contraindicated due to prolongation of apnea. (Note—Pralidoxime reverses echothiophate-induced muscle paralysis.)†[111]
Lithium Carbonate	Lithium may substitute for sodium at neuromuscular junction and impede presynaptic transmission; delays onset of succinylcholine and prolongs neuromuscular blockade. (4)	Reduce dose of NMBA.†[154,169]

Drug	Description	Action
Local Anesthetics—procaine, lidocaine	Inhibit the release of acetylcholine at neuromuscular junction, potentiating neuromuscular blockade. (4)	Reduce dose of NMBA.†[153]
Magnesium Sulfate	(Possible with succinylcholine, but reported only with d-tubocurarine.)	Reduce dose of NMBA.‡[99]
Neostigmine	Reverses neuromuscular blockade by inhibiting cholinesterase activity. (5)	Appropriate therapy for reversal and desensitization of neuromuscular blockade.†[144]
Pancuronium	Selective succinylcholine–pancuronium interaction: inhibition of plasma cholinesterase, which increases acetylcholine levels. (5)	Prolongs neuromuscular blockade and delays onset of direct antagonism.†[170]
Propanidid	Propanidid is hydrolyzed by plasma cholinesterase; competes with succinylcholine for metabolism, prolonging neuromuscular blockade. (5)	Reduce dose of NMBA.†[171]
Quinidine	Quinidine (IV) produces neuromuscular blockade alone; concomitant use potentiates neuromuscular blockade. (4)	Caution—May potentiate neuromuscular blockade‡[172]
Tetrahydroaminacridine—THA, tacrine	Inhibits plasma cholinesterase, prolonging succinylcholine activity. (5)	Reduce dose of NMBA.†[173]
Thiopental	Agent's alkaline solution liberates free base from muscle relaxants (amine base). (5)	Avoid mixture—incompatible.†[8,135,136]

*Group 1: Physical/chemical incompatibilities
Group 2: Alterations in absorption and receptor site uptake
Group 3: Alterations in protein binding
Group 4: Modification of drug activity at the receptor site
Group 5: Acceleration or retardation of metabolism
Group 6: Alterations in elimination

†Clinically significant

‡Possibly clinically significant

CPK = creatine phosphokinase; IV = intravenous

Table 36-5. Drug Interactions with General Anesthetics

Interacting Agent(s)	Pharmacologic Mechanism (Group)*	Dose Recommendation
Alcohol–Barbiturates, Alcohol–Inhalational Anesthetics	Acute intoxication: Additive CNS depressant effects with anesthetic. (4) Chronic alcoholism: Induction of hepatic microsomal enzymes increases metabolism of anesthetic agents. (5)	Acute enhanced CNS depression. Chronic increased anesthetic dose requirements.†[174]
Antiarrhythmics–halothane (phenytoin, lidocaine)	Additive depressant effect on atrioventricular conduction may result in re-entry-type arrhythmias. (4) Lidocaine lowers minimum alveolar concentration for halothane, nitrous oxide.	Caution—May cause arrhythmias. Lidocaine reduces dose of anesthetic.†[175]
Antibiotics–methoxyflurane (aminoglycosides, tetracycline)	Additive nephrotoxicity with agents; methoxyflurane produces nephrotoxicity by accumulation of fluoride metabolite. (4,5)	Avoid potential nephrotoxic drugs with methoxyflurane.†[74,80,81,85,86]
Anticoagulants–barbiturates	Induction of hepatic microsomal enzymes by barbiturates increases metabolism of warfarin; no interaction with heparin. (5)	Avoid warfarin. Use heparin cautiously during anesthesia—monitor PTT, bleeding complications.†[176]
Antihypertensives– inhalational anesthetic (methyldopa, clonidine, reserpine, guanethidine, propranolol)	Reserpine depletes central and peripheral catecholamine stores. Methyldopa has central activity. Clonidine has central activity; stimulates postsynaptic and adrenoreceptors. Guanethidine blocks postganglionic adrenergic neurons; no effect on halothane requirements. Propranolol causes beta blockade (see below).	Caution—Reserpine, methyldopa, clonidine decrease halothane requirement for induction; potentiate direct pressure. Do not abruptly discontinue clonidine or propranolol, may result in severe rebound hypertension.†[177–181]
Beta-Blockers–inhalational anesthetics		
propranolol (halothane, enflurane, isoflurane, trichlorethylene)	Has minimal additive cardiodepressant effect. (4)	Safe combinations. Caution—Propranolol in angina patients may result in MI.†[182–185]
practolol (methoxyflurane)	Markedly reduce cardiac output and contractility. (4)	Avoid combinations.†[186]

Interactant	Mechanism	Recommendation
Carbon Dioxide—inhalational anesthetics	If patient can increase ventilation in response to increased PCO_2, there is increased rate of elimination (or increased uptake during induction). (6)	Useful to hasten recovery (or induction) with inhalational anesthetics.†[187]
Diazepam—halothane	Diazepam reduces minimum alveolar concentration for halothane (diazepam half-life, about 10–15 hr). (6)	Decreased halothane requirement.†[188]
Digitalis—halothane	Halothane reduces the cardiotoxicity of digitalis through myocardial depressant activity. (4)	Caution—Although adequate digitalis dose may be inadequate during halothane anesthesia, do not increase dose of digitalis preoperatively.†[166,187]
Epinephrine—halogenated anesthetics	Reduce intrasurgical bleeding. Epinephrine produces dose-related ventricular irritability; varies with halogenated anesthetic. (4)	Caution—Utilize lower doses of epinephrine with halogenated anesthetic.†[189]
Epinephrine—local anesthetics (vasoconstrictor)	Local vasoconstrictor-diminished regional blood flow delays absorption of anesthetic. (2)	Prolongs anesthetic effect.†[36]
Levodopa—halogenated anesthetics	Dopamine, metabolite of levodopa, produces varying responses on blood vessels and blood pressure. Low-dose (1–2 g) beta-adrenergic effect: direct cardiac stimulation, vasodilation. High-dose (> 3 g) alpha-adrenergic effect: vasoconstriction, hypertension. (4)	Caution—Due to levodopa's short duration of action, continue until night before surgery and resume immediately postoperatively.†[190]
butyrophenones	Haloperidol, droperidol antagonize dopamine. (4)	Avoid combination within 4 hr of levodopa administration.†[190]
Lithium—barbiturates	Lithium increases duration of pentobarbital narcosis—mechanism unknown.	Caution—May potentiate CNS depression.‡[191]
Monoamine Oxidase Inhibitors (MAOI)—barbiturates (phenelzine, nialamide, isocarboxazid, pargyline tranylcypromine)	Inhibition of hepatic enzymes possibly delays elimination of barbiturates, potentiating their effect. (5)	Caution—Discontinue MAOI two weeks prior to surgery.†[192–194]

(Continued)

Table 36-5. Drug Interactions with General Anesthetics (Continued)

Interacting Agent(s)	Pharmacologic Mechanism (Group)*	Dose Recommendation
meperidine	Concomitant use produces excitation, sweating, rigidity, hyper/hypotension, coma.	Avoid combination. Substitute morphine cautiously.†[193,194]
Indirectly acting sympathomimetic (amphetamine)	MAOI inhibits metabolism of catecholamines, additive CNS excitation with sympathomimetic. (5)	Exaggerated pressure response.†[193,195]
Narcotics—barbiturates	Additive CNS depression. (4)	Caution—Potentiates CNS depression.†[6-8]
naloxone	A pure narcotic antagonist. (4)	Antagonizes respiratory and CNS depression of narcotics (opiates).†[57]
Nitrous Oxide—halothane, enflurane	"Second gas effect": rapid nitrous oxide uptake concentrates other agent in alveoli. (2)	Caution—More rapid induction.†[138]
Steroids²—general anesthesia (hydrocortisone)	Prolonged steroid therapy depresses hypothalamic–pituitary–adrenocortical (HPA) function; abrupt discontinuation of steroids may produce adrenal crisis.	Caution—In patients with HPA axis depression, give hydrocortisone 25 mg IV during induction and 100 mg IV postoperatively every 24 hr.†[13,15,196]
Theophylline—halothane	Arrhythmogenic potential increased with combination. (4)	
Thiopental		
Ketamine	Thiopental precipitates ketamine solution. (1)	Avoid mixture—incompatible.†[8,135,136]
Meperidine	Meperidine's acidic solution (pH 3.5) precipitates thiopental's alkaline solution (pH 10.8). (1)	Avoid mixture—incompatible.†[8,135,136]
NMBAS	Thiopental's alkaline solution liberates insoluble free base from muscle relaxants (amine salts). (1)	Avoid mixture—incompatible.†[8,135,136]
Sulfonamides (sulfisoxazole)	Occupy albumin binding sites, decreasing thiopental's protein binding. (3)	Caution—Reduce dose of thiopental for induction.[197]

*Group 1: Physical/chemical incompatibilities
Group 2: Alterations in absorption and receptor site uptake
Group 3: Alterations in protein binding
Group 4: Modification of drug activity at the receptor site
Group 5: Acceleration or retardation of metabolism
Group 6: Alterations in elimination

†Clinically significant

‡Possibly clinically significant

PTT = partial thromboplastin time; MI = myocardial infarction; IV = intravenous

Alterations in serum concentrations of potassium or magnesium increase the sensitivity of neuromuscular receptors to blocking agents.[60] Hypokalemia of less than 2.5 mEq/liter produces membrane hyperpolarization and increases the sensitivity of the receptor to nondepolarizing agents.[98,147,148] Changes in pH produce ion shifts that may potentiate the activity of NMBAs. For example, antagonism of d-tubocurarine by neostigmine is decreased in the presence of severe metabolic alkalosis and resulting hypokalemia.[148] Although succinylcholine only minimally elevates serum potassium concentration by 0.5 to 1.0 mEq/liter, instances of hyperkalemia, ventricular arrhythmias, and muscle fasiculation have been reported following its administration in patients with severe burns, massive trauma, and hemiplegia.[60,168] Pretreatment with pancuronium or diazepam usually attenuates hyperkalemia and muscle fasiculations in these patients.[165] Hyperkalemia with the combination of pancuronium and succinylcholine has also been observed in patients with head trauma and parkinsonism.[100,101] Hypermagnesemia has been associated with the potentiation of nondepolarizing agents, but only at toxic levels of magnesium greater than 7 mEq/liter.[99]

Drug interactions associated with general anesthetics most commonly involve the barbiturates, primarily thiopental. Numerous physical and chemical incompatibilities have been observed with thiopental because of its highly alkaline pH of 10.8[6–8] Concomitant administration of thiopental with narcotics, NMBAs or ketamine should be avoided. Additionally, the CNS effects and respiratory depression that are observed with thiopental can also be potentiated by concomitant use of other depressant agents, such as opiates.

Attention should also be focused on drug interactions between inhalational anesthetic agents and antihypertensive agents. As outlined in Chapter 6. many authors recommend that antihypertensive therapy not be withdrawn prior to anesthesia. Although blood pressure commonly decreases during anesthesia, the reduction is not usually clinically significant even in patients on antihypertensive therapy.[181] Moreover, rebound hypertension has been observed in patients abruptly withdrawn from antihypertensives such as clonidine and propranolol.[179,180,185]

Methyldopa and reserpine are centrally acting antihypertensives that increase the minimal alveolar concentration of halothane and consequently decrease the required dose of halothane for induction.[178] In contrast, guanethidine does not reduce anesthetic requirements, presumably because of its minimal penetration of the blood-brain barrier.[178] Patients taking propranolol can be safely anesthetized with halothane, isoflurane, or enflurane, all of which have only minimal additive cardiodepressant effects.[182,185] In contrast, trichloroethylene and metho-oxyflurane should be avoided in patients on beta-blockers because of their profound effect in reducing cardiac output and contractility.[186]

Drug interactions between local anesthetics and anticholinergics are rare. The only significant interactions involve the concomitant use of regional vasoconstrictors such as epinephrine or depolarizing NMBAs with local anesthetics.[36,153]

DRUG–DISEASE INTERACTIONS

Many surgical patients suffer from diseases that can adversely affect the phar-

Table 36-6. Drug–Disease Interactions with Neuromuscular Blocking Agents (Nondepolarizing and Depolarizing)

Disease State	Anesthetic Dose Recommendation
Asthma	Increased sensitivity to histamine-liberating muscle relaxants, producing bronchospasm. Histamine-liberating potential: tubocurarine > metocurarine.[60,61,96]
Eaton–Lambert syndrome	Increased sensitivity at neuromuscular junction, producing flaccid muscle paralysis; decrease dose of muscle relaxant.[60]
Hypothermia	Increased intensity of neuromuscular blockade; decrease dose of muscle relaxant.[198,199]
Malignant hyperthermia	Specific with succinylcholine, pancuronium; increased calcium release, producing muscle contractions, fasiculations, hyperthermia; *Avoid* muscle relaxants (see text).[195,200–205]
Myasthenia gravis	Increased sensitivity at neuromuscular junction, producing flaccid muscle paralysis (d-tubocurarine test in myasthenia).[60]
Myotonia	Specific with depolarizing agents; increased sensitivity at neuromuscular junction; generalized muscle spasms alleviated with quinine, *not* d-tubocurarine.[60]
Parkinsonism	Specific with depolarizing agents; increased sensitivity due to hyperkalemia potentiation.[101]
Plasma cholinesterase deficiency	Specific with succinylcholine; prolonged apnea. *Avoid* succinylcholine (see text).[206,207]
Renal dysfunction	Gallamine, 70–90% renal excretion; *Avoid* in renal dysfunction. Pancuronium, 35–45% renal excretion; succinylcholine hydrolyzed by plasma cholinesterase.[208,209]
Trauma—head trauma, massive burns, hemiplegia	Specific with succinylcholine; increased sensitivity due to hyperkalemia potentiation.[60,100]

macokinetics of anesthetic agents. The anesthetic agents most frequently involved in drug–disease interactions are the NMBAs (Table 36-6). Two underlying disease states that are especially important in the administration of anesthetic agents are pseudocholinesterase deficiency and the propensity for developing malignant hyperthermia.

Malignant Hyperthermia

Malignant hyperthermia is a disease of skeletal and cardiac muscle that occurs in 1 in 14,000 patients who undergo anesthesia.[200] Susceptibility to malignant hyperthermia is inherited as an autosomal dominant trait. All potent inhalational an-

esthetics, succinylcholine, curare, pancuronium, amide-type local anesthetics, and stress can produce malignant hyperthermia.[195] Each of these agents can initiate the release of calcium from sarcoplasmic reticulum in muscle, producing generalized muscle contractions and fasiculations, which result in the generation of heat.[195] A history of hyperthermia, muscle rigidity during previous general anesthesia, or family history of malignant hyperthermia is useful in the identification of susceptible patients, but a negative history does not guarantee safety. Some physicians suggest that a muscle biopsy be performed in patients and family members to test for susceptibility.[201] Muscle from a susceptible patient contracts significantly *in vitro* on exposure to caffeine, halothane, or succinylcholine.[202]

The clinical manifestations of malignant hyperthermia are usually evident during anesthesia but may not appear until several hours after surgery. Rigidity of the jaw at the onset of anesthesia is a valuable early warning sign but need not be always present. Tachycardia and arrhythmias occur early, followed by tachypnea, respiratory and metabolic acidosis, hypercapnia, hyperkalemia, and hyperglycemia. Hyperthermia, pulmonary edema, consumption coagulopathy, and acute renal failure secondary to myoglobinuria follows.[195]

Therapeutic management consists of immediate cessation of anesthesia, vigorous core and surface cooling, correction of metabolic acidosis, and adequate oxygenation.[203,204] Procainamide or dantrolene sodium is effective in the treatment of malignant hyperthermia.[203,204] Procainamide acts to lower intracellular calcium by affecting sarcoplasmic reticulum calcium efflux, whereas dantrolene acts directly on the contractile mechanism of skeletal muscle to dissociate excitation–contraction coupling.[203] Both agents should be given intravenously immediately.

General anesthetic agents that are suitable as induction agents in patients susceptible to malignant hyperthermia include thiopental, fentanyl, diazepam, and nitrous oxide. If local anesthesia is required, ester-type local anesthetics should be used.[202] Administration of oral dantrolene prior to anesthesia is effective as prophylaxis.[205]

Pseudocholinesterase Deficiency

Cholinesterases may be divided into true cholinesterase which is present at nerve endings and in erythrocytes, and pseudocholinesterase, which is found in liver and serum. Succinylcholine is usually rapidly inactivated by serum pseudocholinesterase, but, in patients with pseudocholinesterase deficiency, ineffective inactivation of succinylcholine results in prolonged postoperative apnea.[206] This enzymatic defect is inherited as an autosomal recessive trait in approximately 1 in 3000 individuals. An alterations in any of five alleles at the genetic locus may produce a change in enzyme structure.[206]

Therapeutic management of succinylcholine-induced apnea consists of mechanical ventilatory support until the respiratory depressant effects of the succinylcholine disappear. A highly purified concentrate of the enzyme cholinesterase can be given to terminate succinylcholine-induced apnea.[207]

Serum cholinesterase activity can be measured in patients suspected of pseudocholinesterase deficiency. Persons are classified as normal, intermediate (heterozygous for the defective gene), or atypical (homozygous for the abnormal gene), according to their level of enzyme.[210] In patients categorized as atypical, succinylcholine must be avoided; however, pancuronium can be substituted. Although pancuronium inhibits cholinesterase by 40%, it has no clinical effect on respiration.[206] Patients classified as either normal or intermediate may receive succinylcholine without risk.

SUMMARY

1. **Drug reactions as well as drug–drug and drug–disease interactions can occur with almost all agents used perioperatively. The physician can detect potential hazards by taking a careful**

medication history, perusing the list of the patient's current medications, and analyzing concomitant drug effects(s) on the patient's underlying disease(s).

2. Particular attention should be focused on inhalational anesthetics and NMBAs in an attempt to identify potential problems.

3. Specific drug effects are presented in Tables 36-1 through 36-6.

REFERENCES

1. Miller RR: Drug surveillance utilizing epidemiologic methods: A report from the Boston Collaborative Drug Surveillance Program. Am J Hosp Pharm 30:584, 1973

2. May FE, Stewart RB, Cluff LE: Drug use in the hospital: Evaluation of determinants. Clin Pharmacol Ther 16:834, 1974

3. Weinberger, Hudgel D, Spector S et al: Inhibition of theophylline clearance by troleandomycin. J Allergy Clin Immunol 59:228, 1977

4. Cummins L, Kozak P, Gillman S: Letter. Erythromycin's effect on theophylline blood level. Pediatrics 59:144, 1977

5. Rolzen MF, Stevens WC: Multiform ventricular tachycardia due to the interaction of aminophylline and halothane. Anesth Analg (Cleve) 57:738, 1978

6. Hansten DH (ed): Drug Interactions, 4th ed. Philadelphia, Lea & Febiger, 1979

7. American Pharmaceutical Association (eds): Evaluation of Drug Interactions, 2nd ed. Washington DC, American Pharmaceutical Association 1976

8. Hartshorn E: Handbook of Drug Interactions, 3rd ed. Hamilton, IL, Drug Intelligence Publications, 1976

9. Adverse interactions of drugs. Medical Letter 21:5, 1979

10. Covington TR: Interviewing and advising the Patient. In Francke DE, Whitney HA (eds): Perspectives in Clinical Pharmacy, Hamilton, IL, Hamilton Press, 1972

11. Levine B: Antigenicity and cross reactivity of penicillins and cephalosporins. J Infect Dis 128:S364, 1973

12. Barza M, Miao P: Cephalosporins. Am J Hosp Pharm 34:621, 1977

13. Byyny R: Withdrawal from glucocorticoid therapy. N Engl J Med 295:30, 1976

14. Fauci A, Dale D, Balow J: Glucocorticosteroid therapy: Mechanisms of action and clinical considerations. Ann Intern Med 84:304, 1976

15. Axelrod L: Glucocorticoid therapy. Medicine 55:39, 1976

16. Lowenstein J: Drugs five years later: Clonidine. Ann Intern Med 92:74, 1980

17. Mizgala H, Counsell J: Acute coronary syndromes following abrupt cessation of oral propranol therapy. Can Med Assoc J 114:1123, 1976

18. Packham M, Mustard J: Clinical pharmacology of platelets. Blood 50:555, 1977

19. Leist E, Banweil J: products containing aspirin. N Engl J Med 291:710, 1974

20. Powell J, Vozeh S, Hopewell P et al: Theophylline disposition in acutely ill hospitalized patients. Am Rev Respir Dis 118:229, 1978

21. Gordon B: Essentials of Immunology, 2nd ed. Philadelphia, F.A. Davis, 1976

22. Fisher M: Severe histamine mediated reactions to intravenous drugs used in anesthesia. Anaesth Intensive Care 3:180, 1975

23. Martin DW et al: Drug fever. Medical Staff Conference, Univ of Calif, San Francisco. West J Med 129:321, 1978

24. Cluff LE, Johnson JE: Drug fever Prog Allergy 8:149, 1964

25. DeLucca P, Rapp R, Bivins B et al: Filtration and infusion phlebitis: A double-blind prospective clinical study. Am J Hosp Pharm 32:1001, 1975

26. Hodges JR, Klainer AS: Pentazocine fever. JAMA 215:1504, 1971

27. Murray H, Mann J: Goal post fever. Ann Intern Med 83:84, 1975

28. Musher DM, Fainstein V, Young E et al: Fever patterns: Their lack of clinical sig-

nificance. Arch Intern Med 139:1225, 1978

29. Reidenberg M, Lowenthal D: Adverse Non-drug reactions. N Engl J Med 279:678, 1968
30. Covino B: Local anesthesia. N Engl J Med 286:975, 1972
31. DeJong R: Toxic effects of local anesthetics. JAMA 239:1166, 1978
32. Adriani J, Naraghi M: Etiology and management of adverse reactions to local anesthetics. J Am Med Wom Assoc 33:367, 1978
33. Covino B: Systemic toxicity of local anesthetic agents. Anesth Analg (Cleve) 57:387, 1978
34. Siegal S: Local allergic edema induced by injected procaine. J Allergy 29:329, 1958
35. American Dental Association: Local anesthetics. In Accepted Dental Therapeutics, 37th ed. Chicago, American Dental Association, 1977
36. Verrill P: Adverse reactions to local anesthetics and vasoconstrictor drugs. Practitioner 214:380, 1975
37. Adriani J, Naraghi M: The pharmacologic principles of regional pain relief. Ann Rev Pharmacol Toxicol 17:223, 1977
38. Aellig W, Laurence D, O'Neill R et al: Cardiac effects of adrenaline and felypressin as vasoconstrictors in local anesthesia for oral surgery with diazepam. Br J Anaesth 42:174, 1970
39. Elliot G, Stein E: Vasoconstrictors in local anesthesia for oral surgery. JAMA 227:1403, 1974
40. deShazo R, Nelson H: An approach to the Patient with a history of local anesthetic hypersensitivity: Experience with 90 patients. J Allergy Clin Immunol 63:387, 1978
41. Gaul E: Cross-sensitization from para-aminobenzoate sunburn preservatives. Anesthesiology 16:606, 1955
42. Incaudo G, Schatz M, Patterson R et al: Administration of local anesthetics to patients with a history of prior adverse reactions. J Allergy Clin Immunol 61:339, 1978

43. Aldrete J, Nicholson J, Sada T et al: Cephalic kinetics of intra-arterially injected lidocaine. Oral Surg 44:167, 1977
44. Olson M, McEvoy G: Methemoglobinemia induced by local anesthetics. Am J Hosp Pharm 38:89, 1981
45. Ngai SH: Current concepts in anesthesiology: Effect of anesthetics on various organs. N Engl J Med 302:564, 1980
46. Merin RG: Effect of anesthetic drugs on myocardial performance in man. Annu Rev Med 28:75, 1977
47. Sonntag H, Donath U, Hillebrand W et al: Left ventricular function in conscious man and during halothane anesthesia. Anesthesiology 48:320, 1978
48. Filner BE, Karliner JS: Alterations in normal left ventricular performance by general anesthesia. Anesthesiology 45:610, 1976
49. Eger EI, Smith NT, Cullen DJ et al: A comparison of the cardiovascular effects of halothane, fluroxene, ether, and cyclopropane in man. Anesthesiology 34:25, 1971
50. Black GW: Enflurane. Br J Anaesth 51:627, 1979
51. Smith NT, Calverly RK, Prys-Roberts C et al: Impact of nitrous oxide on the circulation during enflurane anesthesia in man. Anesthesiology 48:320,1978
52. Stanley TH, Bidwai AV, Lunn JK et al: Cardiovascular effects of nitrous oxide during meperidine infusion in the dog. Anesth Analg (Cleve) 56:836, 1977
53. Stoelting RK, Gibbs PS: Hemodynamic effects of morphine and morphine–nitrous oxide in valvular heart disease and coronary disease. Anesthesiology 38:45, 1973
54. Lowenstein E, Hallowell P, Levine F et al: Cardiovascular response to large doses of intravenous morphine in man. N Engl J Med 281:1389, 1969
55. Tweed WA, Minuck M, Mymin D: Circulatory responses to ketamine anesthesia. Anesthesiology 37:613, 1972
56. Abel RM, Staroscik RN, Reis RL: Effects of diazepam on left ventricular function

and systemic vascular resistance. J Pharmacol Exp Ther 173:364, 1970

57. Martin W: Naloxone. Ann Intern Med 88:765, 1976

58. Gairola RL, Gupta PK, Dandoley K: Antagonists of morphine-induced respiratory depression. Anaesthesia 35:17, 1980

59. Harper MH, Winter PM, Johnson BH et al: Naloxone does not antagonize general anesthesia in rats. Anesthesiology 49:3, 1978

60. Ali H, Savarese J: Monitoring of neuromuscular function. Anesthesiology 45:216, 1976

61. Neigh J: Neuromuscular blockade. Surg Clin North Am 55:837, 1975

62. Ward BE: Decrease in dose requirement of d-tubocurarine by volatile anesthetics. Anesthesiology 51:298, 1979

63. Hughes F, Payne JP: Interacting of halothane with non-depolarizing neuromuscular blocking drugs in man. Br J Clin Pharmacol 7:485, 1979

64. Vitez T: Potency of metocurine during halothaine–nitrous oxide and nitrous oxide narcotic anesthesia. Anesth Analg (Cleve) 57:116, 1978

65. Batchelder BM, Cooperman LH: Effects of anesthetics of splanchnic circulation and metabolism. Surg Clin North Am 55:787, 1975

66. Linde HW, Berman ML: Non-specific stimulation of drug-metabolizing enzymes by inhalation anesthetic agents. Anesth Analg (Cleve) 50:565, 1971

67. Berman ML, Green OL, Calverly RK et al: Enzyme induction by enflurane in man. anesthesiology 44:496, 1976

68. Brown BR, Sipes IG, Sagalyn AM: Mechanism of acute hepatic toxicity: Chloroform, halothane and glutathione. Anesthesiology 41:554, 1974

69. Inman WH, Mushin WW: Jaundice after repeated exposure to halothane: A further analysis of reports to the committee on safety of medicine. Br Med J 2:1455, 1978

70. Wright R, Chisholm M, Lloyd B et al: Controlled prospective study of the effect on liver function of multiple exposure to halothane. Lancet 1:821, 1975

71. McLain GE, Sipes IG, Brown BR: An animal model of halothane hepatotoxicity. Anesthesiology 51:321, 1979

72. Miller DJ, Dwyer J, Klatskin G: Halothane hepatitis: Benign resolution of a severe lesion. Ann Intern Med 89:212, 1978

73. Thompson DS, Friday CD: Changes in liver enzyme values after halothane and enflurane for surgical anesthesia. South Med J 71:779, 1978

74. Joshi PH, Conn HO: The syndrome of methoxyflurane-associated hepatitis. Ann Intern Med 80:395, 1974

75. Cousins MJ: Halothane hepatitis: What's new? Drugs 19:1, 1980

76. Ona FV, Patanella H, Ayub A: Hepatitis associated with enflurane anesthesia. Anesth Analg (Cleve) 59:146, 1980

77. Sharp JH, Trudell JR, Cohen EN: Volatile metabolites and decomposition products of halothane in man. Anesthesiology 50:2, 1979

78. Widger LA, Gandolfi AJ, Van Dyke RA: Hypoxia and halothane metabolism in vivo: Release of inorganic fluoride and halothane metabolite binding to cellular constituents. Anesthesiology 44:197, 1976

79. Deutsch S: Effects of anesthetics on the kidney. Surg Clin North Am 55:775, 1975

80. Churchili D, Knaack J, Chirito E et al: Persisting renal insufficiency after methoxyflurane anesthesia. Am J Med 56:575, 1974

81. Urgena RB, Sergis SD: Nephrotoxicity from methoxyflurane anesthesia: Six-year retrospective study. Br J Anaesth 45:358, 1973

82. Mazze RI, Calvarley RK, Smith NT: Inorganic fluoride nephrotoxicity: Prolonged enflurane and halothane anesthesia in volunteers. Anesthesiology 46:265, 1977

83. Bentley B, Vaughan RW, Miller MS et al:

Serum inorganic fluoride levels in obese patients during and after enflurane anesthesia. Anesth Analg (Cleve) 58:409, 1979

84. Dooley JR, Mazze RI, Rice SA et al: Is enflurane defluorination inducible in man? Anesthesiology 50:213, 1979

85. Mazze RI, Cousins JM: Combined nephrotoxicity of gentamicin and methoxyflurane anesthesia in man. Br J Anaesth 45:394, 1973

86. Cousins MJ, Mazze RI: Tetracycline, methoxyflurane anesthesia and renal dysfunction. Lancet 1:751, 1972

87. Kripke BJ, Talario L, Shah NK et al: Hematologic reaction to prolonged exposure to nitrous oxide. Anesthesiology 47:342, 1977

88. Nunn JF, Sturrock JE, Howell A: Effect of inhalational anesthetics on division of bone marrow cells. Br J Anaesth 48:75, 1976

89. Green C: Toxicity of nitrous oxide. In Eastwood D (ed): Clinical Anesthesia, p 38. Philadelphia, F.A. Davis, 1964

90. Whitwam JG: Adverse reactions to IV induction Agents. Br J Anaesth 50:677, 1978

91. Evans JM, Keough JAM: Adverse reactions to intravenous anesthetic induction agents. Br Med J 2:735, 1977

92. Watkins J, Clark A, Appleyard TN et al: Immune-mediated reactions to althesin. Br J Anaesth 48:881, 1976

93. Watt JM: Anaphylactic reactions after use of CT (1341) althesin. Br Med J 3:207, 1975

94. Coote N, Abeysiri LU: Skin depigmentatioh with intravenous anesthesia induction agents. Anaesthesia 34:336, 1979

95. Savarese J, Ali H, Antonio R: The clinical pharmacology of metocurarine. Anesthesiology 47:277, 1977

96. Roizen M, Feeley T: Pancuronium bromide. Ann Intern Med 88:64, 1978

97. Waterman D, Smith R: Tobramycin–curare interaction. Anesth Analg (Cleve) 56:587, 1977

98. Vaughan R, Lunn J: Potassium and the anesthetist. Anaesthesia 28:118, 1973

99. de Silva A: Magnesium intoxication: An uncommon cause of prolonged curarization. Br J Anaesth 45:1228, 1973

100. Stevenson P, Birch A: Succinylcholine-induced hyperkalemia in patients with closed head injury. Anesthesiology 51:89, 1979

101. Gravlee G: Succinylcholine-induced hyperkalemia in patients with Parkinson's disease. Anesth Analg (Cleve) 59:444, 1980

102. Eisele J, Marta J, Davis H: Quantitative aspects of chronotropic and neuromuscular effects of gallamine in anesthetized man. Anesthesiology 35:630, 1971

103. Grossman E, Jacobi A: Hemodynamic interaction between pancuronium and morphine. Anesthesiology 40:299, 1974

104. Miller R, Eger E, Stevens W et al: Pancuronium-induced tachycardia in relation to alveolar halothane, dose of pancuronium and prior atropine. Anesthesiology 42:352, 1975

105. Tammisto T, Welling I: The effect of alcuronium and d-tubocurarine on blood pressure and heart rate: A clinical comparison. Br J Anaesth 41:317, 1969

106. Perez H: Cardiac arrhythmias after succinylcholine. Anesth Analg (Cleve) 49:33, 1970

107. Walts L, McFarland W: Effect of vagolytic agents on ventricular rhythm during cyclopropane anesthesia. Anesth Analg (Cleve) 44:429, 1965

108. Anderson E, Rosenthal M: Pancuronium bromide and tachyarrhythmias. Crit Care Med 3:13, 1975

109. Stoelting R: Influence of pancuronium or d-tubocurarine on circulatory response during thiamylal-N_2O-halothane anesthesia. Anesth Analg (Cleve) 55:485, 1976

110. Fraley D, Lemoncelli G, Coleman A: Severe hypertension associated with pancuronium. Anesth Analg (Cleve) 57:265, 1978

111. Pantuck E: Ecothiopate iodide eye drops and prolonged response to suxamethonium. Br J Anaesth 38:406, 1968

112. Mongar J, Whelan R: Histamine release by adrenaline and d-tubocurarine in human subjects. J Physiol 120:146, 1953

113. Chan C, Yeung M: Anaphylactic reaction to alcuronium. Br J Anaesth 44:103, 1972

114. Buckland R, Avery A: Histamine release following pancuronium. Br J Anaesth 45:518, 1973

115. Clark R: Reaction to pancuronium? Br J Anaesth 45:997, 1973

116. Mandappa J, Chandrasekhara P, Nelvigi R: Anaphylaxis to suxamethonium. Br J Anaesth 47:523, 1975

117. Moore W, Watson R, Summary J: Massive myoglobinuria precipitated by halothane and succinylcholine in a member of a family with elevation of serum creatinine phosphokinase. Anesth Analg (Cleve) 55:680, 1976

118. Mirakhur R: Anticholinergic drugs. Br J Anaesth 51:671, 1979

119. Middleton M, Zitzer J, Urbach K: Is atropine always necessary before general anesthesia? Anesth Analg (Cleve) 46:51, 1967

120. Mirakhur R, Clarke R, Dundee J et al: Anticholingeric drugs in anesthesia: A survey of their present position. Anaesthesia 33:133, 1978

121. Shutt L, Bower J: Atropine and hyoscine anesthesia. Anaesthesia 34:476, 1979

122. Carrow D, Aldrete J, Masden R et al: Effects of large dose of IV atropine on heart rate and arterial pressure of anesthetized patients. Anesth Analg (Cleve) 54:262, 1975

123. Elkard B, Andersen J: Arrhythmias during halothane anesthesia: Influence of atropine. Acta Anaesthesiol Scand 21:245, 1977

124. Jones R, Deutsch S, Turndorf H: Effects of atropine in cardiac rhythm in conscious and anesthetized man. Anesthesiology 22:67, 1961

125. Mirakhur R, Dundee J, Jones C: Evaluations of the anticholinergic actions of glycopyrronium bromide. Br J Clin Pharmacol 5:77, 1978

126. Mirakhur R, Clarke R, Elliott J et al: Atropine and glycopyrronium premedication. Anaesthesia 33:906, 1978

127. Brock-Utre J, Rubin J, Welman S et al: The effect of glycopyrrolate on the lower esophageal sphincter. Can Anaesth Soc J 25:144, 1978

128. Detmer M, Pandit S, Cohen P: Prophylactic single-dose oral antacid therapy in the preoperative period—Comparison of cimetidine and mallox. Anesthesiology 51:270, 1979

129. DeFalque R, Miller D: Visual disturbances during transurethral resection of prostate. Can Anesth Soc J 22:620, 1975

130. Gooding J, Holcomb M: Transient blindness following IV Administration of atropine. Anesth Analg (Cleve) 56:872, 1977

131. Smith D, Orkin F, Gardner S et al: Prolonged sedation in the elderly after intraoperative atropine administration. Anesthesiology 51:348, 1979

132. Perry P, Wilding D, Juhl R: Anticholinergic psychosis. Am J Hosp Pharm 35:725, 1978

133. Turner K, Keep V, Bartholomaeus N: Anaphylaxis induced by propanidid and atropine. Br J Anaesth 44:211, 1972

134. Hull CJ: Pharmacokinetics and pharmacodynamics. Br J Anaesth 51:579, 1979

135. Kramer W, Inglott A, Cluxton R: Physical and chemical incompatibilities of drugs for IV administration. Drug Intell Clin Pharmacol 5:211, 1971

136. Parker E: Compatibility digest. Am J Hosp Pharm 26:653, 1969

137. Ingallinera TS, Kapadia AJ, Hagman D et al: IV incompatibilities with glycopyrrolate. Am J Hosp Pharm 36:508, 1979

138. Stoelting R, Eger E: An additional explanation for the second gas effect. Anesthesiology 30:273, 1969

139. MacLeod S, Sellers E: Pharmacodynamic and pharmacokinetic drug interactions with coumarin anticoagulants. Drugs 11:461, 1976

140. Lasser E, Elizondo-Martel G, Granke R: Potentiation of pentobarbital anesthesia by competitive protein binding. Anesthesiology 24:665, 1963

141. Lee C, de Silva A: Interaction of neuromuscular blocking effects of neomycin and polymixin B. Anesthesiology 50:218, 1979

142. Oderda G: Clinical Toxicology. J Am Pharm Assoc 14:626, 1974

143. Pittinger C, Adamson R: Antibiotic blockade of neuromuscular function. Annu Rev Pharmacol 12:169, 1972

144. VanNyhuis L, Miller R, Fogdall R: Interaction between d-tubocurarine, pancuronium, polymixin B, and neostigmine on neuromuscular function. Anesth Analg (Cleve) 55:224, 1976

145. Albiero L, Ongini E, Parravicini L: The Neuromuscular blocking activity of a new aminoglycoside antibiotic—netilmicin sulfate. Eur J Pharmacol 50:1, 1970

146. Hashimato Y, Shima T, Matsukawa S et al: A possible hazard of prolonged neuromuscular blockade by amikacin. Anesthesiology 49:219, 1978

147. Miller R, Roderick L: Diuretic-induced hypokalemia, pancuronium, neuromuscular blockade and its antagonism by neostigmine. Br J Anaesth 50:541, 1978

148. Miller R, Sohn Y, Matteo R: Enhancement of d-tuborcurarine neuromuscular blockade by diuretics in man. Anesthesiology 45:442, 1976

149. Deacock AR, Davis TD: The influence of certain ganglionic blocking agents on neuromuscular transmission. Br J Anaesth 30:217, 1958

150. Meyers EF: Partial Recovery from pancuronium neuromuscular blockade following hydrocortisone administration. Anesthesiology 46:148, 1977

151. Stoelting RK, Longnecker DE: Influence of end-tidal halothane concentration on d-tubocurarine hypotension. Anesth Analg (Cleve) 51:364, 1972

152. Stanski D, Ham J, Miller R et al: Pharmacokinetics and pharmacodynamics of d-tubocurarine during nitrous oxide narcotic and halothane in man. Anesthesiology 51:235, 1979

153. Matsuo S, Rao D, Chaudry T et al: Interaction of muscle relaxants and local anesthetics at neuromuscular junction. Anesth Analg (Cleve) 57:580, 1978

154. Amaki Y, Nagashima H, Radnay P et al: Ketamine interaction with neuromuscular blocking agents in phrenic nerve— Hemidiaphragm preparation of rat. Anesth Analg (Cleve) 57:238, 1978

155. Hill G, Wong K, Hodges M: Lithium carbonate and neuromuscular blocking agents. Anesthesiology 46:122, 1977

156. Glisson S, El-Etr A, Lim R: Prolongation of pancuronium-induced neuromuscular blockade by intravenous infusion of nitroglycerin. Anesthesiology 51:47, 1979

157. Glisson S, Sanchez M, El-Etr A et al: Nitroglycerin and the neuromuscular blockade produced by gallamine, succinycholine, d-tubocurarine, and pancuronium. Anesth Analg (Cleve) 59:117, 1980

158. Miller RD, Way WL, Katzung BG: The potentiation of neuromuscular blocking agents by quinidine. Anesthesiology 28:1036, 1967

159. Ivankovic AD, Sidell N, Cairoli VJ et al: Dual action of pancuronium on succinylcholine block. Can Anaesth Soc J 24:228, 1977

160. Doll D, Rosenberg H: Antagonism of neuromuscular blockage by theophylline. Anesth Analg (Cleve) 58:139, 1979

161. Edwards RP, Miller RD, Roizen MF, et al: Cardiac response to imipramine and pancuronium during anesthesia with halothane or enflurane. Anesthesiology 50:421, 1979

162. Glisson SN, Fajardo L, El-Etr AA: Amitriptyline therapy increases changes during reversal of neuromuscular blockade. Anesth Analg (Cleve) 57:77, 1978

163. Zsigmond EK, Robins G: The effect of a series of anticancer drugs on plasma cholinesterase activity. Can Anaesth Soc J 19:75, 1972

164. Collier CB: Dantrolene and suxamethon-

ium. The effect of preoperative dantrolene on the action of suxamethonium. Anaesthesia 34:152, 1979

165. Fahmy N, Malek N, Lappas D: Diazepam prevents some adverse effects of succinylcholine. Clin Pharmacol Ther 26:395, 1979

166. Strong MJ, Keats AS: Digitalis and heart disease. Anesthesiology 31:583, 1969

167. Archer TL, Ganowsky EC: Plasma pseudocholinesteron deficiency associated with diethylstilbesteral therapy. Anesth Analg (Cleve) 57:726, 1978

168. Bourke D, Rosenberg M: Changes in total serum Ca^+, Na^+, K^+ with administration of succinylcholine. Anesthesiology 49:361, 1978

169. Hill GE, Wong KC, Hodges MR: Potentiation of succinylcholine neuromuscular blockade by lithium carbonate. Anesthesiology 44:439, 1976

170. Baraka A: Suxamethonium–neostigmine interaction in patients with normal or atypical cholinesterase. Br J Anaesth 49:479, 1977

171. Monks PS, Normal J: Prolongation of suxamethonium-induced paralysis by propanidid. Br J Anaesth 44:1303, 1972

172. Manzin E, Novello E, Comelli LF: Interference by quinidine on neuromuscular block produced by succinylcholine. Ann Med Psychol (Paris) 103:603, 1972

173. Benveniste D, Hemmingsen L, Joul P: Tacrine inhibition of serum cholinesterase and prolonged succinylcholine action. Acta Anaesthesiol Scand 11:297, 1961

174. Johnstone RE, Kulp RA, Smith TC: Effects of acute and chronic ethanol administration on isoflurane requirements in mice. Anesth Analg (Cleve) 54:277, 1975

175. Attee JL, Hower LD, Tobey RE: Diphenylhydantoin and lidocaine modification of AV conduction in halothane-anesthesized dogs. Anesthesiology 43:49, 1975

176. Pachter HL, Riles TS: Low dose heparin: Bleeding and wound complications in the surgical patient. Ann Surg 186:669, 1977

177. Goldberg LI: Anesthetic management of patients treated with antihypertensive agents or Levodopa. Anesth Analg (Cleve) 51:625, 1972

178. Miller RD, Way WL, Eger EI: Effect of alpha-methyldopa, resperine, guanethidine, iproniazid on minimum alveolar requirements (MAC). Anesthesiology 29:1153, 1968

179. Brodsky JB, Vravo JJ: Acute postoperative clonidine withdrawal syndrome. Anesthesiology 44:519, 1976

180. Bruce DL, Croley TF, Lee JS: Clonidine withdrawal presenting postoperatively. Anesthesiology 51:90, 1979

181. Prys-Roberts C, Meloche R, Foex P et al: Studies of anesthesia in relation to hypertension: Cardiovascular responses of treated and untreated patients. Br J Anaesth 43:122, 1971

182. Robert JG, Foex P, Clarke TNS et al: Hemodynamic interactions of high-dose propranolol pretreatment and anesthesia in the dog. Br J Anaesth 48:315, 403, 411 1976

183. Horan BF, Prys-Roberts C, Hamilton WK et al: Interaction of enflurane anesthesia, beta-receptor blockade, and blood loss in the dog. Br J Anaesth 48:817, 1976

184. Diaz RG, Somberg J, Freeman E et al: Myocardial infarction after propranolol withdrawal. Am Heart J 88:257, 1974

185. Kaplan JA, Dunbar RW: Propranolol and surgical anesthesia. Anesth Analg (Cleve) 55:1, 1976

186. Saner CA, Foex P, Roberts JG et al: Methoxyflurane and practolol: A dangerous combination. Br J Anaesth 47:1025, 1975

187. Avery GS: Check list to potentially clinically important interactions. Drugs 5:187, 1973

188. Perisho JA, Buechel DR, Miller RD: Effect of diazepam on minimal alveolar anesthetic requirement in man. Can Anaesth Soc J 18:536, 1971

189. Johnston RR, Eger EI, Wilson GA: Comparative interaction of epinephrine with enflurane, isoflurane and halothane in man. Anesth Analg (Cleve) 55:709, 1976

190. Ngai SH: Parkinsonism, levodopa, anesthesia. Anesthesiology 37:344, 1972

191. Diamond BI, Hardala HS, Borison RL: Potential of lithium as an anesthetic premedicant. Lancet 2:1229, 1977

192. Brown TC, Cass NM: Beware—The use of MAO inhibitors is increasing again. Anaesth Intensive Care 7:65, 1979

193. Sjogvist F: Psychotic Drugs: Interaction between monoamine oxidase inhibitors and other substances. Proc R Soc Med 58:967, 1965

194. Vickens MD: Anesthesia and MAO inhibitors. Br Med J 1:1126, 1965

195. Britt BA: Etiology and pathophysiology of malignant hyperthermia. Fed Proc 38:44, 1979

196. Kohler H: A rational approach to dosage and preparation of parenteral glucocorticoid substitution therapy during surgical procedures. Acta Anaesthesiol Scand 19:260, 1975

197. Osogor SI, Kerek SF: Enhancement of thiopental anesthesia by sulphafurazole (sulfisoxazole). Br J Anaesth 42:988, 1970

198. Lam HS, Brown TC, Lampard DG: d-Tubocurarine requirement during hypothermia. Anaesth Intensive Care 7:222, 1979

199. Miller RP, Van Nyhis LS, Eger EI: The effect of temperature on a d-Tubocurarine neuromuscular blockade and its antagonism by neostigmine. J Pharmacol Exp Ther 195:237, 1975

200. Waterman PM, Albin MS, Smith RB: Malignant hyperthermia: A case report. Anesth Analg (Cleve) 59:220, 1980

201. Halsoll PJ, Ellis FR: Screening test for malignant hyperpyrexia phenotype using suxamethonium-induced contracture of muscle treated with caffeine and its inhibition by dantrolene. Br J Anaesth 51:753, 1979

202. Relton JE: Anesthesia for elective surgery in patients susceptible to malignant hyperthermia. Int Anesthesiol Clin 17:141, 1979

203. Ryan JF: Treatment of acute hyperthermia crisis. Int Anesthesiol Clin 17:153, 1979

204. Gronert GA, Thompson RL, Onofrio BM: Human malignant hyperthermia: Awake episodes and correction by dantrolene. Anesth Analg (Cleve) 59:377, 1980

205. Pandit K, Kothany S, Cohen P: Orally administered dantrolene for prophylaxis of malignant hyperthermia. Anesthesiology 50:156, 1979

206. Whittaker M: Plasma cholinesterase variants and the anesthetist. Anaesthesia 35:174, 1980

207. Scholler KL, Goedde HW, Benkmann HG: The use of serum cholinesterase in succinylcholine apnea. Can Anaesth Soc J 24:396, 1977

208. Sirotzky L, Lewis EJ: Anesthesia-related muscle paralysis in renal failure. Clin Nephrol 10:38, 1978

209. Gibaldi M, Levy G, Hyton WL: Tubocurarine and renal failure. Br J Anaesth 44:163, 1972

210. Whitby LG: Biochemical screening tests for the anesthetist. Br J Anaesth 46:564, 1974

37

Alcohol and Drug Abuse in the Surgical Patient

WILLIAM K. LEVY

Alcoholism and drug addiction, serious and widespread health problems, increase surgical risk and lead to sequelae that frequently require operative intervention. Treatment of alcohol and drug abusers requires close collaboration between internist and surgeon. The internist should understand the risks of surgery and anesthesia, anticipate common medical complications of addiction that affect surgical outcome, and help manage perioperative withdrawal syndromes. Alcoholism and drug addiction are discussed in separate sections in this chapter but often coexist in the clinical setting.

ALCOHOLICS AND SURGERY

Alcoholism is a common problem among hospitalized medical and surgical patients, with a prevalence varying from 8.5% to 17%.[1-3] One estimate reports the rate in hospitalized men to be as high as 27%. The criteria for the diagnosis of alcoholism established by the National Committee on Alcoholism include a history of excessive intake, physical dependence as indicated by the development of tolerance and withdrawal, psychologic dependence, and alcohol-related illness.[4]

The physician evaluating a preoperative alcoholic patient must not only identify excessive and habitual use of alcohol but also determine the extent of physiologic dependence and organ damage. The patient should be specifically asked about withdrawal symptoms, quantity consumed without intoxication, and history of hepatic, cardiac, hematologic, or neurologic problems associated with alcoholism.

There are few carefully controlled studies that prove that alcoholism constitutes a significant risk for surgery. Common sense and experienced medical opinion support the contention that a high incidence of organ damage, associated metabolic abnormalities, anesthetic difficulties, and the threat of delirium tremens increase surgical morbidity and mortality.[5-8] Alcoholic and acute nonalcoholic hepatitis have been clearly shown to increase perioperative mortality.[9,10] Although it is commonly believed that the same is true for alcohol-induced cardiomyopathy, serious hematologic abnormalities, and withdrawal states, formal studies have not been done.

Lee and co-workers examined the effect of alcohol ingestion on morbidity and mortality in patients undergoing surgery for trauma.[11] No significant difference in mortality was found retrospectively between 530 patients with no ingestion and 169 trauma patients with heavy alcohol intake. In the second prospective part of the study, blood-alcohol levels were measured in 102 patients just prior to induction of anesthesia. There was no increase in morbidity or mortality in patients with levels of less than 250 mg/dl. Mortality for emergency surgery was 15% in 13 patients with blood-alcohol levels of greater than 250 mg/dl as compared to 6% in patients with lower levels. Of 3 patients with levels greater than 400 mg/dl, 1 died and 1 became hypotensive intraoperatively. Although flawed by small numbers and lack of analysis of alcohol-related complications, this study suggests that high blood-alcohol levels at the time of surgery increase operative risk. No study has adequately examined the effect of chronic alcoholism on surgical morbidity and mortality.

The medical complications of alcoholism require careful preoperative evaluation. Acute alcoholism without sequelae of chronic ingestion alters cardiovascular function. Dogs treated with alcohol prior to surgery are more prone than control animals to shock following blood loss.[12,13] Nonalcoholic human subjects with blood-alcohol levels as low as 75 mg/dl demonstrate diminished myocardial contractility. This effect is mild, but it can be potentiated by other myocardial depressants, including anesthetics and barbiturates commonly used in the surgical setting.[14] Patients with minor trauma and acute alcoholism occasionally present with hypotension in excess of that expected from amount of blood loss.[15] The mechanisms for this are unclear but may involve a combination of mild cardiac depression, vasodilatation, and mild hypovolemia.

Chronic alcoholism may lead to signif-

icant cardiac dysfunction and progression to endstage cardiomyopathy. Even chronic alcoholics with no signs or symptoms of congestive heart failure have been shown to have abnormal myocardial contractility. Those with cardiomyopathy generally have a 10- to 15-year history of alcohol abuse and, in the early stages, may show only unexplained tachycardia, significant ventricular or atrial ectopy, or conduction system abnormalities.[16–19] Typical congestive cardiomyopathy is not seen until more advanced stages of the disorder. Alcoholic cardiomyopathy often occurs in patients without evidence of other complications of chronic alcoholism such as cirrhosis, neuropathy, or withdrawal.[19] It is important that this condition be recognized before surgery and that monitoring be done for intraoperative congestive failure or cardiac arrhythmias. Surgery should be postponed when possible for treatment of clinically apparent congestive failure or arrhythmias. Prolonged abstinence from alcohol in patients with early cardiomyopathy may significantly improve cardiac function.[16]

The most common medical complication of alcohol is liver disease. As discussed in Chapter 21, cirrhosis and alcoholic hepatitis can have profound effects on surgical outcome.[9,10,20] Active alcoholic hepatitis is a strong contraindication to surgery; in one study of 12 patients with alcoholic hepatitis undergoing laparotomy, the mortality rate was 58%.[9] The presence of encephalopathy, ascites, or varices and the degree of abnormality in serum albumin, bilirubin, and prothrombin time measurements correlate with surgical morbidity and mortality. Surgery should be delayed, if possible, and these abnormalities ameliorated.

Hematologic disorders such as anemia, thrombocytopenia, abnormal platelet function, and prolonged prothrombin time are common in alcoholic patients and should be corrected preoperatively.[21–23] Leukopenia and abnormal leukocyte chemotaxis may lead to poor wound healing and postoperative infections.[24,25] Metabolic abnormalities, including hypoglycemia, alcoholic ketoacidosis, lactic acidosis, hypomagnesemia, and hypophosphatemia should be corrected preoperatively, when possible.[26–28]

The most difficult perioperative management problem in the alcoholic patient is withdrawal. Tremors and irritability may appear within hours of the last alcohol ingestion, and seizures may occur within 24 hr to 48 hr. Delirium tremens, characterized by fever, tachycardia, global confusion, and hallucinations, usually occur 48 hr to 72 hr after ingestion but may be delayed for as long as 7 to 10 days.[29,30] The mortality rate for delirium tremens alone is 12% to 15%, increasing to 25% when withdrawal is associated with medical or surgical illness.[20,31,32] The leading cause of death is vascular collapse preceded by marked hyperthermia.[32] Ventricular tachyarrhythmias resulting in sudden death have been documented in several patients with delirium tremens.[33]

On a male surgical service in a city hospital, 33 patients developed delirium tremens after admission; the 33 comprised 1.8% of all patients and 20% of all alcoholics admitted. Predictors of delirium tremens included cirrhosis or hepatomegaly, previous history of delirium tremens, consumption of more than 1 pint of whiskey a day for 10 of the 14 days preceding admission, and symptoms of withdrawal on admission. Of 11 patients who developed delirium tremens postoperatively, 3 (27%) died. Mays and associates reported a mortality rate of 45% in a group of 11 patients who developed delirium tremens after surgery.[35] However, neither

study examines morbidity or mortality when surgery is delayed until delirium tremens has resolved, although most authors agree that surgery should be postponed if the disorder is present or anticipated.[31,34,36] Resolution usually requires 2 to 3 days but may take as long as 1 week.[30]

The treatment of alcohol withdrawal is similar for surgical and medical patients. Benzodiazepines are used orally when possible and intravenously in high doses for more severe episodes.[29,37] Paraldehyde can be used only orally or rectally and may be more toxic than benzodiazepines.[37] Phenothiazines are less effective and may carry a higher incidence of seizures.[38] Alcohol itself is effective but has a narrow margin between therapeutic and lethal doses.[34] A recommended approach to the treatment of alcohol withdrawal is shown in Table 37-1.

Withdrawal seizures are self-limited and often do not require therapy.[29,39] However, in patients with a history of withdrawal seizures, prophylactic phenytoin therapy is effective and may be particularly helpful in preventing seizures in the immediate postoperative period.[40]

The effect of acute and chronic alcohol ingestion on anesthesia is complex and unpredictable. Alcohol depresses the reticular activating system and potentiates the effects of general anesthetics, barbiturates, and narcotics. Dose reduction is therefore necessary in the acutely intoxicated patient.[40] Liver disease may also slow the rate of drug metabolism and enhance depressant action. However, chronic alcoholics often require higher than normal quantities of anesthetic agents for both induction and maintenance.[4,6,7,41] Increased requirements for halothane, thiopental, fentanyl, and meperidine have been demonstrated.[42–45] Explanations for

Table 37-1. Treatment of Alcohol Withdrawal States

Clinical Problem	Drug	Route	Dose (mg)	Interval	Comment
Mild to severe agitation, anxiety, tremor	Chlordiaz-epoxide Diazepam	Oral	25–100 5–20	Every 6 hr	Initial dose can be increased or repeated every 2 hr if a satisfactory effect is not observed
Extreme agitation	Chlordiaz-epoxide Diazepam	Intravenous	12.5/min 2.5/min	Slow infusion	Give until patient is calm; subsequent doses must be individualized on basis of clinical picture
History of seizure disorder or previous withdrawal seizures	Phenytoin	Oral	If phenytoin detected in blood: maintenance dose, 100 If no phenytoin detected in blood: loading dose, 200–300; maintenance dose, 100	Every 8 hr Every 8 hr	—
Repeated seizures requiring acute therapy	Phenytoin	Intravenous Oral	Loading dose, 1 g in 250–500 ml of normal saline Maintenance dose, 100	Infuse over 1–4 hr Every 8 hr	Exact loading dose, 10 mg/kg
Hallucinosis	Haloperidol	Intramuscular	0.5–2.0	Every 2 hr	Until patient controlled, or to maximum of 5 doses

(After Sellers EM, Kalart H: N Engl J Med 294:757, 1976)

this resistance include increased sympathetic activity during surgery, induction of microsomal enzymes, and increased volume of distribution due to vasodilatation.[44,46] The most widely accepted theory maintains that cellular adaptation in the central nervous system allowing tolerance to alcohol is responsible for cross-tolerance to other central nervous system depressants.[47]

In addition, variable responses to muscle relaxants may be seen in chronic alcoholics. Resistance to curare develops in patients with liver disease because of increased binding of the agent to gamma-globulins and because of a relative deficiency of pseudocholinesterase.[6,7] Increased sensitivity to depolarizing agents such as succinlycholine may also arise because of a deficiency of pseudocholinesterase. Although anesthesia is the domain of the anesthesiologist, familiarity with the variability of response in the alcoholic may help the internist to explain and manage complications in the perioperative period.

DRUG ADDICTS AND SURGERY

Drug addicts frequently undergo surgery for trauma and infections due to unsterile parenteral injections, including skin abcessses, endocarditis, mycotic aneurysms, and osteomyelitis.[48–51] The internist is often consulted to aid in assessing operative risk and evaluating and managing these complications. Anesthetic and surgical risks in the addict vary with the severity of the complications of addiction. Many of these complications are related not to the drug itself but to the use of unsterilized needles and diluents. Surgical risk may therefore be higher in patients addicted to parenteral agents than in patients using oral preparations. Surgical studies of patients taking oral methadone demonstrate few perioperative problems.[51,52] However, when the course of 10 heroin addicts admitted for surgical treatment of acute trauma was compared to that of 30 nonaddicted patients with comparable trauma, mortality was equivalent, but morbidity was higher in the addicted population.[53] Pulmonary edema developed in the perioperative period in 30% of the addicts and in none of the controls. The incidence of wound infection was 30% and 3%, respectively. Although evidence is scanty, it is reasonable to conclude that the addict using parenteral drugs has an increased risk of surgical complications and perhaps death as well.

Medical complications of drug addiction are listed below:[54–57]

Infectious
  Soft tissue infection—skin abscess, cellulitis, necrotizing fascitis
  Endocarditis
  Osteomyelitis—septic arthritis
  Malaria
  Tetanus
Pulmonary
  Pulmonary edema
  Septic and foreign body emboli
  Aspiration pneumonia—lung abscess
  Pulmonary hypertension
Renal
  Glomerular sclerosis
  Nephrotic syndrome
  Renal failure
Gastrointestinal
  Acute and chronic hepatitis
  Intestinal "pseudo-obstruction"
Neurologic
  Peripheral nerve injury
  Transverse myelitis
  Rhabdomyolysis
Other
  Thrombophlebitis
  Necrotizing vasculitis

Most of the above complications occur in patients taking parenteral drugs, and some are particularly relevant to the perioperative period. Narcotics may be associated with functional small-bowel obstruction.[48–50] Such obstruction is due to a marked increase in the resting tone of the large and small bowels, resulting in areas of spasm and cessation of effective peristalsis. The small bowel is most commonly affected, and the condition may mimic a mechanical small-bowel obstruction, with obstructive bowel sounds and dilated loops of small bowel on radiograph. This functional obstruction usually resolves with conservative management and nasogastric tube decompression.

Pulmonary edema is a common cause of death in patients who have taken a heroin overdose. It has also been reported in methadone and, rarely, in barbiturate ingestion.[58,59] Following heroin injection, patients may present in coma, with physical examination and chest film yielding findings of noncardiac pulmonary edema. The edema is probably caused by damage to the alveolocapillary membrane with subsequently increased permeability, but the precise mechanism of the process is unclear. Unexplained pulmonary edema has also been reported in addicts in the perioperative period.[53] It is unclear whether the same process is involved, because fluid overload may contribute to edema formation in surgical patients.

Liver function tests are abnormal in 75% to 90% of heroin addicts admitted to hospitals or treatment programs.[60,61] Factors that contribute to liver dysfunction include acute or chronic hepatitis secondary to hepatitis B, coexistent alcohol use, and the effects of adulterants used in street preparations of heroin. Liver biopsy may reveal acute hepatitis, chronic hepatitis, and, occasionally, cirrhosis. In most cases, the liver abnormalities are mild and require no special preoperative management.

The possibility of withdrawal must be considered in every drug addict. Withdrawal syndromes and their treatments differ for narcotics, barbiturates and other sedative–hypnotics, and amphetamines and other stimulants. The narcotic abstinence syndrome begins 8 hr to 12 hr after the last dose, with symptoms of yawning, diaphoresis, lacrimation, and rhinorrhea. Later signs and symptoms include restlessness, tremors, dilated pupils, and piloerection. Peak withdrawal occurs after 2 to 3 days, with myalgias, muscle spasm, abdominal cramps, vomiting, diarrhea, tachycardia, and hypertension predominating. The narcotic withdrawal syndrome is dramatic but rarely fatal and is less dangerous than that of alcohol or barbiturates.[62,63] Narcotic withdrawal can be reversed immediately by administration of an appropriate dose of a substitute narcotic.

It has been suggested that drug addicts or patients on methadone maintenance be withdrawn from their drugs prior to surgery.[52,64] This is often not possible, except in preparation for completely elective procedures. It is therefore generally agreed that these patients may be safely maintained on substitute narcotics in the perioperative period.[6,51,65] Methadone is the agent of choice, and most addicted patients can be maintained on 10 to 40 mg/day in divided doses. For patients in whom narcotic addiction is suspected but not clearly documented, it is reasonable to allow early withdrawal symptoms to develop before treating with narcotics, thereby avoiding the possibility of unnecessary new addiction. One protocol suggests giving a dose of 10 mg to 15 mg of methadone after withdrawal symptoms develop and repeating the dose every 2 hr to 6 hr if symptoms persist or recur.[63] The total dose required daily, often less than 40 mg, represents the approximate maintenance dose. In patients undergoing emergency surgery, more frequent doses of a shorter-acting agent such as morphine can be used before and during surgery. Methadone is substituted postoperatively.

Patients on chronic methadone maintenance should receive their usual dose of methadone prior to surgery. If medication cannot be taken by mouth, two-thirds of the daily maintenance dose can be administered intramuscularly or subcutaneously in divided doses.[61] Some physicians hold the dose on the day of surgery, because methadone has a 24- to 36-hr duration of action, and restart it the next day. It is probably safer to give at least part of the maintenance dose on the day of surgery.[52,61]

In addition to maintenance methadone, parenteral narcotics are often needed for analgesia after surgery. Standard narcotics such as morphine, meperidine, or hydromorphine are used for this purpose, although larger and more frequent doses than usual may be required. Pentazocine (Talwin) should not be used postoperatively, since it is a narcotic antagonist and may precipitate a withdrawal reaction.[6,61]

The barbiturate withdrawal syndrome usually begins within 24 hr of the last dose. Initial symptoms include agitation, tremulousness, and diaphoresis, progression to postural hypotension, abdominal cramps, vomiting, and muscle spasms. After 2 to 8 days of seizures, hallucinations and delirium tremens may develop. Withdrawal can be treated acutely with pentobarbital or any other short-acting barbiturate.

A patient may be maintained on a substitute barbiturate through surgery and detoxified when stable postoperatively. Maintenance and detoxification is probably best accomplished with phenobarbital in doses equivalent to those of the abused barbiturate with the daily dose decreased gradually.[63,66] Serious withdrawal states, including seizures and delirium, have been reported with the abrupt withdrawal of the frequently abused benzodiazepines; substitute benzodiazepines or barbiturates may be necessary in this situation.[67]

Stimulant drugs such as amphetamines and cocaine cause relatively little physiologic dependence. Withdrawal produces prolonged sleep and depression requiring no therapy.[62,65] More commonly, the amphetamine addict exhibits a toxic psychosis after prolonged use that may persist for several days after the last dose of amphetamine and may cause postoperative delirium if the patient is undergoing emergency surgery.[65]

Anesthetic problems in drug addicts are less common than in alcoholics. Narcotic addicts are, however, unusually prone to intraoperative hypotension, which may be due to an overdose of narcotics or to withdrawal.[48,64,68] Appropriate treatment consists of administration of either a narcotic antagonist or an appropriate narcotic. Other explanations for intraoperative hypotension include diminished intravascular volume and catecholamine depletion, which respond to volume and pressor agents.

Tolerance to anesthetic agents in addicts is variable and depends on the type of drug used. In general, patients addicted to narcotics require large doses of narcotics for premedication and analgesia but relatively normal anesthetic doses.[51,64,65] Infrequent abusers of barbiturates and other sedative–hypnotics need lower than usual anesthetic doses, but chronic abusers often develop a tolerance to these agents and may require more than usual.[65] Use of amphetamines usually dictates only minor variations in anesthetic dose. Acute limited use may increase anesthetic requirements, but, with chronic use, anesthetic requirements are reduced, perhaps owing to catecholamine depletion.[65]

SUMMARY

1. **The chronic alcoholic should be treated as a high-risk surgical candidate.**
2. **Preoperative evaluation should include a careful physical exam; complete blood and platelet counts, pro-**

thrombin time; measurement of electrolytes, phosphate, magnesium, and liver function tests; chest x-ray; and electrocardiogram. The presence of cardiomyopathy, alcoholic hepatitis, cirrhosis, electrolyte disorders, or hematologic abnormalities may necessitate postponement of surgery.

3. Surgery should be delayed, when possible, until withdrawal is complete.

4. The effect of anesthesia in the alcoholic patient is variable. In general, acutely intoxicated patients require less anesthesia than normal, and chronic alcoholics require more anesthesia than normal.

5. The drug abuser requires careful medical evaluation prior to surgery.

6. Important preoperative tests include chest x-ray, urinalysis, and measurement of blood urea nitrogen, creatinine, liver function, and hepatitis B antigen.

7. Detoxification of patients addicted to narcotics or barbiturates should generally be postponed until after surgery, and such patients should be maintained on appropriate substitution therapy through the perioperative period. Accepted agents for this purpose include methadone for the narcotic addict and phenobarbital for the abuser of sedative–hypnotics.

8. Intraoperative complications in the narcotic addict include unexpected hypotension and pulmonary edema.

9. Anesthetic management is usually uncomplicated, although dosage requirements may vary. Pentazocine should be avoided.

REFERENCES

1. Barchha R, Stewart MA, Guze SB: The prevalence of alcoholism among general hospital ward patients. Am J Psychiatry 125:681, 1968

2. Nolan JP: Alcohol as a factor in the illness of university service patients. Am J Med Sci 249:135, 1965

3. Kearney TR, Bonime H, Cassimatis G: The impact of alcoholism on a community general hospital. Community Ment Health J 3:373, 1967

4. Criteria Committee, National Council on Alcoholism: Criteria for the diagnosis of alcoholism. Ann Intern Med 77:249, 1972

5. Lowenfels AB: The Alcoholic Patient in Surgery. Baltimore, Williams & Wilkins, 1971

6. Orkin LR, Chen C: Addiction, alcoholism and anesthesia. South Med J 70:1172–1174, 1977

7. Keilty SR: Anesthesia for the alcoholic patient. Anesth Analg (Cleve) 48:659, 1969

8. Orloff MJ: Surgical consequences of alcoholism. Ann NY Acad Sci 252:159, 1975

9. Greenwood DS, Leffler C, Minkowitz S: The increased mortality rate of open liver biopsy in alcoholic hepatitis. Surg Gynecol Obstet 134:600, 1972

10. Stone HH: Preoperative and postoperative care. Surg Clin North Am 57:409, 1977

11. Lee JF, Giesecke AH, Jenkins MT: Anesthetic management of trauma: Influence of alcohol ingestion. South Med J 60:1240, 1967

12. Knott DH, Beard JD: The effect of chronic ethanol administration on the response of the dog to repeated acute hemorrhage. Am J Med Sci 254:178, 1967

13. Moss LK, Chenault OW, Gaston FA: Effect of alcohol in experimental hemorrhagic shock. Surg Forum 10:390, 1959

14. Regan TJ: Ethyl alcohol and the heart. Circulation 44:957, 1971

15. Swan KG, Vidaver RM, LaVigne JE et al: Acute alcoholism, minor trauma and "shock." J Trauma 17:215, 1977

16. Demakis JG, Proskey A, Rahimtoola SH et al: The natural course of alcoholic cardiomyopathy. Ann Intern Med 80:293, 1974

17. Burch GE, DePasquale NP: Alcoholic cardiomyopathy. Am J Cardiol 23:723, 1969

18. Goodwin JF: Congestive cardiomyopathy. In Hurst JW (ed): The Heart. New York, McGraw-Hill, 1978

19. Regan TJ, Ettinger PO, Hauder B et al: The role of ethanol in cardiac disease. Ann Rev Med 28:393, 1977

20. Strunin L: Anaesthesia for patients with diminished hepatic function. In Gray TC, Utting JE, Nunn JF (eds): General Anaesthesia. London, Butterworth & Co, 1980

21. Eichner ER: The hematologic disorders of alcoholism. Am J Med 54:621, 1973

22. Strauss DJ: Hematologic aspects of alcoholism. Semin Hematol 10:183, 1973

23. Hart MJ, Cowan DH: The effect of ethanol on hemostatic properties of human blood platelets. Am J Med 56:22, 1974

24. Liu YK: Leukopenia in alcoholics. Am J Med 54:605, 1973

25. Gluckman SJ, Dvorak VC, MacGregor RR: Host defenses during prolonged alcohol consumption in a controlled environment. Arch Intern Med 137:1539, 1977

26. Isselbacher KJ: Metabolic and hepatic effects of alcohol. N Engl J Med 296:612, 1978

27. Levy LJ, Duga J, Girgis M et al: Ketoacidosis associated with alcoholism in nondiabetic subjects. Ann Intern Med 78:213, 1973

28. Miller PD, Heinig RE, Waterhouse C: Treatment of alcoholic acidosis. Arch Intern Med 138:67, 1978

29. Sellers EM, Kalant H: Alcohol intoxication and withdrawal. N Engl J Med 294:757, 1976

30. Thompson WL: Management of alcohol withdrawal syndromes. Arch Intern Med 138:278, 1978

31. Helmus C, Spahn J: Delirium tremens in head and neck surgery. Laryngoscope 84:1479, 1974

32. Tavel ME, Davidson W, Balterton TD: A critical analysis of mortality associated with delirium tremens. Am J Med Sci 242:18, 1961

33. Fisher J, Abrams J: Life-threatening ventricular tachyarrhythmias in delirium tremens. Arch Intern Med 137:1238, 1977

34. Glickman L, Herbsman H: Delirium tre-mens in surgical patients. Surgery 64:882, 1968

35. Mays ET, Ransdell HT, DeWeese BM: Metabolic changes in surgical delirium tremens. Surgery 67:780, 1970

36. Lowenfels AB, Rohman M, Shibatam K: Surgical consequences of alcoholism. Surg Gynecol Obstet 131:129, 1970

37. Thompson WL, Johnson AD, Maddrey WL et al: Diazepam and paraldehyde for treatment of severe delirium tremens. Ann Intern Med 82:175, 1975

38. Kaim SC, Klett CJ, Rohfeld B: Treatment of the acute alcohol withdrawal state: A comparison of four drugs. Am J Psychiatry 125:1640, 1969

39. Josephson GW, Sabatier HS: Rational management of alcohol withdrawal seizures. South Med J 71:1095, 1978

40. Sampliner R, Iber FL: Diphenylhydantoin control of alcohol withdrawal seizures. JAMA 230:1430, 1974

41. Johnstone RE, Kulp RA, Smith TC: Effects of acute and chronic ethanol administration on isoflurane requirement in mice. Anesth Analg (Cleve) 54:277, 1975

42. Han YH: Why do chronic alcoholics require more anesthesia? (Abstr) Anesthesiology 30:341, 1969

43. Tammisto T, Tigerstedt T: The need for halothane supplementation of N_2O-O_2 relaxant anesthesia in chronic alcoholics. Acta Anaesth Scand 21:17, 1977

44. Tammisto T, Tigerstedt T: The need for fentanyl supplementation of N_2O-O_2 relaxant anesthesia in chronic alcoholics. Acta Anaesth Scand 21:216, 1977

45. Mather LE, Tucker GT, Plug A et al: Meperidine kinetics in man. Clin Pharmacol Toxicol 17:21, 1975

46. Tammisto T, Tigerstedt T: The effect of operative stress on plasma catecholamine levels in chronic alcoholics. Acta Anaesth Scand 18:127, 1974

47. Anton AH: Pharmacology of ethanol. Int Anesthesiol Clin 68:299–317, 1968

48. Eiseman B, Lam RC, Rush B: Surgery on the narcotic addict. Ann Surg 159:748, 1964

49. Geelhoed GW, Joseph WL: Surgical se-

quelae of drug abuse. Surg Gynecol Obstet 139:749, 1974

50. Butterfield WC: Surgical complications of narcotic addiction. Surg Gynecol Obstet 134:237, 1972

51. Rubinstein RB, Spira I, Wolff WI: Management of surgical problems in patients on methadone maintenance. Am J Surg 131:566, 1976

52. Cushman P: Methadone maintenance therapy for heroin addiction. Am J Surg 123:267, 1972

53. Camer SJ, King N, Gianelli S et al: Inappropriate response of drug addicts to cardiothoracic surgery. NY State J Med 72:1718, 1972

54. Louria DB, Hensle T, Rose J: The major medical complications of heroin addiction. Ann Intern Med 67:1, 1967

55. Sapira JD: The narcotic addict as a medical patient. Am J Med 45:555, 1968

56. Cherubin CE: The medical sequelae of narcotic addiction. Ann Intern Med 67:23, 1967

57. Becker CE: Medical complications of drug abuse. Adv Intern Med 24:183, 1979

58. Frand VI, Shim CS, Williams MH: Heroin-induced pulmonary edema. Ann Intern Med 77:29, 1972

59. Williams MH: Pulmonary complications of drug abuse. In Fishman AP (ed): Pulmonary Diseases and Disorders. New York, McGraw-Hill, 1980

60. Stimmel B, Vernace S, Tobias H: Hepatic dysfunction in heroin addicts. JAMA 222:811, 1972

61. Fultz JM, Senay EC: Guidelines for the management of hospitalized narcotic addicts. Ann Intern Med 82:815, 1975

62. Jaffe JH: Drug addiction and drug abuse. In Goodman LS, Gilman A (eds): The Pharmacological Basis of Therapeutics. New York, Macmillan, 1975

63. Khantzian EJ, McKenna GJ: Acute toxic and withdrawal reactions associated with drug use and abuse. Ann Intern Med 90:361, 1979

64. Giuffrida JG, Bizarri DV, Saure AC et al: Anesthesia for drug abusers. Anesth Analg (Cleve) 49:272, 1970

65. Elliott HW: Effects of street drugs on anesthesia. Int J Clin Pharmacol 12:134, 1975

66. Smith DE, Wessor DR: Phenobarbital technique for treatment of barbiturate dependence. Arch Gen Psychiatry 24:56, 1971

67. Preskorn SH, Denner JL: Benzodiazepines with withdrawal psychosis. JAMA 237:36, 1977

68. Organ CH: Surgical procedures upon the drug addict. Surg Gynecol Obstet 134:947, 1972

38

Surgery in the Elderly

JERRY C. JOHNSON

The elderly comprise an increasing proportion of surgical patients and frequently receive preoperative evaluation by the internist. More than 40% of operative patients are over 60 years of age and 22% are over 70.[1] In 1973, 40% of the elderly patients under general hospital care in the United States were admitted for surgical treatment.[2]

This chapter discusses the special issues raised by the elderly patient regarding (1) the risk of surgery; (2) the physiology of aging as it relates to clinical decision-making; (3) clinical pharmacology; (4) the assessment of disease; and (5) perioperative management.

RISK OF SURGERY

Studies from 1940 to 1956 reporting higher than normal surgical risk in the elderly rarely separated chronologic age from other confounding variables.[3] More recent studies have demonstrated no clear association between age and surgical risk.[4-9] Although Boushy and co-workers reported increased mortality following lung resection in patients over 60 with a forced expiratory volume in 1 sec (FEV_1) of less than 2 liters, no attempt was made to separate decreased FEV_1 itself from

age.[10] In 1971, Lewin and associates found a mortality rate of 29% in elderly patients following elective abdominal surgery. Mortality was related to pathology, type of surgery, and duration of anesthesia but not to advancing age.[6] Djokovic and Hedley–Whyde studied surgical outcome in 500 consecutive patients over the age of 80 between 1975 and 1977. The overall postoperative mortality rate was 6.2%, and the mortality rate of patients over age 95 was 13%. The authors concluded that age up to 95 was not a significant factor affecting mortality.[4] It is important to note that these patients were managed as aggressively as younger patients, when necessary, with mechanical ventilation, Swan–Ganz catheters, and intra-arterial monitoring. Several other studies of elderly patients undergoing specific types of surgery, such as herniorrhaphy, total hip replacement, and cholecystectomy, have shown no association between chronologic age and mortality rate.[11-16]

Fishman and Roe found no difference in mortality rate following cardiac valve replacement between 104 patients over age 66 and 650 younger adults.[17] Mortality once again correlated with severity of disease rather than with age. Chaitman and colleagues, in a study of operative risk factors in patients with left main coronary artery disease, found no independent age effect.[18] Similar conclusions regarding the effect of age on the risk of cardiovascular surgery have been reached by others.[19–22]

Although the risk of emergency surgery is probably common to young and old, the number of emergency procedures undergone increases with age.[1] Blake and Lynn reported the results of 375 emergency abdominal operations performed between 1969 and 1975 on patients aged 75 to 97. The overall mortality rate of 31.7% showed no correlation with chronologic age.[24]

The majority of deaths in elderly surgical patients are due to cardiovascular and pulmonary complications.[4,5,7,24] Although several studies document an increased incidence of postoperative pulmonary emboli with advancing age, the association of respiratory complications with age is controversial.[25–32] In a prospective survey of the incidence of postoperative pulmonary complications excluding pulmonary emboli, Wightman found no statistically significant difference between the incidence of 16.5% in 85 patients over the age of 70 and that of 8.9% in 700 patients below the age of 70.[32] Latimer and co-workers reported that 42% of patients over the age of 55 with impaired preoperative forced vital capacity and FEV_1 had a higher incidence of postoperative respiratory complications than the remaining 58%.[33] Kitamura and associates found that postoperative hypoxemia and fall in functional residual capacity (FRC) were directly related to advancing age.[34] However, despite these age-related changes, pulmonary reserve, as measured by the usual criteria for preoperative evaluation, is adequate in elderly patients without lung disease.[35] An average 90-year-old man with a height of 5 ft 10 inches has an FEV_1 of 2.5 liters,

well above the level shown to significantly increase pulmonary risk.

Cardiac response to the stresses of exercise, hypoxemia, and hypercapnia is limited even in normal elderly patients. This limitation, along with a high prevalence of organic heart disease, make elderly patients particularly susceptible to perioperative cardiovascular complications.[36–39] The most common cardiovascular complications in noncardiothoracic surgery are myocardial infarction, congestive heart failure, and arrhythmias. In a survey of 1001 patients over the age of 40, Goldman found age greater than 70 to be an independent risk factor for the development of cardiovascular complications.[40] However, pulmonary spirometric and lung volume measurements were not included as variables, and many of the cardiac variables were subject to variation between observers.

For the internist evaluating a healthy elderly patient facing surgery, accurate assessment of physiologic status in light of the stress of the proposed procedure is crucial. It is often difficult to separate normal aging effects from the effects of disease. Furthermore, existing guidelines have often been derived from studies of younger patients. The predictive indices in current use are discussed further in the section on Perioperative Management.

PHYSIOLOGY OF AGING

Recent gerontology textbooks contain comprehensive reviews of the physiologic changes of aging.[41,42] This section reviews those changes that are relevant to the management of the surgical patient.

Knowledge of changes in body composition and renal physiology with age allows for more accurate management of fluid and electrolytes. Whereas approximately 60% of total body weight is water in the young adult, the figure is 54% for the elderly man and 46% to 50% for the elderly woman. This is due to an increase in total body fat.[43,44] Rowe and colleagues showed a dramatic fall in creatinine clearance from 140 ml/min in patients aged 20 to 97 ml/min in patients aged 80. This was associated with a negligible rise in serum creatinine due to decreased muscle mass.[45] Serum blood urea nitrogen (BUN), unlike creatinine, has been reported to increase substantially with age to approximately 35 mg/dl by age 75, but it is unclear whether this increase is due to occult disease.[46] The BUN:creatinine ratio as an index of hydration may therefore be misleading.

Other changes in renal physiology include a decrease in maximal urinary concentrating ability and a slight decrease in the efficiency of acid–base regulation.[47] An increase in the tubular threshold for glucose makes glycosuria an unreliable method of diagnosing and managing diabetes mellitus.[47] Cystometric studies on both men and women show an increase in residual volume with age, a decreased urge to void with bladder-filling, and an increase in number of uninhibited contractions.[47] These changes increase the risk of urinary retention and incontinence in the postoperative period.

Most investigators have noted a small decrease in resting cardiac output and stroke volume with advancing age.[36,48,49] More impressive changes occur in response to exercise: cardiac output decreases, stroke volume decreases, pulmonary artery pressure increases, left ventricular end-diastolic pressure increases, and right ventricular end-diastolic pressure increases. The decrease in cardiac output is attributable to pulmonary and systemic vascular effects, peri-cardial changes with age, prolonged relaxation, sympathetic nervous system control and receptor sensitivity, changes in cardiac contractility, and occult disease. Attributing a decrease in cardiac output at rest or in response to exercise as an age-related decrease in contractility is controversial.[37,38] Even with changes in response to stress, cardiac output in most aging persons can increase considerably above resting level.[50,51]

Population studies in many parts of the world have shown that systolic and diastolic blood pressure rise progressively with age, with few exceptions.[52–54] The prevalence of hypertension among the elderly, defined as a blood pressure of 160/95, is 25% to 50%.[52,55] There is a higher than normal incidence of cardiovascular disease among elderly, hypertensive subjects, and both systolic and diastolic blood pressures vary directly with morbidity and mortality.[52,56,57] Pharmacologic treatment of elderly persons with elevated systolic and diastolic blood pressures reduces the incidence of cardiovascular effects.[52,53,58] The benefits and risks of the treatment of purely systolic hypertension in the elderly have not been adequately studied.[52,59,60]

The influence of aging on the lungs has been extensively studied.[61] Muiesan and associates reported no change in total lung capacity, a fall in vital capacity, increases in residual volume and functional residual capacity, and decreases in flow rates with age.[62] The increase in closing volume may result in significant airway closure during tidal ventilation. This results in ventilation–perfusion mismatch, a fall in arterial PO_2, and an increase in alveolar–arterial oxygen difference.[62,63] Despite the many changes in pulmonary function, pH, P_{CO_2}, and bicarbonate are unaffected by age.[64]

Age differences in endocrine physiology are reviewed by Andres and Tobin.[65] Glucose tolerance clearly decreases with age. Although fasting blood glucose increases only 1 mg/dl per decade, the 2-hr postprandial glucose increases 5 mg/dl and the 1-hr rises 10 mg/dl per decade. Although the serum total T_4 is unaffected by age, basal serum triiodothyronine levels decrease with age. Serum T_3 may therefore be an unreliable indicator of hyperthyroidism in the elderly. Adrenal response to stress remains intact.[65]

Serum albumin decreases with age even with apparently normal nutrition. In a report from the Boston Collaborative Drug Surveillance Program, mean serum albumin concentration fell progressively with each decade of life from 3.97 g/dl at age 40 to 3.58 g/dl over age 80.[66] Anemia is not normal in the aged, but the erythrocyte sedimentation rate does increase to the range of 35 to 40.[67]

CLINICAL PHARMACOLOGY

Prescribing drugs for the elderly can be difficult because of the physiologic changes noted above.[68,69] The factors affecting drug disposition and response in the elderly are listed in Table 38-1. Change in drug absorption with age is not a significant clinical factor, but changes in hepatic metabolism, perhaps secondary to decreased hepatic blood flow or decreased liver size, may be important. Serum creatinine and creatinine clearance decrease with age, and drugs excreted by the kidneys must be used carefully. Classes of drugs commonly used in elderly surgical patients are discussed below.

Analgesics

Several factors should be considered in the prescription of analgesics for the el-

derly. Pain relief may reduce postoperative complications by allowing earlier mobilization, enhancing deep breathing, and improving pulmonary function.[70] Dosage adjusted to age rather than to body size correlates best with pain relief. A progressive, age-related increase in pain relief was reported in patients over the age of 40 who received 5- and 10-mg doses of morphine or 20 mg of pentazocine.[71] The frequency of side-effects did not increase with age. The serum half-life of morphine was independent of age.[72]

Anticoagulants

Elderly individuals are more sensitive than younger persons to the effects of heparin and warfarin.[73,74] Smaller than normal doses may therefore suffice for therapeutic anticoagulation.

Antimicrobials

As long as creatinine clearance is appropriately estimated in accordance with age-related standards, the physician may follow dosage guidelines established for renal function irrespective of age.[69]

Bronchodilators

The maintenance dose for intravenous aminophylline should be reduced 25% to 50% in the elderly for plasma levels to be maintained in the therapeutic range.[75] The loading dose remains the same (6 mg/kg).[76]

Cardiovascular Agents

The half-life of digoxin increases by as much as 40% in the elderly because of the decline in creatinine clearance.[77] How-

Table 38-1. Factors Affecting Drug Disposition and Response in the Elderly

Effect	Altered Physiology	Clinical Importance
Absorption	Elevated gastric pH Reduced Gl blood flow ? Reduced number of absorbing cells ? Reduced Gl motility	Not sufficiently studied

Distribution	Body composition
	   Reduced total body water
	   Reduced lean body mass/kg body
	     weight
	   Increased body fat
	Protein binding
	   Reduced serum albumin
		Higher concentration of drugs
		   distributed in body fluids
		?Longer duration of action of fat soluble
		   drugs
		
		Higher free fraction of highly protein-
		   bound drugs

Elimination	Hepatic metabolism
	   Reduced enzyme activity
	   Reduced hepatic mass
	   Reduced hepatic blood flow
	Renal excretion
	   Reduced glomerular filtration rate
	   Reduced renal plasma flow
	   Altered tubular function
		Apparently slower biotransformation of
		   some drugs
		Influenced by environmental factors
		   (e.g., nutrition and smoking)
		Slower excretion of some drugs

Response	Multiple disease states Multiple drug use common Altered receptor sensitivity Organ-specific age differences	More variation in dose response Adverse drug reactions common

GI = gastrointestinal (Vestal RE: Drugs 16:358, 1978)

ever, elderly patients are not more sensitive than usual to the therapeutic or toxic effects of digitalis at equivalent drug levels.[68] Noncardiac symptoms of digitalis toxicity are common, including fatigue, anorexia, visual diorders, nausea, agitation, and drowsiness.[78] Digoxin can be safely discontinued in elderly patients who are in sinus rhythm and do not exhibit signs of congestive failure.[79–81]

Antihypertensive Agents

Many antihypertensive agents may cause postural hypotension and central nervous system depression in the elderly.[82–84] Alternatively, elderly patients may be less sensitive than younger patients to pro-pranolol despite higher plasma levels after a single dose of 40 mg.[85]

Antiarrhythmic Agents

Toxicity to lidocaine is twice as common in elderly than in young persons, perhaps because of an increased incidence of congestive heart failure.[86] Nation and coworkers demonstrated a significantly longer half-life for lidocaine in elderly than in younger subjects, but plasma levels were equivalent in the two groups because of a change in the distribution of the drug.[87] The half-life of quinidine is also prolonged to an average of 9.7 hr in elderly patients, partly owing to reduced renal clearance.[88]

Sedatives

The response of elderly patients to sedatives may vary from mild restlessness to frank psychosis.[89] This is particularly true of barbiturates, in which the half-life has been shown to increase significantly in persons over the age of 70.[68] Advancing age has variable effects on the pharmacologic disposition of the benzodiazepines.[90–95] Diazepam, lorazepam, flurazepam, and chlordiazepoxide have significantly prolonged plasma half-lives, but the disposition of oxazepam is unaffected by age.[68] Reidenberg and colleagues have shown increased sensitivity of the elderly to the depressant effects of diazepam.[90] An initial test dose of these agents followed by reduced maintenance dosage is recommended for the elderly.[96,97]

Antidepressants and Antipsychotic Drugs

Elderly patients achieve higher plasma levels of tricyclic antidepressants than younger patients.[98] With equivalent doses of antipsychotic drugs, the incidence of drug-induced akinetic parkinsonism is higher in the older patient, peaking in the seventh decade of life.[98] Choreiform movements, akathisia, and tardive dyskinesia in the elderly patient on antipsychotic drugs may develop insidiously and be misdiagnosed. Extrapyramidal symptoms occur in 50% of patients between the ages of 60 and 80 on antipsychotic medications.[97] They are most common with butyrophenones such as haloperidol; sedation and hypotension are most often seen with chlorpromazine and thioridazine. Both tricyclics and antipsychotic preparations may cause confusion, cardiotoxicity, sedation, and urinary retention. Dosages of these agents should be reduced in the elderly.[96]

ASSESSMENT OF DISEASE

A comprehensive assessment is the foundation for perioperative management of the elderly patient.[3] Multiple chronic diseases occur with increasing frequency. Underlying coronary artery disease and chronic obstructive pulmonary disease are often precipitants of postoperative medical complications and death. Mental illness, either organic or psychiatric, is common. Automatic nervous system dysfunction causing hypothermia and hypotension is becoming increasingly recognized. The akinesia of Parkinson's disease can lead to dysphagia and increase the potential for aspiration if necessary medication is discontinued. Prostatic hypertrophy commonly precipitates urinary obstruction postoperatively. Malnutrition may be secondary to socioeconomic factors or medical, surgical, or dental disease.

Acute illnesses in the elderly can present insidiously with nonspecific symptoms such as decreased activity, malaise, or refusal to eat or drink.[99] Myocardial infarction, acute abdominal catastrophe, pneumonia, and urinary tract infection are examples of acute illness in which change in mental status may be the dominant clinical sign. Pain is less commonly a sympton of acute illness in the elderly patient than normal, and acute myocardial infarctions or acute abdominal conditions may present with little or no pain.[100,101] Acute infection may cause only minimal increases in temperature and white blood cell counts. Hyperthyroidism may present as a cardiac arrhythmia or congestive heart failure, and depression may mimic somatic illness.[99]

Any acute illness in an elderly person is more likely than normal to result in serious sequelae. These include venous thrombosis, dehydration, electrolyte imbalances, constipation, urinary incontinence, contractures, and changes in mental status.[3] Serious pressure sores can develop within 1 week.

Eliciting historical data and performing physical examinations in the elderly may be difficult.[3,49] Hearing deficits and intellectual dysfunction are common impediments. Inelasticity of the skin and decreased periorbital fat may mimic dehydration. Deformities of the chest wall may cause displacement of the apical impulse. A tortuous aorta may interfere with assessment of jugular venous pulse elevation, particularly on the left side of the neck. An S_4 gallop is often heard regardless of clinically apparent heart disease. Respiratory splitting of the second heart sound may be less marked in elderly than in younger patients. A systolic ejection murmur at the base is present in 60% of patients over the age of 70 and may be due to aortic ring calcification, aortic sclerosis, or stenosis. Crepitations may be heard at the lung bases in bedridden patients, even when there is no disease. Feces may cause a palpable abdominal mass. Symmetric loss of vibration sense and ankle jerks are common. Minimal bilateral muscle wasting, particularly in the hands, may occur without weakness or other neurologic signs.

All correctable problems should be ameliorated before elective surgery. This is particularly important in the elderly because of their decreased physiologic reserve. The emergency surgical patient requires as complete an evaluation as possible and as many corrective measures as time will allow.

PERIOPERATIVE MANAGEMENT

Specific recommendations for preoperative assessment of the elderly patient have been made by several authors and are similar to those for younger adults covered in Chapter 2.[43,67] An accurate evaluation of cardiac and pulmonary status is imperative, since diseases of the heart and lungs represent major risk factors for postoperative decompensation. Acute myocardial infarction within 6 months of surgery, obstructive lung disease, and congestive heart failure have been shown repeatedly to increase morbidity and mortality significantly.[1,3,35,40] The presence of an asymptomatic carotid bruit does not increase the risk of postoperative stroke, and recent studies have suggested that preoperative invasive studies are not warranted.[102–104]

Electrocardiograms should be done preoperatively, and arterial blood gas analysis and spirometry should be considered.[6] Because of age-associated changes in the electrocardiogram, Simonson has suggested that the upper limit of the PR interval be 220 msec, that the normal limit of the QRS axis be 30° in persons over the age of 50, and that poor R-wave progression in the anterior leads be considered a normal age trend in this group.[105] The pulmonary function criteria for estimating surgical risk are the same as those for younger adults.[35] Factors indicating increased risk include a P_{CO_2} of greater than 50, a maximum voluntary ventilation (MVV) of less than 50%, an FEV_1 of less than 2 liters, and a vital capacity of less than 1 liter. The glomerular filtration rate should be estimated by direct measurement of creatinine clearance or by nomograms and formulas designed to correct for age.[106]

Several authors have attempted to develop indices of operative risk in the elderly that might direct perioperative management.[6,107,108] In 1980, Del Guercio developed a preoperative staging system for elderly patients based on right-heart catheterization and arterial sampling in 148 patients at an average age of 67.3 years.[107] Although some of the patients were younger than 65, they were considered physiologically older because of illness. Primary and derived variables included cardiac index, pulse rate, peripheral vascular resistance, arterial PO_2, arteriovenous oxygen difference, pulmonary wedge pressure, and Sarnoff-type ventricular function curves. These variables were plotted on a preprinted format, the automatic physiologic profile (APP), previously described by Cohn and Del Guercio in 1975.[109] The profile was then used to establish four levels of perioperative management. Stage 1 patients had normal variables and were managed in the routine manner. Stage 2 patients had mild functional deficits requiring interoperative and postoperative right-heart catheterization and arterial blood sampling but not requiring postponement of surgery. Stage 3 patients had mild to moderate deficits, and recommendations were made for postponement of surgery while corrections were made. Stage 4 patients had moderate to advanced deficits that could not be corrected, and it was recommended that major elective surgery under anesthesia be avoided. These patients were offered alternative treatment of operation under local anesthesia.

None of the 20 stage 1 patients died postoperatively. Of the 94 patients in stages 2 and 3, 8 died. Of the 34 stage 4 patients, 7 underwent less extensive operations than originally planned and survived, 8 underwent the originally planned procedure and died, and 19 were not taken to surgery.[7]

Although this study measures functional deficits and provides guidelines for preoperative correction, there are problems with interpretation of the data. First, the staging criteria are described qualitatively (no deficits, mild deficits, moderate to advanced deficits), and it is unclear whether all of the variables are needed for staging. Second, the normal range for the variables comprising the APP was defined by the authors as the mean ± 1 standard deviation for healthy young men. These norms may be inaccurate for elderly patients. Clearly, values for normal PO_2 and ventricular function decrease with age, and norms for other variable may also change. Third, conclusions on the usefulness of the staging system were based on the same patient sample that had been used to establish the staging system. Fourth, because there was no control group, we do not know whether management and outcome for unstaged patients would have differed. Fifth, the mortality rate was not given for the 19 stage 4 patients for whom surgery was cancelled. These patients constitute a control group within stage 4 for whom the mortality rate would be instructive. Sixth, the average age of only 67.3 years and the inclusion of patients below the age of 65 suggest the presence of significant chronic disease in this study group. Routine preoperative invasive monitoring and physiologic profiling for patients over age 65 cannot be recommended on the basis of this study. The usual indications for invasive monitoring should continue to apply for the elderly as for younger surgical patients. Invasive measures should not be denied any patient simply because of age once the decision to operate has been made.

Recommendations for preoperative preparation are directed toward the prevention of venous thrombosis, treatment of congestive heart failure, amelioration of obstructive lung disease, and decrease in pulmonary secretions. Breathing exercises, cessation of smoking, correction of fluid and electrolyte imbalances, correction of significant anemia, and replacement of essential nutrients are important. Prevention and management of other chronic complications should begin in the preoperative period. Although there are pads and mattresses especially designed to prevent pressure sores, these are no substitute for frequent position changes for immobile patients.

Postoperative management involves a continuation of the principles applied during the preoperative period. The goals are to stimulate the patient both physically and mentally, to encourage family members that the patient is recovering, and to prevent the complications that are common in the elderly. Urinary incontinence, pressure sores, atelectasis, venous thrombosis, and constipation may be precipitated by sedative drugs, anesthesia, immobility, and pain. Changes in mental status may be due to isolation, a new environment, drugs, or acute illness. Blundell reported such deficits lasting up to 5 days in 30% of elderly postoperative patients.[110] Aspiration secondary to postoperative ileus may be increasingly common with advancing age, and nasogastric suctioning should be readily instituted, if necessary. Pain relief and sitting position improve vital capacity. Early mobilization, judicious use of analgesic medication, and an aggressive team approach do much to hasten the postoperative recovery of the elderly patient.

SUMMARY

1. **Do not deny surgery simply because of chronologic age.**
2. **Obtain a good history from the patient. If decreased intellectual function is a problem, speak with a family member or other care provider.**
3. **Physical examination should focus on the cardiovascular and respiratory systems. Baseline mental status and neurologic evaluation are also important.**
4. **Preoperative screening tests should include hematocrit, urinalysis, electrolytes, creatinine, fasting blood glucose, electrocardiogram, and chest x-ray. Arterial blood gas and spirometry (vital capacity, FEV$_1$, maximal midexpiratory flow rate, and MVV) are suggested for all individuals over the age of 70. Age-adjustment to normal is important in most tests.**
5. **Preoperative preparation may require more time in the elderly than in younger patients for correction of as many problems as possible before elective procedures.**
6. **Adjust medications to account for changes in drug metabolism with age. This includes decreasing dosages according to creatinine clearance, discontinuing unnecessary drugs, and continuing antiparkinsonism medications.**
7. **Aggressive postoperative support is important in the elderly. Encourage early ambulation and provide sufficient analgesia for pain-free movement and breathing.**
8. **Repeat an electrocardiogram within 5 days of surgery.**
9. **Altered mental status is common postoperatively in the elderly and should prompt a search for disease.**

REFERENCES

1. Powers JH: Coexisting debilitating and degenerative diseases. In Powers JH (ed): Surgery of the Aged and Debilitated Patient, p 209. Philadelphia, W.B. Saunders, 1968

2. Glenn F: Pre- and postoperative management of elderly surgical patients. J Am Geriatr Soc 21:385, 1973

3. Mason JH, Gall FC, Byrne MP: General surgery. In Steinberg FU (ed): The Care of the Geriatric Patient, 5th ed., p 217. St. Louis, C.V. Mosby, 1976

4. Djokovic TL, Hedley-Whyde J: Prediction of outcome of surgery and anesthetics in patients over 80. JAMA 242:2301, 1974

5. Burnett W, McCaffrey J: Surgical procedures in the elderly. Surg Gynecol Obstet 134:221, 1972

6. Lewin I, Lerner A, Green S et al: Physical class and physiologic status in the prediction and operative mortality. Ann Surg 174:217, 1971

7. Young HD, Tanga M, Wellington J et al: Major abdominal surgery in the elderly: A review of 172 consecutive patients. Can J Surg 14:324, 1971

8. Ziffren SE: Comparison of mortality rates for various surgical operations according to age groups, 1951–1977. J Am Geriatr Soc 27:433, 1979

9. Robins RE, Budden MK: Major abdominal surgery in patients over 70 years of age: Results during 1962 to 1966 compared with those during 1950 to 1959. Abd Surg Elderly 15:73, 1972.

10. Boushy S, Billy DM, Worth L et al: Clinical course related to preoperative and postoperative pulmonary function in patients with bronchogenic carcinoma. Chest 59:383, 1971

11. Esselatyn DB: Aneurysmectomy in the aged? Surgery 67:34, 1970

12. Anderson L, Kammerer W, Greer R: Risk factor assessment in 101 total hip arthroplasties. Clin Orthop 141:50, 1979

13. Guillen J, Aldrete J: Anesthetic factors influencing morbidity and mortality of elderly patients undergoing inguinal herniorrhaphy. Am J Surg 120:760, 1970

14. Steiger E, Seltzer M, Rosato F: Cholecystectomy in the aged. Ann Surg 174:142, 1971

15. Panayiotis G, Ellenbogen A, Grunstein S: Major gynecological surgical procedures in the aged. J Am Geriatr Soc 26:459, 1974

16. Stewart I, Millac P, Shephard R: Neurosurgery in the older patient. Postgrad Med J 51:453, 1975

17. Fishman WH, Roe BB: Cardiac valve replacement in patients over 65 during a 10-year period. J Gerontol 33:676, 1978

18. Chaitman BR, Rogers WT, Davis K et al: Operative risk factors in 18 patients with left main coronary artery disease. N Engl J Med 303:953, 1980

19. Barnhorst DA, Giuliani E, Pluth J et al: Open heart surgery in patients more than 65 years old. Ann Thorac Surg 18:81, 1974

20. Quinlan R, Cohn L, Collins J: Determinants of survival following cardiac operations in elderly patients. Chest 68:498, 1975

21. Berman ND, David T, Lipton I et al: Surgical procedures involving cardiopulmonary bypass in patients aged 70 or older. J Am Geriatr Soc 28:29, 1980

22. Gann P, Colin C, Hildner F et al: Coronary artery bypass surgery in patients 70 years of age and older. J Thorac Cardiovasc Surg 73:237, 1977

23. Stahlgren LH: An analysis of factors which influence mortality following extensive abdominal operations upon geriatric patients. Surg Gynecol Obstet 113:283, 1961

24. Blake R, Lynn J: Emergency abdominal surgery in the aged. Br J Surg 63:956, 1976

25. Kakkar VV, Howe C, Nicolaides A et al: Deep vein thrombosis of the leg. Is there a "high risk" group? Am J Surg 120:527, 1978

26. Tsapogas MJ, Goussous H, Peabody R et al: Postoperative venous thrombosis and the effectiveness of prophylactic measures. Arch Surg 103:561, 1971

27. Morrell MT, Dunnill MS: The postmortem. Incidence of pulmonary embolism in a hospital population. Br J Surg 55:347, 1968

28. Dripps R, Dennings MW: Postoperative

atelectasis and pneumonia. Ann Surg 124:94, 1966

29. Myers JR, Lembeck L, O'Kane H et al: Changes in functional residual capacity after operation. Arch Surg 110:576, 1975

30. Marshall WH, Fahey PJ: Operative complications and mortality in patients over 80 years of age. Arch Surg 88:896, 1964

31. Thoren L: Postoperative pulmonary complications: Observations on their prevention by means of physiotherapy. Acta Clin Scand 107:193, 1954

32. Wightman JAK: A postoperative survey of the incidence of postoperative pulmonary complications. Br J Surg 55:85, 1968

33. Latimer RG, Dickman M, Day WC et al: Ventilatory patterns and pulmonary complications after upper abdominal surgery, determined by preop and postop computerized spirometry and blood gas analysis. Am J Surg 122:622, 1971

34. Kitamura H, Sawa T, Ikezona E: Postoperative hypoxemia: The contribution of age to the maldistribution of ventilation. Anesthesiology 36:244, 1972

35. Tisi GM: Preoperative evaluation of pulmonary function. Am Rev Respir Dis 119:293, 1979

36. Gerstenblith G, Lakatta EG, Weisfeldt M: Age changes in myocardial function and exercise response. Prog Cardiovasc Dis 19:1, 1976

37. Weisfeldt ML: Aging of the cardiovascular system. N Engl J Med 303:1172, 1980

38. Port S, Cobb F, Coleman E et al: Effect of age on the response of the left ventricular ejection fraction to exercise. N Engl J Med 303:1133, 1980

39. Kronenberg RS, Drage CW: Attenuation of the ventilatory and heart rate responses to hypoxia and hypercapnia with aging in normal men. J Clin Invest 52:1812, 1973

40. Goldman L, Caldera D, Nussbaum S et al: Multifactorial index of cardiac risk in noncardiac surgical procedures. N Engl J Med 297:845, 1977

41. Brocklehurst JH (ed): Textbook of Geriatric Medicine and Gerontology, 2nd ed. Edinburgh, Churchill Livingstone, 1978

42. Finch CF, Hayflick L: Handbook of the Biology of Aging. New York, Van Nostrand Reinhold, 1977

43. Rossman I: Anatomic and body composition changes with aging. In Finch CF, Hayflick L (eds): Handbook of the Biology of Aging, p 189. New York, Van Nostrand Reinhold, 1977

44. Womersley J, Durnin JVCA, Boddy K et al: Influence of muscular development, obesity and age on the fat-free mass of adults. J Appl Physiol 41:223, 1976

45. Rowe JW, Andres R, Tobin V et al: The effect of age on creatinine clearance in men: A cross-sectional and longitudinal study. J Gerontol 31:155, 1976

46. Milne J, Williamson J: Plasma urea concentrations in older people. Gerontol Clin 14:32–35, 1972

47. Goldman R: The aging of the excretory system: Kidney and bladder. In Finch CF, Hayflick L (eds): Handbook of the Biology of Aging, p 409. New York, Van Nostrand Reinhold, 1977

48. Weisfeldt ML (ed): The Aging Heart: Its Function and Response to Stress. New York, Raven Press, 1980

49. Gerstenblith G: Noninvasive assessment of cardiac function in the elderly. In Weisfeldt ML (ed): The Aging Heart: Its Function and Response to Stress, p 260. New York, Raven Press, 1980

50. Strandell T: Circulatory studies on healthy old men. Acta Med Scand (Suppl) 175 (414):1, 1964

51. Conway J, Wheeler R, Sannerstedt R: Sympathetic nervous activity during exercise in relation to age. Cardiovasc Res 5:577, 1971

52. Dyer AR, Stamler J, Shekelle R et al: Hypertension in the elderly. Med Clin North Am 61:513, 1977

53. O'Malley K, O'Brien E: Management of hypertension in the elderly. N Engl J Med 302:1397, 1980

54. Page LB: Hypertension and atherosclerosis in primitive and acculturating societies. In Summit L (ed): Cardiovascular Risk Factors and Consequences of Hy-

pertension, Vol 1, p 1. Bloomfield, NJ, Health Learning Systems, 1979

55. Ostfeld AM: Elderly hypertensive patient: Epidemiologic review. NY State J Med 78:1125, 1978

56. Kannel WB, Gordon T: Evaluation of the cardiovascular risk in the elderly: The Framingham Study. Bull NY Acad Med 54:573, 1978

57. Veterans' Administration Cooperative Study Group on Antihypertensive Agents: Effects of treatment on morbidity in hypertension. III. Influence of age, diastolic pressure, and prior cardiovascular disease; further analysis of side effects. Circulation 45:991, 1972

58. Koch–Weser J: Treatment of hypertension in the elderly. In Crooks J, Stevenson IH (eds): Drugs and the Elderly, p 247. London, Macmillan, 1979

59. Seligmann AW, Alderman MH, Davis TK: Systolic hypertension: Occurrence and treatment in a defined community. J Am Geriatr Soc 27:135, 1979

60. Koch–Weser J: The therapeutic challenge of systolic hypertension. N Engl J Med 289:481, 1973

61. Klocke RA: Influence of aging on the lung. In Finch CF, Hayflick L (eds): Handbook of the Biology of Aging, p 432. New York, Van Nostrand Reinhold, 1977

62. Muiesan G, Sorbini CA, Grassi V et al: Respiratory function in the aged. Bull Physiopath Respir 7:973, 1971

63. Leblanc P, Ruff F, Milic-Emili J: Effects of age and body composition on airway closure in man. J Appl Physiol 28:448, 1970

64. Sorbini CA, Grassi V, Solenas E et al: Arterial oxygen tension in relation to age in healthy subjects. Respiration 25:3, 1968

65. Andres R, Tobin JD: Endocrine systems. In Finch CF, Hayflick L (eds): Handbook of the Biology of Aging, p 357. New York, Van Nostrand Reinhold, 1977

66. Greenblatt DJ, Koch–Weser J: Adverse reaction to propranolol in hospitalized medical patients: A report from the Boston Collaborative Drug Surveillance Program. Am Heart J 86:478, 1973

67. Anderson WF: Practical Management of the Elderly, 3rd ed, p 28. Oxford, Blackwell Scientific Publications, 1976

68. Vestal RE: Drug use in the elderly: A review of problems and special considerations. Drugs 16:358, 1978

69. Richey DP, Bender AD: Pharmacokinetic consequences of aging. Annu Rev Pharmacol Toxicol 17:49, 1977

70. Bromage PR: Extradural analgesia for pain relief. Br J Anaesth 39:721, 1967

71. Belville JW, Forrest W, Miller E et al: Influence of age on pain relief from analgesics: A study of postoperative patients. JAMA 217:1835, 1971

72. Berkowitz BA, Ngai S, Yang J et al: The disposition of morphine in surgical patients. Clin Pharmacol Ther 17:629, 1975

73. Jick H, Slone D, Borda I et al: Efficacy and toxicity of heparin in relation to age and sex. N Engl J Med 279:284, 1968

74. O'Malley K, Stevenson, I, Ward C et al: Determinants of anticoagulant control in patients receiving warfarin. Br J Clin Pharmacol 4:309, 1977

75. Jusko WL, Koup J, Vance J et al: Intravenous theophylline: Normogram guidelines. Ann Intern Med 86:400, 1977

76. Nielson-Kudsk F, Magnussen I, Jakobsen P: Pharmacokinetics of theophylline in ten elderly patients. Acta Pharmacol Toxicol (Copenh) 42:226, 1978

77. Ewy GA, Kapadia G, Yao L et al: Digoxin metabolism in the elderly. Circulation 39:449, 1969

78. Lely AH, Van Enter CHJ: Non-cardiac symptoms of digitalis intoxication. Am Heart J 83:149, 1972

79. Dall JLC: Maintenance digoxin in elderly patients. Br Med J 2:703, 1970

80. Johnston GD, McDevitt DG: Is maintenance digoxin necessary in patients with sinus rhythm? Lancet 1:507, 1979

81. Spector R: Digitalis therapy in heart failure: A rational approach. J Clin Pharmacol 19:692, 1979

82. Gribbon B, Pickering T, Sleight P et al: Effect of age and high blood pressure on

baroreflex sensitivity in man. Circ Res 29:424, 1971

83. Caird FL, Andrews G, Kennedy R: Effect of posture on blood pressure in the elderly. Br Heart J 35:527, 1973

84. Dollery CT, Harrington J: Methyldopa in hypertension: Clinical and pharmacological studies. Lancet 1:754, 1962

85. Castleden CM, Kaye CM, Parsons RL: The effect of age on plasma levels of propranolol and practolol in man. Br J C Pharmacol 2:303, 1975

86. Pfeifer HJ, Greenblatt DJ, Koch-Weser J: Clinical use and toxicity of intravenous lidocaine. Am Heart J 92:168, 1976

87. Nation RL, Triggs E: Lignocaine kinetics in cardiac patients and aged subjects. Br J Clin Pharmacol 4:439, 1977

88. Ochs HR, Greenblatt DJ, Woo E et al: Reduced guideline clearance in elderly persons. Am J Cardiol 42:481, 1978

89. Bender AD: Pharmacologic aspects of aging. A survey of the effect of increasing age on drug activity in adults. J Am Geriatr Soc 12:114, 1964

90. Reidenberg MM, Levy M, Warner H et al: Relationship between diazepam dose, plasma level, age and central nervous system depression. Clin Pharmacol Ther 23:371, 1978

91. Shader RI, Greenblatt D, Harmatz J et al: Absorption and disposition of chlordiazepoxide in young and elderly male volunteers. J Clin Pharmacol 17:709, 1977

92. Klotz U, Avant G, Hoyumpa A et al: The effects of age and liver disease on the disposition and elimination of diazepam in adult man. J Clin Invest 55:347, 1975

93. Castleden CM, George C, Marcer D et al: Increased sensitivity to nitrazepam in old age. Br Med J 1:10, 1977

94. Kyriakopoulos AA: Bioavailability of lorazepam in humans. In Gottschalk LA, Merlis S (eds): Pharmacokinetics of Psychoactive Drugs, p 45. New York, Spectrum, 1976

95. Wilkinson GR: The effect of aging on the disposition of benzodiazepines in man (abstr). Presented at the Symposium on Drugs and the Elderly, Ninewalls Hospital, Dundee, Scotland, 1977

96. Levenson A (ed): Neuropsychiatric Side-Effects of Drugs in the Elderly. New York, Raven Press, 1979

97. Holloway: Drug Intell Clinical Pharm 8:632, 1974

98. Nies A et al: Relationship between age and tricyclic antidepressant plasma levels. Am J Psychiatry 134:790, 1977

99. Hodkinson HM: Non-specific presentations of illness. Br Med J 4:94, 1973

100. Pathy MS: Clinical presentation of myocardial infarction in the elderly. Br Haematol J 29:190, 1967

101. Vowles LDL: Surgical Problems in the Aged, pp 1–11. Bristol, England, John Wright & Sons, 1979

102. Corman L: The preoperative patient with an asymptomatic cervical bruit. Med Clin North Am 63:1335, 1979

103. Trieman R et al: Carotid bruit significance in patients undergoing an abdominal aortic operation. Arch Surg 106:803, 1973

104. Evans WE, Cooperman M: The significance of asymptomatic unilateral carotid bruits in preoperative patients. Surgery 83:521, 1978

105. Simonson E: The effect of age on the electrocardiogram. Am J Cardiol 29:64, 1972

106. Gral T, Young M: Measured versus estimated creatinine clearance in the elderly as an index of renal function. J Am Geriatr Soc 28:492, 1980

107. Del Guercio LRM, Cohn JD: Monitoring operative risk in the elderly. JAMA 243:1350, 1980

108. Gudwin AL, Goldstein CR et al: Estimation of ventricular mixing volume for prediction of operative mortality in the elderly. Ann Surg 168:183, 1968

109. Cohn JD, Engler PE, Del Guercio LRM: The automated physiologic profile. Crit Care Med 3:51, 1975

110. Blundell E: A psychological study of the effects of surgery on 86 elderly patients. Br Soc Clin Psychol 6:297, 1967

Index

Note: Page numbers in *italics* indicate illustrations; those followed by *t* indicate tables.

/